KT-498-494

Atlas of Multiplane Transesophageal Echocardiography

Volume 2

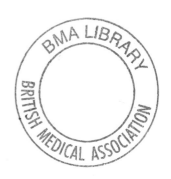
BMA LIBRARY
BRITISH MEDICAL ASSOCIATION

Dedication

Clare, Eleanor Isabelle, Eugenie Alice

Christina Marie, Jennifer Ann, Jacqueline Michelle, Alycia Yvonne, Dan, Laura Nicole, Alan III, Maria

Atlas of Multiplane Transesophageal Echocardiography

Volume 2

Martin G St John Sutton MB BS FRCP
John Bryfogle Professor of Cardiovascular Diseases and
Director, Cardiac Imaging Program
Cardiovascular Division
University of Pennsylvania Medical Center
Philadelphia PA
USA

Alan R Maniet DO FAAIM
St Louis University Medical Center
Cardiology Division
St Louis MO
USA

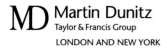
Martin Dunitz
Taylor & Francis Group
LONDON AND NEW YORK

© 2003 Martin Dunitz, a member of the Taylor & Francis Group

First published in the United Kingdom in 2003
by Martin Dunitz, Taylor & Francis Group plc, 11 New Fetter Lane, London EC4P 4EE

Tel.:   +44 (0) 20 7583 9855
Fax: +44 (0) 20 7842 2298
E-mail: info@dunitz.co.uk
Website: http://www.dunitz.co.uk

All rights reserved. No part of this publication may be reproduced, stored in a retrieval system, or transmitted, in any form or by any means, electronic, mechanical, photocopying, recording, or otherwise, without the prior permission of the publisher or in accordance with the provisions of the Copyright, Designs and Patents Act 1988 or under the terms of any licence permitting limited copying issued by the Copyright Licensing Agency, 90 Tottenham Court Road, London W1P 0LP.

Although every effort has been made to ensure that all owners of copyright material have been acknowledged in this publication, we would be glad to acknowledge in subsequent reprints or editions any omissions brought to our attention.

A CIP record for this book is available from the British Library.

ISBN 1 85317 217 0

Distributed in the USA by
Fulfilment Center
Taylor & Francis
10650 Toebben Drive
Independence, KY 41051, USA
Toll Free Tel.: +1 800 634 7064
E-mail: taylorandfrancis@thomsonlearning.com

Distributed in Canada by
Taylor & Francis
74 Rolark Drive
Scarborough, Ontario M1R 4G2, Canada
Toll Free Tel.: +1 877 226 2237
E-mail: tal_fran@istar.ca

Distributed in the rest of the world by
Thomson Publishing Services
Cheriton House
North Way
Andover, Hampshire SP10 5BE, UK
Tel.:   +44 (0)1264 332424
E-mail: salesorder.tandf@thomsonpublishingservices.co.uk

Composition by Scribe Design, Gillingham, Kent, UK
Printed and bound in Spain by Grafos S.A. Arte Sobre Papel

Contents

Preface

Over the past few years transesophageal echocardiography has become one of the most exciting imaging modalities available today in modern clinical cardiology. Transesophageal echocardiography through its portability, relatively inexpensive equipment and semi-noninvasive nature is currently available and readily accessible to almost every cardiac patient in comparison to other radiographic techniques. Multiplane transesophageal echocardiography is the result of the technologic evolution of echocardiography from single plane and biplane transducers over the past decade. Multiplane transesophageal echocardiography provides high resolution cardiac images in an infinite number of planes which, combined with conventional color Doppler modalities, offers a superlative diagnostic tool for evaluating cardiac structure and function. In addition to enhanced diagnostic capabilities, multiplane technology allows for greater patient safety with less discomfort because transducer manipulation is minimized. The advantages of multiplane transesophageal echocardiography are that it provides an array of multiplane images in real time which offers a three-dimensional perspective of cardiac anatomy that cannot be appreciated even by the cardiac pathologist.

The aim of this atlas is to provide medical students, anesthesiologists, cardiac surgeons and cardiologists with a concise but in-depth analysis of cardiac imaging from an experience of over 10,000 transesophageal echocardiograms performed by the authors. This atlas may also serve as a reference for diagnostic examples of cardiac pathology physicians who practice transesophageal echocardiography. The format of each chapter is consistent throughout, starting with normal cardiac structure and function, followed by abnormalities of structure and function. Chapters include evaluation of prostheses, interventional cardiology techniques and intraoperative transesophageal echocardiography. A concise explanation of measurements of cardiac chamber sizes and function and Doppler are provided only for transesophageal echocardiographic applications. Transesophageal echocardiographic images are juxtaposed with correlative anatomic specimens to provide a clear understanding of normal and abnormal cardiac anatomy.

Martin G St John Sutton
Alan R Maniet

Acknowledgements

The authors are indebted to the sonographers, cardiology fellows and secretaries of the laboratories of Thomas Jefferson University Hospital, Hospital of the University of Pennsylvania and the Episcopal Hospital for their assistance in the preparation of this textbook. It is hoped that the readers of this book will obtain as much enjoyment and knowledge as went into its preparation.

Technical expertice, Norman (Ali) Alexander, Harry Kutner, Florence Orsini, Maureen McDonald, Lois Nitka.
Photographic assistance Frederick Ross
Editorial assistance Alan Burgess, Clive Lawson
With special thanks to Ted Plappert

6

Evaluation of the cardiac chambers and pericardium: structure and function

Multiplane transesophageal echocardiography demonstrates the intricate details of cardiac structural anatomy through its ability to provide multiple imaging planes with a high-resolution transducer.[1–3] The major advantage of transesophageal echocardiography is the visualization of the posterior anatomic structures. Due to their close proximity to the esophagus, the atria and the pulmonary veins are particularly well visualized with greater image resolution than may be obtained from transthoracic windows. Transesophageal echocardiography also provides excellent visualization of the ventricular endocardium for demonstrating wall motion abnormalities and assessing global ventricular function. In these regards it is extremely important that the physician performing transesophageal echocardiography possess an intimate knowledge of normal cardiac anatomy, and is familiar with the anatomic variants, with congenital abnormalities, and with the structural changes produced by cardiac diseases.[4]

Normal anatomy

Right atrium and vena cavae

The right atrium may be visualized from multiple windows with multiplane transesophageal echocardiography. In the deep transgastric view, the body of the right atrium is visualized in the far field, with the ventricles displayed towards the apex of the image sector. This view provides full visualization of the right atrium in contrast to other views where only portions of the right atrium are visualized when displayed in the near field. The deep transgastric window provides an oblique orientation for visualizing the ventricles; however, a true plane is obtained for the body of the right atrium with a vertical projection from 0 to 15 degrees and from 95 to 125 degrees. Minor rightward to leftward rotation of the probe produces a scan of the right atrium from the origin of the superior vena cava to the inferior vena cava.

Withdrawal of the probe to the lower esophageal junction, maintaining a rightward probe orientation, visualizes the posterior portion of the right atrium, tricuspid valve, atrial septum and the origin of the coronary sinus in the superior and central part of the image. Multiple levels of the right atrium may be visualized from the lower esophageal window. From the lower esophageal position and neutral orientation of the probe at 0 degrees, a four-chamber view of the heart is obtained, with the atrium in the superior portion and the ventricles in the inferior portion of the image sector. Slow advancement of the probe, with clockwise or rightward rotation, directs the ultrasound beam towards the right heart, producing a two-chamber orientation. Slow rightward rotation of the probe visualizes the whole body of the right atrium in a 'breadloaf' manner in transverse planes. Initially from the four-chamber view, the right atrium and ventricle are presented in a vertical orientation with the orifice of the inferior vena cava cut in an oblique fashion in the most superior portion of the image and the coronary sinus entering the right atrium in a more longitudinal orientation, inferior and to the right of the inferior vena cava. The septal and anterior tricuspid valve leaflets are visualized along with the basal portion of the right ventricle. With further advancement of the probe the two-chamber right heart is presented in a more horizontal orientation, with the coronary sinus becoming the most superior structure in the image. With slow rightward rotation of the probe, various levels of the right atrium, through the inferior vena cava and the right atrial appendage to the superior vena cava, are visualized in the far field of the image sector. In contrast to the smooth walls of the main body of the right atrium, the right atrial appendage is readily identified by the trabeculation pattern of the pectinate muscles, with a broad based orifice.

Further withdrawal of the probe to the midesophageal position transects the central portion of the right atrium and the atrial septum at the level of the foramen ovale. In the upper to mid-esophageal window, near the base of the heart, longitudinal planes of the right atrium are obtained from 90 to 115 degrees. The inferior and superior vena cava is demonstrated simultaneously in a bicaval view, with the left atrium and atrial septum in the superior portion of the image sector and the right atrium centered in the image. With slow advancement of the probe the body of the right atrium is visualized through various levels of the atrial septum until reaching the level of the tricuspid valve annulus as demonstrated in the inferior portion of the image sector. The whole atrial septum may be interrogated with minor manipulation of the transesophageal probe, specifically demonstrating the foramen ovale in the central area of the image sector. A significant portion of either the inferior or superior vena cava in long axis may be imaged as they enter the right atrium, at an intermediate probe level obtained with clockwise to counterclockwise rotation of the probe and steering the ultrasound beam to the specific level of each vena cava. At the level of the inferior vena cava, minor manipulation of the probe visualizes the orifice of the coronary sinus in relatively the same position as the inferior vena cava but in a more inferior plane. The orifice of the inferior vena cava is readily demonstrated by its larger opening and frequent association with the Eustachian valve. Occasionally, a small, less prominent, vestigial Thebesian valve is demonstrated at the junction of the coronary sinus and the right atrium.

Remnants of the embryological development of the right atrium define many of the anatomical structures that may be seen in the right atrium with various techniques. The right atrium is formed embryologically by the union of the sinus venosus and the primitive atrium. During fetal development, the union of the two structures is demarcated by the sinus venosus valve, which extends vertically from the inferior vena cava to the superior vena cava and serves to direct blood flow from the vena cava to the foramen ovale. During maturation the sinus venosus valve regresses, essentially denoting the vestigial Eustachian valve originating from the inferior orifice of the inferior vena cava extending to the septum primum and the crista terminalis, and frequently produces a protuberance or ridge on the atrial surface extending from the junction of the superior vena cava over the posterior and lateral right atrial wall. Various degrees of abnormal persistence of the sinus venosus valve, is manifest in several variants that may be confused with or interpreted

as abnormal masses within the right atrium with various image modalities which are readily identified with transesophageal echocardiography.[5] If re-absorption is incomplete, the resultant echo-dense membrane extends from the inferior vena cava to the superior vena cava, and delegates the right atrial appendage and the tricuspid valve to a separate lower chamber resulting in a two-chambered right atrium, denoted as cor triatriatum dexter and may be associated with flow obstruction to the right ventricular inflow tract.[6-8] A Chiari network is produced when a filamentous or fishnet remnant remains, and is visualized as a non-obstructive membrane undulating with the cardiac cycle within the right atrium, originating from the inferolateral portion of the atrial wall and extending to the limbus region of the fossa ovalis.[9] A lesser remnant form is denoted as a prominent Eustachian valve, which may be visualized as a highly mobile ligamentous echodense structure at the junction of the inferior vena cava and the right atrium.[10]

Lipomatous hypertrophy represents accumulation of non-encapsulated adipose tissue in the atrial septum contiguous with subendocardial fat.[11-13] Lipomatous hypertrophy appears as brighter echogenic protuberances of the atrial septum usually above, below, and sometimes surrounding the foramen ovale, which has led to the transthoracic echocardiographic description of a 'dumbbell' appearance of the atrial septum. Lipomatous hypertrophy is rarely greater than 2 to 3 cm in diameter, thus differentiating hypertrophy from a true lipoma of the atrial septum. Prominent accumulations of tissue may occur at the primum atrial septum and near the crista terminalis, where the superior vena cava enters the right atrium and joins the right atrial appendage. Occasionally, prominent pectinate muscles in the atrium may be confused with thrombus.

In the upper esophageal horizontal views at 0 degrees, a cross-section of the superior vena cava is demonstrated lying adjacent to the ascending aorta and below the right pulmonary artery seen in long axis projection. Slow withdrawal and mild anteflexion of the probe provides interrogation of a significant length of the superior vena cava in cross-section along with the ascending aorta.

A significant portion of the inferior vena cava in long axis may be visualized in the distal gastric probe position. The transesophageal probe is rotated directly posterior to visualize the descending aorta in cross-section at 0 degrees at a level that approximates the level of the diaphragm and the depth of the image sector is increased to approximately 16 cm. The transducer is rotated to 90 degrees to visualize the aorta in long axis and the probe is slowly advanced with mild retroflexion to visualize the maximum obtainable extent of the aorta. The transesophageal probe is then rotated in a counterclockwise manner until the inferior vena cava is demonstrated lying inferior in the image sector with the same orientation as the aorta, at an approximate level of the superior pole of the right kidney. Color flow Doppler demonstrates low velocity flow in the inferior vena cava in the opposite direction of the aortic flow, with numerous branches at the level of the liver. The probe is slowly withdrawn, with minor manipulation to keep the inferior vena cava central in the image sector until it is seen entering the right atrium.

Left atrium

The left atrium is also visualized in many views with transesophageal echocardiography, but due to its posterior position and close approximation to the esophagus and thus the transducer, only portions of the left atrial cavity are demonstrated within the image sector. Therefore, measurement of the left atrial dimension or area is not feasible by transesophageal echocardiography, requiring the construction of a mental image of the left atrial dimension obtained from multiple views during the examination.[14,15] Each wall segment of the left atrium may be visualized with high resolution, however, by various views and windows.

The body of the left atrium is visualized from the midesophageal window in the four-chamber view. The left atrium is visualized in the apex of the image sector closest to the transducer. The left atrium is visualized in its broadest appearance and full extent with mild retroflexion of the probe and with rotation of the transducer from 0 to 90 degrees. The left atrium may also be visualized with slightly lower resolution from the deep transgastric windows from 15 to 45 degrees, which displays an obliquely cut left ventricle towards the apex of the image sector, with a long axis cut of the body of the left atrium in the center of the image sector. The pulmonary veins are frequently seen entering the posterior wall of the left atrium in these views with minor manipulation of the probe. In the mid-esophageal basal short-axis view at the level of the aortic valve, the left atrium is visualized in a broad extent in transverse planes from 30 to 60 degrees and at longitudinal planes from 120 to 150 degrees. Block et al have proposed this view for measuring the left atrial systolic dimension.[15] In this view, transesophageal imaging produced the best correlation (r = 0.759) of left atrial dimensions determined by standard transthoracic echocardiographic measurement, however this view underestimated the left atrial dimension by 9%. Of particular interest, the imaging position of the patient also influenced the measurement of the left atrium with transesophageal echocardiography, with the best measurement obtained with the patient in the left lateral decubitus position rather than the supine position that is usually encountered in the operative arena.

A prominent fold of tissue may appear emanating from the junction of the left atrial appendage with the left superior pulmonary vein and coursing through the left atrial cavity to the superior limbus of the foramen ovale representing the demarcation of the embryological remnant of the junction of primitive atrium with the pulmonary atrial chamber. Persistence of a membrane with obstruction at the junction of the embryologic atria is cor triatriatum.[16-21]

Left atrial appendage

In contrast to the body of the left atrium, the full extent of the left atrial appendage is demonstrated in multiple planes with transesophageal echocardiography and is the best diagnostic method for visualizing the appendage.[22-24] The left atrial appendage arises from the anterolateral border of the left atrium and lies in the left atrioventricular groove above the proximal portion of the left circumflex coronary artery. The left atrial appendage varies considerably in size and shape, according to age and sex. The orifice of the left atrial appendage is elliptical with a curvilinear shape to the body of the appendage. In greater than 80% of patients the appendage is multilobed with between 2 to 5 side lobes, with a spiraling tail section. Thus the left atrial appendage frequently lies in more than one examining plane. On average the appendage has an orifice diameter of 1.5 to 2.1 cm, a maximal body width of 1.5 to 3.1 cm and a length of 2.5 to 3 cm. In the adult appendage, the pectinate muscles are slightly larger than 1 mm in width.

The left atrial appendage is visualized in short-axis views of the basal heart from the mid-esophageal window adjacent to the left atrium in a transverse plane from 0 to 45 degrees at the level of the aortic valve. With further rotation of the transducer between 75 and 90 degrees the left atrial appendage is visualized in a longitudinal plane from a two-chamber view of the heart. Visualization of the full extent of the left atrial appendage usually requires moving from the transverse plane to the longitudinal plane, with minor rotation of the probe to the left and mild antegrade flexion of the probe with or without lateral rotation. In these positions, the left atrial appendage is visualized adjacent to the left upper pulmonary vein. A prominent accumulation of tissue may be seen at the site where the left pulmonary vein enters the left atrium near the superior margin of the left atrial appendage, demonstrated as a bulbous protrusion known as the Q-tip sign. The left atrial appendage protrudes from the body of the left atrium with a triangular morphology in the long axis. The endocardial surface of the appendage is lined with muscular ridges or pectinate muscles, which appear as multiple small refractile echogenicities that move in unison with the cardiac cycle. Echocardiographically the size, morphology and function of the left atrial appendage may thus be determined.[24,25]

The size of the left atrial appendage may be measured in area or dimension but this does not add considerably to the overall visual assessment of the appendage size. Typically the orifice dimension may be measured from the junction of the left superior vein to the junction of the left atrial appendage and the left atrium. The morphology of the appendage is noted in multiple continuous planes in order to determine the number of lobes present and to differentiate pectinate muscles from thrombi. Thrombi, when present, usually are larger, produce a filling defect to the appendage and demonstrate texture distinct from the surrounding muscle and frequently exhibit chaotic motion during the cardiac cycle. Spontaneous echocardiographic contrast when present is noted, and shares an association with thrombi, which should be excluded through a meticulous examination.[26–28]

Left atrial appendage function is assessed with color and pulsed Doppler techniques. Color Doppler provides visualization of the maximum flow velocity within the left atrial appendage to provide optimum alignment of the pulsed Doppler sample. In addition, color Doppler helps in determining the morphology of the appendage by delineating its shape when filled with color flow. Color Doppler may also help define thrombi from pectinate muscles as a result of the color flow outline produced in the cavity of the appendage. Once the site of the maximal flow velocity is determined the pulse Doppler sample volume is directed to the proximal third of the appendage.[24,29] Lower filter settings in conjunction with smaller sample size settings may be required to produce a clear envelope for the spectral analysis of the appendage flow. The appendage flow pattern recorded will differ according to the underlying cardiac rhythm and heart rate.[30] In patients with normal sinus rhythm, left atrial appendage flow has four components.[31–33] The first component is a contraction wave, denoted as a large positive deflection (towards the transducer) in late diastole following the electrocardiographic P wave. Velocities have been determined between 50 and 65 cm/s in normal patients. The second component is the filling wave, which again is a large deflection (46 to 58 cm/s) in a negative direction following the contraction wave denoting systolic filling of the atrium and appendage. The third component is the systolic reflection wave, which consists of alternating positive and negative deflections between 20 and 38 cm/s that gradually decrease in size, and which are determined by the cardiac cycle length. The fourth component is the early diastolic outflow wave, denoted by a low velocity positive deflection, which follows the mitral Doppler E wave and the electrocardiographic T wave. The early diastolic outflow wave is thought to coincide with passive emptying of the left atrial appendage during rapid ventricular filling in early diastole. With faster heart rates, the contraction wave and the early diastolic outflow wave are frequently merged. During atrial fibrillation, rapid fibrillatory flow waves are recorded, with higher velocity waves recorded during diastole in contrast to systole, with higher overall velocities recorded with longer RR intervals and slower ventricular response rates. In atrial flutter, the flutter flow waves produced in the appendage have a higher overall velocity than atrial fibrillation, showing a two-fold increase, and are usually slower corresponding to the slower and more regular ventricular response.[24,30]

The determination of atrial appendage function may provide insight for overall left atrial function and other cardiac hemodynamics. Although left atrial appendage function is not entirely understood, various observations regarding left atrial appendage function have been described. Left atrial appendage flow velocities, predominately the early diastolic outflow velocity, become depressed with the normal aging process. Left atrial appendage function appears to be affected by loading conditions, where increases in left atrial pressure increases left atrial appendage contraction, initially and then decreases when the pulmonary capillary wedge pressure is increased to pathologic levels.

There appears to be a strong correlation between left atrial appendage dysfunction and the formation of left atrial thrombi, and risk of future thromboembolic events, especially in patients with atrial fibrillation and atrial flutter.[26–28,34] Left atrial appendage dysfunction denoted by low velocity flows in the appendage are associated with spontaneous echocardiographic contrast, which is indicative of stagnant blood flow in the left atrial cavity and left atrial appendage, and is a precursor to thrombus formation. In a subset of the SPAF III trial for determining the risk of thromboembolic events in atrial fibrillation patients, transesophageal echocardiographic determination of left atrial appendage dysfunction helped predict spontaneous echocardiographic contrast, presence of left atrial thrombus and thromboembolic events associated with ischemic stroke and peripheral systemic embolization.[34] Spontaneous echocardiographic contrast was associated with left atrial contraction velocities < 20 cm/s in 75% with left atrial appendage thrombus identified in 17% of patients with atrial fibrillation. In patients with higher velocities the incidence of spontaneous echocardiographic contrast was detected in only 58% and thrombus in only 5% of patients. In the patients with low atrial contraction velocities there was also a 2.6 times greater incidence of ischemic stroke.

The short-term success for the conversion of atrial fibrillation to sinus rhythm may be predicted by left atrial appendage velocities of greater than 20 cm/s before cardioversion.[35,36] After cardioversion of atrial fibrillation and atrial flutter, left atrial dysfunction or stunning may be detected with the measurement of left atrial appendage flow velocities. Stunning, or temporary decline in left atrial mechanical function, as denoted by a further reduction in already low appendage flow velocities with transesophageal echocardiography, occurs immediately after cardioversion of atrial fibrillation despite the return of sinus rhythm. Stunning of the left atrial function may predispose to spontaneous echocardiographic contrast and thrombus formation, and may result in thromboembolic events that have been observed in patients after spontaneous, pharmacological and electrical cardioversion. The occurrence of atrial stunning substantiates the need for anticoagulation during the recovery period and the return of mechanical atrial function.

Pulmonary veins

Usually all four pulmonary veins may be readily demonstrated with transesophageal echocardiography.[37–39] In order to consistently demonstrate all four pulmonary veins, variations in pulmonary vein anatomy must be appreciated in relationship to the orientation of the posterior wall of

the left atrium in the chest cavity (Figure 6.1). The superior pulmonary veins enter the superior portion of the left atrium in an anteroposterior direction in relation to the transesophageal transducer as it lies in the neutral position within the esophagus. In addition the esophagus lies closer to the longitudinal axis of the right pulmonary veins than the left pulmonary veins. The inferior pulmonary veins enter the right atrium in either a posteroanterior direction or a near parallel plane coinciding to the true frontal plane of the left atrium and the heart as visualized from the esophagus. In addition, to the spatial orientation of the pulmonary veins, variations in the connections to the left atrium commonly occur. The left pulmonary veins frequently exhibit a common opening for the superior and inferior vein, whereas the right pulmonary veins may demonstrate separate openings with an additional accessory vein.

In the mid to upper esophageal short-axis basal view of the heart from 0 to 45 degrees, the left superior

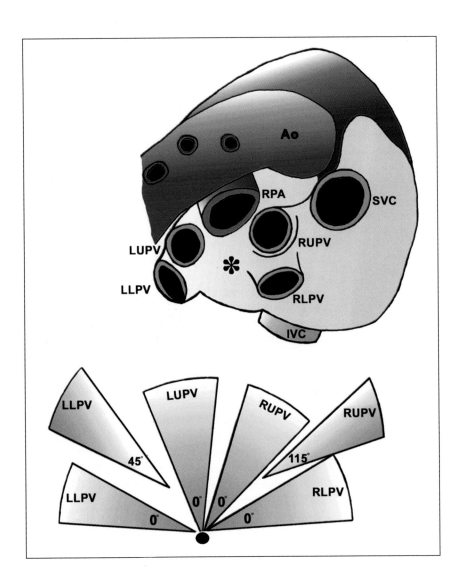

Figure 6.1
Pulmonary vein anatomy. Artist's rendition of the posterior aspect of the heart in respect to the transesophageal echocardiographic probe position depicting the position of the pulmonary veins and the imaging planes obtained for each pulmonary vein.

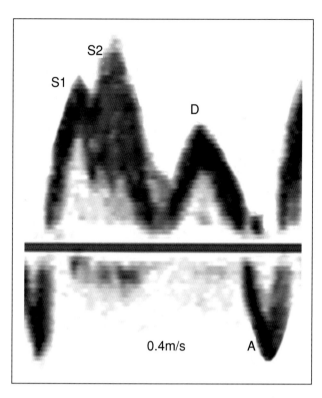

Figure 6.2

Normal pulmonary venous flow. Normal pulsed-wave Doppler recording of pulmonary venous flow. Sampling of pulmonary venous flow is easily performed with transesophageal echocardiography, which provides excellent quality tracings in the majority of cases. Sampling may be performed from all four pulmonary veins. The pulmonary venous flow profile consists of a dominate systolic (S) wave followed by a less dominate diastolic (D) wave and a small retrograde (AR) wave which corresponds to atrial systole. The systolic wave in a good recording is usually notched with the initial component (S1) corresponding to atrial relaxation and the second component (S2) related to the normal motion of the mitral annular descent during the cardiac cycle. S1, first systolic flow wave; S2, second systolic flow wave; D, diastolic flow wave; A, atrial reversal flow wave.

pulmonary vein is identified lateral to the orifice of the left atrial appendage. The left superior pulmonary vein may be better visualized with anteflexion and slight leftward rotation of the probe. To visualize the left lower pulmonary vein requires further leftward or counterclockwise rotation with or without slight advancement of the probe, which visualizes the orifice of the inferior pulmonary vein as the left atrial appendage disappears from view. The left pulmonary veins may also be visualized from the longitudinal plane with rotation of the transducer from 90 to 110 degrees, in the mid-esophageal

window. With leftward rotation of the probe, frequently both the left superior and inferior pulmonary veins will be seen simultaneously joining the left atrium.

The right pulmonary veins may be visualized in the mid-esophageal short-axis basal view at 0 degrees with slight rotation of the probe to the right of the midline. The right superior pulmonary vein again is readily visualized entering the left atrium adjacent to the interatrial septum, in close proximity to the origin of the superior vena cava. With further rightward rotation of the probe the right inferior pulmonary vein may be visualized entering the left atrium in close approximation to the apex of the image sector, frequently allowing simultaneous visualization of the right superior pulmonary vein. In the bicaval view of the right atrium at 90 degrees, the superior and inferior vena cava are visualized with vertical orientation of the superior vena cava to the right atrium adjacent to a cross-section of the right pulmonary artery. Rightward rotation of the probe visualizes the right superior pulmonary vein entering from a superior direction to the left atrium adjacent to the interatrial septum. Further rotation of the probe visualizes the right inferior pulmonary vein entering the left atrium in an inferior direction. Improved visualization may require rotating the transducer closer to 60 degrees.

After imaging each pulmonary vein, minor manipulation of the transesophageal probe, usually allows orientation of the pulmonary vein in the image sector to provide a parallel plane for the pulsed Doppler interrogation of pulmonary venous flow (Figure 6.2).

Ventricular function

Two-dimensional echocardiography is an excellent tool for evaluating regional and global systolic ventricular function. Improvements in echocardiography technology have improved overall image quality. In addition, newer methods including harmonic imaging, automated border detection, Doppler tissue imaging and echocardiographic contrast agents (Figure 6.3), allow the assessment of ventricular function with transthoracic echocardiography in the majority of patients. Therefore transesophageal echocardiography has a limited role in the evaluation of systolic ventricular function. Transesophageal echocardiography is ideal, however, for monitoring systolic function during both cardiac and non-cardiac surgery or in critical care environment.

Echocardiography assesses regional systolic function through the demonstration of segmental wall motion and global function through ventricular size and volume determinations. Studies have shown excellent correlation between transesophageal and transthoracic echocardiography for ventricular function evaluation.

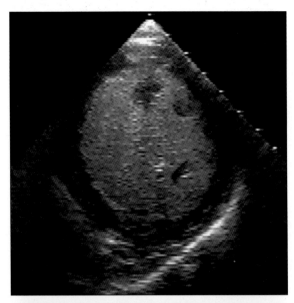

a

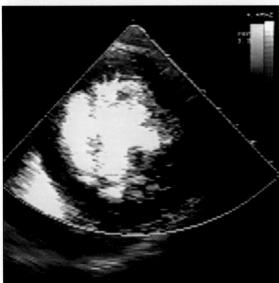

b

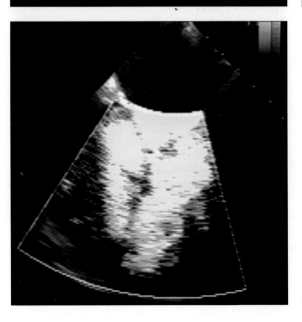

c

Figure 6.3
Myocardial contrast. A. Myocardial contrast agents are currently available that when injected peripherally through a vein cross the pulmonary bed and highlight the blood pool of the left ventricle and define the endocardial myocardial border in great detail for the evaluation of regional and global ventricular function. Power Doppler with harmonic imaging and myocardial contrast agents provide assessment of wall motion through the definition of the endocardial borders, and myocardial contrast uptake. B. Short axis left ventricle. C. Longitudinal axis left ventricle obtained from the four-chamber view in the lower esophageal window.

Regional ventricular function

Transesophageal echocardiography provides direct visualization of left and right systolic ventricular wall thickening and endocardial motion for the assessment of regional ventricular function (Figures 6.4 and 6.5). Regional wall motion abnormalities are visually assessed in a qualitative manner as to the degree of thickening of the ventricular walls during systole.[40–45] Myocardial ischemia is identified by illustrating a decrease in myocardial contraction and is shown echocardiographically as regional wall motion abnormalities. The normal myocardium demonstrates systolic thickening of greater than 40%. Wall thickening is greater in the free wall segments than the ventricular septum and gradually decreases from the apex to the base of the heart. Wall motion abnormalities are labeled as hypokinetic when there is less than 30% systolic wall thickening, akinetic with less than 10% systolic thickening, and dyskinetic when there is no detectable motion and there is systolic thinning. It is important to remember that the size of the regional wall motion abnormality may be overestimated due to tethering of the margins of abnormal motion to normal segments.[46] The borders of the abnormal segment will be dragged along with the motion of the normal segment. Although both transesophageal and transthoracic echocardiography are subjective assessments good correlation is obtained with either technique compared with assessments of myocardial perfusion.

Guidelines for the assessment of regional wall motion have been recommended by the ASE/SCA for transesophageal echocardiography.[47] These guidelines are based on a 16-segment model of the left ventricle as was originally recommended by the Subcommittee on Quantification of the ASE Standards Committee for transthoracic echocardiography (Figures 6.4 and 6.5).[48] The 16-segment model divides the left ventricle into three levels, consisting of the basal, mid and apical levels as visualized from short-axis mitral annular, mid papillary muscle, and

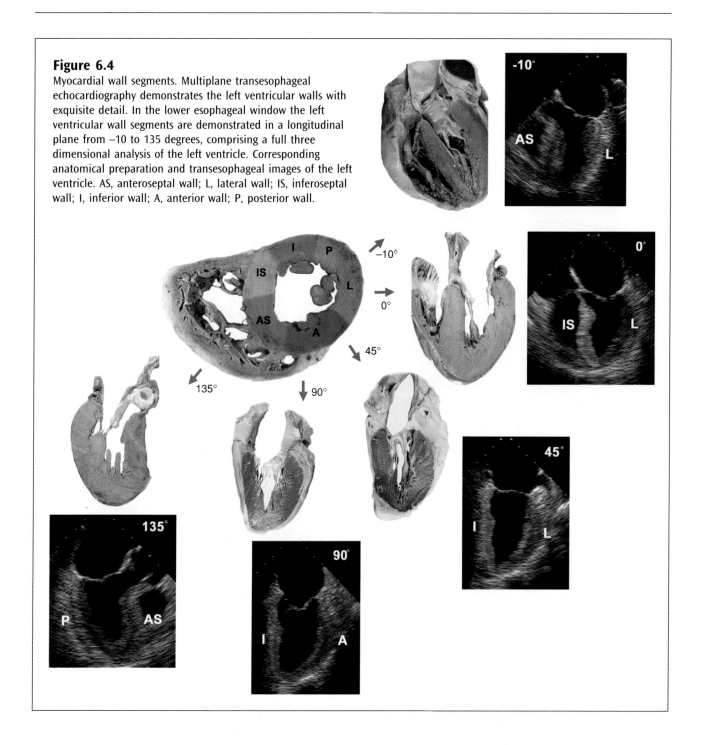

Figure 6.4
Myocardial wall segments. Multiplane transesophageal echocardiography demonstrates the left ventricular walls with exquisite detail. In the lower esophageal window the left ventricular wall segments are demonstrated in a longitudinal plane from −10 to 135 degrees, comprising a full three dimensional analysis of the left ventricle. Corresponding anatomical preparation and transesophageal images of the left ventricle. AS, anteroseptal wall; L, lateral wall; IS, inferoseptal wall; I, inferior wall; A, anterior wall; P, posterior wall.

apical views obtained from the transgastric window. Each level is further divided into segments around its circumference, with the basal and mid levels comprising six segments (anteroseptal, anterior, lateral, posterior, inferior, septal) and the apical level four segments (anterior, lateral, inferior, septal). The percentage degree of wall thickening during systole for each segment is assessed as normal (greater than 30% thickening), mild hypokinesis (10% to 30% thickening), severely hypoki-

netic (less than 10% thickening), akinetic (demonstrating lack of detectable thickening) and dyskinetic or paradoxical endocardial motion. Additionally, a score may be assigned to each wall segment: 1, normal; 2, mildly hypokinetic; 3, severely hypokinetic; 4, akinetic; 5, dyskinetic, which has been utilized in various degrees in the literature. It must be emphasized however that the delineation of the posterior and inferior walls used in this scheme does not coincide with traditional anatomic or

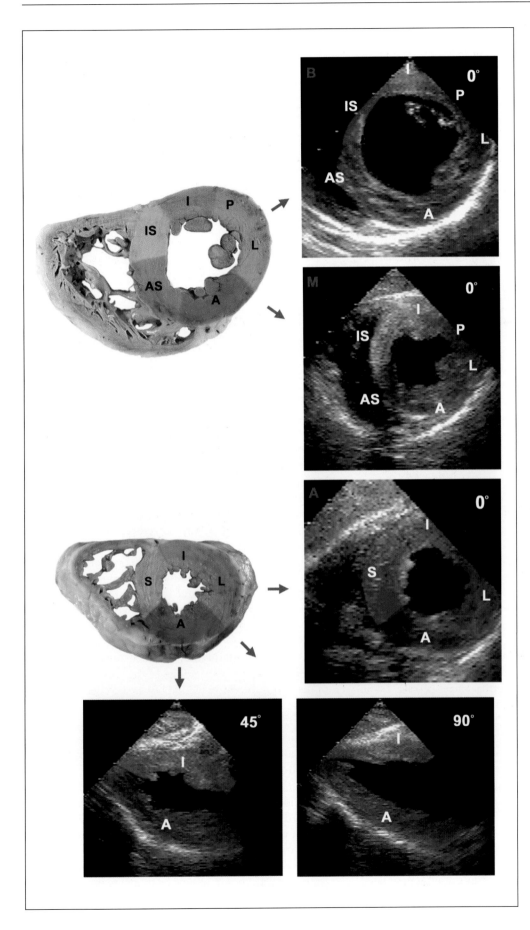

Figure 6.5
Myocardial wall segments. Multiplane transesophageal echocardiographic images of the left ventricle obtained from the transgastric window. Corresponding anatomical images and echocardiographic images obtained from the base, mid-papillary and apical areas of the left ventricle at 0 degrees. Longitudinal images of the left ventricle are obtained from 45 to 90 degrees. AS, anteroseptal wall; L, lateral wall; IS, inferoseptal wall; I, inferior wall; A, anterior wall; P, posterior wall.

surgical nomenclature utilizing strict posterior and inferior labels for wall segments, which may produce confusion or discrepancies when describing these segments. The wall motion score for each segment is added together and divided by 16 to provide a wall motion score index, with an increasing score denoting severe regional systolic function. A score of greater than 1.7 has been correlated with greater than a 20% defect in myocardial perfusion.[49]

Global ventricular function

Global ventricular function is primarily assessed echocardiographically by changes in ventricular size and volume through quantitative or qualitative analysis. Left ventricular cavity volume measurements may be obtained echocardiographically using either the modified Simpson's method or the single plane method. Currently the ASE recommends measurement of ventricular volume with biplane or paired orthogonal longitudinal views of the left ventricle, which are easily provided by transesophageal echocardiography from the four-chamber (0 degree) and two-chamber (90 degree) views as obtained from the mid-esophageal window.[48] The summation of disks or the modified Simpson's algorithm is frequently used in these views to provide an echocardiographic volumetric analysis. The technique involves tracing the endocardial border of the ventricle at end-diastole and end-systole, excluding the papillary muscles and determining the maximal long axis dimension in each view. The tracings and dimensions are then used to essentially break up the left ventricular cavity into a consecutive series of volumetric disks starting at the level of the mitral annulus and progressing through the ventricular apex, incorporating the sum of each volumetric disc into a single ventricular volume. In this manner, a truer volumetric shape is obtained in difference to other formulas, which frequently make assumptions about the shape of the ventricle.[50,51] This is particularly important when regional wall motion abnormalities are present. Ejection fraction is then calculated as EF = EDV − ESV/EDV with normal values of 70 ± 7% in male and 65 ± 10% in female patients.[52] Fractional shortening may be determined as FS = EDD-ESD/EDD and fractional area change as FAC = EDA-ESA/EDA.

Doppler echocardiography can also be utilized to determine stroke volume and cardiac output.[53–55] The flow rate through a circular orifice with a cross-sectional area is obtained by multiplying that area by the time-velocity integral of the blood flow through an orifice. The left ventricular outflow tract is the orifice usually utilized for calculating stroke volume. The stroke volume is calculated as SV cm^3 = A (cm^2) × velocity (cm/s) × time (s), where A = (orifice diameter)^2 × π/4. Cardiac output is calculated as CO = SV × HR.

Global left ventricular myocardial contractility can also be determined with Doppler interrogation of the mitral regurgitant jet.[56,57] This is particularly useful when systolic function visually appears normal. The dP/dt is the time taken for the mitral regurgitant velocity to rise from 1 to 3 m/s. In this time period the left atrial pressure does not increase significantly and the rise in ventricular pressure is approximately 32 mmHg. Therefore myocardial contractility can be determined independently as LV dP/dt = 32/t (ms) × 100 mmHg/s. Normal values for dP/dt are usually 1,200 mmHg/s or greater. Initial studies have demonstrated good correlation for ventricular dP/dt measured with echocardiography and obtained in the cardiac catheterization laboratory.

Acoustic quantification (automated border detection)

Acoustic quantification assists in the detection of global cardiac function echocardiographically.[58–62] Acoustic quantification incorporates the process of automated border detection, which allows the ultrasonic distinction between the blood and tissue interface (Figure 6.6). Automated border detection is provided by an algorithm that analyzes acoustic data using an integrated backscatter analysis according to the power of the returning ultrasound signal in reference to a fixed threshold. Returning signals above the threshold represent tissue signals and signals below the threshold are related to the blood pool. The data is collected from every scan line within the image sector frame by frame, and the interface difference between the two thresholds is denoted as the endocardial border and is tagged by the computer. The number of samples identified as blood within a user-defined region of interest denotes the area or volume of the blood pool.

In real time, the two-dimensional image is displayed simultaneously with an outline of the endocardial border or display of the entire blood pool area. When a region of interest such as the left ventricle is defined in a single plane, the blood area or blood volume is calculated and presented in a variety of formats, including real-time wave forms and/or averaged composite waveforms for changes in end-systolic and end-diastolic areas or volumes. Automatic calculations of ejection fraction and fractional area change are done. In addition, a rate-of-change waveform (dA/dt or dV/dt) may be displayed for calculating peak ejection rate, peak rapid filling rate and atrial filling fraction rate.[63,64]

Color kinesis uses automatic border detection to define the endocardial border, frame by frame, to indicate border excursion or contraction during the cardiac cycle.[65–71]

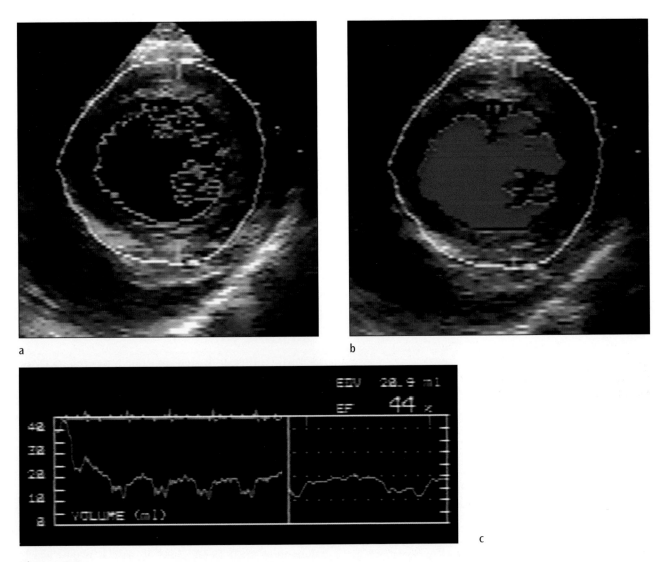

Figure 6.6

Acoustic quantification. Acoustic quantification incorporates the process of automated border detection, which allows the ultrasonic distinction between the blood and tissue interface. Automated border detection is provided by an algorithm that analyzes acoustic data using the principal of integrated backscatter analysis according to the power of the returning ultrasound signal in reference to a fixed threshold. Returning signals above the threshold represent tissue signals and signals below the threshold are related to the blood pool. The data are collected from every scan line within the image sector frame by frame and the interface difference between the two thresholds is denoted as the endocardial border and is tagged by the computer. The number of samples identified as blood within a user-defined region of interest denotes the area or volume of the blood pool.

In real time, the two-dimensional image is displayed simultaneously with outline of the endocardial border (A) or display of the entire blood pool area (B). When a region of interest such as the left ventricle is defined in a single plane, the blood area or blood volume is calculated and presented in a variety of formats, including real-time wave forms and/or averaged composite waveforms for changes in end-systolic and end-diastolic areas or volumes (C). Automatic calculations of ejection fraction and fractional area change are performed.

With real-time imaging the endocardial border excursion is color-coded during systole, diastole or in a user defined time interval, and the coded color is displayed simultaneously with the two-dimensional cardiac image (Figure 6.7). Color kinesis may be used for the global and regional assessment of left ventricular systolic function as well as in the assessment of global left ventricular diastolic function.

The accuracy of acoustic quantification has been substantiated with other established methods for determining left ventricular function. However it is also highly dependent on the quality of the image obtained making it

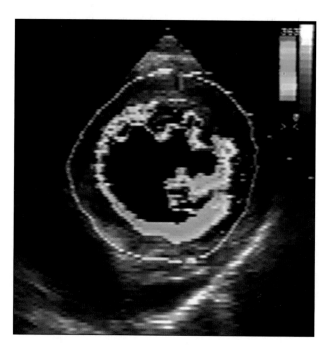

Figure 6.7
Color kinesis. Color kinesis uses automatic border detection to define the endocardial border, frame by frame to indicate border excursion or contraction during the cardiac cycle. With real-time imaging, the endocardial border excursion is color-coded during systole, diastole or in a user defined time interval and displayed simultaneously with the two-dimensional cardiac image. Color kinesis may be used for the global and regional assessment of left ventricular global and regional systolic function as well as in the assessment of global left ventricular diastolic function.

extremely attractive in conjunction with transesophageal imaging.[72–84] Technical factors for adjusting the overall echocardiographic gain (transmitted and received acoustic signals), time gain compensation (amplification of returning signals at a specific range) and lateral gain control (amplification of returning signals within a specific vertical region) dramatically influence image quality and differentiates real cardiac structures from echocardiographic artifact which would obviously effect the accuracy of the technique.

Accuracy of acoustic quantification is also determined by the proper definition of the region of interest, which should include the maximum and minimum blood areas with the entire left ventricular endocardium, excluding extraneous blood pools from the other cardiac chambers during the cardiac cycle and translational motion of the heart within the chest. With these considerations acoustic quantification has been delegated to the role of prolonged monitoring of left ventricular function in critical care, or in conjunction with anesthesia monitoring during surgery.[85,86] Standard acoustic quantification and color

kinesis have also been used for research purposes with both transthoracic and transesophageal echocardiography.

Doppler tissue imaging may be also used for determining the velocity of the myocardium during systole[87,88] (Figure 6.8). Conventional color-flow Doppler recording is modified from its standard form to detect the low wall motion velocity of the myocardium during systole. Ventricular wall motion towards the transducer is color-coded in shades of red, and ventricular wall motion away from the transducer is color-coded in shades of blue, simultaneously with the two-dimensional image. The absence of motion (akinesis) appears as black, with the brightest shades of color representing the higher velocities of motion. With two-dimensional (and especially M-mode recording) wall motion velocity can be assessed over time during the cardiac cycle.

Diastolic function

Normal ventricular diastolic function is a necessary factor in maintaining normal hemodynamics and cardiac function during rest and exercise. Although heart failure is usually equated with abnormal ventricular systolic function, most cases of heart failure result from a combination of systolic and diastolic dysfunction. Simply stated, myocardial disease may affect the relaxation quality of the ventricular myocardium resulting in the abnormal elevation of diastolic pressure promoting abnormal cardiac performance and eventually heart failure. In the presence of normal systolic function, heart failure may be precipitated by pathologies promoting diastolic dysfunction alone in as many as one-third of cases. It is now widely appreciated that abnormal diastolic function is particularly relevant in elderly patients, as a result of the normal aging process of the heart irrespective of the presence of other cardiac pathology.

The maintenance of a normal forward stroke volume with each cardiac cycle, as defined by the Frank-Starling Law, is provided by the ability of the heart to properly fill and contract without incurring elevated ventricular end-diastolic pressure. The hearts filling ability is promoted largely by the dynamics of myocardial relaxation during diastole, and thus defines diastolic function. The elastic recoil of the ventricle, the rate of relaxation of the ventricular myocardium, the compliance or stiffness of the myocardium and the driving pressure for filling as reflected in the atrial pressure characterize the determinants of ventricular filling.

Echocardiography and Doppler flow indices may be used to describe diastolic function, non-invasively. It must be remembered that many of the traditional parameters for determining diastolic function invasively with cardiac catheterization are not directly measured

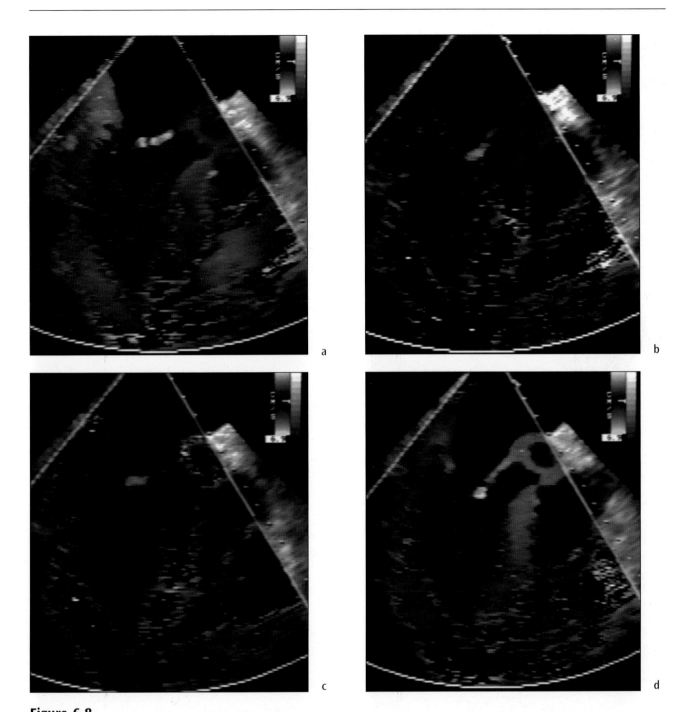

a

b

c

d

Figure 6.8

Tissue Doppler. Doppler tissue imaging may also be used for determining the velocity of the myocardium during systole and diastole. Conventional color-flow Doppler recording is modified from its standard form to detect the low wall motion velocity of the myocardium during systole. A–H. Ventricular wall motion towards the transducer is color-coded in shades of red, and ventricular wall motion away from the transducer is color-coded in shades of blue, simultaneously with the two-dimensional image. The absence of motion (akinesis) appears as black with the brightest shades of color representing the higher velocities of motion. With two-dimensional, and especially m-mode recording, wall motion velocity can be assessed over time during the cardiac cycle.

I. Doppler tissue imaging may also be used to assess diastolic function. Tissue Doppler displays the excursion of mitral annular motion during the cardiac cycle and most notably does not appear to be influenced by the preload state. The displacement and velocity of the mitral annulus along the longitudinal axis of the left ventricular is examined from the four-chamber view either along the septal or the lateral longitudinal axis of the mitral annulus and corresponds to the myocardial diastolic velocities induced by myocardial relaxation. Myocardial velocities recorded with tissue Doppler consist of the peak systolic velocity (S_m), the peak early diastolic (E_m) and late diastolic (A_m) myocardial expansion velocities. A–H. Tissue Doppler recording throughout the cardiac cycle. I. Normal tissue Doppler tracing. S_m, peak systolic velocity; E_m, peak early diastolic; A_m, late diastolic myocardial expansion velocities. *continued*

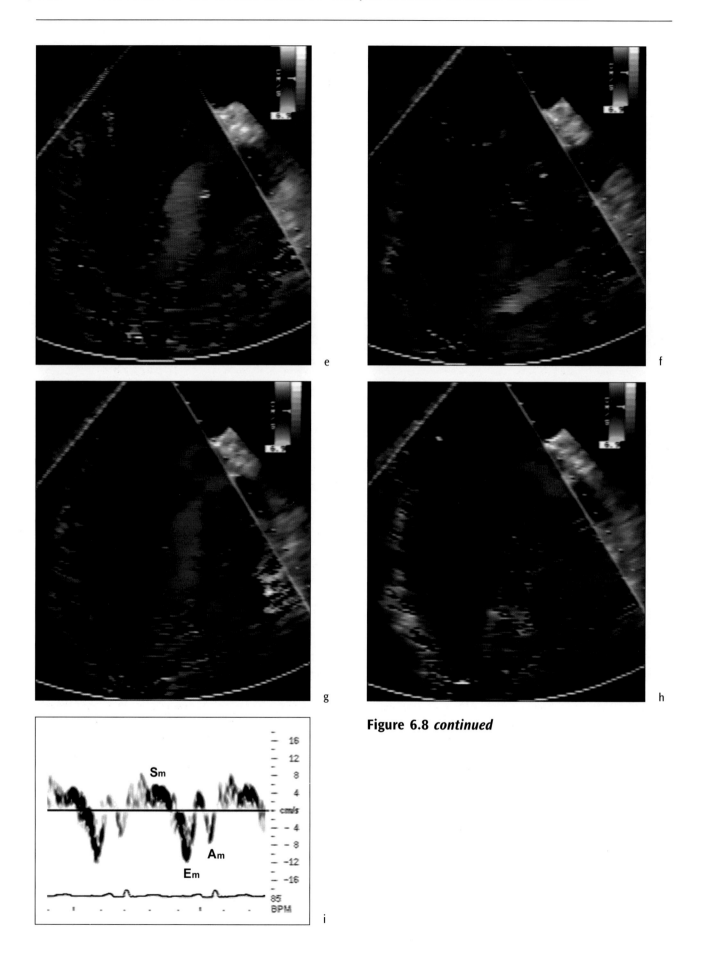

e

f

g

h

Figure 6.8 *continued*

i

with echocardiography and Doppler but largely are inferred from specific observations and measurements. Diastolic function may be difficult to assess in many cases for a number of reasons. Primarily, diastolic function may be influenced by one or multiple pathologies in the same patient, in addition to the normal changes in myocardial relaxation or diastolic properties that occur due to the normal myocardial aging process. Individual pathologies may be responsible for producing a variety of abnormalities. Doppler flow indices utilized to assess diastolic function may be influenced by heart rate, after-load, preload, and intravascular volume and therefore may not adequately represent the true cardiac hemodynamics. Lastly, the parameters for assessing diastolic function for many of the Doppler technologies are still evolving.

Despite these limitations, transesophageal echocardiography is extremely useful for obtaining and evaluating the Doppler flow indices utilized in determining left ventricular relaxation disorders or abnormal diastolic function, especially when transthoracic imaging does not provide adequate diagnostic information. Recently, tissue Doppler and color m-mode technologies have become available for use with transesophageal probes increasing the armamentarium of transesophageal echocardiography. Transesophageal echocardiography is therefore well suited for providing an overall accurate assessment of cardiac performance, to help distinguish particularly difficult cases.

Doppler interrogation of the mitral inflow velocity and pulmonary venous flow velocity provides a semiquantitative, indirect assessment for left ventricular filling pressure and thus provides assessment for diastolic dysfunction,[89–92] in the absence of mitral valvular disease (Figure 6.9). Transesophageal echocardiography is particularly useful for assessing pulmonary venous flows. Good alignment of the Doppler beam for the mitral flow velocity is obtained in the midesophageal window from the four-chamber view. The Doppler sample size is appropriately adjusted for the mitral orifice and recordings are obtained from the level of the mitral valve leaflet tips for determining maximum flow velocities and intervals and at the mitral valve annulus for determining volumetric flow indices. The normal flow profile recorded at the leaflet tips consist of a prominent early rapid diastolic filling wave or E wave and late diastolic wave or A wave associated with atrial contraction.[93] In normal patients, the majority of filling occurs during the early rapid filling phase, with approximately 15 to 20% of filling occurring in late diastole during atrial contraction. This is reflected in the larger E wave and small A wave appearance. The components of the E wave correspond to the left atrial and left ventricular hemodynamic pressure crossover points during the cardiac cycle. The E wave starts when the ventricular pressure initially falls below the atrial pressure

during relaxation, and reaches its peak when the left ventricular pressure rebounds above atrial pressure as a result of the inertial forces of the flow of blood, which leads to the gradual deceleration of the E wave when the left atrial and ventricular pressures equilibrate.[94] The demonstration of a normal E wave deceleration time has been described as a useful parameter for assessing normal filling and is usually between 160 to 240 ms. The A wave occurs with atrial systole and is generated by the increase of atrial pressure during atrial contraction. The E/A velocity ratio provides an index describing the normal left atrial and ventricular pressure relationship, and is normally greater than 1.

To properly interpret the E and A wave velocities and the corresponding E/A velocity ratio the normal effects of aging must be recognized.[95] In younger patients, the E/A ratio is usually greater than 1 by a significant degree. With advancing age the E/A ratio decreases with the E/A ratio gradually approaching 1. With further advancement in age the E/A ratio becomes less than 1 at around age 65 to 70 years old.

Diastolic dysfunction is associated with higher left ventricular diastolic pressures, which influence the mitral profile for the E wave and A wave velocity.[96] Relaxation abnormalities impede early filling and thus decrease the E wave velocity in addition to prolonging the E wave deceleration. To maintain stroke volume, there is a corresponding increase in atrial contractions contribution to filling and thus A wave velocity.[97,98] Therefore, initially in diastolic dysfunction the E/A ratio is less than 1. As the disease process progresses, restrictive physiology develops and the ratio gradually becomes greater than 1 as exhibited by a marked increase in E wave amplitude and shortening of the E deceleration and diminishing of the A wave amplitude. A pseudonormal pattern of mitral inflow may be demonstrated with the development of restrictive physiology in the later phases of diastolic dysfunction, denoted by increased left ventricular end-diastolic and left atrial pressures, with the left atrial pressure greater than the left ventricular end-diastolic pressure. The pseudonormal pattern is represented as an intermediate pattern during progressive change from an E/A ratio initially less than 1 with milder dysfunction to an E/A ratio greater than 1 with the development of restrictive physiology,[99] limiting the use of the mitral inflow velocities exclusively. Many physiological factors may alter the left ventricular and left atrial pressure relationship, thus affecting the mitral flow profile,[100–102] these include heart rate, atrioventricular block, preload and afterload, as well as intravascular volume. Similarities between the normal effects of aging and the presence of disease may also occur which may produce a confusing picture, highlighting the need for incorporating additional variables for determining normal versus abnormal diastolic dysfunction.[103,104]

The isovolumic relaxation time is determined by the rate of ventricular relaxation, which is impaired with

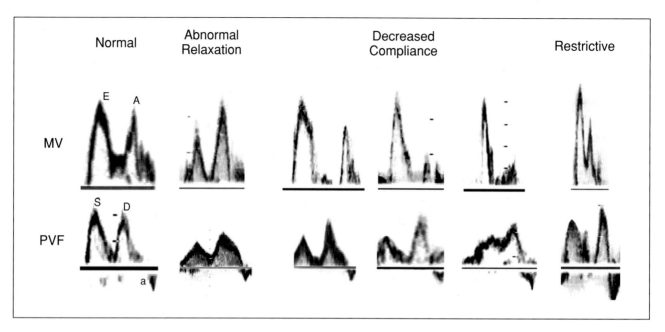

Figure 6.9

Assessment of diastolic function. Mitral inflow and pulmonary venous pulsed Doppler flow recordings depicting the normal relationship of the mitral and pulmonary flows, during abnormal relaxation, decreased diastolic compliance and with restrictive physiology. The normal flow profile recorded at the leaflet tips consist of a prominent early rapid diastolic filling wave or E wave and late diastolic wave or A wave associated with atrial contraction. Diastolic dysfunction is associated with higher left ventricular diastolic pressures, which influences the mitral profile for the E wave and A wave velocity. Relaxation abnormalities impede early filling and thus decrease the E wave velocity in addition to prolonging the E wave deceleration. To maintain stroke volume there is a corresponding increase in atrial contraction contribution to filling and thus A wave velocity. Therefore, initially in diastolic dysfunction the E/A ratio is less than 1. As the disease process progresses, restrictive physiology develops and the ratio gradually becomes greater than 1 as exhibited by a marked increase in E wave amplitude and shortening of the E deceleration and decrease of the A wave amplitude. A pseudonormal pattern of the mitral inflow may be demonstrated with the development of restrictive physiology in the later phases of diastolic dysfunction, denoted by increased left ventricular end-diastolic and left atrial pressures, with the left atrial pressure greater than the left ventricular end-diastolic pressure. The pseudonormal pattern is represented as an intermediate pattern during the progressive change from an E/A ratio initially less than 1 with milder dysfunction to an E/A ratio greater than 1 with the development of restrictive physiology, limiting the use of the mitral inflow velocities exclusively.

The amplitude of the pulmonary venous systolic wave is dependent on overall atrial function, as determined by the elastic properties of the left atrium, degree of annular descent and the driving pressure of the pulmonary veins, and is reduced with left ventricular dysfunction among other factors. The diastolic wave corresponds to the mitral E wave and, similar to the E wave, the amplitude of the diastolic wave is affected by the age of the patient, being more prominent in younger patients and gradually decreasing with age. The retrograde atrial wave corresponds to the mitral inflow A wave recorded during atrial contraction. With atrial contraction the majority of blood flow is directed towards the mitral orifice with a small amount flowing in a retrograde fashion into the pulmonary veins since their orifice is not protected with a remnant valve. The amplitude of the retrograde atrial contraction is smaller and its duration is less in comparison to the mitral inflow A wave. In cases of left ventricular diastolic dysfunction associated with a stiff ventricle and a raised left ventricular end-diastolic pressure, both the amplitude and duration of the retrograde atrial contraction wave increases in relation to the mitral inflow A wave.

diastolic dysfunction and thus is prolonged.[105–107] The isovolumic relaxation time usually exhibits a strong correlation with the E wave deceleration time. The normal isovolumic relaxation time is 70 to 90 ms. The isovolumic relaxation time is demonstrated echocardiographically as the interval between the aortic valve closure and the mitral valve opening. The isovolumic relaxation time may be measured with Doppler echocardiography by placing the Doppler sample volume in-between the left ventricular outflow tract and the anterior mitral valve and measuring the flow interval from the end of the outflow velocity to the beginning of mitral inflow.

The pulmonary venous flow profile may be recorded with pulsed Doppler techniques from any one of the pulmonary veins with transesophageal echocardiography (Figure 6.2). Although not fully standardized, the pulsed sample volume is placed in the proximal third or 1–2 cm from the orifice of the pulmonary vein, and the sample size is adjusted to accommodate the vein dimension in order to obviate artifact from the venous walls during the cardiac cycle. The pulmonary venous flow profile consists of a predominate systolic (S) wave followed by a less dominate diastolic (D) wave and a small retrograde (AR) wave which corresponds to atrial systole.[108–113] The systolic wave in a good recording is usually notched with the initial component (S1) corresponding to atrial relaxation and the second component (S2) related to the normal motion of the mitral annular descent during the cardiac cycle. The amplitude of the systolic wave is dependent on overall atrial function, as determined by the elastic properties of the left atrium, degree of annular descent and the driving pressure of the pulmonary veins and is reduced with left ventricular dysfunction among other factors. The diastolic wave corresponds to the mitral E wave and, similar to the E wave, the amplitude of the diastolic wave is affected by the age of the patient, being more prominent in younger patients and gradually decreases with aging.

The retrograde atrial wave corresponds to the mitral inflow A wave recorded during atrial contraction. With atrial contraction the majority of blood flow is directed towards the mitral orifice with a small amount flowing in a retrograde fashion into the pulmonary veins since their orifice is not protected with a remnant valve. The amplitude of the retrograde atrial contraction is smaller and its duration is less in comparison to the mitral inflow A wave. In cases of left ventricular diastolic dysfunction associated with a stiff ventricle and a raised left ventricular end-diastolic pressure, both the amplitude and duration of the retrograde atrial contraction wave increases in relation to the mitral inflow A wave. When the duration of the retrograde atrial contraction wave exceeded the duration of the mitral A wave the left ventricular end-diastolic pressure was greater than 15 mmHg with a sensitivity of 85% and a specificity of 79% in a study by Oki et al.[114]

Doppler tissue imaging may also be used to assess diastolic function as demonstrated in Figure 6.8. Tissue Doppler displays the excursion of mitral annular motion during the cardiac cycle and most notably does not appear to be influenced by the preload.[115–125] The displacement and velocity of the mitral annulus along the longitudinal axis of the left ventricular is examined from the four-chamber view either along the septal or the lateral longitudinal axis of the mitral annulus and corresponds to the myocardial diastolic velocities induced by myocardial relaxation. Myocardial velocities recorded with tissue Doppler consist of the peak systolic velocity (S_m), the peak early diastolic (E_m) and late diastolic (A_m) myocardial expansion velocities. Normal values suggested for myocardial velocities: S_m 11 cm/s, E_m 13 cm/s, A_m 11 cm/s and E_m/A_m 1.5. The rate of deceleration (E_mDT) and acceleration (E_mAT) of the

early peak diastolic excursion may be determined, as well as the duration of the time to deceleration E_mD – t which correlates with the early mitral diastolic filling acceleration time. The late diastolic myocardial expansion time A_m – t is measured as the total duration of the late diastolic wave.

With normal diastolic function the early diastolic annulus velocity (E_m) is greater than the late diastolic annulus velocity (A_m). The peak early diastolic expansion (E_m) appears to be substantially related to ventricular relaxation. The index of annular expansion velocity (E_m)/mitral inflow peak E velocity has been shown to correlate well with mean pulmonary capillary wedge pressure and its calculation serves to normalize for the possible effects of preload.[124]

In all grades of abnormal ventricular relaxation the peak early diastolic annulus velocity (E_m) is less than the peak late diastolic annulus velocity (A_m), which makes it useful for distinguishing cases of pseudonormalization obtained with the mitral inflow velocities. Generally, the E_m and the A_m coincide with the mitral inflow E and A wave velocities. The ratio of the mitral annulus motion during atrial systole to the total diastolic annular motion velocity is increased in cases of abnormal ventricular relaxation. The E_mDT has also been shown to increase corresponding to increasing early diastolic filling acceleration time associated with mitral inflow E/A ratios less than 1. Sohn et al, have demonstrated that the mitral annulus velocity demonstrates a reduced early diastolic annulus velocity in relation to the late diastolic annulus velocity, despite a pseudo-normal mitral inflow pattern in the presence of diastolic dysfunction and is independent of preload.[124] With the severest forms of abnormal ventricular relaxation associated with increased filling pressures and restrictive physiology, the peak early and late diastolic annular velocities are markedly reduced. Dagdelen et al demonstrated that tissue Doppler parameters provide estimates of left ventricular end-diastolic pressure with a high sensitivity and specificity. A left ventricular end-diastolic pressure of greater than 15 mmHg was associated with a E_mDT > 120 ms, A_m – t > 110 ms, E_m/A_m ratio < 0.5.[125]

Color M-mode Doppler provides a spatial and temporal velocity map for the analysis of the diastolic filling pattern for left ventricular relaxation and is also independent of preload (Figure 6.10).[126–135] The propagation of peak early filling flow is visualized by placing the color m-mode cursor between the mitral valve opening and the ventricular apex in four-chamber views, and recording early and late diastolic flows. The flow propagation velocity (V_p) is determined from the velocity of the leading edge of the early-filling wave as determined from the transition from no color to color in the recording. The time delay of the mitral propagation velocity (V_pDT) is measured from the interval between the beginning to the peak point of the color convergence. The rate of propagation of flow is determined by the distance/time ratio between two sampling points, the origin of flow at the mitral

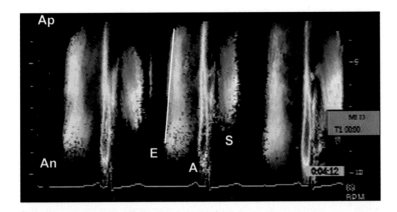

a

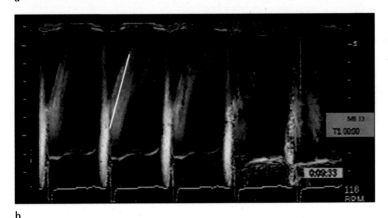

b

Figure 6.10
Color m-mode Doppler tracing. Color m-mode Doppler provides a spatial and temporal velocity map for the analysis of the diastolic filling pattern for left ventricular relaxation and is also independent of preload. The propagation of peak early filling flow is visualized by placing the color m-mode cursor between the mitral valve opening and the ventricular apex in four-chamber views, and recording early and late diastolic flows. The flow propagation velocity (V_p) is determined from the velocity of the leading edge of the early-filling wave as determined from the transition from no color to color in the recording. The time delay of the mitral propagation velocity (V_pDT) is measured from the interval between the beginning to the peak point of the color convergence. The rate of propagation of flow is determined by the distance/time ratio between two sampling points the origin of flow at the mitral orifice and the mid left ventricular level. A. Color m-mode tracing obtained from the mitral inflow tract demonstrating a normal pattern of left ventricular relaxation. Note the rapid acceleration in the early and late diastolic flow waves toward the ventricular apex. B. Color m-mode tracing of impaired ventricular relaxation demonstrating a delayed integral of foward flow. An, annulus; Ap, apex; S, systolic flow wave; E, early diastolic flow wave; A, late diastolic flow wave.

orifice and the mid left ventricular level. Pai et al found the rate of propagation of flow in the left ventricle is determined by early diastolic stiffness of the left ventricular.[126] The flow propagation (V_p) exhibits an inverse relationship to left ventricular relaxation and left ventricular end-diastolic pressure. The time delay of the mitral propagation velocity is prolonged with myocardial ischemia. Brun et al have demonstrated that early left ventricular filling patterns correlated with the time constant for left ventricular relaxation and left ventricular end-diastolic pressure.[127] Dagdelen et al have demonstrated the relationship of V_pDT with left ventricular end-diastolic pressure.[125] In patients with catheterization measured left ventricular end-diastolic pressure of less than 10 mmHg the V_pDT was less than 45 ms with a sensitivity of 73% and a specificity of 89%. When the left ventricular end-diastolic pressure was greater than 15 mmHg, the V_pDT was greater than 60 ms with a sensitivity of 78% and a specificity of 86%.

Myocardial infarction

Echocardiography has become instrumental in the evaluation of myocardial infarction.[136–138] In addition to

diagnosing myocardial infarction in chest pain syndromes that do not present with the classical findings of myocardial infarction, echocardiography is beneficial in assessing the size and location of infarction and in some degree predicting the prognosis of myocardial infarction.[139–141] Wall motion abnormalities are present in the majority of cases of transmural myocardial infarction on initial presentation. The lack of demonstrable regional wall motion abnormalities, coupled with normal or near normal ejection fraction, denotes small infarctions with good prognosis with the lack of developing complications. Echocardiography, especially transesophageal echocardiography, is particularly helpful in excluding myocardial infarction in the setting of chest pain with the absence of wall motion abnormality. In cases of pulmonary embolus, congestive heart failure, pericardial disease, aortic dissection, valvular disease etc., transesophageal echocardiography frequently demonstrates the specific etiology for chest pain and/or hemodynamic instability. Akinetic or dyskinetic wall motion is associated with a high sensitivity for myocardial infarction, but the positive predictive value is low since regional wall motion abnormalities are also associated with other disease entities including those that do not include coronary artery disease. In cases of myocardial infarction, echocardiography assesses the amount of myocardium at risk and determines the results of reperfusion. True aneurysm formation, ventricular thrombus, pericardial effusion and right ventricular infarction are frequently demonstrated with echocardiography.

The mechanical complications of myocardial infarction are frequently responsible for producing hemodynamic instability and cardiogenic shock.[142–147] Cardiogenic shock complicating myocardial infarction carries a high morbidity and mortality, if not diagnosed promptly. When diagnosed early, many of the structural abnormalities responsible for producing cardiogenic shock may be corrected with surgery or interventional catheterization techniques thus substantially decreasing the morbidity and mortality of myocardial infarction in many patients. Transesophageal echocardiography is extremely useful for evaluating the complications of myocardial infarction, particularly related to the cause of cardiogenic shock. Numerous reports in the literature have described the transesophageal echocardiographic diagnosis of partial or complete papillary muscle rupture, acquired ventricular septal defect, free wall myocardial rupture, pseudo and true aneurysmal formation of the ventricle, intraventricular obstruction, ventricular thrombus formation, pericardial tamponade and right ventricular infarction.

Papillary muscle partial or complete rupture, producing severe mitral regurgitation, is an infrequent complication of myocardial infarction however is associated with cardiogenic shock and high mortality.[148–158] When diagnosed early, prompt surgical intervention is associated with a good prognosis. Transesophageal echocardiography permits a rapid assessment for papillary muscle rupture as discussed in chapter 2.

Free wall rupture of the myocardium in the setting of myocardial infarction is a rare but usually lethal complication that requires a high index of suspicion for the rapid diagnosis in order to offer prompt surgical repair in most cases.[159–164] Free wall rupture is a late cause of hemodynamic collapse, occurring in days 4 to 9 of acute myocardial infarction, and appears to occur more frequently in women and elderly patients. Historically, free wall rupture of the infarcted myocardium was noted to occur around day 9 in the pathologic literature. However, with advent of thrombolysis and the potential for creating a hemorrhagic infarct with reperfusion, free wall rupture now typically occurs earlier around day 4.[161] Free wall rupture may produce exsanguination or hemopericardium with pericardial tamponade when blood directly enters and fills the pericardial space. In a lesser form, partial rupture of the myocardial wall segment may result in a subepicardial hematoma or 'partial aneurysm'. Transesophageal echocardiography frequently demonstrates the site of rupture by direct visualization or by the demonstration of free flow within the myocardium with color flow Doppler.[162–164] Pericardial effusion is almost always present

and is associated with the presence of a thrombus in the pericardial sac near the vicinity of the ruptured myocardial segment, after echocardiographic and Doppler findings of pericardial tamponade. Although pericardial effusion with or without rupture is frequently associated with an acute myocardial infarction, the absence of pericardial effusion virtually excludes the diagnosis of free wall rupture. In cases with pericardial effusion that are not definitive for myocardial free wall rupture, pericardiocentesis may be helpful for demonstrating a hemopericardium associated with a small rupture.

Acquired or post-myocardial infarction ventricular septal defect is similar to free wall rupture, with the rupture occurring between the ventricles creating a left to right shunt instead of allowing free rupture to the pericardium. Similar to papillary muscle rupture, ventricular septal rupture is associated clinically with a new loud systolic murmur in the setting of hemodynamic deterioration with acute myocardial infarction. Numerous reports have described the rapid and accurate detection of ventricular septal rupture with transesophageal echocardiography especially in the setting of acute hemodynamic collapse.[165–171] Ventricular septal rupture occurs with an incidence of 1 to 3% and is associated with death in 5% of all acute myocardial infarctions. Ventricular septal rupture usually occurs in the first week of the infarction and appears to be more frequent in women and the elderly. Early diagnosis is paramount, since in patients that develop ventricular septal rupture, mortality is approximately 90% when not treated surgically. Ventricular septal rupture frequently occurs in the setting of single vessel disease.

With echocardiography, ventricular septal rupture is suggested by a new regional wall motion abnormality consistent with myocardial infarction and the protrusion of the ventricular septum at the site of infarction towards the right ventricle. Transesophageal echocardiography directly demonstrates the site of septal rupture in conjunction with color flow Doppler demonstration of a high velocity left-to-right ventricular shunt in nearly all, if not in all, cases. Ventricular septal rupture in the setting of inferoseptal infarction is frequently related to right ventricular infarction, and the rupture site is located closer to the basal septal segment. Ventricular septal ruptures associated with anterior wall infarction typically occur closer to the ventricular apex. Similar to free wall rupture, ventricular septal rupture appears as a serpiginous oblique tear through the myocardial infarction site.

Pseudoaneurysm may result from free wall rupture and produce a more stable lesion initially, but is associated with a substantial risk for spontaneous rupture in the long term. In pseudoaneurysm, the parietal pericardium becomes adherent to the epicardial surface of the segment of infarcted myocardium as a result of inflammation produced in the infarction process. With subsequent rupture of the myocardial wall blood flow is restrained by the pericardium, which usually expands in a ballooning fashion producing a pseudoaneurysm. This may be difficult to distinguish from true aneurysm after acute myocardial infarction. Pseudoaneurysms are detected by echocardiography, especially with transesophageal echocardiography, and are differentiated from true aneurysm through the demonstration of a small narrow neck and blood flow demonstrated with color flow Doppler in a to-and-fro motion through the defect.[172,173] Filling of the pseudoaneurysm occurs during systole, and is illustrated by expansion of the pseudoaneurysm during systole. Due to stasis of blood flow in the pseudoaneurysm, they are frequently filled with thrombus, which may be detected echocardiographically as a laminated layer adjacent to the pericardial margin. Studies have shown the ratio of the origin of the pseudoaneurysm to the maximal diameter of the body of the out pouching to be less than 0.5 in distinction to true aneurysm that have a broad neck at the origin of the aneurysm. Transesophageal echocardiography is particularly useful for differentiating true from pseudo aneurysms that occur in the posterior and inferior walls that appear to have a small neck at their origin, by delineating the walls of the aneurysm as composed of muscle or pericardium and demonstrating the blood flow characteristics within the aneurysmal sac.[174–177]

Cardiomyopathy

Dilated cardiomyopathy

Dilated cardiomyopathy is characterized by cardiac enlargement accompanied by impaired systolic function of unknown cause.[178] Although ventricular enlargement and contractile dysfunction often heralds the onset of congestive heart failure, it is not uncommon to find patients who are relatively asymptomatic when initially diagnosed with echocardiography. Anatomically all four cardiac chambers are dilated, with greatest enlargement occurring in the ventricular chambers in comparison to the size of the atria. Left ventricular dilatation is accompanied with eccentric hypertrophy of the ventricular walls. The degree of hypertrophy is inadequate however, in comparison to the degree of dilatation. Ventricular wall motion demonstrates global hypokinesis as exhibited by decreased systolic thickening and reduced endocardial border excursion. Regional wall motion abnormalities may be demonstrated in 60% of cases with echocardiography, despite the absence of significant coronary artery disease.[179] Either the left or right ventricle may be predominately involved. Cardiac chamber enlargement, especially of the left ventricle is frequently associated with

spontaneous echocardiographic contrast and thrombus formation.[180–184]

The primary role of echocardiography is to demonstrate impaired systolic function and to rule out specific correctable causes of heart failure such as valvular disease or ischemic heart disease.[185] Systolic function may be assessed through measurements of stroke volume, cardiac output and ejection fraction obtained from the calculations of ventricular volume and area. Doppler echocardiography demonstrates diastolic dysfunction and provides estimates of left atrial filling pressure through the evaluation of the transmitral pressure gradient and pulmonary venous flows.[185–193] Patients with compensated physiology and dilated cardiomyopathy exhibit echocardiographic/Doppler findings of reduced ejection fraction with near normal stroke volume, cardiac output and early grades of diastolic dysfunction. Decompensated dilated cardiomyopathy is suggested by decreased stroke volume and cardiac output with restrictive physiology and pulmonary hypertension by Doppler echocardiography. Restrictive physiology and pulmonary hypertension determined by high velocity tricuspid regurgitation (TR velocity greater than 3 m/s) carry the worst prognosis with dilated cardiomyopathy.[191] Echocardiography also provides assessment of mitral and tricuspid valvular regurgitation resulting from annular dilation that accompanies atrioventricular enlargement.[194–196] Annular dilatation may be associated with moderate to severe mitral regurgitation, irrespective of the degree of dilated cardiomyopathy as discussed in chapter 2. Pulmonary hypertension may be estimated from the tricuspid regurgitant jet, using the modified Bernoulli formula. Left atrial pressure may be estimated in the setting of mitral regurgitation as $LA_{press} = SBP - 4(MR_V)^2$ with SBP as the systolic arm blood pressure and MR_V as the peak velocity of the mitral regurgitant jet. Left ventricular end-diastolic pressure may be estimated by $LVEDP = DBP - 4(AR\text{-}EDV)^2$ with DBP as the diastolic arm blood pressure and AR-EDV as the velocity of the aortic regurgitant jet at end-diastole. Echocardiography has been utilized to assess the results of therapy and predict prognosis.

Hypertrophic cardiomyopathy

Hypertrophic cardiomyopathy is a genetic disorder characterized by severe myocardial hypertrophy. Hypertrophic cardiomyopathy is usually associated with a dynamic gradient in the outflow tract, but the presence of the gradient is not mandatory for the diagnosis. Echocardiography provides a visual demonstration of the pattern of hypertrophy, which may be concentric or eccentric.[196] Hypertrophic cardiomyopathy is suggested with ventricular wall thickness greater than 15 mm and significantly increased left ventricular mass. Although the pattern of asymmetric septal hypertrophy is the most widely recognized pattern as originally described in idiopathic hypertrophic subaortic stenosis, various patterns may be demonstrated with echocardiography.[197] Diffuse hypertrophy of the anteroseptal and anterolateral wall occurs in 70 to 75% of cases, basal septal hypertrophy in 10 to 15%, concentric hypertrophy in 5%, apical hypertrophy in less than 5%, and lateral hypertrophy in 1 to 2%. Hypertrophic cardiomyopathy must be differentiated from the variant of sigmoid septum (discreet proximal septal hypertrophy) in the elderly that does not demonstrate the other features of obstructive hypertrophic cardiomyopathy.[198]

Echocardiographically, hypertrophic cardiomyopathy demonstrates ventricular hypertrophy with increased echogenicity to the myocardial walls, often in a bright granular pattern. The left ventricular end-diastolic dimension is normal to small. Ventricular wall motion appears hyperdynamic with obliteration or near cavity obliteration of the ventricular cavity during systole.[199–201] Left atrial enlargement is associated with mitral regurgitation and atrial fibrillation. The aortic valve may demonstrate early mid systolic closure. Systolic anterior motion of the mitral valve (SAM) frequently denotes the site of ventricular obstruction.[202,203] Excessive systemic anterior motion of the mitral apparatus has been attributed to the Venturi and Bernoulli effects as a result of the ventricular flow obstruction, abnormal papillary muscle placement and function, and abnormal mitral annular displacement and leaflet configuration associated with a decreased aortomitral angle and abnormal ventricular geometry.[204–208] Various degrees of mitral regurgitation are associated with hypertrophic cardiomyopathy. High velocity mitral regurgitation is frequently demonstrated along the posterior lateral wall of the left atrium but may occur in any direction, especially when associated with enlargement of the posterior leaflet and lack of apposition during closure. Mitral regurgitation may predominate in late systole, as a result of 'relief valve' regurgitation in the setting of high intraventricular pressure that overcomes the normal function of the mitral apparatus associated with an abnormal ventricular configuration during systole. Transesophageal echocardiography is extremely helpful for detecting mitral valvular chordal rupture that occasionally occurs with hypertrophic cardiomyopathy. Chordal rupture in hypertrophic cardiomyopathy produces severe mitral regurgitation and a sudden deterioration in hemodynamics, frequently necessitating mitral repair or mitral valve replacement.[209]

Conventional and color flow Doppler demonstrates the site of intraventricular obstruction when present.[210–214] Pulsed and continuous-wave Doppler demonstrate a late peaking or 'dagger' systolic flow profile at the site of obstruction. Continuous-wave Doppler interrogation of the obstruction is estimated by the modified Bernoulli formula. Care must be taken not to confuse a mitral regurgitation jet with an intraventricular flow gradient, which is usually easily accomplished with transesophageal echocardiography through visualization of the narrowed orifice at the site of obstruction distinct from the mitral regurgitation jet. Pulsed Doppler interrogation of the mitral inflow and pulmonary venous flow demonstrates marked impairment in ventricular relaxation by demonstrating an increased isovolumic relaxation time and early diastolic deceleration time, with a decreased E/A ratio.[215,216]

The major role of transesophageal echocardiography in hypertrophic cardiomyopathy is in assessing the results of surgical myectomy or interventional septal ablation.[217–221] Initially, echocardiography demonstrates the septal anatomy and provides the thickness of the septum and the exact site of obstruction. The mitral valve apparatus is assessed to help determine its role in the obstructive process, as well as demonstrating the severity of mitral regurgitation and associated abnormalities of the valvular apparatus, which may require mitral valvular repair in addition to septal myectomy. The anatomy of the ventricular septum is readily visualized for the success of reducing septal tissue with either technique, with widening of the left ventricular outflow tract as the predominate finding. Multiplane transesophageal echocardiography accurately assesses the flow velocity and residual pressure gradient of the left ventricular outflow tract in the deep transgastric at 0 to 15 degrees or transgastric view at 125 degrees. When a substantial residual gradient is detected, echocardiography is extremely useful for determining the site for further removal of tissue, considering the limited view provided during surgical exposure. Although systolic anterior motion of the mitral valve apparatus may initially persist following either technique, it usually resolves if the left ventricular outflow tract gradient is substantially decreased.

Following surgical myectomy, complications of aortic regurgitation, anterior mitral leaflet perforation and ventricular septal defect, which may occur during surgery, are excluded. With high magnification, color flow Doppler may detect abnormal flow within the resected portion of the septal muscle and this should not be confused with a ventricular septal defect created during the resection. Following alcohol septal ablation of the ventricular septum the size and location of the 'new' regional wall motion abnormality created is assessed; the parameters of ventricular function are measured in addition to determining the residual gradient. Mitral regurgitation is assessed when present and compared to preintervention state. With either technique, surgical or interventional, it is not expected that the gradient will be totally relieved. However, it has generally been adopted that a residual gradient

> 50 mmHg is an unacceptable result requiring a second cardiopulmonary pump run and a reduction to approximately 20 mmHg denotes a successful result. It also appears that the initial residual gradient persists in the short-term, however this needs to be further substantiated.

Restrictive cardiomyopathy

The least common form of cardiomyopathy is restrictive cardiomyopathy. Restrictive cardiomyopathy is a condition characterized by reduced diastolic ventricular filling as a result of primary myocardial disease.[222, 223] Restrictive cardiomyopathy is frequently implicated in cases of heart failure of unknown cause. In moderate to severe cases, restrictive cardiomyopathy produces severe refractory congestive heart failure with both pulmonary and/or systemic venous congestion. Many cases of restrictive cardiomyopathy result from infiltrative myocardial disease as associated with amyloidosis, sarcoidosis, hemochromatosis, endomyocardial fibrosis, endocardial fibroelastosis, glycogen storage disease, mucopolysaccharidosis, scleroderma and Loffler endocarditis.[224, 225] When the cause for the myocardial disease is unknown the restrictive cardiomyopathy is designated as idiopathic. Histologically, the idiopathic form is defined by interstitial fibrosis of the myocardium without the presence of inflammatory cells. In all cases of restrictive cardiomyopathy, a degree of fibrosis results in stiffness or reduction of the normal compliance and elasticity of the ventricular myocardium.

The hallmark of restrictive cardiomyopathy, anatomically and echocardiographically, is the demonstration of significant atrial enlargement with normal or small ventricular dimensions. Atrial enlargement and failure occur as a result of the back-pressure produced from the impedance to ventricular filling provided the stiff ventricles. Initially in the disease process, the systolic function is preserved and thus the ventricles are normal in size. In some cases with infiltrative involvement, there may be thickening of the ventricular walls. This atrial and ventricular configuration resembles a double scoop ice cream cone with echocardiography in the four-chamber view. The diagnosis of restrictive cardiomyopathy represents a clinical challenge, since it shares many of the clinical, hemodynamic and echocardiographic findings of constrictive pericarditis.

Amyloidosis may result in an infiltrative cardiomyopathy due to the myocardial deposition of amyloid fibrils. Increased myocardial wall thickness usually occurs without ventricular dilatation and frequently results in a restrictive Doppler filling pattern.[226] Amyloid deposits within the heart may occur in the ventricular myocardium, cardiac valves and interatrial septum. Echocardiographically, these deposits may produce an increased echogenicity and a ground glass appearance to a thickened ventricular myocardium and marked thickening with a bulbous appearance to the atrial septum. Valvular deposits may be suggested by non-specific leaflet thickening and valvular regurgitation.

Restrictive cardiomyopathy demonstrates an abnormal diastolic filling pattern with Doppler echocardiography.[227–230] In most cases of restrictive cardiomyopathy, the myocardial pathology is diffuse and is responsible for producing a global decrease in myocardial expansion and therefore abnormal relaxation dynamics are present throughout diastole. In addition to the lack of expansion, ventricular filling in restrictive cardiomyopathy is not dramatically influenced by the normal changes in intrathoracic pressure during the phases of respiration. Demonstration of these findings with Doppler echocardiography helps to distinguish restrictive cardiomyopathy from other causes of abnormal ventricular relaxation.

The stiff or non-compliant myocardium of restrictive cardiomyopathy results in a high ventricular end-diastolic pressure, which produces a high atrial pressure and subsequently decreases venous flow velocity during systole necessitating an increase in venous flow during diastole. With pulsed-wave Doppler the mitral and tricuspid inflow demonstrate an increased early rapid diastolic inflow velocity or E wave due to the increased transvalvular pressure gradient. The contribution of atrial systole is diminished due to the high ventricular end-diastolic pressure which is exhibited by both a decreased A wave velocity and duration. Typically this alteration in E and A wave results in a marked increase in the E/A ratio usually ≥2.0. Respiration demonstrates no variation in the E wave velocity in the mitral inflow and only mild variation in the E wave velocity in the tricuspid inflow. The higher left atrial pressure results in a decrease in both the intraventricular relaxation time and deceleration time. The pulmonary and hepatic venous flows demonstrate diminished flow velocity during systole in comparison to diastolic flow velocities in reference to normal, with increased atrial flow reversal duration and velocity in the pulmonary veins, and decreased diastolic flow reversal in the hepatic veins with inspiration.

Early studies suggest that both tissue Doppler and color m-mode Doppler echocardiography may play a significant role in demonstrating abnormal left ventricular relaxation in restrictive cardiomyopathy, particularly when the usual Doppler indices of ventricular filling are not helpful.[118,119,128,129] The major advantage of tissue Doppler and color m-mode Doppler is that they both appear to be independent of the filling pressure. Tissue Doppler recordings at the lateral mitral annulus demonstrate decreased longitudinal expansion and contraction motion compared to normal myocardium. Tissue Doppler demonstrates decreases in early peak diastolic expansion velocity (E_m), the mean rates of acceleration and deceleration of the early diastolic expansion and in late peak diastolic velocity (A_m). Color m-mode Doppler echocardiography may be helpful for demonstrating a significant delay for the progression of the maximal velocity of diastolic blood flow from the mitral annulus to the apex in restrictive cardiomyopathy.

Pericardial disease

The pericardium comprises a fibrous sac, which surrounds the heart and the proximal portion of the great arteries and veins.[231,232] The pericardium is composed of two layers, the visceral and parietal pericardium. The visceral pericardium is closely adherent to the epicardial surface of the heart and consists of a thin layer of loose fibrous tissue covered by a serous layer of mesothelial cells. The parietal pericardium is formed as a reflection of the serous layer of the visceral pericardium and an outer fibrous layer, which encloses the entire heart and attaches to the adventitia of the aorta and pulmonary artery, creating a potential space or pericardial cavity, which usually contains 15 to 20 cc of clear fluid under normal circumstances. The normal thickness of the pericardium is approximately 3 mm. comprising all layers and demonstrated with most standard imaging techniques. Due to the reflection of the pericardium around the great vessels of the heart, two separate cul-de-sac spaces or sinuses are created. The oblique sinus lies behind the left atrium in between the pulmonary veins. The transverse sinus is formed from the space created between the aorta and the pulmonary artery anteriorly and the atria posteriorly.

Injury or inflammation of the pericardium often results in the accumulation of pericardial fluid, which may produce detrimental affects to cardiac hemodynamics. Pericardial effusions are frequently asymptomatic; but depending on the clinical scenario, may produce profound hemodynamic collapse. Normally, intrapericardial pressure approximates zero, and corresponds to diastolic pressures as a reflection of the intrathoracic pressure. With the accumulation of pericardial fluid, pressure may build within the pericardial sac and effectively overcome the intracardiac pressures. Large pericardial effusions that accumulate over a longer time may be better tolerated than smaller effusions that rapidly accumulate over a shorter time, due to the relative compliance of the pericardial sac.

Echocardiography serves as the best imaging technique for demonstrating pericardial effusions, due to its high sensitivity and specificity. It reliably detects pericardial fluid in quantities of greater than 25 cc.[233–235] Echocardiographically, a pericardial effusion is demonstrated by a relatively echo-free space that persists during the cardiac cycle and which separates the heart from the surrounding pericardium. The amount of fluid is determined by the size of the echo-free space. Smaller effusions are denoted by a posterior echo-free space predominately occurring during systole, without the presence of an anterior free space. Due to the lack of restraint in the posterior and lateral portions of the pericardial sac, pericardial fluid primarily fills these areas initially, and the heart rises due to the effects of buoyancy, obliterating the anterior pericardial space. The increasing accumulation of pericardial effusion gradually reduces parietal pericardial motion and ultimately surrounds the entire heart. As pericardial fluid accumulates, the anterior free space enlarges as the heart assumes a posterior position in the pericardial sac, effectively decreasing the posterior free space. Transesophageal echocardiography is usually relegated to the demonstration of effusions that are not adequately detected with transthoracic echocardiography when there is a high index of suspicion for effusions, especially when loculation of fluid may occur secondary to the presence of pericardial adhesions.[236–250] The greatest role for transesophageal echocardiography is in the diagnosis of pericardial effusion following cardiac surgery or catheterization interventions when cardiac perforation is suspected, and transthoracic imaging may not be possible.

Pericardial tamponade occurs when pericardial effusions accumulate under pressure and exert restriction on the cardiac structures. Due to lack of correlation between the size of the pericardial effusion and presence of pericardial tamponade, the quantification of pericardial effusion is less important than its identification. Reduction in the venous return to the heart results in a reduction in stroke volume, resulting in decreased cardiac output and hypotension. Pericardial tamponade is not an echocardiographic diagnosis but the presence of pericardial tamponade is often suggested by a variety of echocardiographic findings. Echocardiography demonstrates a pericardial effusion with two-dimensional imaging, and with large pericardial effusion the heart is noted to swing in the pericardial sac during the cardiac cycle with inspiration. Various degrees of cardiac collapse may be denoted by late diastolic right atrial collapse, early right ventricular diastolic collapse, left atrial collapse, left ventricular diastolic collapse (rarely), exaggerated ventricular septal motion and marked inspiratory changes in ventricular dimensions and/or a lack of inferior vena cava luminal dimension change during respiration.

Doppler findings suggest the hemodynamic consequences of pericardial tamponade, and are similar to the findings with constrictive pericarditis.[251,252] With cardiac tamponade intrapericardial pressure remains high despite a fall in intrathoracic pressure with respiration, resulting in a decrease in left ventricular filling pressure gradient with inspiration with reciprocal changes in the right heart hemodynamics. In addition, the increased atrial pressure induced by the increased ventricular filling pressure gradient is reflected by the venous inflow patterns to each respective atrium. These hemodynamic changes result in a decrease in rapid diastolic filling or Doppler mitral inflow E-wave velocity and prolonged isovolumic relaxation time after inspiration, with opposite effects on tricuspid inflow parameters. The pulmonary venous inflow pattern shows a decrease in diastolic forward flow with inspiration. After expiration the mitral inflow E-wave velocity increases and the tricuspid inflow E-wave velocity decreases, with a reduction in diastolic forward flow and an increase in diastolic flow reversal compared with normal physiology. Most noticeable is the influence of respiratory variation produced to the mitral inflow pattern, along with exaggeration of the mitral tricuspid inflow patterns between inspiration and expiration. With normal physiology, the respiratory variation in the E wave velocity is generally less than 10%, which is not easily detected by casual observation. However, when tamponade is present this is readily demonstrated and highlighted with the use of a respirometer tracing.

Pericardial constriction

Constrictive pericarditis results from disease that alters the normally compliant pericardium and produces constriction of the heart within the pericardial sac.[253,254] In constrictive pericarditis the pericardium becomes thickened as the result of fibrosis and/or calcification, and is frequently associated with a pericardial effusion. The constriction of the heart imposes a structural restraint to ventricular expansion during the ventricular filling phase of diastole. Initially the restraint is limited to the later two-thirds of diastole. These findings are manifest echocardiographically by right atrial enlargement, dilatation of the inferior vena cava, and abnormal interventricular septal motion in the presence of normal left ventricular size and systolic function.[255] The thickness of the pericardium can be measured with echocardiography, with better results obtained with the transesophageal technique.[256] Computed tomography and magnetic resonance imaging are the best imaging methods for determining pericardial thickening. The treatment of constrictive pericarditis is surgical removal of the pericardium or pericardiectomy.

In constrictive pericarditis, alterations to hemodynamics are produced through two mechanisms. The thickened pericardium dampens the transmission of the intrathoracic pressure to the cardiac chambers. Secondly, the diseased pericardium restrains cardiac expansion during diastolic filling, thus limiting total cardiac capacity and promoting the physiological phenomenon of ventricular

coupling, whereby the expansion distensibility for each ventricular chamber is influenced by the other. This is illustrated by the abnormal septal motion that accompanies constrictive pericarditis.[257,258] During inspiration, the fall in intrathoracic pressure is reflected with a drop in pulmonary venous pressure which is not accompanied by a corresponding drop in left ventricular diastolic pressure. This produces an abnormal gradient between the two, which results in the reduction of the transmitral filling which serves to dampening pulmonary venous diastolic forward flow.[259–262] Reduced transmitral filling subsequently produces an increase in transtricuspid filling. This is represented by a reduced mitral E wave velocity and pulmonary venous diastolic velocity, with an increased tricuspid E wave velocity in the first complex following inspiration. During expiration, the opposite occurs – an increase in mitral E wave velocity and a decrease in tricuspid E wave velocity, with an increase in diastolic flow reversal in the hepatic veins. In constrictive pericarditis, there is marked respiratory variation in mitral (>25%) and tricuspid flow velocities, which has been shown to distinguish constrictive pericarditis from other entities responsible for producing abnormal ventricular relaxation. Similar to restrictive cardiomyopathy, tissue Doppler and color m-mode Doppler are useful techniques for demonstrating a pattern of abnormal relaxation for constrictive pericarditis.

The differentiation of restrictive cardiomyopathy from constrictive pericarditis can present a diagnostic challenge due to the similarities between clinical, hemodynamic and echocardiographic findings. Often patients present with mixed pathology, demonstrating qualities of restrictive and constrictive pathologies further compounding the problem of making a diagnosis. It is important to diagnose constrictive pericarditis when present since surgical treatment often yields good results.

With transesophageal echocardiography, the identification of a thickened pericardium with or without calcification suggests a diagnosis of constrictive pericarditis. In cases of infiltrative cardiomyopathy, transesophageal echocardiography may demonstrate abnormal myocardial echogenicity suggesting a restrictive cardiomyopathy, but in cases of non-infiltrative types the myocardium appears normal. The echocardiographic demonstration of dilated atria in comparison to small ventricles and normal systolic function suggests restrictive cardiomyopathy.

Pulsed wave Doppler of the indices of left ventricular filling have been helpful in differentiating restrictive cardiomyopathy from constrictive pericarditis by demonstrating differences in respiratory variation patterns and ventricular interdependence.[263–265] An increased mitral inflow E wave velocity, a mitral inflow E/A ratio greater than 2.0 and a short E wave deceleration velocity are demonstrated in both constrictive pericarditis and restrictive cardiomyopathy. Hatle et al have demonstrated the marked changes and reciprocal pattern between mitral and tricuspid flow velocities during respiration that occurs with constrictive pericarditis and the lack of significant respiratory variation in inflow velocities with restrictive cardiomyopathy.[263] Oh et al have shown a greater than a 25% change between the inspiratory and expiratory mitral inflow E wave velocity with constrictive cardiomyopathy, although no significant change in E wave velocity was detected with restrictive cardiomyopathy unless the patient also had chronic obstructive pulmonary disease.[259] In addition, hepatic vein flow reversals are more prominent with inspiration in restrictive cardiomyopathy. In constrictive pericarditis there was a greater than 25% increase in diastolic hepatic vein flow reversal during expiration. Klein et al studied the respiratory changes of pulmonary venous flow patterns with transesophageal echocardiography between constrictive pericarditis and restrictive cardiomyopathy.[264] In patients with constrictive pericarditis, pulmonary venous systolic flows during inspiration and expiration were greater than exhibited in patients with restrictive cardiomyopathy. In the same patients, pulmonary venous diastolic flows during inspiration were also reduced in patients with constrictive cardiomyopathy. In constrictive pericarditis the difference with respiration in pulmonary venous diastolic flow is greater than the difference noted in peak mitral inflow E wave velocity. This is different in restrictive cardiomyopathy, where similar changes occur between the pulmonary venous and mitral inflow. Both typically demonstrate a lack of significant variation with respiration.[264,265]

Using tissue Doppler and color m-mode Doppler to differentiate constrictive pericarditis from restrictive cardiomyopathy, Rajagopalan et al[265] demonstrated that respiratory variation of the mitral inflow E wave of >10% predicted constrictive pericarditis with a sensitivity of 84% and a specificity of 91%. Respiratory variation in the pulmonary venous peak diastolic flow velocity of >18% detected constrictive pericarditis with a sensitivity and specificity of 79% and 91% respectively. Using tissue Doppler a peak early velocity of longitudinal expansion (E_m) of >8.0 cm/s distinguished constrictive pericarditis from restrictive cardiomyopathy with a sensitivity of 89% and a specificity of 100%. With color m-mode determination of the first aliasing contour of flow propagation a slope of >100 cm/s predicted patients with constrictive pericarditis with a sensitivity of 74% and a specificity of 91%. Although further studies are needed to validate these findings, both tissue Doppler and color m-mode Doppler appear to be promising techniques for distinguishing constrictive pericarditis from restrictive cardiomyopathy, especially when equivocal findings are demonstrated with other techniques.[266]

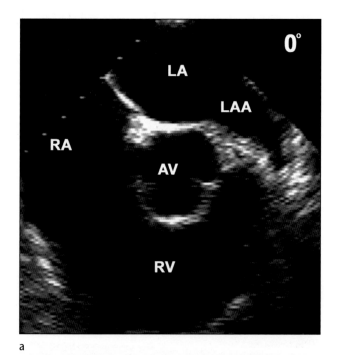

a

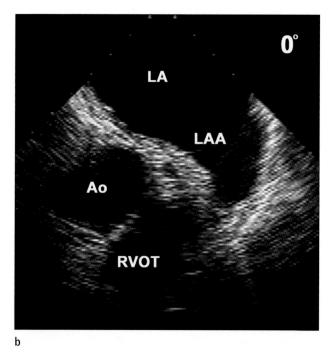

b

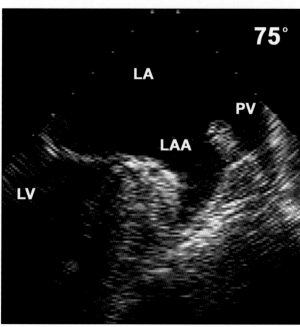

c

Case 6.1

Left atrial appendage. A–C. The full extent of the left atrial appendage is demonstrated in multiple planes with transesophageal echocardiography and is the diagnostic method of choice for visualizing the appendage. The left atrial appendage arises from the anterolateral border of the left atrium and lies in the left atrioventricular groove above the proximal portion of the left circumflex coronary artery. The left atrial appendage varies considerably in size and shape, according to age and sex. The orifice of the left atrial appendage is elliptical with a curvilinear shape to the body of the appendage. Color Doppler provides visualization of the maximum flow velocity within the left atrial appendage to provide optimum alignment of the pulsed Doppler sample. In addition color Doppler helps in determining the morphology of the appendage by delineating its shape when filled with color flow. Color Doppler may also help define thrombi from pectinate muscles as a result of the color flow outline produced to the cavity of the appendage.

continued

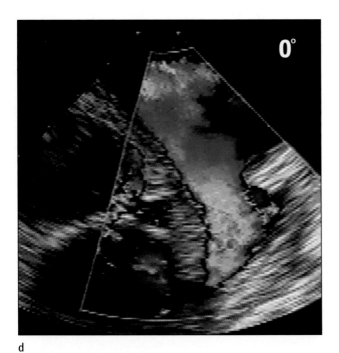

d

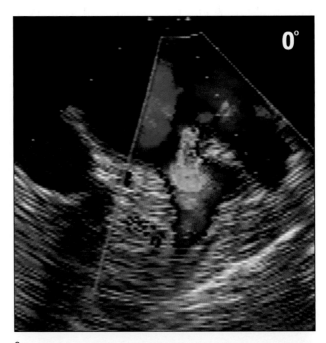

e

Case 6.1 *continued*

D, E. Color-flow Doppler interrogation of normal left atrial appendage flow. F. Pulsed-wave Doppler of normal left atrial appendage flow. In patients with normal sinus rhythm, left atrial appendage flow exhibits four components. The first component is contraction wave denoted as a large positive deflection (towards the transducer) in late diastole following the electrocardiographic P wave. Velocities have been determined between 50 to 65 cm/s in normal patients. The second component is the filling wave, which again is a large deflection (46 to 58 cm/s) in a negative direction following the contraction wave denoting systolic filling of the atrium and appendage. The third component is the systolic reflection waves, which consist of alternating positive and negative deflections between 20 to 38 cm/s that gradually decrease in size and are determined by the cardiac cycle length. The fourth component is the early diastolic outflow wave, denoted by a low velocity positive deflection, which follows the mitral doppler E wave and the electrocardiographic T wave. RA, right atrium; LA, left atrium; LAA, left atrial appendage; AV, aortic valve; TV, tricuspid valve; RVOT, right ventricular outflow tract; PV, pulmonary valve; LV, left ventricle; RV, right ventricle; Ao, aorta.

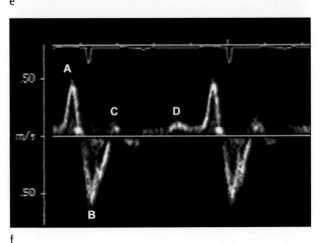

f

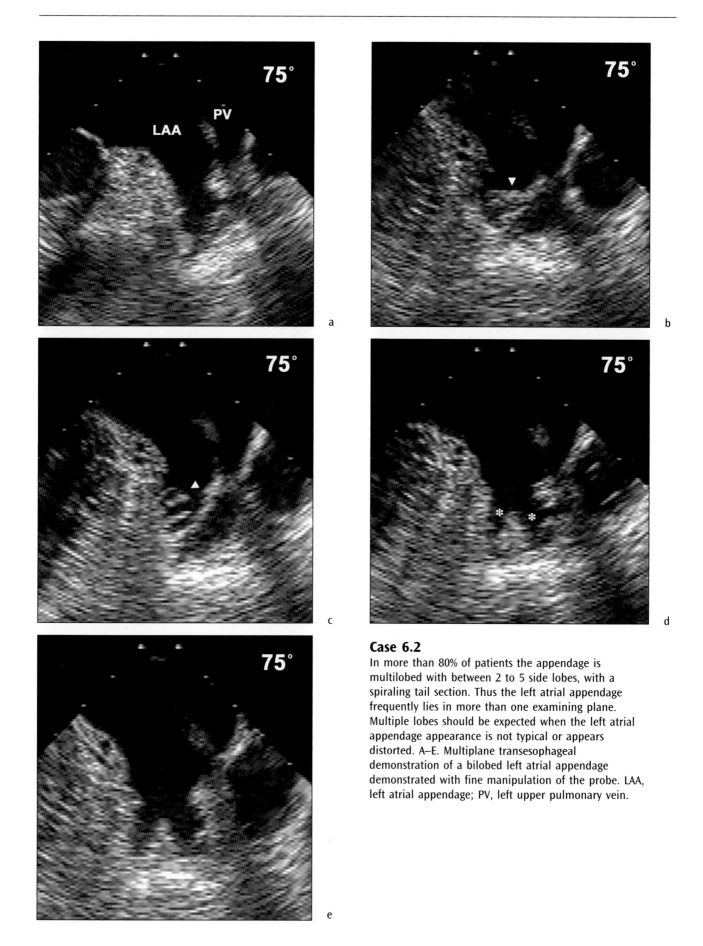

Case 6.2

In more than 80% of patients the appendage is multilobed with between 2 to 5 side lobes, with a spiraling tail section. Thus the left atrial appendage frequently lies in more than one examining plane. Multiple lobes should be expected when the left atrial appendage appearance is not typical or appears distorted. A–E. Multiplane transesophageal demonstration of a bilobed left atrial appendage demonstrated with fine manipulation of the probe. LAA, left atrial appendage; PV, left upper pulmonary vein.

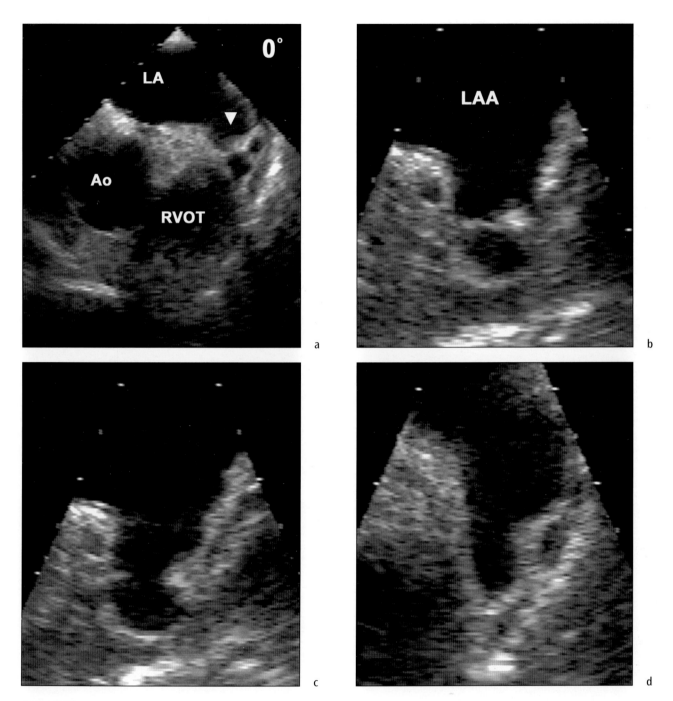

Case 6.3

Prominent pectinate muscle. A–D. In the adult appendage the pectinate muscles are slightly larger than 1 mm in width and may be confused with mass defects within the left atrial appendage. Pectinate muscles generally have the same echo texture as the surrounding myocardium, are frequently linear, and do not exhibit chaotic motion independent of the motion of the atrial appendage. Magnification or zoom mode frequently helps in the identification of prominent pectinate muscles. LA, left atrium; Ao, aorta; RVOT, right ventricular outflow tract.

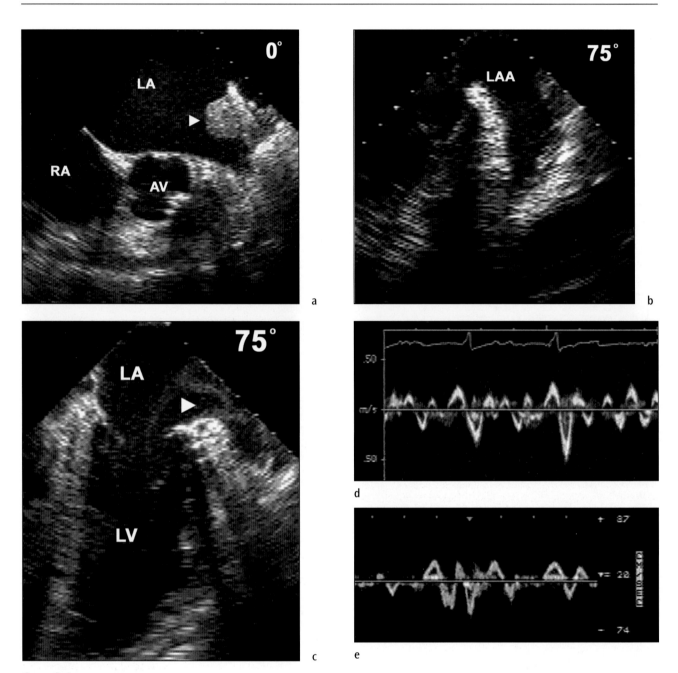

Case 6.4

Left atrial appendage. Thrombi when present usually are larger than pectinate muscles having a propensity for producing a filling defect to the appendage, demonstrate a different echo texture than the surrounding muscle and frequently exhibit chaotic motion during the cardiac cycle. Spontaneous echocardiographic contrast when present is noted, and shares an association with thrombi, which should be excluded through a meticulous examination. A. Thrombus (arrow) attached to the orifice of the left atrial appendage. B. Long tubular left atrial appendage measuring 6.5 cm. On average the appendage has an orifice diameter of 1.5 to 2.1 cm, a maximal body width of 1.5 to 3.1 cm and a length of 2.5 to 3 cm. C. Spontaneous contrast filling the left atrial appendage. Left atrial appendage function is assessed with color and pulsed Doppler examination techniques. During atrial fibrillation, rapid fibrillatory flow waves are recorded, with higher velocity waves recorded during diastole in contrast to systole, with higher overall velocities recorded with longer RR intervals and slower ventricular response rates. D. Pulsed wave Doppler recording of high velocity left atrial appendage blood flow in the setting of atrial fibrillation. E. Pulsed wave Doppler recording of low velocity left atrial appendage blood flow in the setting of atrial fibrillation. Left atrial appendage dysfunction denoted by low velocity flows in the appendage are associated with spontaneous echocardiographic contrast which is indicative of stagnant blood flow in the left atrial cavity and left atrial appendage, and is a precursor to thrombus formation. There appears to be a strong correlation between left atrial appendage dysfunction and the formation of left atrial thrombi and the risk for future thromboembolic events, especially in patients with atrial fibrillation and atrial flutter. LA, left atrium; RA, right atrium; AV, aortic valve; LAA, left atrial appendage; LV, left ventricle.

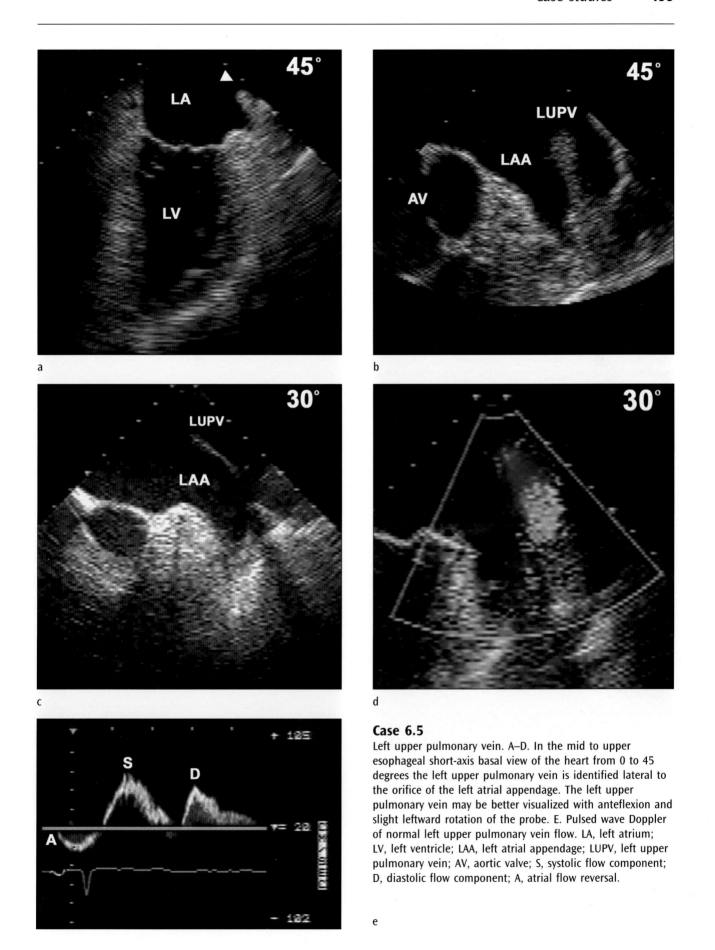

Case 6.5

Left upper pulmonary vein. A–D. In the mid to upper esophageal short-axis basal view of the heart from 0 to 45 degrees the left upper pulmonary vein is identified lateral to the orifice of the left atrial appendage. The left upper pulmonary vein may be better visualized with anteflexion and slight leftward rotation of the probe. E. Pulsed wave Doppler of normal left upper pulmonary vein flow. LA, left atrium; LV, left ventricle; LAA, left atrial appendage; LUPV, left upper pulmonary vein; AV, aortic valve; S, systolic flow component; D, diastolic flow component; A, atrial flow reversal.

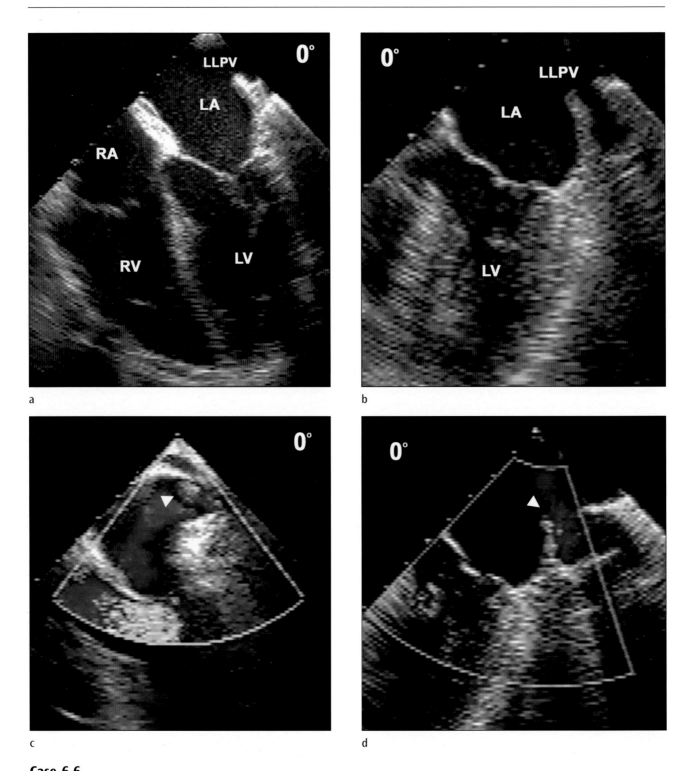

Case 6.6

A–F. Left lower pulmonary vein. To visualize the left lower pulmonary vein (arrow) requires further leftward or counterclockwise rotation with or without slight advancement of the probe, which visualizes the orifice of the inferior pulmonary vein as the left atrial appendage disappears from view. RA, right atrium; RV, right ventricle; LA, left atrium; LV, left ventricle; LLPV, left lower pulmonary vein; AV, aortic valve.

continued

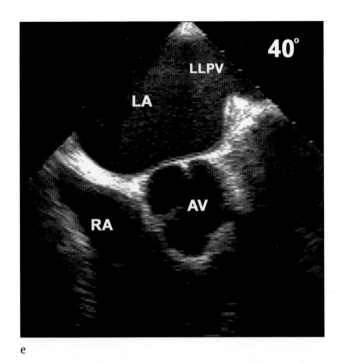

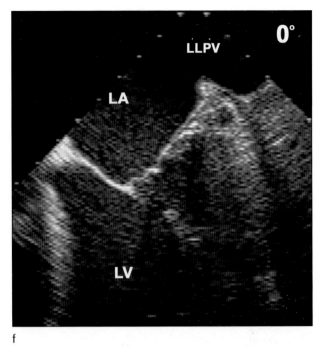

e

f

Case 6.6 *continued*

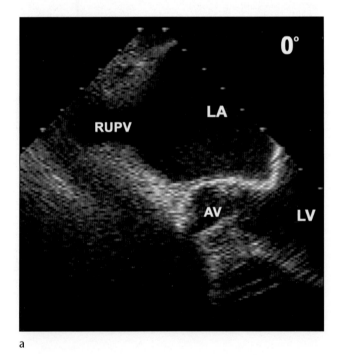

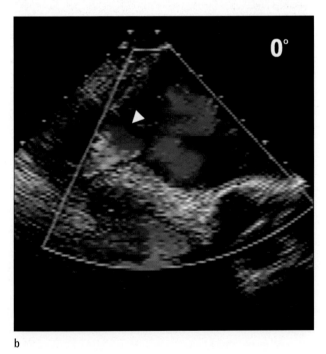

a

b

Case 6.7

Right upper pulmonary vein. The right pulmonary veins may be visualized in the mid esophageal short-axis basal view at 0 degrees with slight rotation of the probe to the right of the midline. A, B. The right upper pulmonary vein again is readily visualized entering the left atrium adjacent to the interatrial septum, in close proximity to the origin of the superior vena cava.

continued

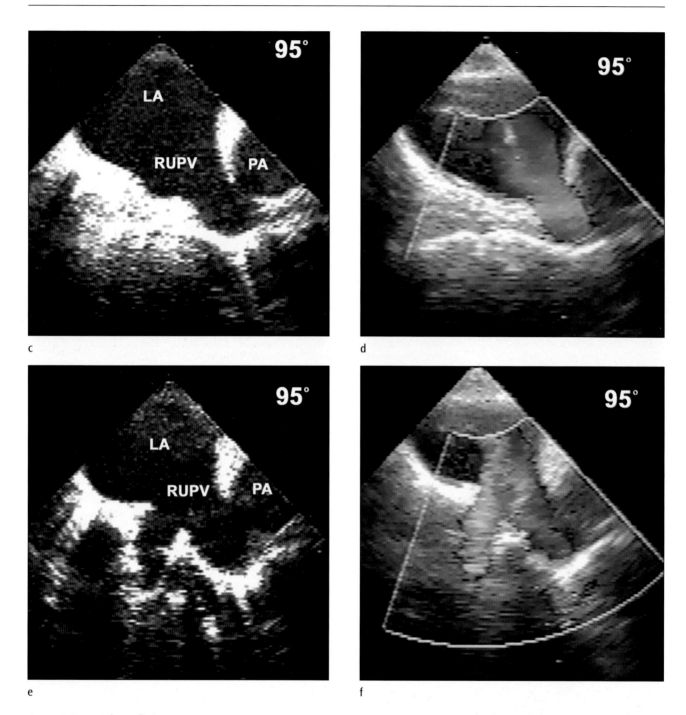

c   d

e   f

Case 6.7 *continued*

C–F. Rightward rotation of the probe visualizes the right superior pulmonary vein entering from a superior direction to the left atrium adjacent to the interatrial septum. RUPV, right upper pulmonary vein; LA, left atrium; AV, aortic valve; LV, left ventricle; PA, pulmonary artery.

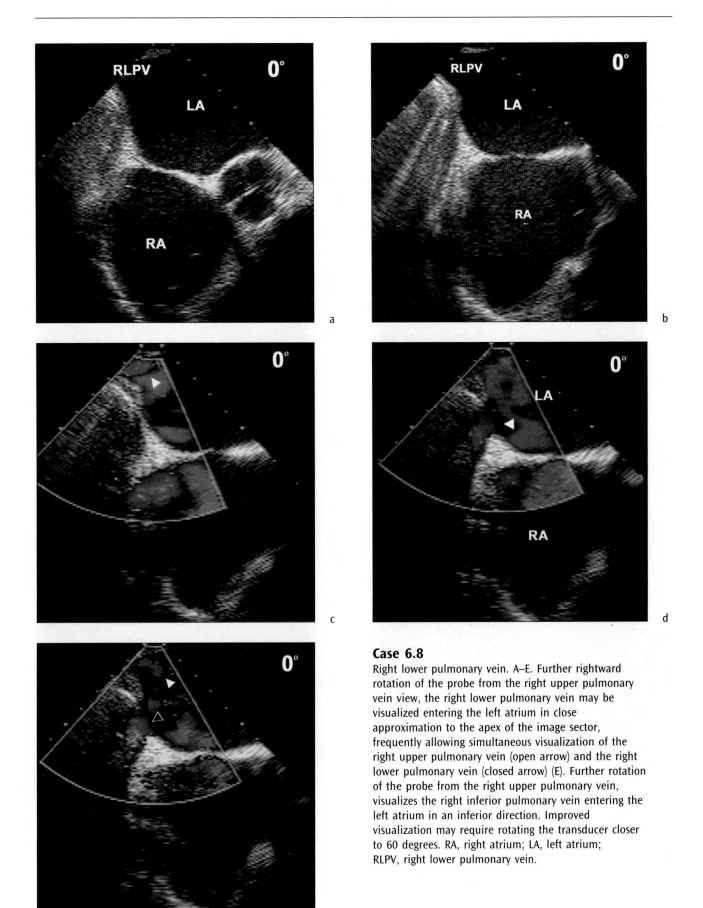

Case 6.8

Right lower pulmonary vein. A–E. Further rightward rotation of the probe from the right upper pulmonary vein view, the right lower pulmonary vein may be visualized entering the left atrium in close approximation to the apex of the image sector, frequently allowing simultaneous visualization of the right upper pulmonary vein (open arrow) and the right lower pulmonary vein (closed arrow) (E). Further rotation of the probe from the right upper pulmonary vein, visualizes the right inferior pulmonary vein entering the left atrium in an inferior direction. Improved visualization may require rotating the transducer closer to 60 degrees. RA, right atrium; LA, left atrium; RLPV, right lower pulmonary vein.

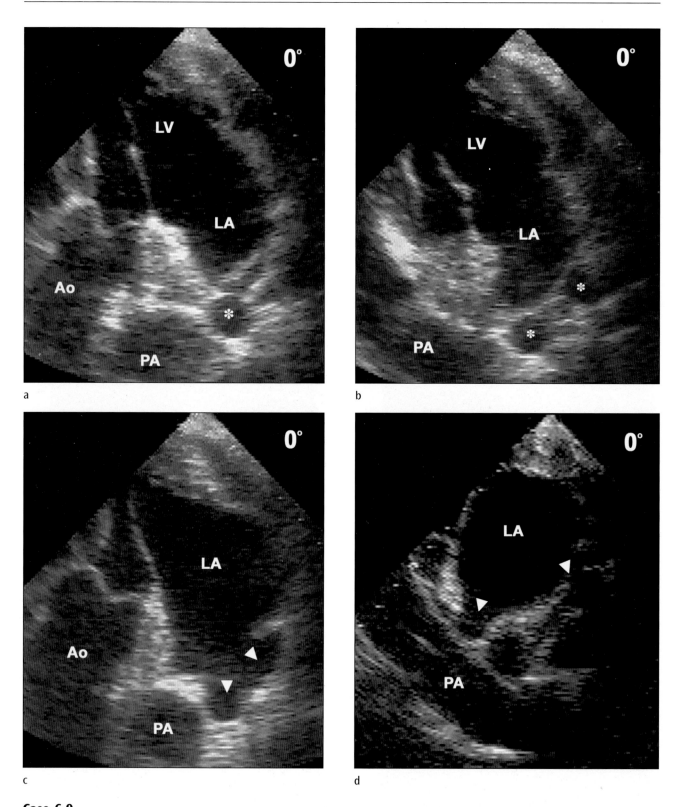

Case 6.9

Pulmonary veins. A–E. The pulmonary veins (star) may also be visualized from the deep transgastric window. These views may be particularly helpful in evaluating congenital disease, and in obtaining a spatial orientation for the pulmonary veins (arrows) since they may be visualized simultaneously. LV, left ventricle; LA, left atrium; Ao, aorta; PA, pulmonary artery; LAA, left atrial appendage; AV, aortic valve.

continued

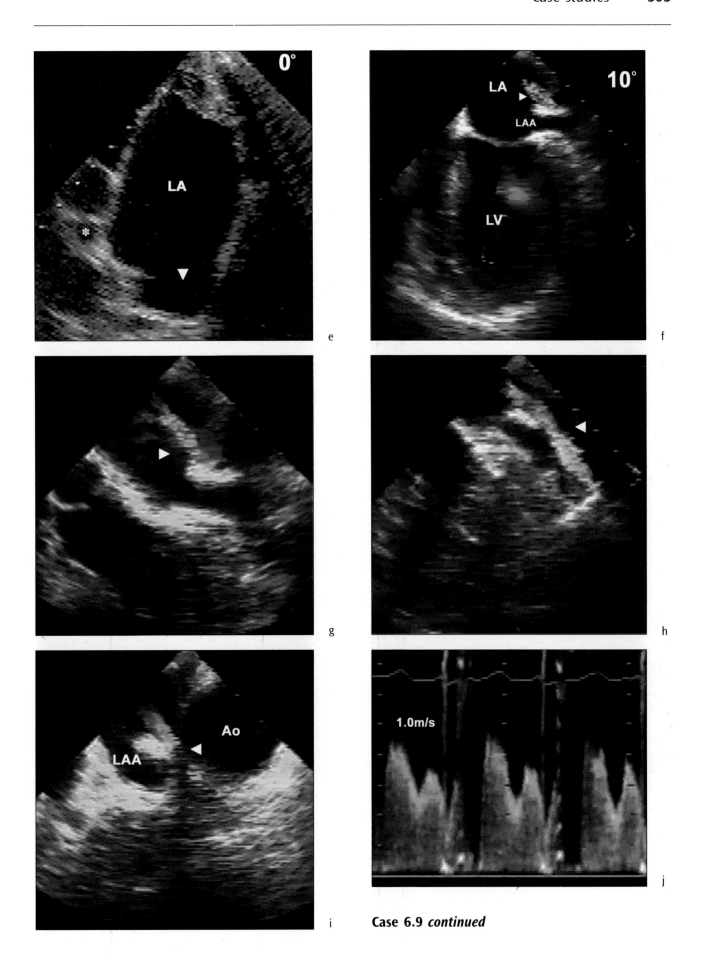

Case 6.9 *continued*

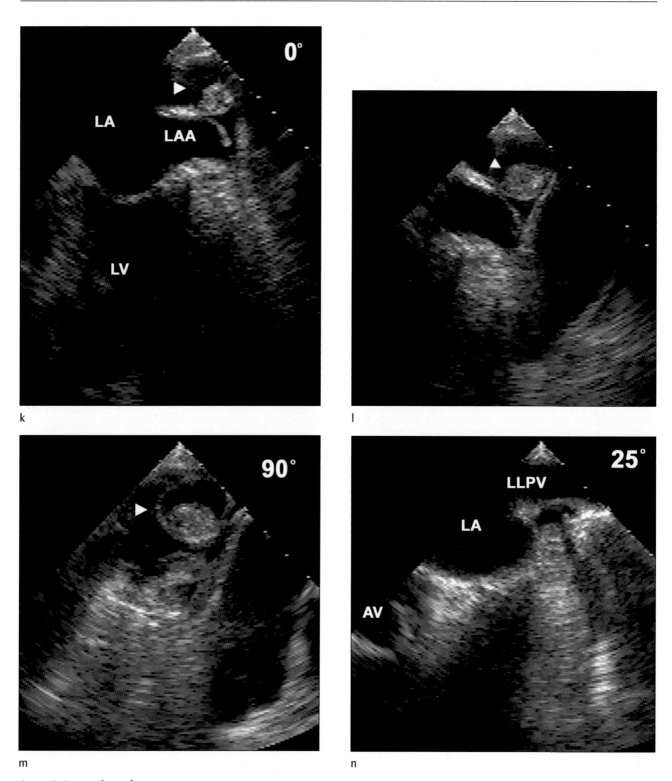

k

l

m

n

Case 6.9 *continued*

F–I. Pulmonary vein stenosis. Longitudinal two-chamber view (F) of the left heart demonstrating a high velocity flow jet (arrow) entering the left atrium above the left atrial appendage with color flow Doppler. G–I. Magnified views of the left atrium with mild rotation of the probe to the left, concentrating on the ostia of the left pulmonary vein demonstrating venous flow with aliasing which is not expected with venous flow. J. Pulsed-wave Doppler of pulmonary venous flow demonstrating high velocity flow consistent with obstruction to forward flow. K–N. Pulmonary vein stump thrombus. Two-chamber view (A) of the left heart demonstrating a round mass (arrow) near the vicinity of left upper pulmonary vein ostia lateral to the typical q-tip sign, in a patient following lung resection for carcinoma of the lung. L, M. Magnified view of the pulmonary vein ostia demonstrating ligated pulmonary vein filled with thrombus. N. Magnified view of the normal left lower pulmonary vein.

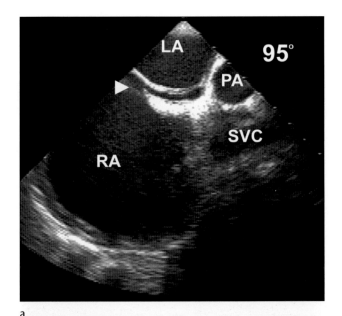

a

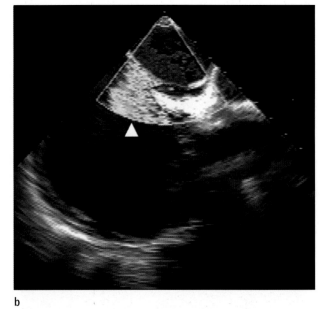

b

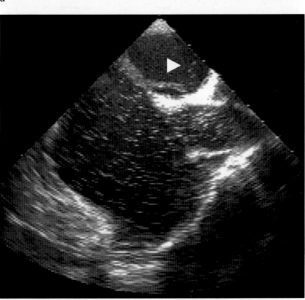

c

Case 6.10

Patent foramen ovale. Transesophageal echocardiographic demonstration of a patent foramen ovale in a standard bicaval view obtained from the upper esophageal window. A. A defect is observed in the atrial septum near the area of the foramen ovale (arrow) in the presence of marked right atrial enlargement. B. Color flow Doppler demonstrates a small shunt flow jet (arrow) emanating from the septal defect. C. Administration of the saline echocardiographic contrast through a peripheral intravenous line fills the right atrium with contrast and bubbles (arrow) are seen crossing the atrial septum and entering the left atrial cavity. LA, left atrium; RA, right atrium; PA, pulmonary artery; SVC superior vena cava.

a

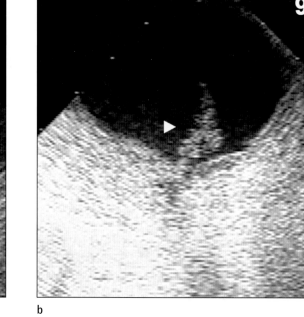

b

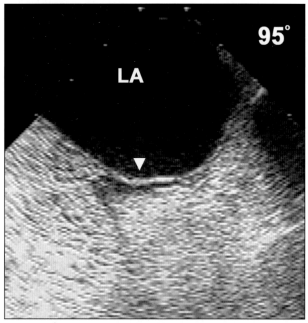

c

Case 6.11

Patent foramen ovale. Magnified bicaval view transesophageal echocardiographic image of the foramen ovale during injection of agitated saline contrast. A. Negative contrast is produced on the right atrial side of the foramen ovale as the right atrium is filled with contrast. B, C. A few cardiac cycles following a Valsalva maneuver, contrast is seen crossing the defect and entering the left atrium. LA, left atrium.

Case 6.12

Atrial septum aneurysm. Multiplane transesophageal demonstration of an atrial septal aneurysm from the lower esophageal window. A–D. Note the atrial septum in the region of the secundum atrial septum (arrow), which is undulating throughout the cardiac cycle. E. Color Doppler demonstration of flow outlining the septum. In many cases there is a patent foramen ovale present with the atrial septum aneurysm. Many debate the issue whether atrial septum aneurysm without a patent foramen ovale is associated with cardiac source of embolism. F. The m-mode cursor is placed through the area of the atrial septal aneurysm, which provides an easy method to measure the excursion of the aneurysm and also describe the motion according to the type of aneurysm. LA, left atrium; RA, right atrium.

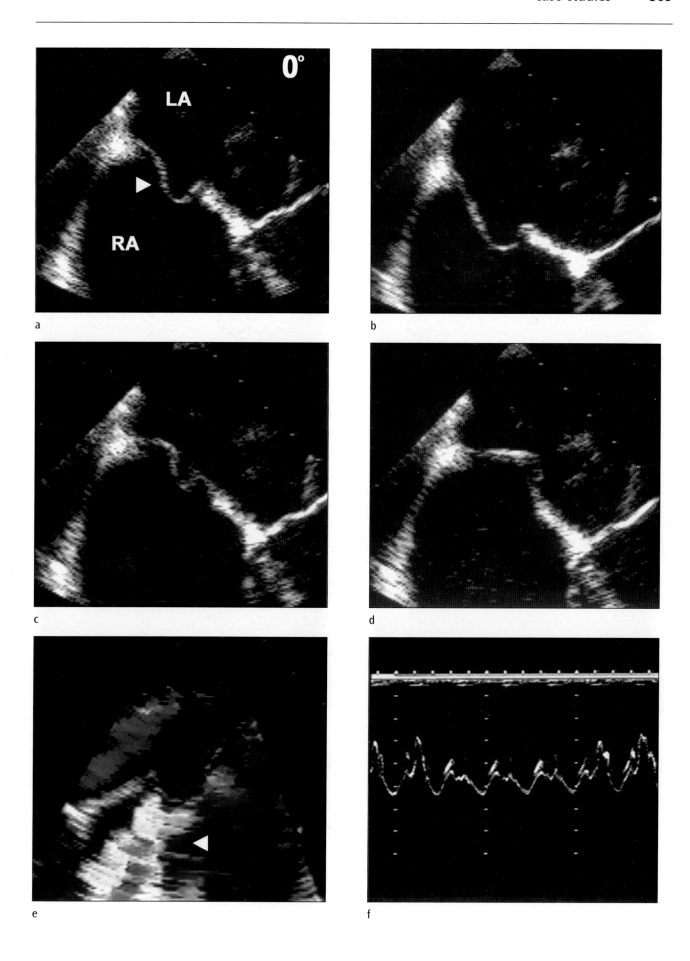

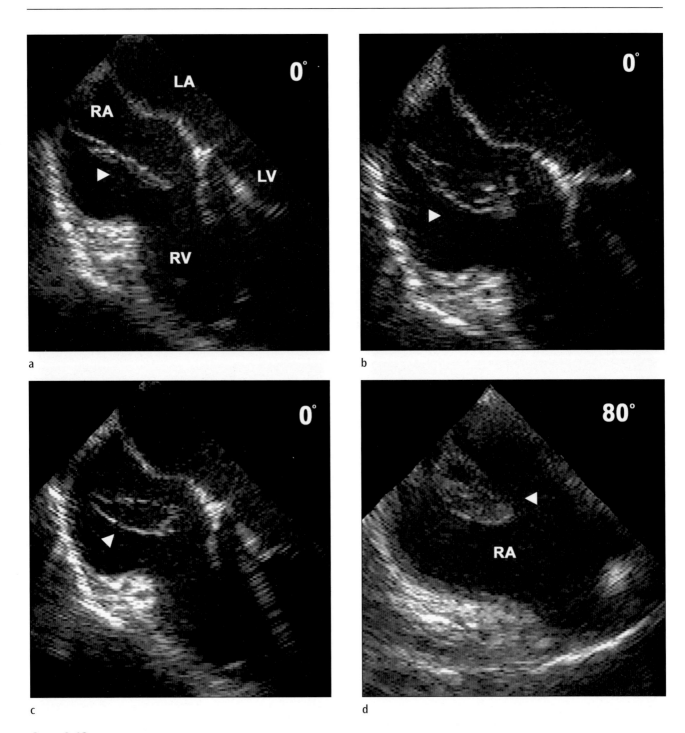

a   b

c   d

Case 6.13

Chiari network. Multiplane transesophageal demonstration of a Chiari network in multiple views. A–D. In views obtained from the lower esophageal window a circular membrane (arrow) is detected originating from the lower region of the inferior vena cava orifice and projects diagonally toward the area of the foramen ovale.

continued

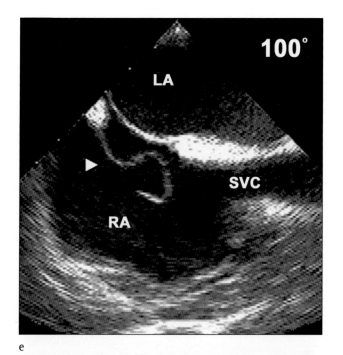

e

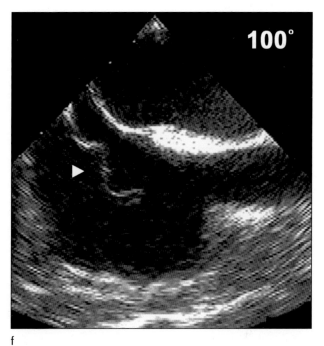

f

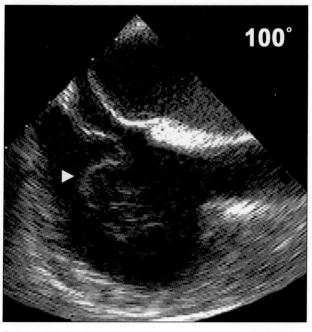

g

Case 6.13 *continued*

E–G. Views obtained from the upper esophageal window in the bicaval view demonstrate the undulating nature of the Chiari network (arrow). Note the difference in appearance between the two views illustrating the limitation of a two-dimensional image, which explains why a Chiari network may be confused with a mass. LA, left atrium; RA, right atrium; SVC, superior vena cava.

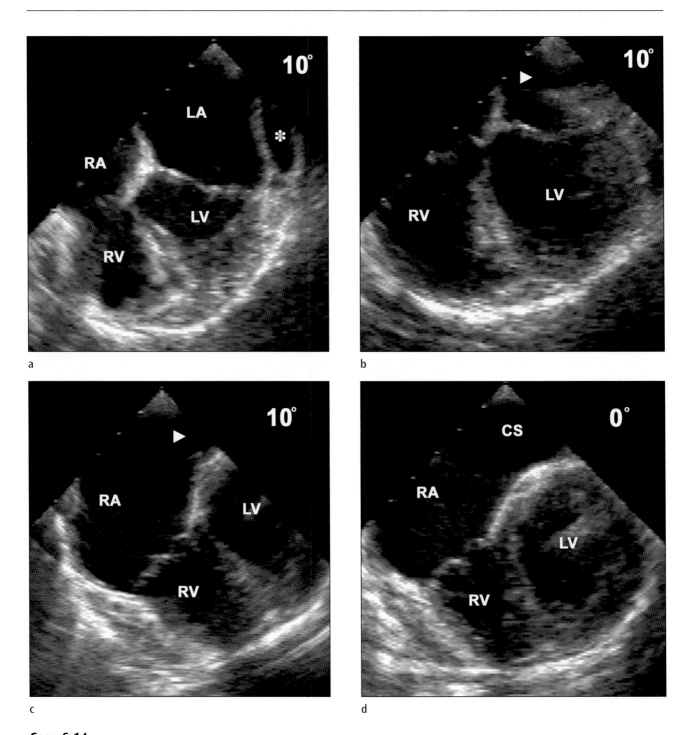

a

b

c

d

Case 6.14

Persistent left superior vena cava. A. A persistent left superior vena cava is visualized in a foreshortened four chamber view obtained from the mid esophageal window. The left vena cava is depicted as a separate circular structure (star) on the lateral portion of the left atrial wall. The left superior vena cava frequently empties into the coronary sinus, as in this case, or may enter directly into the body of the left atrium. B–D. With minor manipulation of the probe an enlarged coronary sinus (arrow) is demonstrated associated with the left vena cava draining into it.

continued

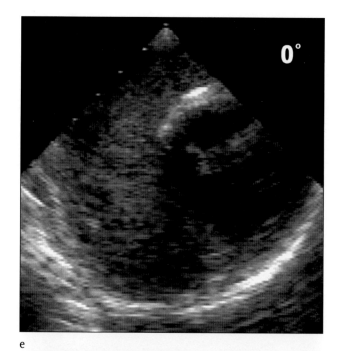

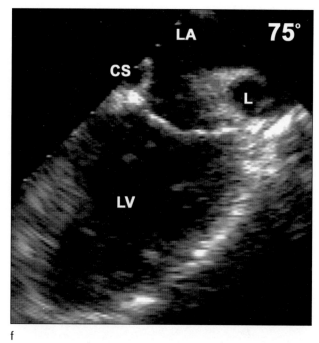

e

f

Case 6.14 *continued*

E. Color flow Doppler demonstrating the flow from the origin of the coronary sinus. F, G. Longitudinal view obtained at 75 degrees demonstrating the enlarged coronary sinus and the left superior vena cava. LA, left atrium; RA, right atrium; RV, right ventricle; LV, left ventricle; CS, coronary sinus; L or star, left superior vena cava.

g

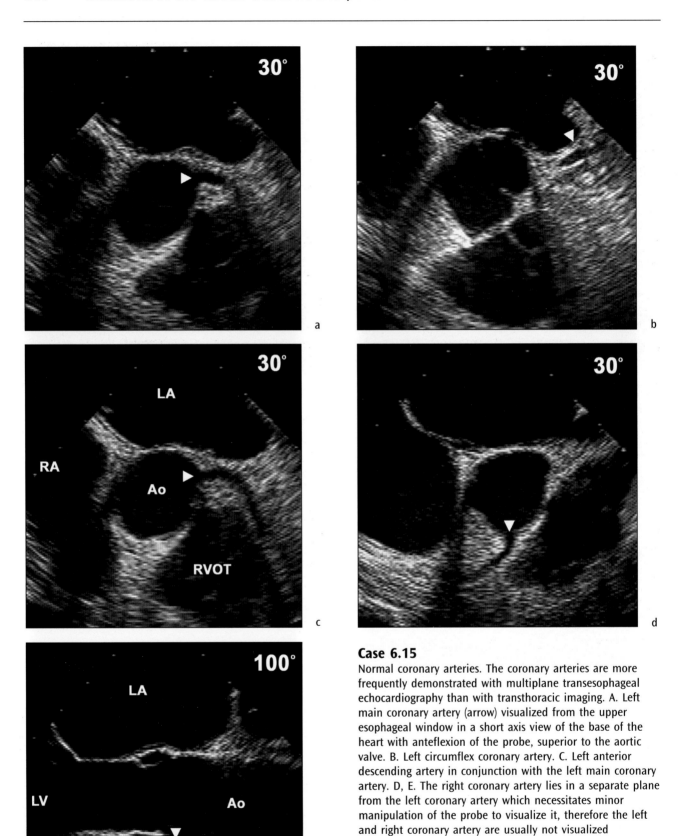

Case 6.15

Normal coronary arteries. The coronary arteries are more frequently demonstrated with multiplane transesophageal echocardiography than with transthoracic imaging. A. Left main coronary artery (arrow) visualized from the upper esophageal window in a short axis view of the base of the heart with anteflexion of the probe, superior to the aortic valve. B. Left circumflex coronary artery. C. Left anterior descending artery in conjunction with the left main coronary artery. D, E. The right coronary artery lies in a separate plane from the left coronary artery which necessitates minor manipulation of the probe to visualize it, therefore the left and right coronary artery are usually not visualized simultaneously. Right coronary artery from the short axis (D) and longitudinal view (E).

continued

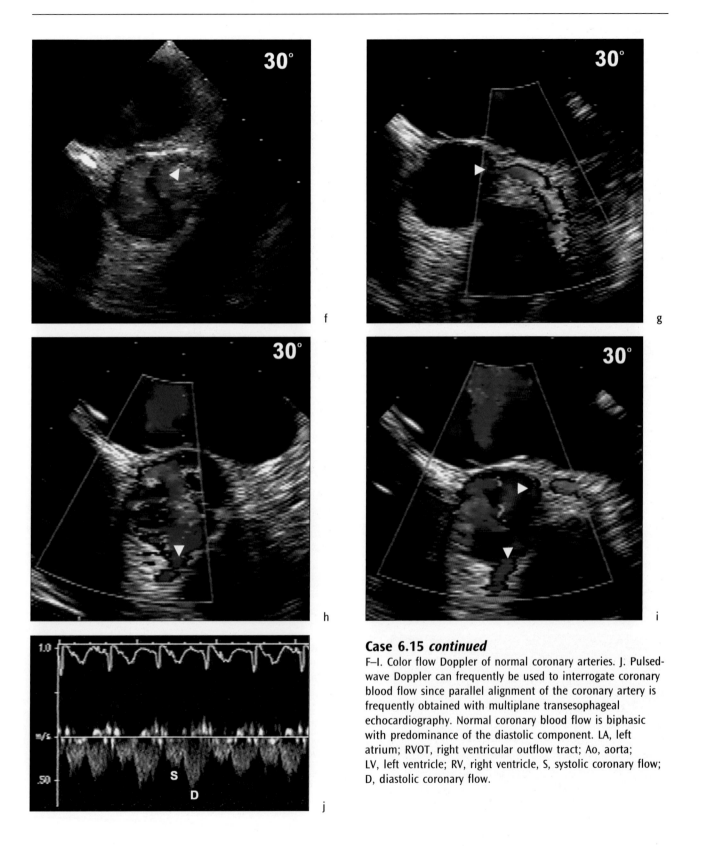

Case 6.15 *continued*

F–I. Color flow Doppler of normal coronary arteries. J. Pulsed-wave Doppler can frequently be used to interrogate coronary blood flow since parallel alignment of the coronary artery is frequently obtained with multiplane transesophageal echocardiography. Normal coronary blood flow is biphasic with predominance of the diastolic component. LA, left atrium; RVOT, right ventricular outflow tract; Ao, aorta; LV, left ventricle; RV, right ventricle, S, systolic coronary flow; D, diastolic coronary flow.

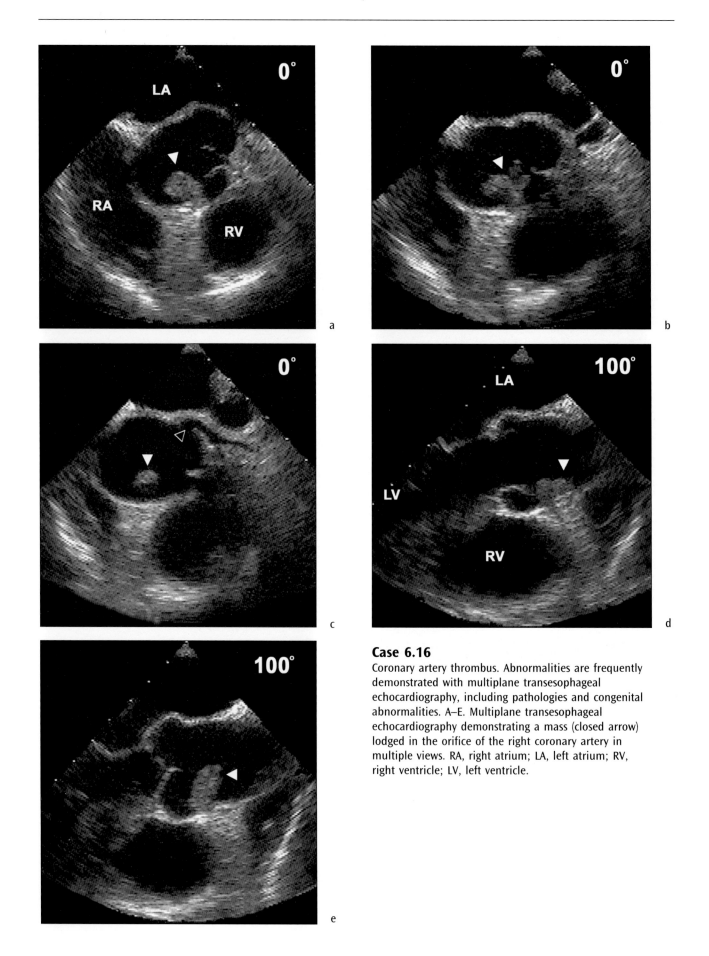

Case 6.16
Coronary artery thrombus. Abnormalities are frequently demonstrated with multiplane transesophageal echocardiography, including pathologies and congenital abnormalities. A–E. Multiplane transesophageal echocardiography demonstrating a mass (closed arrow) lodged in the orifice of the right coronary artery in multiple views. RA, right atrium; LA, left atrium; RV, right ventricle; LV, left ventricle.

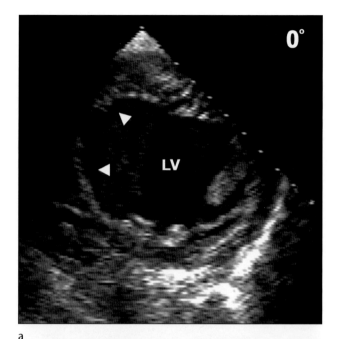

a

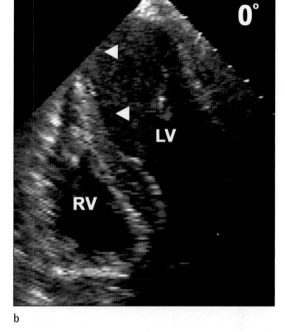

b

c

Case 6.17

Left ventricular aneurysm post-myocardial infarction.
A–C. Multiplane transesophageal echocardiographic
demonstration of a large anteroseptal and anterior
wall myocardial infarction complicated by aneurysmal
formation. A. Transgastric short axis view obtained at
0 degrees demonstrating an obvious deformity of the
septal wall (arrows). B. Deep transgastric view, which
demonstrates thinning of the distal ventricular septal
wall (arrow). C. Transgastric longitudinal view of the
left ventricle demonstrating the out pouching of the
anterior wall (arrows) consistent with aneurysmal
formation following myocardial infarction. LV, left
ventricle; RV, right ventricle.

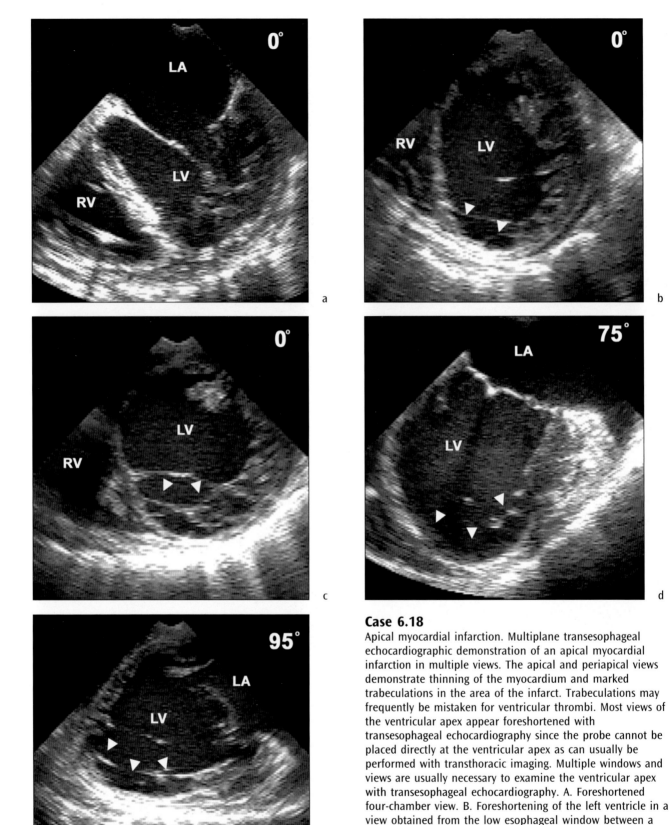

Case 6.18

Apical myocardial infarction. Multiplane transesophageal echocardiographic demonstration of an apical myocardial infarction in multiple views. The apical and periapical views demonstrate thinning of the myocardium and marked trabeculations in the area of the infarct. Trabeculations may frequently be mistaken for ventricular thrombi. Most views of the ventricular apex appear foreshortened with transesophageal echocardiography since the probe cannot be placed directly at the ventricular apex as can usually be performed with transthoracic imaging. Multiple windows and views are usually necessary to examine the ventricular apex with transesophageal echocardiography. A. Foreshortened four-chamber view. B. Foreshortening of the left ventricle in a view obtained from the low esophageal window between a standard four-chamber view and a short axis view. C. Typical short-axis transgastric view. D. Longitudinal view of the left ventricle from the low esophageal window at 75 degrees. E. Transgastric view of the left ventricle at 95 degrees.
LA, left atrium; LV, left ventricle; RV, right ventricle.

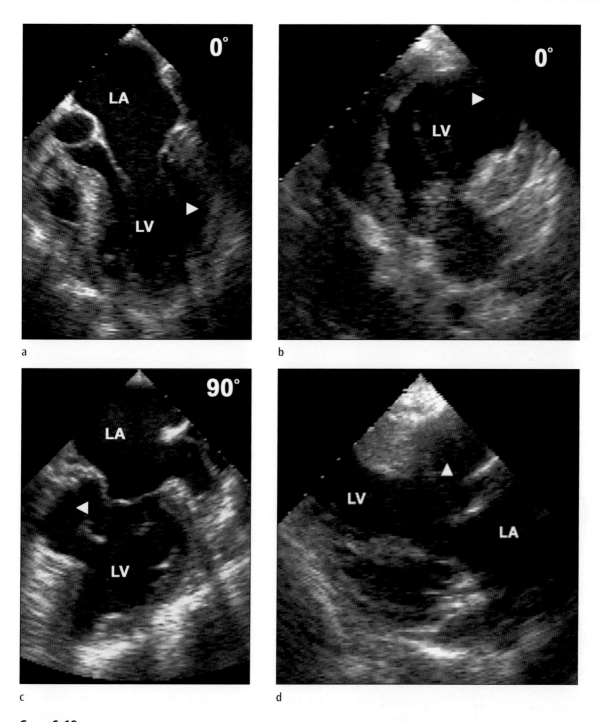

a

b

c

d

Case 6.19

Inferolateral myocardial infarction with inferior aneurysm. A–D. Multiplane transesophageal demonstration of an inferolateral myocardial infarction. A. Five-chamber view from the mid-lower esophageal window with lateral myocardial wall thinning (arrows). Deep transgastric view with a modified short-axis view at 0 degrees demonstrating inferolateral myocardial wall thinning (arrow). C. In the two-chamber longitudinal view at 75 degrees from the mid esophageal window a discreet aneurysm (arrow) is noted in the proximal region of the inferior wall. D. In a modified transgastric view at 95 degrees discreet out pouching of the proximal inferior wall is characteristic of aneurysmal dilatation. LA, left atrium; LV, left ventricle.

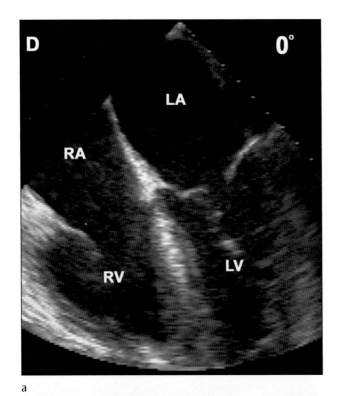

a

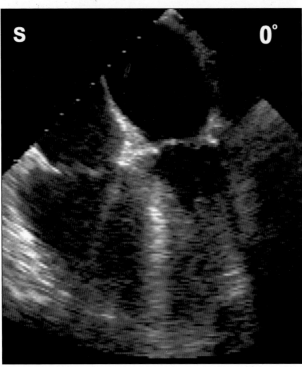

b

Case 6.20

Right ventricular infarct. A, B. Diastolic and systolic frames of a four-chamber view visualizing the right ventricle in the setting of an inferior wall infarction. The right ventricle is dilated with ventricular wall thinning and no demonstrable regional thickening between diastole and systole. LA, left atrium; LV, left ventricle; RA, right atrium; RV, right ventricle.

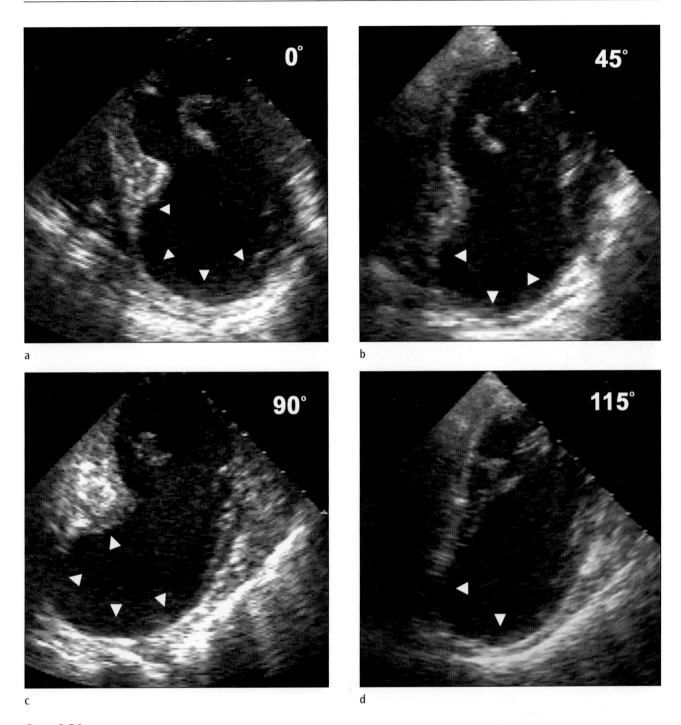

Case 6.21

Anteroapical aneurysm post-myocardial infarction. Visualization of the left ventricular apex may be difficult with transesophageal echocardiography. An anteroapical aneurysm is demonstrated in a modified short-axis view obtained from the lower esophageal window. A–D. The left ventricular apex is imaged from 0 to 115 degrees to demonstrate the full extent of the anterior apical segment and resultant aneurysm after anterior wall infarction.

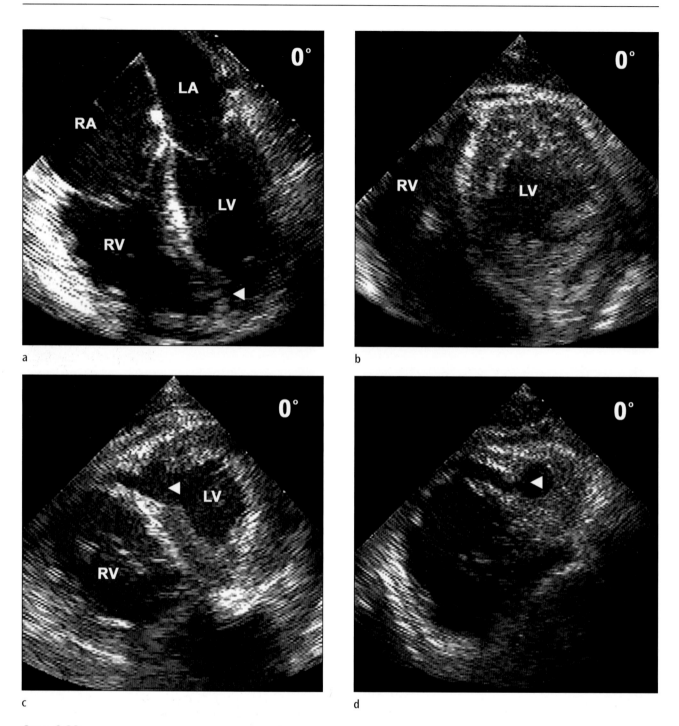

Case 6.22

Acquired ventricular septal defect. Multiplane transesophageal echocardiography is very useful for defining the complications of myocardial infarction, and plays a major role in the preoperative diagnosis and for the determination of postoperative repair results in acquired ventricular septal defect. An inferoseptal post-myocardial ventricular defect is demonstrated in multiple views. A, B. A defect is suggested in the standard four-chamber and two-chamber short axis views in the region of the inferior septum. Note the multiple 'cystic defects' in the ventricular myocardium in the inferoseptal myocardium. C, D. A modified short-axis view obtained from the transgastric window with rotation of the probe to the right demonstrates the defect in the ventricular septum (arrow) at the junction of the septum and the inferior wall of the left and right ventricle. E–F. Color flow Doppler demonstrating a mosaic flow jet in the vicinity of the defect illustrating shunt flow in a left to right direction from the left ventricle to the right ventricle. LV, left ventricle; RV, right ventricle; RA, right atrium; LA, left atrium.

continued

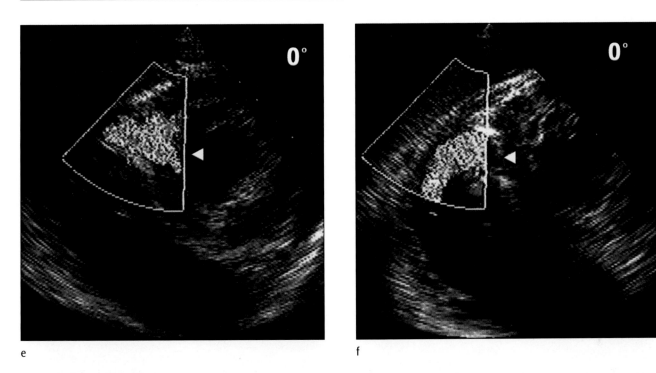

e

f

Case 6.22 *continued*

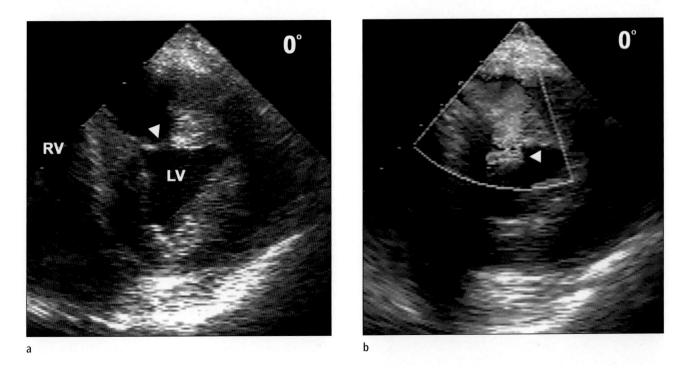

a

b

Case 6.23

Acquired ventricular septal defect. Multiplane transesophageal echocardiography demonstration of a large ventricular septal defect in the setting of cardiogenic shock. A. A large defect is depicted within the inferior ventricular septum near the junction of the inferior walls of the right and left ventricle. Typically a large pocket defect is detected within the septum with a smaller rupture that opens to the right ventricle obliquely to the entry point from the left ventricle. B. Color flow Doppler with blood flow denoted within the defect.

continued

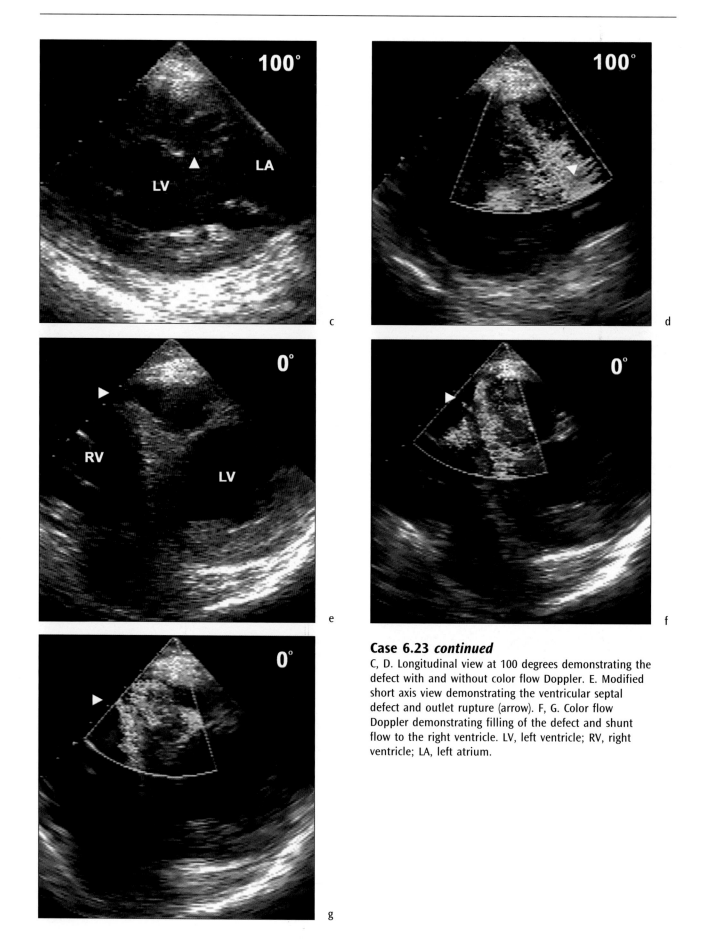

c

d

e

f

g

Case 6.23 *continued*

C, D. Longitudinal view at 100 degrees demonstrating the defect with and without color flow Doppler. E. Modified short axis view demonstrating the ventricular septal defect and outlet rupture (arrow). F, G. Color flow Doppler demonstrating filling of the defect and shunt flow to the right ventricle. LV, left ventricle; RV, right ventricle; LA, left atrium.

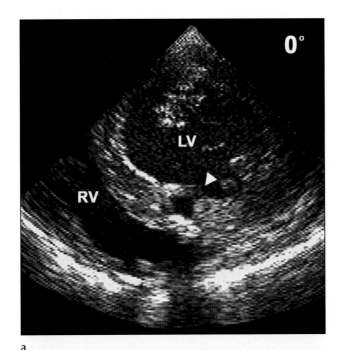

a

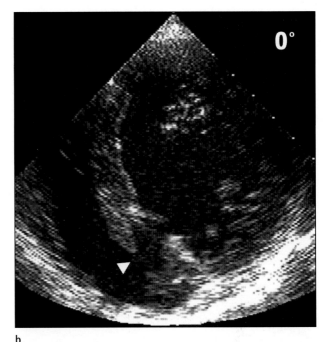

b

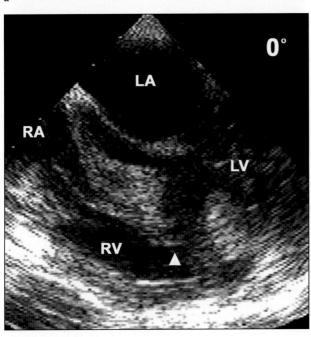

c

Case 6.24

Acquired ventricular septal defect. Multiplane transesophageal echocardiography demonstration of a post myocardial ventricular septal defect. A. Transgastric short-axis view of the left ventricle with a defect in the anteroseptal wall. B. Modified short-axis view obtained by rightward rotation of the probe. The rupture of the defect to the right ventricle is illustrated by the arrow. C. Foreshortened four-chamber view at 0 degrees demonstrating the defect in the distal septum. Note this defect appears to go straight through the septum rather than having an oblique orientation.

continued

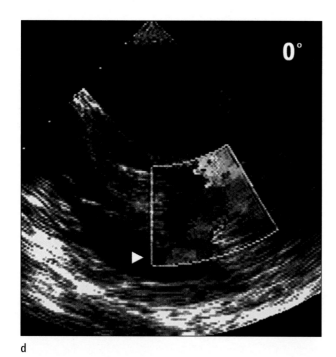

d

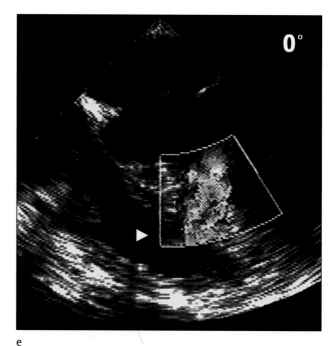

e

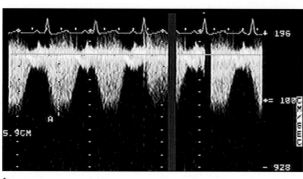

f

Case 6.24 *continued*

D, E. Color flow Doppler demonstrating a continuous shunt jet from the same projection demonstrating low velocity flow during diastole and higher velocity during systole. F. Continuous wave Doppler interrogation of the shunt flow illustrating a 5 m/s flow jet towards the right ventricle and low velocity flow during diastole. LV, left ventricle; RV, right ventricle; LA, left atrium; RA, right atrium.

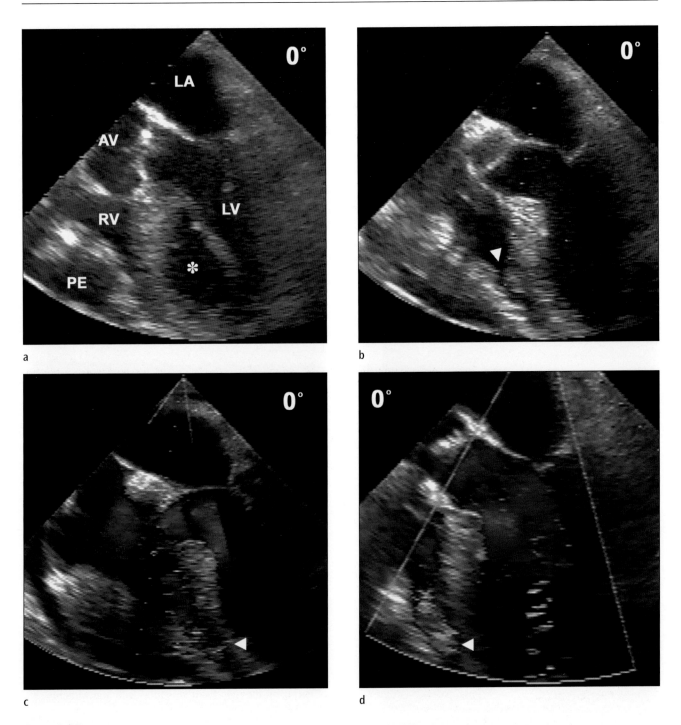

a

b

c

d

Case 6.25

Free ventricular wall rupture. Free wall rupture of the left ventricle is a devastating complication of myocardial infarction that requires a rapid diagnosis and prompt intervention. Mutiplane transesophageal echocardiography is well suited to permit a rapid diagnosis. A–D. Standard four-chamber view demonstrating a large defect in the ventricular septum and filling with color flow Doppler. Note the presence of a pericardial effusion.

continued

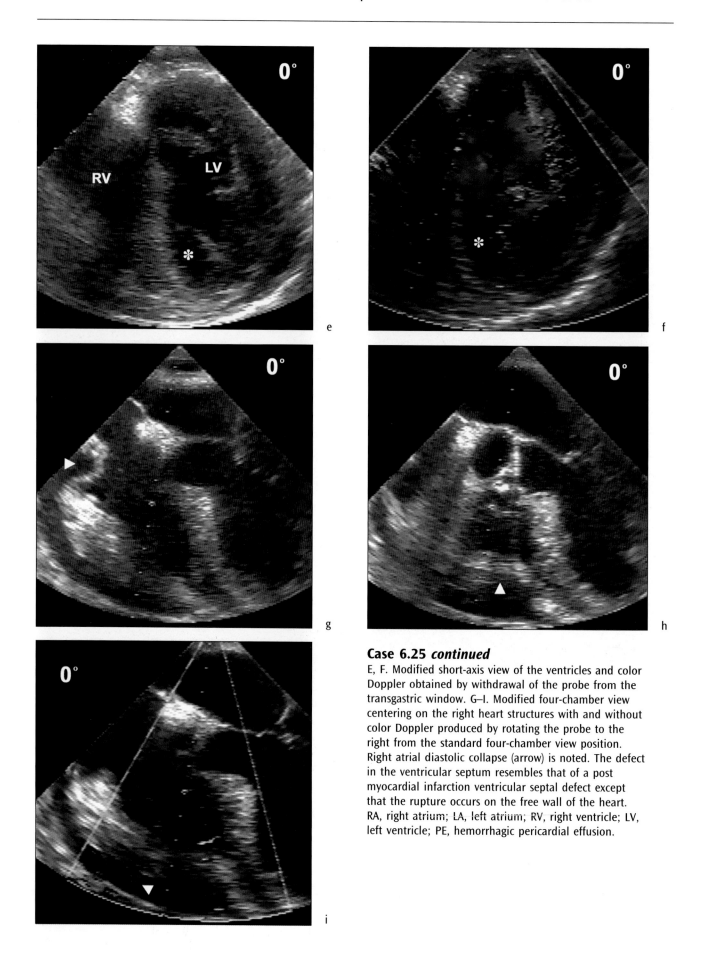

Case 6.25 *continued*

E, F. Modified short-axis view of the ventricles and color Doppler obtained by withdrawal of the probe from the transgastric window. G–I. Modified four-chamber view centering on the right heart structures with and without color Doppler produced by rotating the probe to the right from the standard four-chamber view position. Right atrial diastolic collapse (arrow) is noted. The defect in the ventricular septum resembles that of a post myocardial infarction ventricular septal defect except that the rupture occurs on the free wall of the heart. RA, right atrium; LA, left atrium; RV, right ventricle; LV, left ventricle; PE, hemorrhagic pericardial effusion.

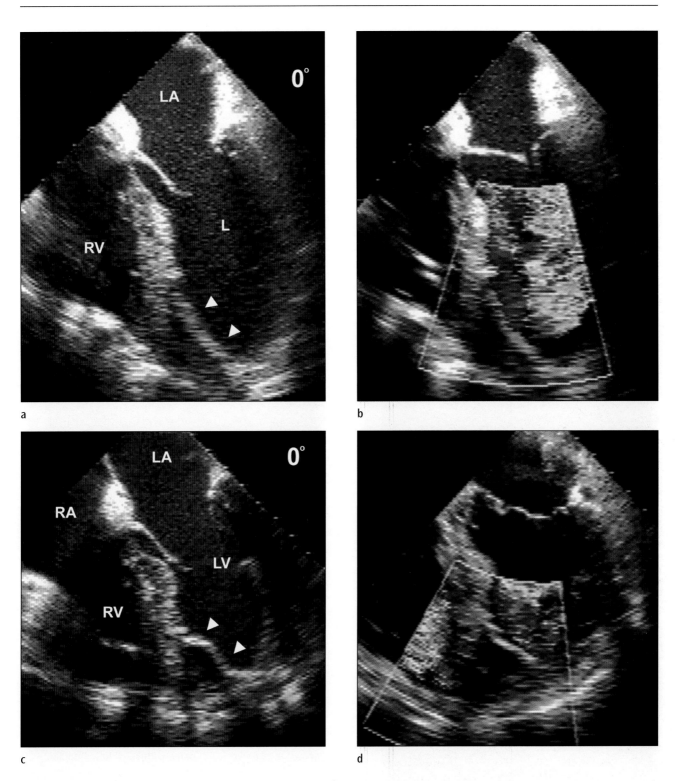

a

b

c

d

Case 6.26

Postoperative VSD repair. Following surgical repair of the ventricular septal defect the ventricles initially appear slightly distorted with evidence of the surgical patch material. The patch will appear to undulate with the cardiac cycle, especially when the ventricles are under-filled. A, B. Four-chamber image and color flow demonstrating an intact surgical patch (arrows) near the ventricular apex. C, D. Modified four-chamber image with rotation of the probe to the right concentrating on the right heart with and without color flow Doppler. Color flow Doppler outlines the patch.

continued

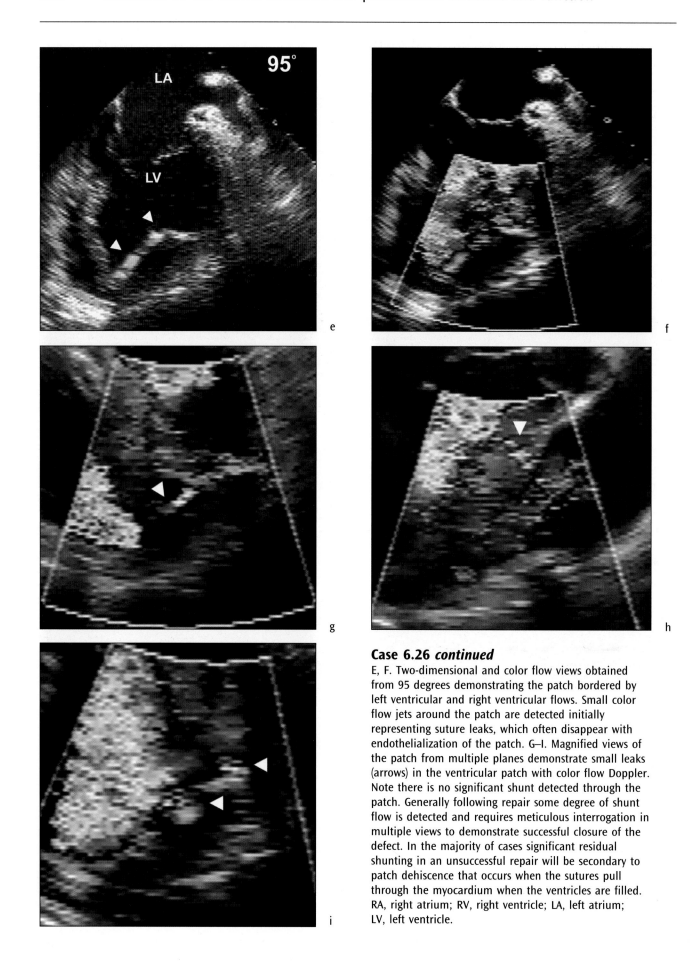

Case 6.26 *continued*

E, F. Two-dimensional and color flow views obtained from 95 degrees demonstrating the patch bordered by left ventricular and right ventricular flows. Small color flow jets around the patch are detected initially representing suture leaks, which often disappear with endothelialization of the patch. G–I. Magnified views of the patch from multiple planes demonstrate small leaks (arrows) in the ventricular patch with color flow Doppler. Note there is no significant shunt detected through the patch. Generally following repair some degree of shunt flow is detected and requires meticulous interrogation in multiple views to demonstrate successful closure of the defect. In the majority of cases significant residual shunting in an unsuccessful repair will be secondary to patch dehiscence that occurs when the sutures pull through the myocardium when the ventricles are filled. RA, right atrium; RV, right ventricle; LA, left atrium; LV, left ventricle.

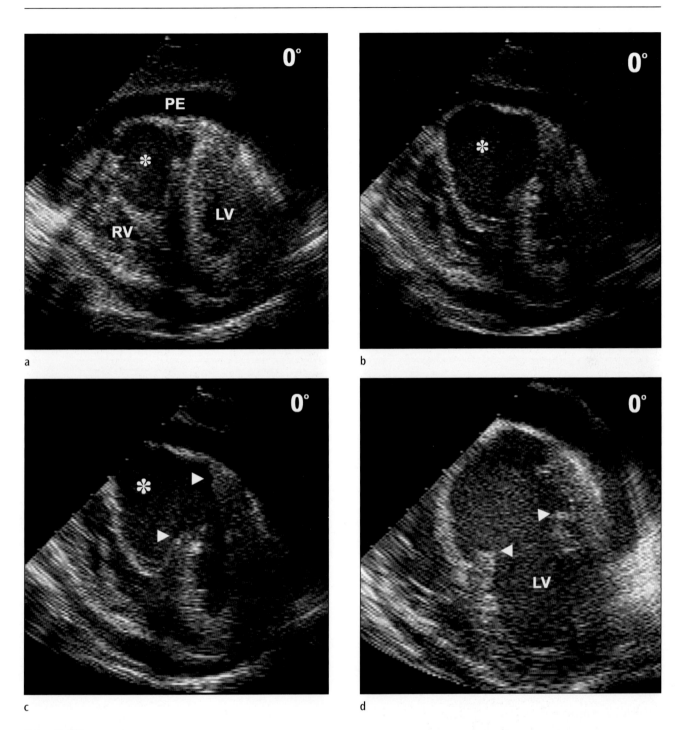

Case 6.27

Pseudoaneurysm post-myocardial infarction. Pseudoaneurysm formation of the left ventricle following myocardial infarction represents a variant of myocardial rupture where the rupture is contained by the pericardium. It has been postulated that the pericardium becomes adherent to the myocardial infarction site due to the inflammation that results. The hallmark of pseudoaneurysm designation is the small neck at the orifice of the aneurysm and the lack of myocardial tissue surrounding the wall of the aneurysm sack. A–D. Short axis view of the left ventricle illustrating the body of the pseudoaneurysm sack. The neck of the pseudoaneurysm is demonstrated in C, D and usually requires manipulation of the probe from standard views to adequately demonstrate its size. Color flow Doppler demonstrates flow in and out of the pseudoaneurysm sac. RV, right ventricle; LV, left ventricle; RA, right atrium; LA, left atrium.

continued

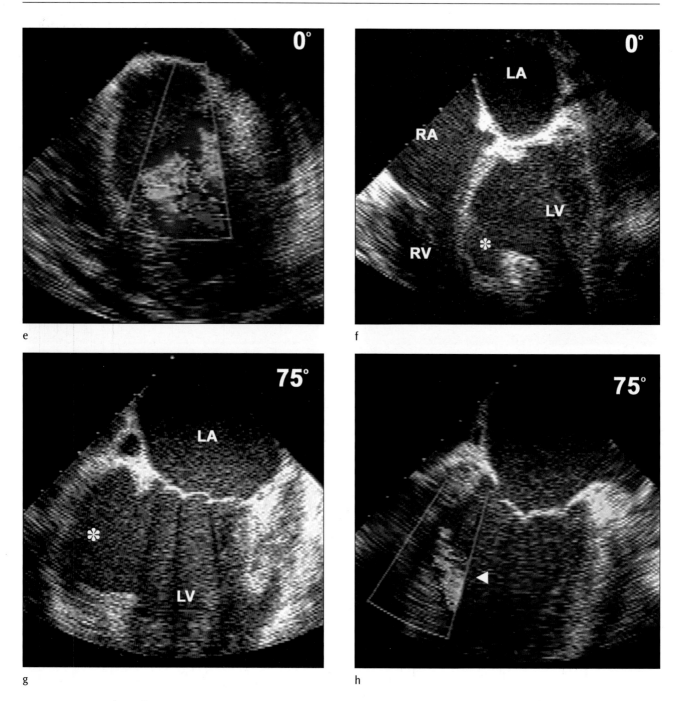

Case 6.27 *continued*

F–K. From the lower esophageal window the pseudoaneurysm may be reconstructed mentally in three-dimensions to appreciate the size and position of the pseudoaneurysm with rotation of the probe from 0 to 135 degrees with and without color flow Doppler.

continued

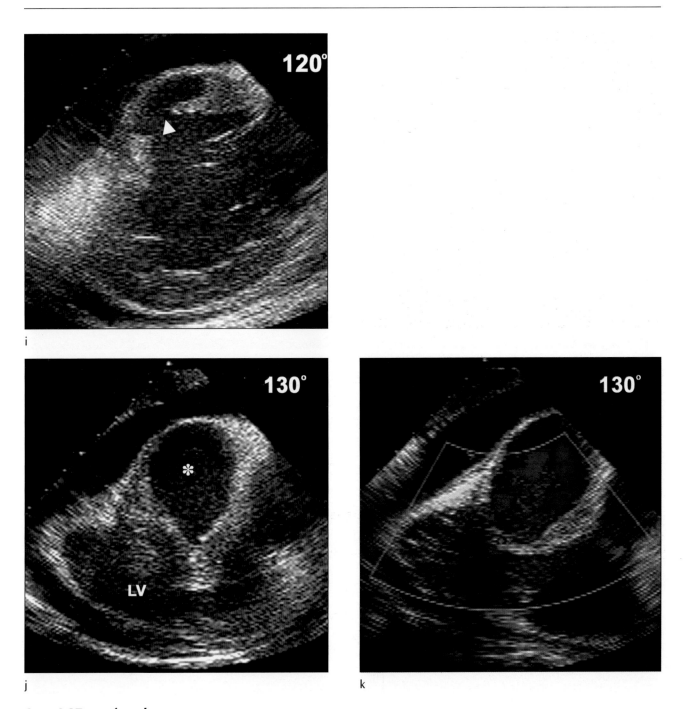

Case 6.27 *continued*

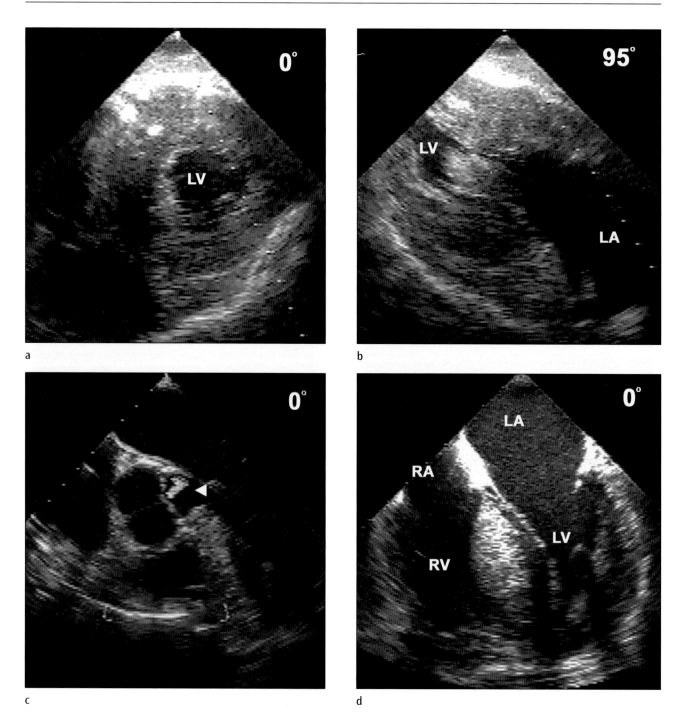

a

b

c

d

Case 6.28

Obstructive hypertrophic cardiomyopathy. Transesophageal echocardiography is generally not necessary for the diagnosis of obstructive or non-obstructive hypertrophic cardiomyopathy. The major role of transesophageal echocardiography is the demonstration and evaluation of associated mitral regurgitation as well as the evaluation of results following surgical correction or interventional septal ablation. A, B. Transgastric short-axis at 0 degrees and long-axis at 95 degrees demonstrating marked thickening of the left ventricular wall predominately of the anterior and septal myocardium with a fine speckled echogenicity texture to the myocardium. C. Five-chamber view from the low esophageal window demonstrating marked enlargement of the ventricular septum that encroaches and produces narrowing of the left ventricular outflow tract. Also note the acuteness of the aorto-mitral angle that is produced by the geometry of the left ventricle.

continued

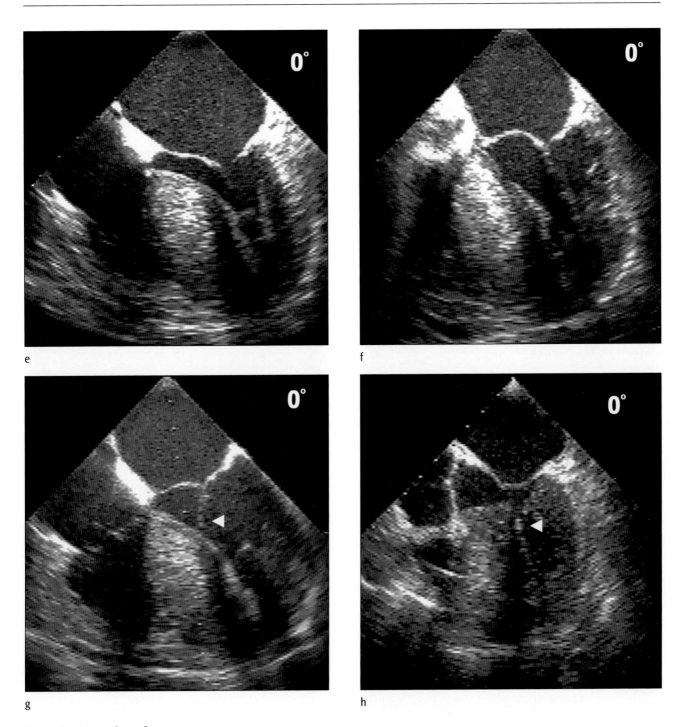

e

f

g

h

Case 6.28 *continued*

D–H. Four-chamber view of the left ventricle illustrating systolic anterior motion (SAM) (arrow) of the mitral apparatus.

continued

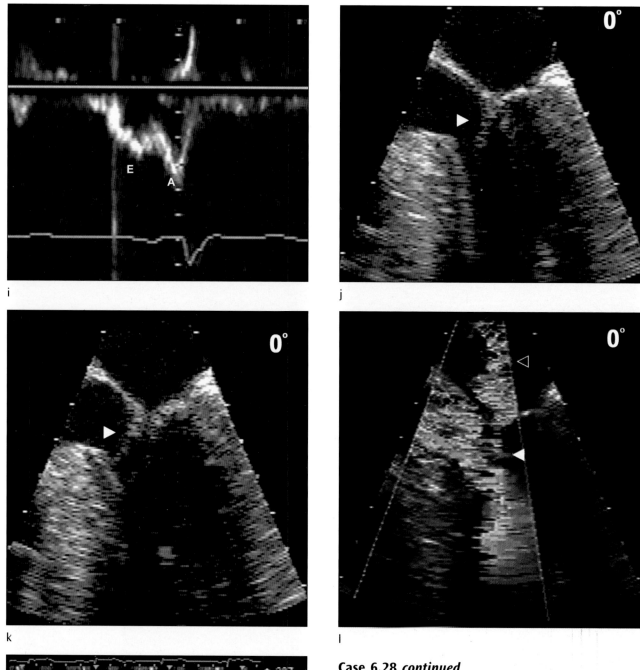

i

j

k

l

m

Case 6.28 *continued*

I. Pulsed wave Doppler interrogation of the mitral inflow demonstrating diastolic dysfunction with a reversed E to A ratio, which is typical of the dysfunction produced by obstructive hypertrophic cardiomyopathy. J–L. Two-dimensional and color flow Doppler of the area of SAM and the correlation with the site of the maximum narrowing and obstruction produced in the left ventricular outflow tract. Mosaic color flow illustrates the highest site of obstruction, which allows precise interrogation with continuous wave doppler (M). The flow contour of the outflow jet exhibits a sabre shape with a maximum velocity of 2 m/s. LA, left atrium; RA, right atrium; LV, left ventricle; RV, right ventricle.

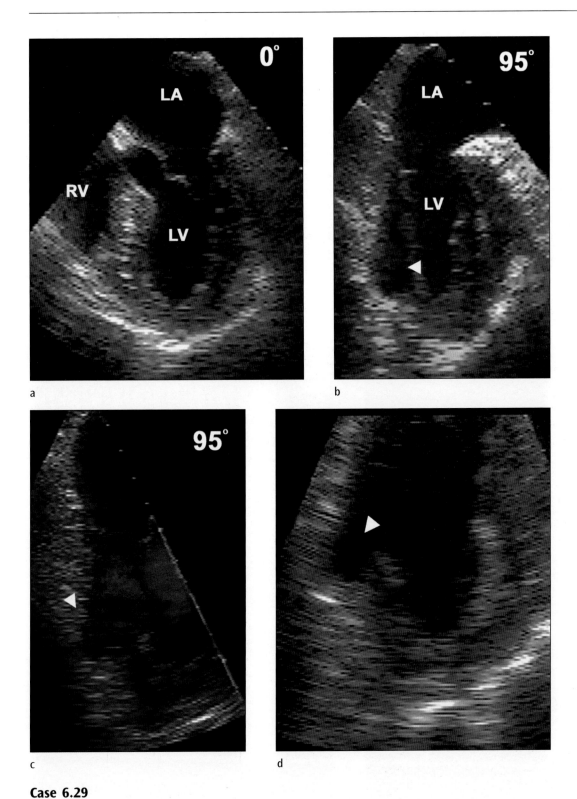

Case 6.29

Left ventricular diverticula. Multiplane transesophageal demonstration of a left ventricular diverticula representing a rare anatomic variant of the left ventricle that may be confused with a ventricular aneurysm. The diverticulum illustrated, which is larger than usually detected, is long and slender with a narrow neck. A. Four-chamber view obtained from the low esophageal window. B. With rotation of the transducer a narrow out-pouching of the left ventricle is recognized, which fills with blood with color flow Doppler (C). D. Magnification mode imaging demonstrating the narrow neck (arrow) of the diverticula. LA, left atrium; LV, left ventricle; RV, right ventricle.

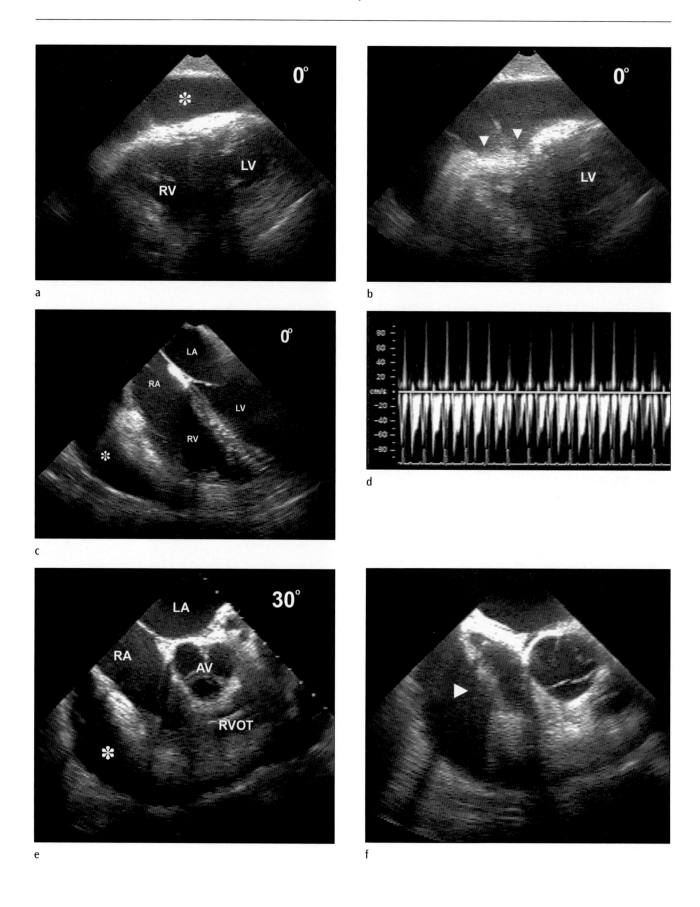

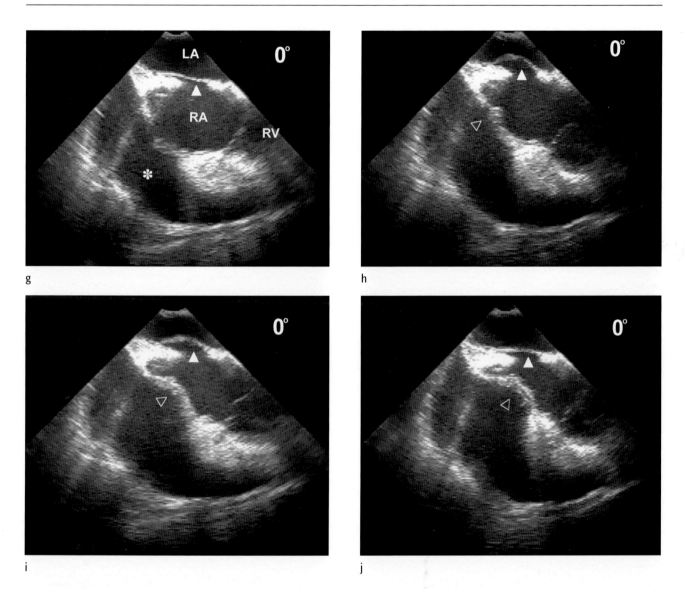

g

h

i

j

Case 6.30

Pericardial tamponade. Transesophageal echocardiography is usually not necessary to evaluate pericardial effusion and/or tamponade. Postoperatively, in the evaluation of cardiac trauma or during the monitoring of certain interventions, transesophageal echocardiography can evaluate pericardial effusion. A–J. Multiplane transesophageal echocardiography demonstration of the development of a pericardial effusion and pericardial tamponade following myocardial perforation. Gastric short-axis view of the ventricles demonstrating an echo free space (star) in the posterior pericardium with right ventricular collapse (arrow) noted during a diastolic frame (B). C. Four-chamber view from the lower esophageal window demonstrating an echo-free space (arrow) on the surface of the right heart. D. Pulsed wave Doppler through the left ventricular inflow tract demonstrating tamponade filling. E, F. Short-axis views of the base of the heart demonstrating pericardial fluid (star) and diastolic collapse (arrow) of the right atrium. G, H. In addition the pericardial effusion (star) and the diastolic collapse of the right atrium (open arrow) note the motion of the atrial septum (closed arrow) bowing towards the left atrium in the opposite direction and out of synch of the atrial collapse during the cardiac cycle. LV, left ventricle; RV, right ventricle; RA, right atrium; LA, left atrium; AV, aortic valve; RVOT, right ventricular outflow tract.

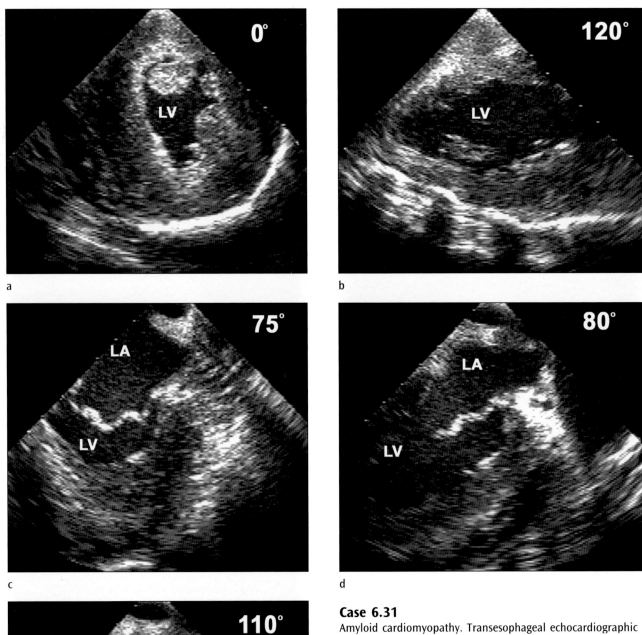

Case 6.31

Amyloid cardiomyopathy. Transesophageal echocardiographic demonstration of amyloid infiltration. A, B. Transgastric short-axis at 0 degrees and long-axis view at 90 degrees of the left ventricle illustrating marked ventricular hypertrophy with a coarse ground glass echogenicity of the ventricular myocardium. C–E. Midesophageal views from 75 to 90 degrees demonstrating marked thickening of the cardiac structures near the base of the heart. Note the prominent pectinate muscles of the left atrial appendage.

continued

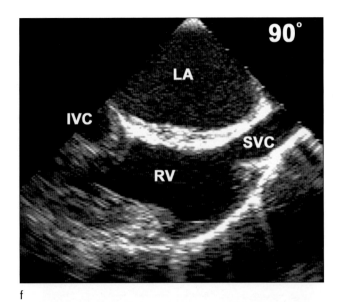

f

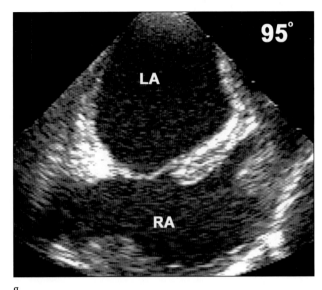

g

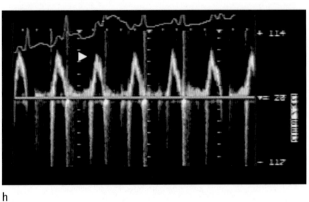

h

Case 6.31 *continued*

F, G. Upper esophageal bicaval views of the atrium demonstrating the marked thickening of the atrial septum consistent with amyloid infiltration. H. Pulsed wave Doppler interrogation of the left ventricular inflow tract demonstrating a merged E–A wave pattern accentuated at atrial contraction. LA, left atrium; LV, left ventricle; RA, right atrium; RV, right ventricle; PA, pulmonary artery; IVC, inferior vena cava; SVC, superior vena cava.

Case 6.32

Constrictive pericarditis. The constriction process in constrictive pericarditis of the heart imposes a structural restraint to ventricular expansion during the ventricular filling phase of diastole. Initially the restraint is limited to the later two-thirds of diastole. A–K. These findings are manifest echocardiographically by right atrial enlargement, dilatation of the inferior vena cava abnormal interventricular septal motion in the presence of normal left ventricular size and systolic function.

continued

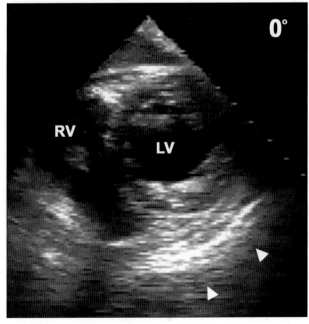

a

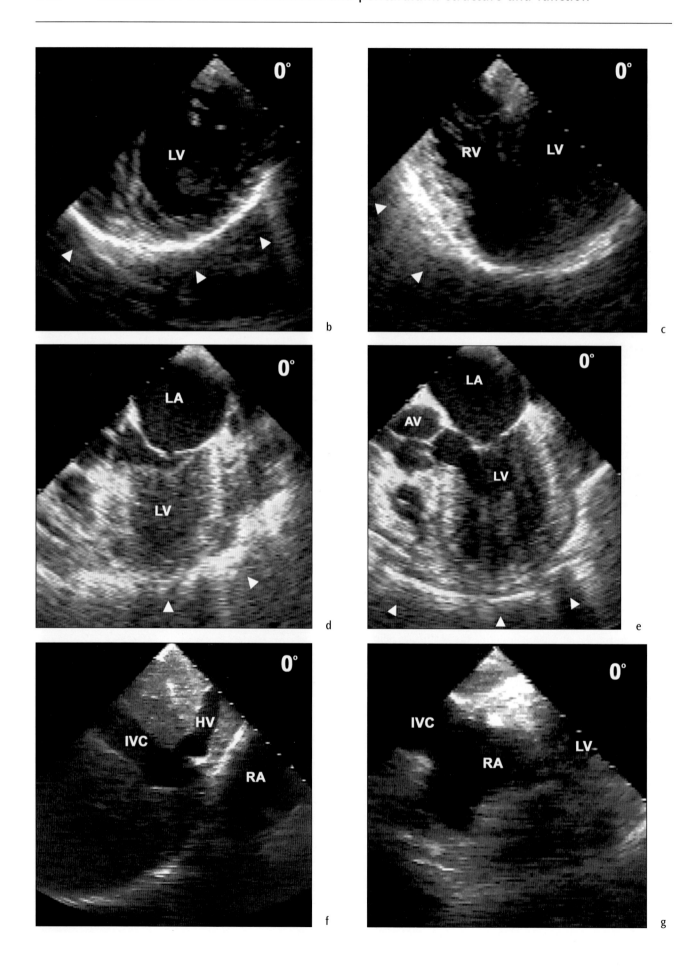

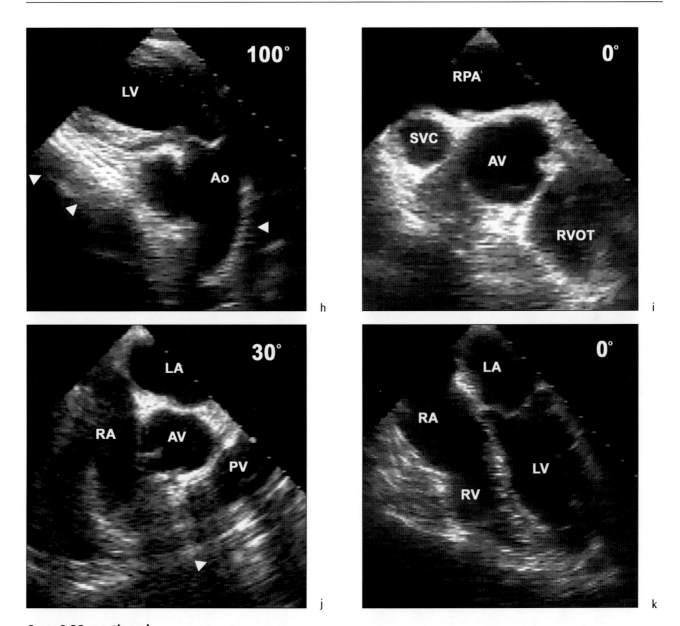

Case 6.32 *continued*

The thickness of the pericardium can be measured with echocardiography, with better results obtained with the transesophageal technique. During inspiration, the fall in intrathoracic pressure is reflected with a drop in pulmonary venous pressure which is not accompanied by a corresponding drop in left ventricular diastolic pressure, producing an abnormal gradient between the two which results in the reduction of the transmitral filling serves to dampening pulmonary venous diastolic forward flow. Reduced transmitral filling subsequently produces an increase in the transtricuspid filling. This is represented by a reduced mitral E wave velocity and pulmonary venous diastolic velocity with an increased tricuspid E wave velocity in the first complex following inspiration. During expiration the opposite occurs, as represented by an increased mitral E wave velocity and a decreased tricuspid E wave velocity with an increase in diastolic flow reversal in the hepatic veins. In constrictive pericarditis, there is marked respiratory variation in mitral (> 25%) and tricuspid flow velocities profiles, which has been shown to distinguish constrictive pericarditis from the other entities responsible for producing abnormal ventricular relaxation.

continued

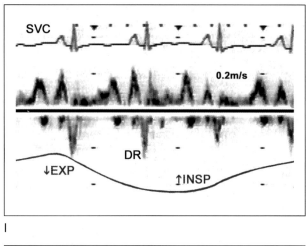

l

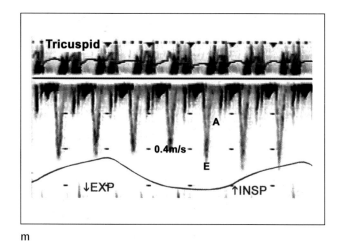

m

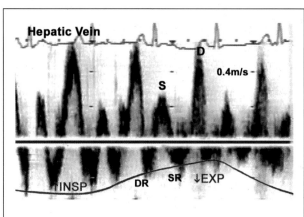

n

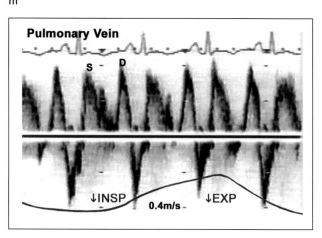

o

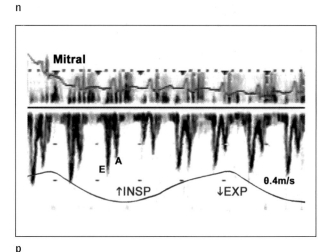

p

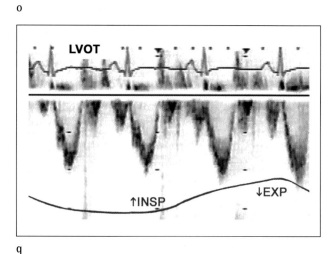

q

Case 6.32 *continued*

L–Q. Pulsed wave Doppler waveforms through the heart from the superior vena cava to the left ventricular outflow tract. See text for further details. RV, right ventricle; LV, left ventricle; LA, left atrium; AV, aortic valve; IVC, inferior vena cava; HV, hepatic vein; RA, right atrium; Ao, aorta; SVC, superior vena cava; RPA, right pulmonary artery; RVOT, right ventricular outflow tract; PV, pulmonary valve; S, systolic; D, diastolic.

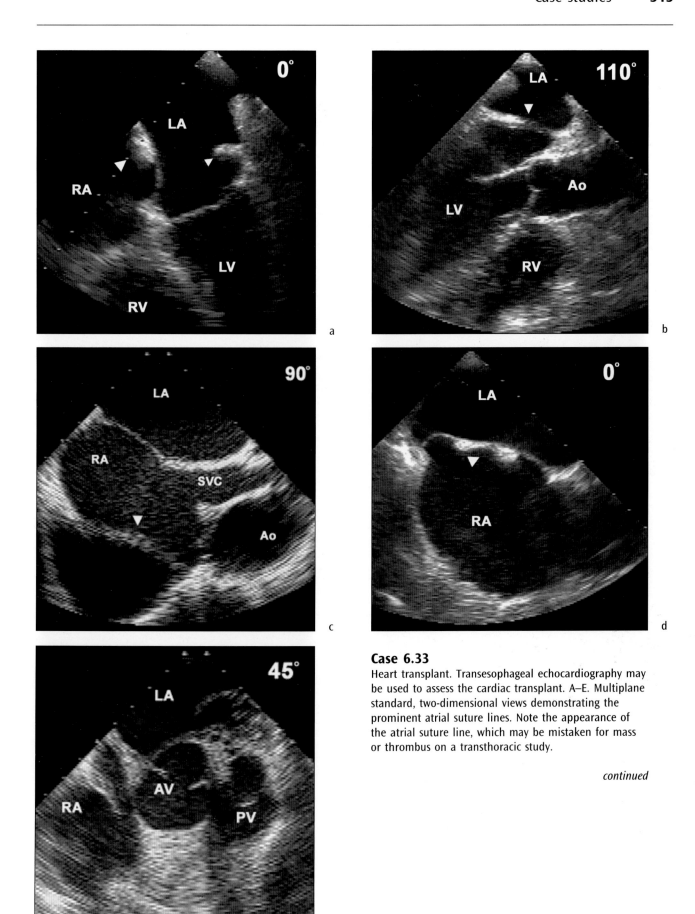

Case 6.33

Heart transplant. Transesophageal echocardiography may be used to assess the cardiac transplant. A–E. Multiplane standard, two-dimensional views demonstrating the prominent atrial suture lines. Note the appearance of the atrial suture line, which may be mistaken for mass or thrombus on a transthoracic study.

continued

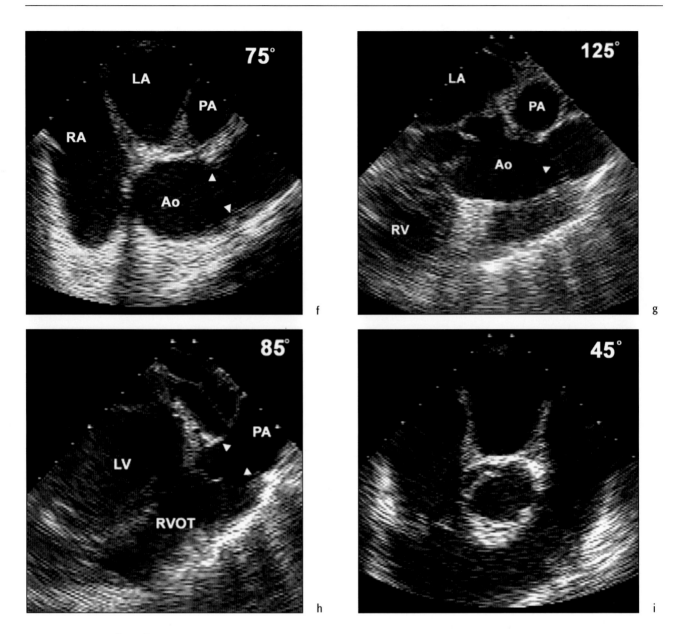

Case 6.33 *continued*

F–I. Multiplane views of the great vessel anastomosis line superior the semilunar valves. In cardiac rejection the typical echocardiographic pattern is a restricted filling pattern, with systolic dysfunction usually occuring late in the rejection process. LA, left atrium; RA, right atrium; LV, left ventricle; RV, right ventricle; Ao, aorta; SVC, superior vena cava; AV, aortic valve; PV, pulmonary valve; PA, pulmonary artery; RVOT, right ventricular outflow tract.

References

1. Pandian NG, Tsui-Lieh H, Schwartz SL, et al. Multiplane transesophageal echocardiography. Imaging planes, echocardiographic anatomy, and clinical experience with a prototype phases array Omniplane probe. *Echocardiography* 1992;9:649–66.
2. Seward JB, Khanderia BK, Freeman WK, et al. Multiplane transesophageal echocardiography: image orientation, examination technique, anatomic correlations, and clinical applications. *Mayo Clin Proc* 1993;11:505.
3. Flachskampf FA, Hoffmann R, Verlande M, et al. Initial experience with a multiplane transesophageal transducer: assessment of diagnostic potential. *Eur Heart J* 1992;13:1201–6.
4. Schluter M, Hinrichs A, Thier W, et al. Transesophageal two-dimensional echocardiography: comparison of ultrasonic and anatomic sections. *Am J Cardiol* 1984;53:1173–8.
5. Roldan FJ, Vargas-Barron J, Espinola-Zavaleta N, et al. Three-dimensional echocardiography of the right atrial embryonic remnants. *Am J Cardiol* 2002;89:99–101.
6. Limacher MC, Gutgesell HP, Vick GW, et al. Echocardiographic anatomy of the Eustachian valve. *Am J Cardiol* 1986;57:363–5.
7. Werner JA, Cheitlin MD, Gross BW, et al. Echocardiographic appearance of Chiari network: differentiation from right heart pathology. *Circulation* 1981;63:1104–9.
8. Savas V, Samyn J, Schreiber TL, et al. Cor triatriatum dexter: recognition and percutaneous transluminal correction. *Cathet Cardiovasc Diagn* 1991;23:183–6.
9. Mahy I, Anderson RH. Division of the right atrium. *Circulation* 1998;98:2352–3.
10. Hansing CE, Young WP, Rowe FF. Cor triatriatum dexter: persistent right sinus venosus valve. *Am J Cardiol* 1972;30:559–64.
11. Schwinger ME, Gindea AJ, Freedberg RS, Kronzon I. The anatomy of the interatrial septum: a transesophageal echocardiographic study. *Am Heart J* 1990;119:1401–5.
12. Fyke FE, Tajik AJ, Edwards WD, Seward JB. Diagnosis of lipomatous hypertrophy of the atrial septum by two-dimensional echocardiography. *J Am Coll Cardiol* 1983;1:1352–7.
13 Pochis WT, Saeian K, Sagar KB. Usefulness of transesophageal echocardiography in diagnosing lipomatous hypertrophy of the atrial septum with comparison to transthoracic echocardiography. *Am J Cardiol* 1992;70:396–8.
14. Stoddard M, Lidell N, Vogel R, et al. Comparison of cardiac dimensions by transesophageal and transthoracic echocardiography. *Am Heart J* 1992;124:675–8.
15. Block M, Hourigan L, Bellows WH, et al. Comparison of left atrial dimensions by transesophageal and transthoracic echocardiography. *J Am Soc Echocardiogr* 2002;15:143–9.
16. Buchholz S, Jenni R. Doppler echocardiographic findings in 2 identical variants of a rare cardiac anomaly, 'subtotal' cor triatriatum: a critical review of the literature. *J Am Soc Echocardiogr* 2001;14:846.
17. Tantibhedhyangkul W, Godoy I, Karp R, Lang RM. Cor triatriatum in a 70–year-old woman: role of transesophageal echocardiography and dynamic three-dimensional echocardiography in diagnostic assessment. *J Am Soc Echocardiogr* 1998;11:837–40.
18. Sadiq M, Sreeram N, Silove ED. Congenitally divided left atrium: diagnostic pitfalls in cross-sectional echocardiography. *Int J Cardiol* 1995;48:99–101.
19. Kacenelenbogen R, Decoodt P. Biplane transesophageal echocardiographic diagnosis of cor triatriatum. *Chest* 1994;105:601–2.
20. Hoffmann R, Lambertz H, Flachskampf FA, Hanrath P. Transesophageal echocardiography in the diagnosis of cor triatriatum; incremental value of colour Doppler. *Eur Heart J* 1992;13:418–20.
21. Vuocolo LM, Stoddard MF, Longaker RA. Transesophageal two-dimensional and Doppler echocardiographic diagnosis of cor triatriatum in the adult. *Am Heart J* 1992;124:791–3.
22 Veinot JP, Harrity PJ, Gentile F, et al. Anatomy of the normal left atrial appendage: a quantitative study of age-related changes in 500 autopsy hearts: implications for echocardiographic examination. *Circulation* 1997;96:3112–15.
23. Ernst G, Stollberger C, Abzieher F, et al. Morphology of the left atrial appendage. *Anat Rec* 1995;242:553–61.
24. Agmon Y, Khandheria BK, Gentile F, Seward JB. Echocardiographic assessment of the left atrial appendage. *J Am Coll Cardiol* 1999;34:1867–77.
25. Hwang JJ, Li YH, Lin JM, et al. Left atrial appendage function determined by transesophageal echocardiography in patients with rheumatic mitral valve disease. *Cardiology* 1994;85:121–8.
26. Black IW, Hopkins AP, Lee LC, Walsh WF. Left atrial spontaneous echo contrast: a clinical and echocardiographic analysis. *J Am Coll Cardiol* 1991;18:398–404.
27. Fatkin D, Kelly RP, Feneley MP. Relations between left atrial appendage blood flow velocity, spontaneous echocardiographic contrast and thromboembolic risk in vivo. *J Am Coll Cardiol* 1994;23:961–9.
28. Mügge A, Daniel WG, Hausmann D, et al. Diagnosis of left atrial appendage thrombi by transesophageal echocardiography: clinical implications and follow-up. *Am J Card Imaging* 1990;4:173.
29. Appleton CP, Jensen JL, Hatle LK, Oh JK. Doppler evaluation of left and right ventricular diastolic function: a technical guide for obtaining optimal flow velocity recordings. *J Am Soc Echocardiogr* 1997;10:271–92.
30. Fatkin D, Feneley MP. Patterns of Doppler-measured blood flow velocity in the normal and fibrillating human left atrial appendage. *Am Heart J* 1996;132:995–1003.
31. Kortz RA, Delemarre BJ, van Dantzig JM, et al. Left atrial appendage blood flow determined by transesophageal echocardiography in healthy subjects. *Am J Cardiol* 1993;71:976–81.
32. Tabata T, Oki T, Fukuda N, et al. Influence of aging on left atrial appendage flow velocity patterns in normal subjects. *J Am Soc Echocardiogr* 1996;9:274–80.
33. Mügge A, Kuhn H, Nikutta P, et al. Assessment of left atrial appendage function by biplane transesophageal echocardiography in patients with nonrheumatic atrial fibrillation: identification of a subgroup of patients at increased embolic risk. *J Am Coll Cardiol* 1994;23:599–607.
34. The Stroke Prevention in Atrial Fibrillation Investigators Committee on Echocardiography. Transesophageal echocardiographic correlates of thromboembolism in high-risk patients with non-valvular atrial fibrillation. *Ann Intern Med* 1998;128:639–47.
35. Verhorst PM, Kamp O, Welling RC, et al. Transesophageal echocardiographic predictors for maintenance of sinus rhythm after electrical cardioversion of atrial fibrillation. *Am J Cardiol* 1997;79:1355–9.
36. Tanabe K, Yoshitomi H, Asanuma T, et al. Prediction of outcome of electrical cardioversion by left atrial appendage flow velocities in atrial fibrillation. *Jpn Circ J* 1997;61:19–24.
37. Pinheiro L, Nanda NC, Jain H, Sanyal R. Transesophageal echocardiographic imaging of the pulmonary veins. *Echocardiography* 1991;8:741–8.
38. Seward JB, Khanderia BK, Edwards WD, et al. Biplanar transesophageal echocardiography: anatomic correlations, image orientation, and clinical applications. *Mayo Clin Proc* 1990;65:1193–213.
39. Nanda NC, Pinheiro L, Sanyal RS, Storey O. Transesophageal biplane echocardiographic imaging: technique, planes, and clinical usefulness. *Echocardiography* 1990;7:771–88.
40. Shah PM, Kyo S, Matsumura M, Omoto R. Utility of biplane transesophageal echocardiography in left ventricular wall motion analysis. *J Cardiothorac Vasc Anesth* 1991;5:316–19.

41. Tennant R, Wiggers CJ. The effect of coronary occlusion on myocardial contraction. *Am J Physiol* 1935;112:351.

42. Kerber RE, Marcus ML, Ehrhardt J, et al. Correlation between echocardiographically demonstrated segmental dyskinesis and regional myocardial perfusion. *Circulation* 1975;52:1097–1104.

43. Kerber RE, Abboud FM. Echocardiographic detection of regional myocardial infarction. *Circulation* 1973;47:997–1005.

44. Jacobs JJ, Feigenbaum H, Corya BC, Phillips JF. Detection of left ventricular asynergy by echocardiography. *Circulation* 1973;48:263–71.

45. Alam M, Khaja F, Brymer J, et al. Echocardiographic evaluation of left ventricular function during coronary angioplasty. *Am J Cardiol* 1986;57:20–5.

46. Weiss JL, Bulkley BH, Hutchins GM, Mason SJ. Two-dimensional echocardiographic recognition of myocardial injury in man. Comparison with postmortem studies. *Circulation* 1981;63:401–8.

47. ASE/SCA Guidelines for performing a comprehensive intraoperative multiplane transesophageal echocardiography examination: Recommendations of the American Society of Echocardiography Council for Intraoperative Echocardiography and the Society of Cardiovascular Anesthesiologists Task Force for Certification in Perioperative Transesophageal Echocardiography. *J Am Soc Echocardiogr* 1999;12:884–900.

48. Schiller NB, Shah PM, Crawford M, et al. Recommendations for Quantitation of the Left Ventricle by Two-Dimensional Echocardiography. American Society of Echocardiography Committee on Standards, Subcommittee on Quantitation of Two-Dimensional Echocardiograms. *J Am Soc Echocardiogr* 1989;2:358–67.

49. Oh JK, Gibbons RJ, Christian TF, et al. Correlation of regional wall motion abnormalities detected by two-dimensional echocardiography with perfusion defect determined by technetium 99m sestamibi imaging in patients treated with reperfusion therapy during acute myocardial infarction. *Am Heart J* 1996;131:32–7.

50. Wahr DW, Wang YS, Schiller NB. Left ventricular volumes determined by two-dimensional echocardiography in a normal adult population. *J Am Coll Cardiol* 1983;1:863–8.

51. Gordon EP, Schnittger I, Fitzgerald PJ, et al. Reproducibility of left ventricular volumes by two-dimensional echocardiography. *J Am Coll Cardiol* 1983;2:506–13.

52. Shiina A, Tajik AJ, Smith HC, et al. Prognostic significance of regional wall motion abnormality in patients with prior myocardial infarction: a prospective correlative study of two-dimensional echocardiography and angiography. *Mayo Clin Proc* 1986;61:254–62.

53. Christie J, Sheldahl LM, Tristani FE et al. Determination of stroke volume and cardiac output during exercise: comparison of two-dimensional and Doppler echocardiography, fick oximetry and thermodilution. *Circulation* 1987;76:539–47.

54. Dittmann H, Voelker W, Karsch K et al. Influence of sampling site and flow area on cardiac output measurements by Doppler echocardiography. *J Am Coll Cardiol* 1987;10:818–23.

55. Nicolosi GL, Pungercic E, Cervesato E, et al. Feasibility and variability of six methods for echocardiographic and Doppler determination of cardiac output. *Br Heart J* 1988;59:299–303.

56. Chen C, Rodriquez L, Lethor J et al. Continuous wave Doppler echocardiography for noninvasive assessment of left ventricular dP/dt and relation time constant from mitral regurgitant spectra in patients. *J Am Coll Cardiol* 1994;23:970–6.

57. Pai RG, Bansal RC, Shah PM. Doppler derived rate of left ventricular pressure rise: its correlation with the postoperative left ventricular function in mitral regurgitation. *Circulation* 1990;82:514–20.

58. Bednarz JE, Marcus RH, Lang RM. Technical guidelines for performing automated border detection studies. *J Am Soc Echocardiogr* 1995;8:293–305.

59. Vandenberg BF, Rath LS, Stuhlmuller P, et al. Estimation of left ventricular cavity area with an on-line, semiautomated echocardiographic edge detection system. *Circulation* 1992;86:159–66.

60. Stewart WJ, Rodkey SM, Gunawardena S, et al. Left ventricular volume calculation with integrated backscatter from echocardiography. *J Am Soc Echocardiogr* 1993;6:553–63.

61. Antonini-Canterin F, Pavan D, Nicolosi GL. Echocardiographic evaluation of the volumes and global systolic function of the left ventricle. *Ital Heart J* 2000;1(Suppl 10):1261–72.

62. Clarkson PB, Wheldon NM, Lim PO, et al. Left atrial size and function: assessment using echocardiographic automatic boundary detection. *Br Heart J* 1995;74:664–70.

63. Tighe DA, James JP, Pohl CA, Cook JR, Huhta JC. Automatic border detection for assessment of left ventricular diastolic function among normal neonates: Comparison with Doppler. *Echocardiography* 1998;15:545–52.

64. Moidl R, Chevtchik O, Simon P, et al. Noninvasive monitoring of peak filling rate with acoustic quantification echocardiography accurately detects acute cardiac allograft rejection. *J Heart Lung Transplant* 1999;18:194–201.

65. Lang RM, Vignon P, Weinert L, et al. Echocardiographic quantification of regional left ventricular wall motion with color kinesis. *Circulation* 1996;93:1877–85.

66. Lau YS, Puryear JV, Gan SC, et al. Assessment of left ventricular wall motion abnormalities with the use of color kinesis: a valuable visual and training aid. *J Am Soc Echocardiogr* 1997;10:665–72.

67. Hartmann T, Kolev N, Blaicher A, et al. Validity of acoustic quantification colour kinesis for detection of left ventricular regional wall motion abnormalities: a transesophageal echocardiographic study. *Br J Anaesth* 1997;79:482–7.

68. Vitarelli A, Sciomer S, Penco M, et al. Assessment of left ventricular dysynergy by color kinesis. *Am J Cardiol* 1998;81:86G–90G.

69. Vitarelli A, Sciomer S, Schina M, Luzzi MF, Dagianti A. Detection of left ventricular systolic and diastolic abnormalities in patients with coronary artery disease by color kinesis. *Clin Cardiol* 1997;20:927–33.

70. Lang RM, Vignon P, Weinert L, et al. Echocardiographic quantification of regional left ventricular wall motion with color kinesis. *Circulation* 1996;93:1877–85.

71. Santoro F, Tramarin R, Colombo E, et al. Evaluation of regional left ventricular wall motion with color kinesis: comparison with two-dimensional echocardiography in patients after acute myocardial infarction. *G Ital Cardiol* 1998;28:984–95.

72. Vandenberg BF, Lindower PD, Lewis J, Burns TL. Reproducibility of left ventricular measurements with acoustic quantification: the influence of training. *Echocardiography* 2000;17:631–7.

73. Spencer KT, Mor-Avi V, Gorcsan J 3rd, et al. Effects of aging on left atrial reservoir, conduit, and booster pump function: a multi-institution acoustic quantification study. *Heart* 2001;85:272–7.

74. Mor-Avi V, Vignon P, Bales AC, et al. Acoustic quantification indexes of left ventricular size and function: effects of signal averaging. *J Am Soc Echocardiogr* 1998;11:792–802.

75. Greim CA, Roewer N, Laux G, et al. On-line estimation of left ventricular stroke volume using transesophageal echocardiography and acoustic quantification. *Br J Anaesth* 1996;77:365–9.

76. Seliem MA, McWilliams ET, Palileo M. Beat-to-beat variability of left ventricular indexes measured by acoustic quantification: influence of heart rate and respiration—correlation with M-mode echocardiography. *J Am Soc Echocardiogr* 1996;9:221–30.

77. Spencer KT, Mor-Avi V, Weinert L, et al. Age dependency of left atrial and left ventricular acoustic quantification waveforms for the evaluation of diastolic performance in left ventricular hypertrophy. *J Am Soc Echocardiogr* 1998;11:1027–35.

78. Jiang L, Morrissey R, Handschumacher MD, et al. Quantitative three-dimensional reconstruction of left ventricular volume with complete borders detected by acoustic quantification underestimates volume. *Am Heart J* 1996;131:553–9.

79. Yvorchuk KJ, Davies RA, Chan KL. Measurement of left ventricular ejection fraction by acoustic quantification and comparison with radionuclide angiography. *Am J Cardiol* 1994;74:1052–6.

80. Chandra S, Bahl VK, Reddy SC, et al. Comparison of echocardiographic acoustic quantification system and radionuclide ventriculography for estimating left ventricular ejection fraction: validation in patients without regional wall motion abnormalities. *Am Heart J* 1997;133:359–63.

81. Vermes E, Leroy G, Soustelle C, et al. Validation of the measurement of cardiac output by acoustic quantification in patients with severe congestive heart failure. *Arc Mal Coeur Vaiss* 2000;93:1089–95.

82. Tsujita-Kuroda Y, Zhang G, Sumita Y, et al. Validity and reproducibility of echocardiographic measurement of left ventricular ejection fraction by acoustic quantification with tissue harmonic imaging technique. *J Am Soc Echocardiogr* 2000;13:300–5.

83. Hultman J, Palmgren I, Landelius J, Andren B. Transesophageal echocardiography and acoustic quantification in assessing regional left ventricular wall motion. *Acta Anaesthesiol Scand* 1994;38:575–9.

84. Zhang GC, Nakamura K, Tsukada T, et al. Impact of presence of abnormal wall motion on echocardiographic determination of left ventricular function with automated boundary detection technique: re-evaluation. *Int J Card Imaging* 1998;14:253–9.

85. Irwin MG. Ng JK. Transesophageal acoustic quantification for evaluation of cardiac function during laproscopic surgery. *Anaesthesia* 2001;56:623–9.

86. Niimi Y, Ichinose F, Saegusa H, et al. Echocardiographic evaluation of global left ventricular function during high thoracic epidural anesthesia. *J Clin Anesth* 1997;9:118–24.

87. McDicken WN, Sutherland GR, Moran CM, et al. Colour Doppler velocity imaging of the myocardium. *Ultrasound Med Biol* 1992;18:651–4.

88. Miyatake K, Ymagishi M, Tanaka N, et al. New method for evaluating left ventricular wall motion by color-coded tissue Doppler imaging: in vitro and in vivo studies. *J Am Coll Cardiol* 1995;25:717–24.

89. Kitabatake A, Inoue M, Asao M, et al. Transmitral blood flow reflecting diastolic behavior of the left ventricle in health and disease—a study by pulsed Doppler technique. *Jpn Circ J* 1982;46:92–102.

90. Appleton CP, Hatle LK, Popp RL. Relation of transmitral flow velocity patterns to left ventricular diastolic function: new insights from a combined hemodynamic and Doppler echocardiographic study. *J Am Coll Cardiol* 1988;12:426–40.

91. Oh JK, Appleton CP, Hatle LK, et al. The noninvasive assessment of left ventricular diastolic function with two-dimensional and Doppler echocardiography. *J Am Soc Echocardiogr* 1997;10:246–70.

92. Quinones MA, Otto CM, Stoddard M, et al. Recommendations for quantification of Doppler echocardiography: A report from the Doppler Quantification Task Force of the Nomenclature and Standards Committee of the American Society of Echocardiography. *J Am Soc Echocardiogr* 2002;15:167–84.

93. Appleton CP, Hatle LK. The natural history of left ventricular filling abnormalities: assessment by two-dimensional and Doppler echocardiography. *Echocardiography* 1992;9:437.

94. Courtois C, Kovacs SJ, Ludbrook PA. Transmitral pressure-flow velocity relation: Importance of regional pressure gradients in the left ventricle during diastole. *Circulation* 1988;78:661–71.

95. Klein Al, Burstow DJ, Tajik AJ, et al. Effects of age on left ventricular dimensions and filling dynamics in 117 normal persons. *Mayo Clin Proc* 1994;69:212–24.

96. Yamamoto K, Nishimura RA, Burnett JC Jr, Redfield MM. Assessment of left ventricular end-diastolic pressure by Doppler echocardiography: contribution of duration of pulmonary venous versus mitral flow velocity curves at atrial contraction. *J Am Soc Echocardiogr* 1997;10:52–9.

97. Pai RG, Suzuki M, Heywood JT, et al. Mitral A wave velocity wave transit time to the outflow tract as a measure of left ventricular diastolic stiffness. *Circulation* 1994;89:553–7.

98. Pai RG, Shah PM. A new Doppler index of left ventricular stiffness based on the principles of flow wave propagation: Mathematical basis and review of the method. *J Heart Valve Dis* 1993;2:167–73.

99. Nishimura RA, Schwartz RS, Holmes DR Jr, Tajik AJ. Failure of calcium channel blockers to improve ventricular relaxation in humans. *J Am Coll Cardiol* 1993;21:182–8.

100. Thomas JD, Newell JB, Choong CYP, Weyman AE. Physical and physiological determinants of transmitral velocity: Numerical analysis. *Am J Physiol* 1991;260:H1718–31.

101. Choong CY, Herrmann HC, Weyman AE, Fifer MA. Preload dependence of Doppler-derived indexes of left ventricular diastolic function in humans. *J Am Coll Cardiol* 1987;10:800–8.

102. Thomas JD, Choong CYP, Flachskampf FA, Weyman AE. Analysis of the early transmitral Doppler velocity curve: Effect of primary physiologic changes and compensatory preload adjustment. *J Am Coll Cardiol* 1990;16:644–55.

103. Appleton CP, Galloway JM, Gonzalez MS, et al. Estimation of left ventricular filling pressures using two-dimensional and Doppler echocardiography in adult patients with cardiac disease. *J Am Coll Cardiol* 1993;22:1972–82.

104. Pearson AC, Labovitz AJ, Mrosek D, et al. Assessment of diastolic function in normal and hypertrophied hearts: Comparison of Doppler and M-mode echocardiography. *Am Heart J* 1987;113:1417–25.

105. Frais MA, Bergman DW, Kingma I, et al. The dependence of the time constant of left ventricular isovolumic relaxation on pericardial pressure. *Circulation* 1990;81:1071–80.

106. Rousseau MF, Pouleur H, Detry JMR, et al. Relationship between changes in left ventricular inotropic state and relaxation in normal subjects and patients with coronary disease. *Circulation* 1981;64:736–43.

107. Craig WE, Murgo JP. Evaluation of isovolumic relaxation in normal man during rest, exercise and isoproterenol infusion. *Circulation* 1980;62(Suppl III):III-22.

108. Nishimura RA, Abel MD, Hatle LK, Tajik AJ. Relation of pulmonary vein to mitral flow velocities by transesophageal Doppler echocardiography. *Circulation* 1990;81:1488–97.

109. Rossvoll O, Hatle LK. Pulmonary venous flow velocities recorded by transthoracic Doppler ultrasound: relation to left ventricular diastolic pressures. *J Am Coll Cardiol* 1993;21:1687–96.

110. Masuyama T, Lee JM, Yamamoto K, et al. Analysis of pulmonary venous flow velocity pattern as assessed with transthoracic pulsed Doppler echocardiography in subjects without cardiac disease. *Am J Cardiol* 1991;67:1396–404.

111. Klein AL, Tajik AJ. Doppler assessment of pulmonary venous flow in healthy subjects and in patients with heart disease. *J Am Soc Echocardiogr* 1991;4:379–92.

112. Keren G, Meisner JS, Sherez J, et al. Interrelationship of middiastolic mitral valve motion, pulmonary venous flow, and transmitral flow. *Circulation* 1986;74:36–44.

113. Chen YT, Kan MN, Lee AYS, et al. Pulmonary venous flow: Its relationship to left atrial and mitral valve motion. *J Am Soc Echocardiogr* 1993;6:387–94.

114. Oki T, Tabata T, Yamada H, et al. Assessment of abnormal left atrial relaxation by transesophageal pulsed Doppler echocardiography of pulmonary venous flow velocity. *Clin Cardiol* 1998;21:753–8.

115. Sutherland GR, Stewart MJ, Groundstroem KWE, et al. Color Doppler myocardial imaging: a new technique for the assessment of myocardial function. *J Am Soc Echocardiogr* 1994;7:441–58.

116. Gorcsan J III, Gulati VK, Mandarino WA, Katz WE. Color-coded measures of myocardial velocity throughout the cardiac cycle by tissue Doppler imaging to quantify regional left ventricular function. *Am Heart J* 1996;131:1203–13.

117. Wilkenshoff UM, Hatle L, Sovany A, et al. Age-dependent changes in regional diastolic function evaluated by color Doppler myocardial imaging: A comparison with pulsed Doppler indexes of global function. *J Am Soc Echocardiogr* 2001;14:959–69.

118. Nagueh SF, Middleton KJ, Kopelen HA, et al. Doppler tissue imaging: a noninvasive technique for evaluation of left ventricular relaxation and estimation of filling pressures. *J Am Coll Cardiol* 1997;30:1527–33.

119. Oki T, Tabata T, Yamada H, et al. Clinical application of pulsed Doppler tissue imaging for assessing abnormal left ventricular relaxation. *Am J Cardiol* 1997;79:921–8.

120. Pai RG, Gill KS. Amplitudes, durations and timings of apically directed left ventricular myocardial velocities: I. Their normal pattern and coupling to ventricular filling and ejection. *J Am Soc Echocardiogr* 1998;11:105–11.

121. Garcia MJ, Rodriquez L, Ares M, et al. Myocardial wall velocity assessment by pulsed Doppler tissue imaging: characteristic findings in normal subjects. *Am Heart J* 1996;132:648–56.

122. Waggoner AD, Bierig SM. Tissue Doppler imaging: A useful echocardiographic; method for the sonographer to assess systolic and diastolic ventricular function. *J Am Soc Echocardiogr* 2001;14:1143–52.

123. Naqvi TZ, Neyman G, Broyde A, et al. Comparison of myocardial tissue Doppler with transmitral flow Doppler in left ventricular hypertrophy. *J Am Soc Echocardiogr* 2001;14:1153–60.

124. Sohn DW, Chai IH, Lee DJ, et al. Assessment of mitral annulus velocity by Doppler tissue imaging in the evaluation of left ventricular diastolic function. *J Am Coll Cardiol* 1997;30:474–80.

125. Dagdelen S, Eren N, Karabulut H, et al. Estimation of left ventricular end-diastolic pressure by color M-mode Doppler echocardiography and tissue Doppler imaging. *J Am Soc Echocardiogr* 2001;14:951–8.

126. Pai RG, Yoganathan AP, Toomes C, et al. Mitral E wave propagation as an index of left ventricular diastolic function. I: Its hydrodynamic basis. *J Heart Valve Dis* 1998;7:438–44.

127. Brun P, Tribouilloy C, Duval AM, et al. Left ventricular flow propagation during early filling is related to wall relaxation: a color M-mode Doppler analysis. *J Am Coll Cardiol* 1992;20:420–32.

128. Takatsuji H, Mikami T, Urasawa K, et al. A new approach for evaluation of left ventricular diastolic function: spatial and temporal analysis of left ventricular filling flow propagation by color M-mode Doppler echocardiography. *J Am Coll Cardiol* 1996;27:365–71.

129. Voon WC, Huang CH, Sheu SH. Role of intraventricular dispersion of early diastolic filling in indicating left ventricular diastolic dysfunction: assessment by color M-mode inflow propagation velocity. *Cardiology* 2001;95:151–5.

130. Garcia MJ, Palac RT, Malenka DJ, et al. Color M-mode Doppler flow propagation velocity is a relatively preload-independent index of left ventricular filling. *J Am Soc Echocardiogr* 1999;12:129 37.

131. Garcia MJ, Smedira NG, Greenberg NL, et al. Color M-mode Doppler flow propagation velocity is a preload insensitive index of left ventricular relaxation: animal and human validation. *J Am Coll Cardiol* 2000;35:201–8.

132. Moller JE, Poulsen SH, Sondergaard E, Egstrup K. Preload dependence of color M-mode Doppler flow propagation velocity in controls and in patients with left ventricular dysfunction. *J Am Soc Echocardiogr* 2000;13:902–9.

133. Garcia MJ, Ares MA, Asher C, et al. An index of early left ventricular filling that combined with pulsed Doppler peak E velocity may estimate capillary wedge pressure. *J Am Coll Cardiol* 1997;29:448–54.

134. Gonzalez-Vilchez F, Ares M, Ayuela J, Alonso L. Combined use of pulsed and color M-mode Doppler echocardiography for the estimation of pulmonary capillary wedge pressure: an empirical approach based on an analytical relation. *J Am Coll Cardiol* 1999;34:515–23.

135. Moller JE, Sondergaard E, Poulsen SH, Egstrup K. Pseudonormal and restrictive filling patterns predict left ventricular dilation and cardiac death after a first myocardial infarction: a

serial color M-mode Doppler echocardiographic study. *J Am Coll Cardiol* 2000;36:1841–6.

136. Peels CH, Visser CA, Kupper AJ, et al. Usefulness of two-dimensional echocardiography for immediate detection of ischemia in the emergency room. *Am J Cardiol* 1990;65:687–91.

137. Sabia P, Afrooktch A, Touschstone DA, et al. Value of regional wall motion abnormality in the emergency room diagnosis of acute myocardial infarction. *Circulation* 1991;84:I-85–92.

138. Oh JK, Miller FA, Shub C, et al. Evaluation of acute chest pain syndromes by two-dimensional echocardiography: its potential application in the selection of patients for acute reperfusion therapy. *Mayo Clin Proc* 1987;62:59–66.

139. Launbjerg J, Berning J, Fruergaard P, et al. Sensitivity and specificity of echocardiographic identification of patients eligible for safe early discharge after myocardial infarction. *Am Heart J* 1992;124:846–53.

140. Horowitz RS, Morganroth J. Immediate detection of early high-risk patients with acute myocardial infarction using two-dimensional echocardiographic evaluation of left ventricular regional wall motion abnormalities. *Am Heart J* 1982;103:814–22.

141. St John Sutton M, Pfeffer MA, Plappert T, et al. Quantitative two-dimensional echocardiographic measurements are major predictors of adverse cardiovascular events after myocardial infarction. *Circulation* 1994;89:68–75.

142. Reeder GS. Identification and treatment of complications of myocardial infarction. *Mayo Clin Proc* 1995;70:880–4.

143. Iga K, Konishi T, Kusukawa R. Intracardiac thrombi in both the right atrium and right ventricle after acute inferior-wall infarction. *Int J Cardiol* 1994;46:169–71.

144. Vargas-Barron J, Romero-Cardenas A, Keirns C, et al. Transesophageal echocardiography and right atrial infarction. *J Am Soc Echocardiogr* 1993;6:543–7.

145. Hilton TC, Pearson AC, Serota H, et al. Right atrial infarction and cardiogenic shock complicating acute myocardial infarction: diagnosis by transesophageal echocardiography. *Am Heart J* 1990;120:427–30.

146. Behnam R, Walter S, Hanes V. Myocardial abscess complicating myocardial infarction. *J Am Soc Echocardiogr* 1995;8:334–7.

147. Haley JH, Sinak LJ, Tajik AJ, et al. Dynamic left ventricular outflow tract obstruction in acute coronary syndromes: an important cause of new systolic murmur and cardiogenic shock. *Mayo Clin Proc* 1999;74:901–6.

148. Patel AM, Miller FA Jr, Khandheria BK, et al. Role of transesophageal echocardiography in the diagnosis of papillary muscle rupture secondary to myocardial infarction. *Am Heart J* 1989;118:1330–3.

149. Chirillo F, Totis O, Cavarzerani A, et al. Transesophageal echocardiographic findings in partial and complete papillary muscle rupture complicating acute myocardial infarction. *Cardiology* 1992;81:54–8.

150. Assi ER, Tak T. Posterior myocardial infarction complicated by rupture of the posteromedial papillary muscle. *J Heart Valve Dis* 1999;8:565–6.

151. Manning WJ, Waksmonski CA, Boyle NG. Papillary muscle rupture complicating inferior myocardial infarction: identification with transesophageal echocardiography. *Am Heart J* 1995;129:191–3.

152. Kozlowski CM, Dorogy ME. Transesophageal echocardiography and concurrent coronary angiography for the rapid assessment of papillary muscle rupture. *Echocardiography* 1994;11:47–50.

153. Kranidis A, Koulouris S, Filippatos G, et al. Mitral regurgitation from papillary muscle rupture: role of transesophageal echocardiography. *J Heart Valve Dis* 1993;2:529–32.

154. Zotz RJ, Dohmen G, Genth S, et al. Diagnosis of papillary muscle rupture after acute myocardial infarction by transthoracic and transesophageal echocardiography. *Clin Cardiol* 1993;16:665–70.

155. Herrera CJ, Gurevicius J, Stecy P, et al. The clinical utility of transesophageal echocardiography in ischemic papillary muscle rupture. *Am J Card Imaging* 1995;9:226–8.

156. Akasaka K, Kawashima E, Yamazaki S, et al. Partial rupture progressing to complete rupture of the left ventricular anterior papillary muscle after acute myocardial infarction: a case report. *J Cardiol* 1996;28:349–54.

157. Christ G, Siostrzonek P, Maurer G, Baumgartner H. Partial papillary muscle rupture complicating acute myocardial infarction. diagnosis by multiplane transesophageal echocardiography. *Eur Heart J* 1995;16:1736–8.

158. Singh A, Breisblatt W, Cutrone M, et al. Transesophageal echocardiography as an important tool in the diagnosis of postinfarction papillary muscle rupture. *Cardiology* 1995;86:417–20.

159. Maeta H, Imawaki S, Shiraishi Y, et al. Repair of both papillary and free wall rupture following acute myocardial infarction. *J Cardiovasc Surg* 1991;32:828–32.

160. Pollak H, Dietz W, Speil R, et al. Early diagnosis of subacute free wall rupture complicating acute myocardial infarction. *Eur Hear J* 1993;14:640–8.

161. Pollak H, Nobis H, Miczocj J. Frequency of left ventricular free wall rupture complicating acute myocardial infarction since the advent of thrombolysis. *Am J Cardiol* 1994;74:184–6.

162. Fein SA, Vargas M. Transesophageal echocardiographic diagnosis of cardiac rupture. *J Am Soc Echocardiogr* 1991;4:415–16.

163. Deshmukh HG, Khosla S, Jefferson KK. Direct visualization of left ventricular free wall rupture by transesophageal echocardiography in acute myocardial infarction. *Am Heart J* 1993;126:475–7.

164. Lopez-Sendon J, Gonzalez A, Lopez E, et al. Diagnosis of subacute ventricular wall rupture after acute myocardial infarction: sensitivity and specificity of clinical, hemodynamic and echocardiographic criteria. *J Am Coll Cardiol* 1992;19:1145–53.

165. Ballal R, Sanyal RS, Nanda NC, Mahan EF. Usefulness of transesophageal echocardiography in the diagnosis of ventricular septal rupture secondary to acute myocardial infarction. *Am J Cardiol* 1993;71:367–70.

166. Zotz RJ, Dohmen G, Genth S, et al. Transthoracic and transesophageal echocardiography to diagnose ventricular septal rupture: importance of right heart infarction. *Coron Artery Dis* 1993;4:911–17.

167. Harpaz D, Shah P, Bezante GP, Meltzer RS. Ventricular septal rupture after myocardial infarction. Detection by transesophageal echocardiography. *Chest* 1993;103:1884–5.

168. Ballal RS, Sanyal RS, Nanda NC, Mahan EF 3rd. Usefulness of transesophageal echocardiography in the diagnosis of ventricular septal rupture secondary to acute myocardial infarction. *Am J Cardiol* 1993;71:367–70.

169. Topaz O, Taylor AL. Interventricular septal rupture complicating acute myocardial infarction: from pathophysiologic features to the role of invasive and noninvasive diagnostic modalities in current management. *Am J Med* 1992;93:683–8.

170. Koenig K, Kasper W, Hofmann T, et al. Transesophageal echocardiography for diagnosis of rupture of the ventricular septum or left ventricular papillary muscle during acute myocardial infarction. *Am J Cardiol* 1987;59:362.

171. Alvarez JM, Brady PW, Ross DE. Technical improvements in the repair of acute postinfarction ventricular septal rupture. *J Card Surg* 1992;7:198–202.

172. Nanda NC, Gatewood RD. Differentiation of left ventricular pseudoaneurysm from true aneurysms by two-dimensional echocardiography. *Circulation* 1979;60:II144.

173. Sutherland GR, Smylie JH, Roelandt JRT. Advantages of colour flow imaging in the diagnosis of left ventricular pseudoaneurysm. *Br Heart J* 1989;61:59–64.

174. Yvorra S, Desfossez L, Panagides D, et al. False pseudoaneurysm of the left ventricle after myocardial infarction. Recognition by transesophageal echocardiography. *Arch Mal Coeur Vaiss* 1994;87:395–8.

175. Esakof DD, Vannan MA, Pandian NG, et al. Visualization of left ventricular pseudoaneurysm with panoramic transesophageal echocardiography. *J Am Soc Echocardiogr* 1994;7:174–8.

176. Halphen C, Bical O, Haiat R, et al. False aneurysm of the left ventricle during the acute phase of myocardial infarction: diagnosis by transesophageal echocardiography. *Ann Cardiol Angeiol* 1992;41:391–4.

177. Stoddard MF, Dawkins PR, Longaker RA, et al. Transesophageal echocardiography in the detection of left ventricular pseudoaneurysm. *Am Heart J* 1993;125:534–9.

178. Corya B, Feigenbaum H, Rasmussen S, Black MJ. Echocardiographic features of congestive cardiomyopathy compared with normal subjects and patients with coronary artery disease. *Circulation* 1974;49:1153–9.

179. Wallis DE, O'Connell JB, Henkin RE, et al. Segmental wall motion abnormalities in dilated cardiomyopathy: a common finding and good prognostic sign. *J Am Coll Cardiol* 1984;4:674–9.

180. Siostrzonek P, Koppensteiner R, Gossinger H, et al. Hemodynamic and hemorheologic determinants of left atrial spontaneous echo contrast and thrombus formation in patients with idiopathic dilated cardiomyopathy. *Am Heart J* 1993;125:430–4.

181. Shen WF, Tribouilloy C, Rida Z, et al. Clinical significance of intracavitary spontaneous echo contrast in patients with dilated cardiomyopathy. *Cardiology* 1996;87:141–6.

182. Vigna C, Russo A, De Rito V, et al. Frequency of left atrial thrombi by transesophageal echocardiography in idiopathic and in ischemic dilated cardiomyopathy. *Am J Cardiol* 1992;170:1500–1.

183. Tsai LM, Chen JH, Tsao CJ. Relation of left atrial spontaneous echo contrast with prethrombotic state in atrial fibrillation associated with systemic hypertension, idiopathic dilated cardiomyopathy, or no identifiable cause (lone). *Am J Cardiol* 1998;81:1249–52.

184. Chen C, Koschyk D, Hamm C, et al. Usefulness of transesophageal echocardiography in identifying small left ventricular apical thrombus. *J Am Coll Cardiol* 1993;21:208–15.

185. Rihal CS, Nishimura RA, Hatle LK, et al. Systolic and diastolic dysfunction in patients with clinical diagnosis of dilated cardiomyopathy. Relation to symptoms and prognosis. *Circulation* 1994;90:2772–9.

186. Vitarelli A, Luzzi MF, Penco M, et al. PVF velocity pattern in patients with heart failure: transesophageal echocardiographic assessment. *Cardiology* 1997;88:585–94.

187. Ito T, Suwa M, Otake Y, et al. Left ventricular Doppler filling pattern in dilated cardiomyopathy: relation to hemodynamics and left atrial function. *J Am Soc Echocardiogr* 1997;10:518–25.

188. St. Goar FG, Masuyama T, Alderman EL, Popp RL. Left ventricular diastolic dysfunction in end-stage dilated cardiomyopathy: simultaneous Doppler echocardiography and hemodynamic evaluation. *J Am Soc Echocardiogr* 1991;4:349–60.

189. Pinamonti B, Zecchin M, Di Lenarda A, et al. Persistence of restrictive left ventricular filling pattern in dilated cardiomyopathy: an ominous prognostic sign. *J Am Coll Cardiol* 1997;29:604–12.

190. Lee D-C, Oh JK, Osborn SL, et al. Repeat evaluation of diastolic filling pattern after treatment of congestive heart failure in patients with restrictive diastolic filling: Implication for long-term prognosis. *J Am Soc Echocardiogr* 1997;10:431.

191. Abramson SV, Burke JF, Kelly JJ, et al. Pulmonary hypertension predicts mortality and morbidity in patients with dilated cardiomyopathy. *Ann Intern Med* 1992;116:888–95.

192. Fellahi JL, Valtier B, Beauchet A, et al. Does positive end-expiratory pressure ventilation improve left ventricular function? A comparative study by transesophageal echocardiography in cardiac and noncardiac patients. *Chest* 1998;114:556–62.

193. Oki T, Fukuda N, Luchi A, et al. Possible mechanisms of mitral regurgitation in dilated hearts: a study using transesophageal echocardiography. *Clin Cardiol* 1996;19:639–43.

194. Flachskampf FA, Chandra S, Gaddipatti A, et al. Analysis of shape and motion of the mitral annulus in subjects with and without

cardiomyopathy by echocardiographic 3-dimensional reconstruction. *J Am Soc Echocardiogr* 2000;13:277–87.

195. Hamilton MA, Stevenson LW, Child JS et al. Sustained reduction in valvular regurgitation and atrial volumes with tailored vasodilator therapy in advanced congestive heart failure secondary to dilated (ischemic or idiopathic) cardiomyopathy. *Am J Cardiol* 1991;67:259–63.

196. Henry WL, Clark CE, Epstein SE. Asymmetric septal hypertrophy. Echocardiographic identification of the pathognomonic anatomic abnormality of IHSS. *Circulation* 1973;47:225–33.

197. Klues HG, Schiffers A, Maron BJ. Phenotypic spectrum and patterns of left ventricular hypertrophy in hypertrophic cardiomyopathy: morphologic observations and significance as assessed by two-dimensional echocardiography in 600 patients. *J Am Coll Cardiol* 1995;26:1699–708.

198. Swinne C, Shapiro EP, Jamart J, Fleg J. Age associated anatomic and functional changes in left ventricular outflow geometry in normal subjects. *Am J Cardiol* 1996;78:1070–3.

199. Frielingsdorf J, Franke A, Kuhl HP, et al. Evaluation of regional systolic function in hypertrophic cardiomyopathy and hypertensive heart disease: a three-dimensional echocardiographic study. *J Am Soc Echocardiogr* 1998;11:778–86.

200. Posma JL, van der Wall EE, Blanksma PK, et al. New diagnostic options in hypertrophic cardiomyopathy. *Am Heart J* 1996;132:1031–41.

201. Memmola C, Iliceto S, Napoli VF, et al. Coronary flow dynamics and reserve assessed by transesophageal echocardiography in obstructive hypertrophic cardiomyopathy. *Am J Cardiol* 1994;74:1147–51.

202. Jiang L, Levine RA, King ME, et al. An integrated mechanism for systolic anterior motion of the mitral valve in hypertrophic cardiomyopathy based on echocardiographic observations. *Am Heart J* 1987;113:633–44.

203. Klues HG, Roberts WC, Maron BJ. Morphologic determinants of echocardiographic patterns of mitral valve systolic anterior motion in obstructive hypertrophic cardiomyopathy. *Circulation* 1993;87:1570–9.

204. Shah PM, Taylor RD, Wong M. Abnormal mitral valve coaptation in hypertrophic obstructive cardiomyopathy proposed role in systolic anterior motion of the mitral valve. *Am J Cardiol* 1981;48:258–62.

205. Schwammenthal E, Nakatani S, He S, et al. Mechanism of mitral regurgitation in hypertrophic cardiomyopathy: mismatch of posterior to anterior leaflet length and mobility. *Circulation* 1998;98:856–65.

206. Manabe K, Oki T, Fukuda N, Luchi A, Tabata T. Transesophageal echocardiographic study on the mechanisms of mitral regurgitation in hypertrophic cardiomyopathy: comparison with sigmoid septum. *J Cardiol* 1995;26:233–41.

207. Yeo TC, Miller FA Jr, Oh JK, et al. Hypertrophic cardiomyopathy with obstruction: important diagnostic clue provided by the direction of the mitral regurgitation jet. *J Am Soc Echocardiogr* 1998;11:61–5.

208. Oki T, Fukuda N, Luchi A, et al. Transesophageal echocardiographic evaluation of mitral regurgitation in hypertrophic cardiomyopathy: contributions of eccentric left ventricular hypertrophy and related abnormalities of the mitral complex. *J Am Soc Echocardiogr* 1995;8:503–10.

209. Zhu WX, Oh JK, Kopecky SL, et al. Mitral regurgitation due to ruptured chordae tendineae in patients with hypertrophic obstructive cardiomyopathy. *J Am Coll Cardiol* 1992;20:242–7.

210. Sasson Z, Yock PG, Hatle LK, et al. Doppler echocardiographic determination of the pressure gradient in hypertrophic cardiomyopathy, *J Am Coll Cardiol* 1988;11:752–6.

211. Schwammenthal E, Block M, Schwartzkopff B, et al. Prediction of the site and severity of obstruction in hypertrophic cardiomyopathy by color flow mapping and continuous wave Doppler echocardiography. *J Am Coll Cardiol* 1992;20:964–72.

212. Yock PG, Hatle L, Popp RL. Patterns and timing of Doppler detected intracavitary and aortic flow in hypertrophic cardiomyopathy. *J Am Coll Cardiol* 1986;8:1047–58.

213. Panza JA, Petrone RK, Fananapazir L. Utility of continuous wave Doppler echocardiography in the noninvasive assessment of left ventricular outflow tract pressure gradient in patients with hypertrophic cardiomyopathy. *J Am Coll Cardiol* 1992;19:91–9.

214. Nishimura RA, Tajik AJ, Reeder GS, Seward JB. Evaluation of hypertrophic cardiomyopathy by Doppler color flow imaging: initial observations. *Mayo Clin Proc* 1986;61:631–9.

215. Maron BJ, Spirito P, Green KJ, et al. Noninvasive assessment of left ventricular diastolic function by pulsed Doppler echocardiography in patients with hypertrophic cardiomyopathy. *J Am Coll Cardiol* 1987;10:733–42.

216. Nishimura RA, Appleton CP, Redfield MM, et al. Noninvasive Doppler echocardiographic evaluation of left ventricular filling pressures in patients with cardiomyopathies: a simultaneous Doppler echocardiographic and cardiac catheterization study. *J Am Coll Cardiol* 1996;28:1226–33.

217. McCully RB, Nishimura RA, Bailey KR, et al. Hypertrophic obstructive cardiomyopathy: preoperative echocardiographic predictors of outcome after septal myectomy. *J Am Coll Cardiol* 1996;27:1491–6.

218. Grigg LE, Wigle ED, Williams WG, et al. Transesophageal Doppler echocardiography in obstructive hypertrophic cardiomyopathy: Clarification of pathophysiology and importance in intraoperative decision making. *J Am Coll Cardiol* 1992;20:42–52.

219. Marwick TH, Stewart WJ, Lever HM, et al. Benefits of intraoperative echocardiography in the surgical management of hypertrophic cardiomyopathy. *J Am Coll Cardiol* 1992;20:1066–72.

220. Widimsky P, Ten Cate FJ, Vletter W, van Herwerden L. Potential applications for transesophageal echocardiography in hypertrophic cardiomyopathies. *J Am Soc Echocardiogr* 1992;5:163–7.

221. Eng J, Nair UR, Scott PJ, Walker DR. Intraoperative transesophageal echocardiography for hypertrophic cardiomyopathy. *Ann Thorac Surg* 1990;50:513–14.

222. Child JS, Perloff JK. The restrictive cardiomyopathies. *Cardiol Clin* 1988;6:289–316.

223. Siegel RJ, Shah PK, Fishbein MC. Idiopathic restrictive cardiomyopathy. *Circulation* 1984;70:165–9.

224. Garcia-Pascual J, Gonzalez-Gallarza RD, Jimenez MP, et al. Loffler's syndrome: pulmonary vein and transmitral Doppler flow analysis by transesophageal echocardiography—report of a case. *J Am Soc Echocardiogr* 2000;13:690–2.

225. Berensztein CS, Pineiro D, Marcotegui M, et al. Usefulness of echocardiography and Doppler echocardiography in endomyocardial fibrosis. *J Am Soc Echocardiogr* 2000;13:385–92.

226. Brooker RF, Farah MG. Postoperative left atrial compression diagnosed by transesophageal echocardiography. *J Cardiothorac Vasc Anesth* 1995;9:304–7.

227. Appleton CP, Hatle LK, Popp RL. Demonstration of restrictive ventricular physiology by Doppler echocardiography. *J Am Coll Cardiol* 1988;11:757–68.

228. Little WC, Ohno M, Kitzman DW, et al. Determination of left ventricular chamber stiffness from the time for deceleration of early left ventricular filling. *Circulation* 1995;92:1933–9.

229. Klein AL, Canale MP, Rajagopalan N, et al. Role of transesophageal echocardiography in assessing diastolic dysfunction in a large clinical practice: a 9-year experience. *Am Heart J* 1999;138:880–9.

230. Cueto-Garcia L, Reeder GS, Kyle RA, et al. Echocardiographic findings in systemic amyloidosis. Spectrum of cardiac involvement and relation to survival. *J Am Coll Cardiol* 1985;6:737–43.

231. Holt JP. The normal pericardium. *Am J Cardiol* 1970;26:455–65.

232. Spodick DH. The pericardium: structure, function and disease spectrum. In *Pericardial Diseases. Cardiovascular Clinics*. DH Spodick ed. Philadelphia FA Davis Co. 1976.

233. Feigenbaum H, Waldhausen JA, Hyde LP. Ultrasound diagnosis of pericardial effusion. *JAMA* 1965;191:107.

234. Tajik AJ. Echocardiography in pericardial effusion. *Am J Med* 1977;63:29–40.

235. Lemire F, Tajik AJ, Giuliani ER, et al. Further echocardiographic observations in pericardial effusion. *Mayo Clin Proc* 1976;51:13–18.

236. Kronzon I, Tunick PA, Freedberg RS. Transesophageal echocardiography in pericardial disease and tamponade. *Echocardiography* 1994;11:493–505.

237. Simpson IA, Munsch C, Smith EEJ, et al. Pericardial haemorrhage causing right atrial compression after cardiac surgery: Role of transesophageal echocardiography. *Br Heart J* 1991;65:355–6.

238. Torelli J, Marwick TH, Salcedo EE, et al. Left atrial tamponade: Diagnosis by transesophageal echocardiography. *J Am Soc Echocardiogr* 1991;4:413–14.

239. Beppu S, Ikegami K, Tanaka N, et al. Cardiac tamponade as a complication of open heart surgery: The clinical significance and diagnostic value of transesophageal echocardiography. *J Cardiol* 1991;21:125–32.

240. Kochar GS, Jacobs LE, Kotler MN. Right atrial compression in postoperative cardiac patients: detection by transesophageal echocardiography. *J Am Coll Cardiol* 1990;16:511–16.

241. D'Cruz IA, Macander PJ, Gross CM, Pai GM. Distention of the oblique pericardial sinus in tamponade due to loculated posterior pericardial effusion. *Am J Cardiol* 1990;65:1520–1.

242. Rosenzweig BP, Stern A, Kronzon I. Transesophageal echocardiography in a case of cardiac compression: was it therapeutic?. *J Am Soc Echocardiogr* 1998;11:494–6.

243. Jadhav P, Asirvatham S, Craven P, et al. Unusual presentation of late regional cardiac tamponade after aortic surgery. *Am J Cardiac Imaging* 1996;10:204–6.

244. Armstrong WF, Bach DS, Carey L, et al. Spectrum of acute dissection of the ascending aorta: a transesophageal echocardiographic study. *J Am Soc Echocardiogr* 1996;9:646–56.

245. LiMandri G, Gorenstein LA, Starr JP, et al. Use of transesophageal echocardiography in the detection and consequences of an intracardiac bullet. *Am J Emerg Med* 1994;12:105–6.

246. Berge KH, Lanier WL, Reeder GS. Occult cardiac tamponade detected by transesophageal echocardiography. *Mayo Clin Proc* 1992;67:667–70.

247. Mitchell MM. Detection of occult hemopericardium using intraoperative transesophageal echocardiography. *Anesthesiology* 1992;76:145–7.

248. Torelli J, Marwick TH, Salcedo EE. Left atrial tamponade: diagnosis by transesophageal echocardiography. *J Am Soc Echocardiogr* 1991;4:413–14.

249. Shapiro MJ, Yanofsky SD, Trapp J, et al. Cardiovascular evaluation in blunt thoracic trauma using transesophageal echocardiography (TEE). *J Trauma* 1991;31:835–9.

250. Delgado C, Duran RM, Serra E, Barturen F. Left ventricular pseudoaneurysm with left atrium tamponade: a rare postinfarction complication. *J Am Soc Echocardiogr* 1997;10:582–7.

251. Appleton CP, Hatle LK, Popp RL. Cardiac tamponade and pericardial effusion: respiratory variation in transvalvular flow velocities studied by Doppler echocardiography. *J Am Coll Cardiol* 1988;11:1020–30.

252. Burstow DJ, Oh JK, Bailey KR, et al. Cardiac tamponade: Characteristic Doppler observations. *Mayo Clin Proc* 1989;64:312–24.

253. White PD. Chronic constrictive pericarditis (Pick's disease). Treated by pericardial resection. *Lancet* 1935;2:539.

254. Wood P. Chronic constrictive pericarditis. *Am J Cardiol* 1961;7:48.

255. Hutchison SJ, Smalling RG, Albornoz M, et al. Comparison of transthoracic and transesophageal echocardiography in clinically overt or suspected pericardial heart disease. *Am J Cardiol* 1994;74:962–5.

256. Ling LH, Oh JK, Tei C, et al. Pericardial thickness measured with transesophageal echocardiography: feasibility and potential clinical usefulness. *J Am Coll Cardiol* 1997;29:1317–23.

257. Gibson TC, Grossman W, McLaurin LP, et al. An echocardiographic study of the interventricular septum in constrictive pericarditis. *Br Heart J* 1976;38:738–43.

258. Candell-Riera J, Garcia del Castillo H, et al. Echocardiographic features of the interventricular septum in chronic constrictive pericarditis. *Circulation* 1978;57:1154–8.

259. Oh JK, Hatle LK, Seward JB, et al. Diagnostic role of Doppler echocardiography in constrictive pericarditis. *J Am Coll Cardiol* 1994;23:154–62.

260. Oh JK, Tajik AJ, Appleton CP, et al. Preload reduction to unmask the characteristic Doppler features of constrictive pericarditis: a new observation. *Circulation* 1997;95:796–9.

261. Sun JP, Abdalla IA, Yang XS, et al. Respiratory variation of mitral and pulmonary venous Doppler flow velocities in constrictive pericarditis before and after pericardiectomy. *J Am Soc Echocardiogr* 2001;14:1119–26.

262. Shapira OM, Connelley GP, Aldea GS, Shemin RJ. Pulmonary venous flow in constrictive pericarditis. *Clin Cardiol* 1995;18:231–3.

263. Hatle LK, Appleton CP, Popp RL. Differentiation of constrictive pericarditis and restrictive cardiomyopathy by Doppler echocardiography. *Circulation* 1989;79:357–70.

264. Klein AL, Cohen GI, Pietrolungo JF, et al. Differentiation of constrictive pericarditis from restrictive cardiomyopathy by Doppler transesophageal echocardiographic measurements of respiratory variations in pulmonary venous flow. *J Am Coll Cardiol* 1993;22:1935–43.

265. Rajagopalan N, Garcia MJ, Rodriguez L, et al. Comparison of new Doppler echocardiographic methods to differentiate constrictive pericardial heart disease and restrictive cardiomyopathy. *Am J Cardiol* 2001;87:86–94.

266. Garcia MJ, Rodriquez L, Ares M, et al. Differentiation of constrictive pericarditis from restrictive cardiomyopathy: assessment of left ventricular diastolic velocities in longitudinal axis by Doppler tissue imaging. *J Am Coll Cardiol* 1996;27:108–14.

7

Prosthetic heart valves

The prosthetic heart valve has played a large role in clinical cardiology over the past 30 years. In many instances prosthetic heart valve replacement represents the last stage of the natural history for cardiac valvular heart disease, and has dramatically improved the lives of many patients. Unfortunately, prosthetic valves are far from perfect, have a limited lifespan and may introduce a different set of problems for the cardiac patient, i.e. substituting one disease process for another.

The ideal artificial heart valve should permit the unimpeded flow of blood from cardiac chamber to chamber, restore near normal hemodynamics and offer the best chance for regression or remodeling from the effects of the primary valvular disease. In addition the ideal prosthetic valves need to be durable and non-thrombogenic. Since the 1950s many prosthetic valves have been introduced in order to overcome the inadequacies of previously designed valve models[1,2] (Figure 7.1). Flaws in performance or in structural integrity have eliminated many former valve designs and new models have been introduced that include refinements to some of the previously successful valves.[3] Trends in surgical management have also changed from routine replacement to valve repair. Prosthetic heart valves require routine evaluation of the physiological function and detection of structural malfunction.

In the past, the non-invasive evaluation of prosthetic valves has included phonocardiography, cinefluoroscopy, and ultrasound. Transthoracic echocardiography has been the routine evaluation of prosthetic heart valves, despite the limitations due to their non-biological components.[4–6] Multiplane transesophageal echocardiography, with its better resolution and ability to provide multiple imaging planes has greatly enhanced the evaluation of prosthetic heart valves.[7–10] However the transesophageal echocardiographic evaluation

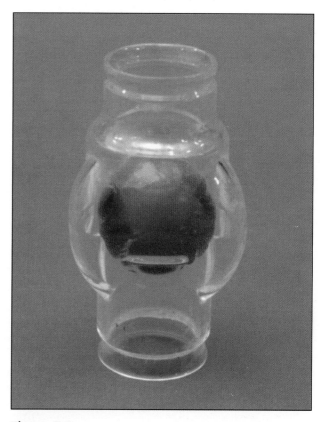

Figure 7.1
Hufnagel caged-ball valve. One of the earliest prosthetic valves of the 1950s implanted in humans; this valve incorporated the bottle stopper principle. The valve consisted of a Lucite tube and a mobile spherical poppet and was sewn into the descending thoracic aorta by a fixation ring in patients with severe aortic regurgitation. With the success of this prosthesis and the development of total cardiopulmonary bypass for intracardiac surgery, the development of prosthetic valves flourished.

of prosthetic valves is often quite a challenging task. In most instances transesophageal echocardiography is performed when the transthoracic study is inconclusive and/or malfunction of the prosthesis is suspected. An accurate diagnosis is important since in most cases mechanical prosthetic valve malfunction can be catastrophic, and re-operation has a significantly higher mortality and morbidity than the initial valve surgery.

To simplify the transesophageal echocardiographic examination it is helpful for the echocardiographer to have a working knowledge of the different prosthetic valve types and their echocardiographic appearances. Prior to performing the transesophageal examination it is important to know the type of prosthetic valve, date of implant, model number if available and anticoagulation status.[11] Most prosthetic valves have specific echocardiographic and structural characteristics, which may differ in the semilunar from the atrioventricular position. In our experience, due to the inherent problems unique to individual types and models of each prosthetic valve, the length of the transesophageal echocardiographic examination is dramatically shortened and the interpretation process is simplified when all of this information is available prior to performing the study.

Types of prosthetic heart valves

Two types of prosthetic valves have been designed in an attempt to reproduce the function of native cardiac valves. Mechanical prosthetic valves have been engineered to promote structural integrity over long periods, and bioprosthetic valves have been made to simulate native value hemodynamics and give less thrombogenicity. Most prosthetic valves are designed for insertion into the semilunar and atrioventricular positions with only minor modifications in the sewing rings.

Mechanical prostheses

Mechanical prosthetic heart valves may be classified by their supporting structure (strut or cage) and type of occluder mechanism (Table 7.1). Mechanical valves comprise the central occluder ball-cage valve, central occluder disk-cage valve, eccentric tilting-monocuspid disk valve, and tilting bileaflet disk valve.

Due to their structural composition, mechanical prosthetic valves inherently produce obstruction and turbulence to blood flow. The first mechanical valves were constructed with a cage mounted in a sewing ring with a ball shaped poppet in the MU position, the cage being oriented such that it protruded into the valvular outflow tract. When

Table 7.1 Mechanical prosthetic valves
Central ball occluder
Starr-Edwards
Smeloff-Cutter (Smeloff-Sutter)
Braunwald-Cutter
Magovern-Cromie
Harken
DeBakey-Surgitool
Hufnagel
Central disk occluder
Beall-Surgitool
Starr-Edwards disk
Cooley-Cutter
Kay-Shiley
Kay-Suzuki
Cross-Jones
Starr-Edwards (models 6500, 6520)
Eccentric monocuspid disk
Bjork-Shiley (standard, convexo-concave, monostrut)
Lillehei-Kaster
Kaster-Hall (Medtronic-Hall)
Wada-Cutter
Omniscience I and II
Bileaflet bicuspid disks
St. Jude
Duromedics
Carbomedics
On-X

the valve was in the open position with the ball at the top of the cage, turbulence occurred. Since the metallic cage had to be mounted in a stiff sewing ring for support, a somewhat bulky valve resulted; with a relatively small effective orifice area to ring circumference. In addition, mechanical valves are thrombogenic resulting from turbulence associated with their non-biological components. Advancements and modifications in mechanical valve technology have largely sought to address problems of thrombogenicity and valve obstruction (Figure 7.2). Increased valve orifice area promotes less turbulence and improved materials have increased durability. In addition, efforts have centred on decreasing the profile of the valve by incorporating tilting disks instead of central occluders, and changing from cages to shorter struts and finally to leaflet disks with only hinge supports. In comparison to tissue valves, mechanical valves are extremely durable and enjoy a long life expectancy.

Bioprosthetic valves

The development of tissue or bioprosthetic cardiac valves was an attempt to manufacture a facsimile of the native

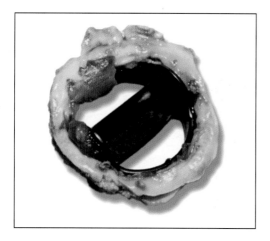

Figure 7.2
Explanted St. Jude bileaflet valve with pannus formation and thrombus which interfered with leaflet opening and closure with protrusion to the orifice of the sewing ring.

cardiac valve (Table 7.2). The first tissue valves were fresh cadaveric aortic homografts. Due to the unavailability of fresh valves, bioprosthetic valves or valves constructed of chemically stabilized biological tissue with metallic or plastic structural support were developed. Bioprosthetic cardiac valves are constructed of human or animal tissue formed as valve leaflets suspended within struts in an orientation, typical to a semilunar cardiac valve, mounted in a sewing ring. Bioprosthetic valves are classified according to their type of valve tissue. Heterograft valves are made from animal tissue (bovine or porcine), homografts are composed of human tissue, and autographs are made of tissue from the same patient. Recently, stentless valves have been introduced, which are composed of porcine tissue. Since the leaflets are composed of tissue, the valve is less bulky and there is some degree of flexibility to the

valve and the sewing ring, in comparison to mechanical valves with rigid sewing rings. Therefore, the obstruction to flow produced is minimal compared with mechanical valves, and thrombogenicity is less of an issue. The main drawback to bioprosthetic valves has been the durability of the tissue used to produce the valves.

Due to the inflammatory response, a form of rejection to the leaflet tissue occurs and bioprosthetic leaflets tend to degenerate and calcify, which may greatly shorten the durability of these valves (Figure 7.3). Initially bioprosthetic tissue valves were composed of animal valve leaflets which were later replaced by animal pericardium which produced better valve flow dynamics and increased strength with less tendency to calcify, degenerate and subsequently tear or rupture. Modifications of the preservation process, with the use of glutaraldehyde fixation of the valve tissue, serves to strengthen the tissue and promote less of a degenerative response.[12] This degenerative and calcification process is accelerated in younger patients, prohibiting the use of bioprosthetic valves in children.

A major problem with porcine valves is the septal shelf or the muscular bar that is naturally associated with the right coronary cusp in the pig. When a porcine valve is removed and prepared, the right coronary cusp cannot be removed without a significant portion of septal muscle which, when mounted in a sewing ring, tends to reduce the valve orifice which impedes blood flow.

Improvements in bioprosthesis technology have addressed the issues of premature degeneration by varying tissue type and fixation methods. Porcine valves have many configurations and sizes closely resembling human valves. The treated valves are nonviable and become stiffer than normal valves. Thrombogenicity is low since flow through the triangular central orifice is less turbulent.[13] In smaller valves, the orifice opening may be asymmetrical at low flow rates, and can produce obstruction to forward flow.[14]

Table 7.2 Bioprosthetic tissue valves

Heterograft
    Porcine aortic leaflet
        Hancock
        Carpentier-Edwards
        St. Jude BioImplant (Liotta)
        Medtronic Intact
        Tascon
        Angell-Shiley
    Bovine pericardium
        Hancock Pericardial
        Carpentier-Edwards Pericardial
        Ionescu-Shiley
        Mitro-flow (Mitral Medical)
Homograft
    Preserved human aortic valve Cryolife
    Dura mater
Autograft
    Fascia lata
Stentless

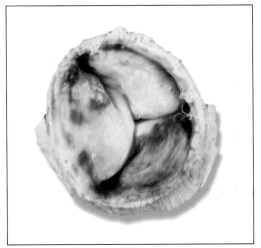

a

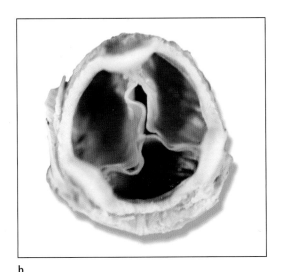

b

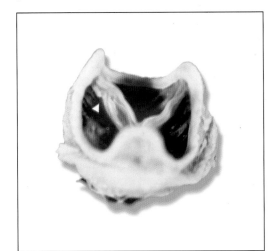

c

Figure 7.3
Explanted porcine bioprosthesis with leaflet thickening and calcification. Degenerative changes in the leaflets frequently result in tears or perforations in the leaflets.

Porcine valves have less regurgitation than mechanical valves with regurgitation occurring in only approximately 10% of valves.[15–17] Dysfunction is usually associated with progressive leaflet thickening and calcification. As the process progresses, the leaflets become more rigid, and tears or progressive stenosis result. Tears most commonly occur in the mitral position due to back-pressure and occur along the site of attachment to the strut. Newer pericardial (bovine) valves, which have been designed to overcome some of these problems, are constructed to resemble a normal human aortic valve.

Human aortic and pulmonary valves harvested from cadaveric human hearts and cyropreserved are also available for implantation with and without a supporting stent (Figures 7.4 and 7.5).[18,19] Homografts placed in the aortic position closely mimic the normal native aortic valve, and are difficult to detect echocardiographically. Homografts have the lowest gradients, a lower incidence of endocarditis and do not require long-term anticoagulation.

Homograft failure is usually the result of progressive aortic incompetence.

Echocardiographic examination of prosthetic heart valves

Prosthetic heart valves require serial examinations on a routine basis, due to the inherent problem of valve malfunction that occurs over the lifetime of the valve. Echocardiographic examinations are routinely performed at 6-month to 1-year intervals depending on various clinical variables. In many hospitals, transesophageal echocardiography is routinely performed during the surgical implantation of the prosthetic valve and establishes the initial valve function which serves as the baseline for comparison of subsequent evaluations. Performing transesophageal echocardiography during

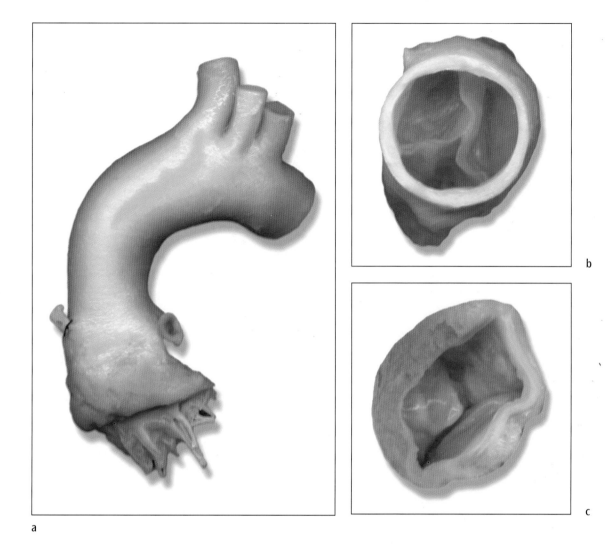

a
b
c

Figure 7.4

Aortic homograft. Human aortic and pulmonary valves harvested from cadaveric human hearts and with cyropreserved are also available for valve replacement and implanted with and without a supporting stent. Homografts placed in the aortic position closely mimic the normal native aortic valve, and are difficult to detect echocardiographically. Homografts present the lowest gradients, with a lesser propensity for the development of endocarditis and do not require long-term anticoagulation. Homograft failure is usually the result of progressive aortic incompetence. Homografts employing stents have not shared the same enthusiasm especially when placed in other valvular positions.

surgery has had a major impact on reducing both early valve malfunctions and perioperative mortality and morbidity.[20] In subsequent routine follow-up examinations, transthoracic evaluations are usually sufficient for follow-up, with transesophageal echocardiography evaluations performed only when questions arise from the transthoracic imaging. In patients with hemodynamic compromise and suspected prosthetic valve malfunction, however, transesophageal echocardiography increasingly is the diagnostic method of choice[21] (Table 7.3). In order to adequately describe echocardiographic findings for prosthetic heart valves it is helpful to fully understand

Table 7.3 Prosthetic valve malfunction

1. Pannus formation, fibrous tissue in growth – obstructive
2. Paravalvular regurgitation
3. Endocarditis
4. Poppet variance, abnormal motion or sticking
5. Disk wear
6. Sewing ring dehiscence
7. Valve outflow turbulence, obstruction
8. Strut fracture
9. Leaflet tear or rupture
10. Annulus abnormality, pseudoaneurysm
11. Thrombogenicity, systemic embolism

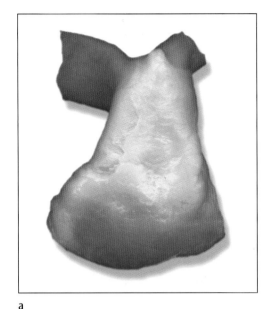

a

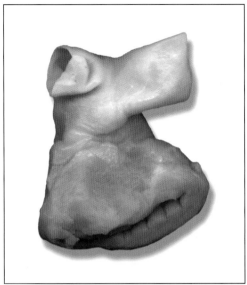

b

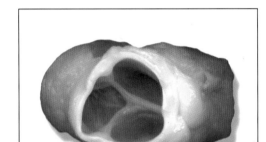

c

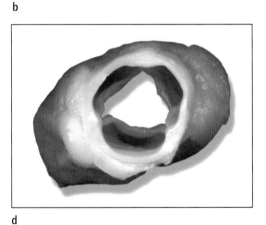

d

Figure 7.5
Pulmonary homograft. Pulmonary homografts may be used in repair of pulmonary atresia and other right ventricular outflow congenital abnormalities as well as in the Ross procedure. There has been a suggestion that pulmonary homografts exhibit a slightly better 5-year freedom from homograft failure.

and know the specific terminology. Table 7.4 summarizes some of the most common terms used with prosthetic valves.

Transesophageal echocardiographic examinations are frequently requested and may provide vital information in patients with thromboembolic events, suspected endocarditis and at the end of life of certain prosthetic valves. As a result, 16% of all transesophageal echocardiographic examinations are performed in our laboratory for prosthetic valve evaluations.

Echocardiographic artifacts such as reverberations and shadowing or ghosting are frequently produced by the non-biological components of the prosthesis. These artifacts prevent the visualization of anatomic structures and prosthetic valve components and frequently attenuate color and conventional Doppler flows that lie posterior to or behind the valve in the far field of the image sector. These artifacts limit transthoracic echocardiographic examinations, especially due to the depth of these structures in the imaging sector and inability to evaluate

the posterior structures of the heart without the prosthetic valve being interposed between those structures and the transducer. Spatial distortion, due to the high acoustic impedance of artificial material, affects both transthoracic and transesophageal echocardiography. To some degree these limitations may be overcome with multiplane transesophageal imaging at higher transducer frequencies and with the better echo windows produced in multiple planes. Optimized planes obtained with rotation of the multiplane transducer improve spatial understanding of both morphological and color Doppler findings, thereby producing a more complete examination. One drawback of transesophageal echocardiography is the inability to provide imaging planes with adequate parallel alignment of cardiac blood flow for conventional Doppler analysis in all patients. Often, Doppler examinations may be better performed with transthoracic imaging. For total echocardiographic analysis of a prosthetic valve in our laboratories, transesophageal and transthoracic imaging are frequently complementary.

Table 7.4 Prosthetic valve definitions

Primary valve orifice – internal diameter of the sewing ring.

Effective valve orifice – the true orifice area of the valve. Due to the geometry of the prosthetic valve and leaflets that are inside the sewing ring the true valve opening is smaller than the internal diameter of the sewing ring.

Stent – mechanical supporting structure for the tissue leaflets in a bioprosthesis

Strut – occluder supporting structures projecting from the ring structure.

Flange – metallic ring which retains the occluder disk or ball.

Occluder – portion of the mechanical valve that simulates the valve leaflet.

Physiological regurgitation – backflow leakage due to the reversal of blood flow pushed backwards as the leaflets close, or normal leak when the valve is closed due to the mechanics of the valve.

Valve profile – height of valve from the sewing ring to the top of the valve.

Paravalvular regurgitation – regurgitation occuring in between the valve sewing ring and the native valve annulus, due to partial or complete dehiscence.

Transvalvular regurgitation – pathological regurgitation through the valve leaflets as a result of valve malfunction.

Primary tissue failure – leaflet calcification or prolapse in a bioprosthesis secondary to tissue degeneration resulting from inflammation, infection or tissue rejection.

Stent creep – the inward migration of the stents towards the valve opening of a prosthetic valve due to tension on the stents produced by thickened and/or restricted leaflets.

Pannus formation – migration of excessive fibrous tissue to the prosthetic valve structures from the native annulus as part of the normal endothelialization process.

Ring abscess – spread of infection in between the sewing ring and the native annulus to the soft tissues of the fibrous skeleton and contiguous cardiac structures.

Ring or valve dehiscence – displacement or excessive motion of the prosthetic sewing ring in relation to the native annulus due to broken sutures or abscess, etc.

Fatigue failure – mechanical failure due to wear and tear over time.

Variance – abnormal occluder motion produced by deformity of the occluder due to wear and tear.

Disk notching – deformity of the occluder disk due to wear and tear.

Ball swelling – enlargement of the occluder ball (silicon rubber) due to absorption of materials, i.e. lipids etc.

Cloth wear – disintegration of the cloth material used to cover the sewing ring and/or struts due to wear and tear.

Strut fracture – mechanical separation of the strut from the valve ring due to material fatigue or a broken weld.

Disk embolization – dislodgment of the occluder device from the valve supporting apparatus due to mechanical failure, usually lethal.

The echocardiographic evaluation of prosthetic heart valves is similar, no matter whether the examination uses the transthoracic or transesophageal approach. To assure a complete assessment, the echocardiographer should apply a systematic approach to evaluating the prosthetic valve, as outlined in Table 7.5. When interpreting prosthetic valve echocardiographic studies it is important to know the specific type of valve being visualized including the model number, the size of the valve, the date it was implanted and also the results of previous echocardiographic analysis. The anticoagulation status of the valve is also important, especially if there have been abrupt alterations in the anticoagulation state. Although prosthetic valves are usually easily identifiable on echocardiography, it may be difficult to establish the exact type of prosthesis other than mechanical versus bioprosthesis, if the type of valve is not known. Each type of prosthetic valve has specific characteristics that require individual attention, before establishing its normality and excluding a diagnosis of malfunction.

Table 7.5 Evaluation of prosthetic valves

1. Two-dimensional evaluation of valve structural integrity
2. Opening and closing ability
3. Fixation of the sewing ring
4. Measure gradient
5. Evaluate physiological regurg, transvalvular regurgitation, or paravalvular regurgitation
6. Individual valve idiosyncrasies

Certain pathologies affect all prosthetic valves, whereas a few structural conditions are more specific to mechanical or bioprosthetic valves. In general, prosthetic valves must be evaluated for obstruction or stenosis, valve regurgitation, endocarditis, and mechanical or structural failure. The complete echocardiographic evaluation often requires the utilization of two-dimensional and M-mode imaging, together with conventional color flow Doppler, to rule out these pathologies.

Transthoracic echocardiographic examination of prosthetic valves has been adequately described in many echocardiographic textbooks, and the physician performing transesophageal echocardiography should be well versed in these techniques, as the principles are identical in transesophageal studies.[22–25]

The multiplane transesophageal echocardiographic examination should include a full evaluation of the heart and, specifically, the prosthetic valves. It is important to identify the appropriate window for visualizing the prosthetic valve. Once identified, the valve should be centered in the field of view and the transducer should be rotated slowly through a full 180 degrees to allow close inspection of the valve. Rotation of the transducer invariably provides an imaging plane that is perpendicular to leaflet motion, allowing direct visualization of the leaflet opening and closing within the sewing ring. The depth of field of the echocardiographic sector should be adjusted to allow full evaluation of the valve, using the zoom feature when necessary. It is frequently helpful to use less gain when visualizing the prosthesis to help reduce echocardiographic artifact, which may be more pronounced with transesophageal echocardiography. After evaluating the valve structure, it is necessary to perform a continuous wave and color Doppler evaluation to correlate abnormal hemodynamics with suspected structural abnormalities.

When visualizing the prosthesis, the appearance of the valve ring should be noted to determine whether the valve is intact and seated properly, orientated normally with the valve annulus. Excessive movement or abnormal rocking of the valve ring shows valvular dehiscence. The location and extent of dehiscence should be noted along with associated abnormal flows detected by color Doppler. In magnified views, suture material or remnants of the native valve may be visible and associated with malfunction. Large thrombi, vegetations or pannus tissue which may interfere with occluder (disk, ball or leaflet) motion velocity and valve opening or closing should be excluded. With bioprosthetic valves, excessive chaotic motion or prolapse suggests flail leaflets. Abnormal or chaotic occluder motion may be better demonstrated with m-mode echocardiography, when performing a transesophageal examination. In addition to observing the prosthesis it is important to note cardiac chamber dimensions and function, which may be the source of hemodynamic dysfunction and not malfunction of the cardiac prosthesis. With multiplane transesophageal echocardiography, multiple windows permit the examination of the cardiac chambers that are obscured with prosthetic valve artifact by transthoracic echocardiographic examinations.

TEE imaging aortic valve prosthesis

Transesophageal echocardiographic imaging of the aortic valve prosthesis can be performed in multiple views from various esophageal windows with excellent resolution. Doppler interrogation of the prosthesis may be difficult, however, with the transesophageal approach, since it may be difficult to obtain parallel imaging planes across the aortic prosthesis.

In the mid to upper esophageal probe position, the aortic valve is visualized obliquely at 0 degrees, similar to the transthoracic parasternal short axis view. The aortic valve prosthesis is displayed in the center of the imaging sector and may be visualized enface from approximately 30 to 60 degrees. Fine adjustment, by withdrawing or advancing of the transesophageal probe within the esophagus, allows the valve profile to be examined from the sewing ring to the superior struts, intermittently visualizing the valve poppet or leaflets. For best visualization of the prosthesis it is helpful to slowly reduce the overall gain to decrease artifact reflections from the valve and employ the zoom option. The sewing ring may be visualized as a circular ring surrounded by an echogenic free space within the aortic root. The sewing ring should appear centered within the root and appears motionless throughout the cardiac cycle. With slight withdrawal of the probe, the valve poppet or leaflets will be visualized with the mechanical prosthesis. Poor detail of the leaflets may be caused by reflection from the valve, but distinct opening and closing motion should be visualized. With bioprostheses, the valve struts and valve leaflets are visualized with the struts, appearing as three small echodense circles in the arrangement of a triangle, with the leaflets within the confines of the struts resembling opening and closure of a native aortic valve. The aortic valve-opening orifice is usually readily assessed, as is leaflet thickness, calcification and motion.

Color Doppler must be used to detect disturbed accelerated flow in systole and regurgitant flow in diastole. Although physiological regurgitation may be difficult to record, pathological regurgitation will be frequently recorded in this view and the exact site of origin may be delineated to within the valve struts and sewing ring or outside the valve between the sewing ring and aortic root. Regurgitant flow around the sewing ring represents paravalvular leaking. Excessive motion of the valve ring or large spaces visualized between the sewing ring and the aortic root may suggest dehiscence or annular aneurysm or abscess. Thrombi or vegetation including suture remnant or valve material degeneration may also be identified in this view by moving in and out of the valve plane during the cardiac cycle with mechanical or bioprosthetic valves. It is often helpful to use the m-mode cursor to interrogate mobile structures attached to the valve ring or leaflets.

Rotation of the probe to 90 degrees from the en-face, short-axis view, enables the aortic prosthesis to be visualized in a longitudinal plane similar to the transthoracic parasternal long axis view. The relationship between the sewing ring and the aortic root and annulus is optimally demonstrated. The magnification or zoom modes permits detailed visualization of the ventricular surface of the prosthetic valve. Poppet motion in mid- and high-profiled mechanical valves is readily demonstrated. With bioprosthetic valves, leaflet motion and amplitude of opening may be assessed as well as leaflet thickness and/or calcifications. Excessive motion of the sewing ring or leaflets may be demonstrated as motion in and out of the valve plane or prolapsing into the left ventricular outflow tract. In the longitudinal views, masses such as thrombi or vegetation may be seen attached to the valve structures.

Color Doppler demonstrates antegrade flow through the valve into the aortic root with the valve open during systole, and the direction and orientation of systolic flow can be defined. Regurgitant flow jets are best identified in this view for assessing size, direction and severity. The exact origin of regurgitant flow may be difficult to identify with mechanical prostheses. With bioprosthetic valves, the width of the regurgitant jet and vena contracta may be demonstrated. Echo-free spaces surrounding the sewing ring should be examined to detect para-aortic communications with filling from the aortic root.

The deep transgastric views, which resemble the transthoracic apical views, are important for assessing the aortic valve prosthesis. This is usually the best and only view for obtaining parallel imaging planes for continuous wave Doppler interrogation of the left ventricular outflow tract and aortic flow. This view is also the best for visualizing the left ventricular outflow tract proximal to the prosthetic valve without the interference of ghosting from the prosthesis. The deep transgastric views are important for assessing the motion of tilting disk prostheses. Additionally, color Doppler readily demonstrates regurgitant flow in this view.

In the gastric view between 90 and 125 degrees, the aortic prosthesis is visualized in an oblique, longitudinal view. Conventional Doppler may be performed if a parallel imaging plane is obtainable.

Intraoperative transesophageal echocardiography is helpful in determining the correct size for aortic homografts and stentless aortic prostheses.[26–34] Measurements are usually performed in longitudinal views for determining the left ventricular outflow tract diameter, aortic annulus diameter, and diameter of the sinotubular junction. Homografts are usually selected that are approximately 1 to 2 mm smaller than the left ventricular outflow tract diameter. The diameter of the sinotubular junction is most useful for determining the appropriate size of stentless valves. In addition the overall aortic root is assessed for aneurysmal dilatation or excessive calcification that may complicate prosthesis implantation.

TEE imaging mitral valve prosthesis

Multiplane transesophageal echocardiography is superior to transthoracic echocardiography for the evaluation of the mitral valve prosthesis when malfunction is suspected. For routine evaluations, transthoracic echocardiography may be sufficient as long as there are no abnormalities detected and no clinical suspicion for malfunction.

The mitral valve prosthesis is visualized in long axis from the mid-esophagus in views similar to the standard transthoracic four and two chamber apical views, except that with transesophageal echocardiography the prosthetic artifacts are projected towards the left ventricle allowing examination of the left atrium and the atrial surface of the valve. Starting with the transducer at 0 degrees and rotating the transducer through 180 degrees, the mitral prosthesis, especially the sewing ring, may be examined in detail. The mitral valve leaflets or poppets open toward the ventricular apex, allowing rapid identification of the type of valve and assessment of the opening and closing motion, allowing the maximum opening excursion to be directly assessed in this view. The orientation of the sewing ring to the annulus is easily demonstrated throughout its circumference. Excessive motion of the sewing ring is visible, as are gaps between the ring and the native annulus. The sewing ring should appear firmly attached to the native mitral annulus and does not move during the cardiac cycle. However, when the posterior leaflet of the mitral valve is preserved, the sewing ring appears to have more motion postoperatively than when the mitral prosthesis is sewn directly to the annulus. Paraprosthetic mitral valve leaks, due to lack of approximation of the sewing ring to the annulus, are commonly visualized with transesophageal echocardiography. Surgical debridement techniques involving the annulus, similar to those used in reparative techniques, have also been described for allowing better seating of the sewing ring. Despite these techniques, small mitral prosthesis paravalvular leaks are most frequently seen in the central portion of the posterior annulus, which is the area most prone to distortion, as discussed in chapter 2. Many newer valves are being developed with deformable sewing rings to address this issue. The mid-esophageal long axis views of the mitral prosthesis enable optimal visualization of masses such as thrombi or vegetations attached to the prosthetic valve components, and clots in the left atrium and the left atrial appendage that may be present with normal prostheses or with prosthetic malfunction.

Color and conventional Doppler is performed in these views since parallel alignment to the antegrade and retrograde flow through the valve is easily obtained. Color flow Doppler determines the direction and orientation of normal and abnormal flows to assist in directing pulsed and continuous lines of interrogation for determining maximum velocities for determining peak and mean gradients, deceleration and pressure half-time measurements and effective valve orifice areas. Posterior orientation of the transesophageal probe ensures that regurgitant jets are rarely missed. Continuous wave Doppler may also be used in the continuity formula or PISA method for determining valve areas and determining valve obstruction.

The mitral prosthesis is also visualized in the short axis view at 0 degrees and in longitudinal views at 90 degrees from the gastric windows, similar to the transthoracic parasternal long and short axis views. The short axis views at 0 to 15 degrees are ideal for evaluating mitral bioprostheses rather than mechanical prostheses. Similar to the mid-esophageal views, the mitral prosthesis type, leaflet or poppet motion, sewing ring stability and approximation to the annulus may be assessed. Thrombi, vegetation and prosthetic valve material degeneration are often demonstrated in these views. Excessive bioprosthesis leaflet motion, suggesting torn or flail leaflet segments as well as limited amplitude excursion, may be recognized in the longitudinal views. Color Doppler should be performed in longitudinal views for determining regurgitant flow jet and vena contracta width.

The deep transgastric view from 10 to 30 degrees provides the optimal images of the mitral valve prosthesis for evaluating the ventricular surface of the valve free of prosthetic valve artifacts.

TEE imaging tricuspid valve prosthesis

Both transthoracic and transesophageal imaging are valuable in the evaluation of tricuspid prosthetic valves. Transesophageal echocardiography has a clear advantage, however, in visualizing small vegetations or thrombi. Tricuspid prosthetic valves are visualized from the mid to lower esophagus. In the lower esophageal views at 0 to 45 degrees, the tricuspid prosthesis is seen in the longitudinal two-chamber view better than in the four chamber views from the mid-esophagus windows. The tricuspid prosthesis type, stability of the sewing ring, and leaflet or poppet motion are easily assessed. Because of the oblique orientation of tricuspid valve, transvalvular flow velocities through the prosthesis may not be obtainable with pulsed or continuous wave Doppler in these views. However, tricuspid prosthetic valve regurgitation is readily appreciated from both the lower and mid-esophagus with color flow Doppler. In addition, the right atrium is well visualized to evaluate tricuspid valve vegetative endocarditis, valvular thrombi, atrial thrombi or spontaneous echocardiographic contrast that frequently occurs with right atrial enlargement.

The tricuspid prosthesis can be visualized from the deep transgastric probe position, in which the ventricular aspect of the valve is demonstrated with the valve struts projected towards the apex. Diastolic antegrade flow through the tricuspid valve is directed towards the transducer and frequently allows a parallel orientation of the Doppler beam for suitable recording of the maximum flow velocity, to determine peak and mean pressure gradients as well as pressure half-time measurements. In addition, regurgitant systolic flow may be recorded for calculating the right atrial/right ventricular gradient.

The tricuspid valve prosthesis may also be visualized from the upper esophagus at 90 degrees from the aspect of the right atrium in the standard bi-caval view. With slight advancement of the transesophageal probe, the tricuspid prosthesis is frequently visualized in the far field to the left of the image sector. Unfortunately, due to the obliquity of the prosthesis, the whole valve may not be entirely imaged in a longitudinal plane. However, prosthetic valvular regurgitation is usually well visualized in a parallel plane for pulsed or continuous wave Doppler interrogation. Systolic retrograde flow through the prosthesis may be interrogated for determining maximum velocity measurements.

TEE imaging pulmonary valve prosthesis

The pulmonary valve prosthesis is imaged in the same views by transesophageal echocardiography as the native pulmonary valve. Doppler techniques are extremely difficult to perform by transesophageal echocardiography since the pulmonary outflow tract is usually orthogonal to the Doppler beam.

The right ventricular outflow tract can be visualized from the deep transgastric view, with the transducer maximally anteflexed with rightward rotation of the probe. The ventricular apex is at the top of the echocardiographic sector, with the right ventricular outflow tract coursing obliquely in the center of the inferior portion of the sector. This view provides the best opportunity for Doppler interrogation, in which the right ventricular outflow tract is close to parallel to the ultrasound beam.

A similar view of the right ventricular outflow tract is obtained from the transgastric transducer position with rightward rotation of the probe, with its imaging plane from 90 to 115 degrees. In this view, the right ventricular inflow and outflow tracts may be visualized in the same echocardiographic sector with foreshortening of the right ventricular apex.

A longitudinal view of the right ventricular outflow tract may be obtained from the lower esophageal position with rightward rotation of the probe and steering the transducer to between 110 and 135 degrees. The infundibulum, pulmonary valve prosthesis and main pulmonary artery are visualized in a longitudinal plane coursing obliquely in the image sector.

From the mid to upper esophagus at 0 degrees, a horizontal plane of the base of the heart is obtained with the right ventricular inflow tract cut obliquely and the right ventricular outflow tract wrapping around the aortic valve. A small portion of the main pulmonary artery is seen before it is obscured by the left atrial appendage. With rotation of the transducer from 75 to 90 degrees, the pulmonary valve prosthesis may be occasionally visualized in short axis.

Doppler interrogation: gradients and prosthetic stenosis

The assessment of blood flow through a prosthetic valve can be measured with transesophageal echocardiography with pulsed wave and continuous wave Doppler techniques with similar accuracy to transthoracic imaging, provided that imaging planes parallel to the prosthetic valve flows are obtained.[35–39] All prosthetic valves are inherently obstructive since their effective valve orifice area is less than the normal native valve area. It is important to take into consideration the specific flow profile through a given prosthesis, and not to assume that Doppler interrogation should be directly perpendicular to the valve plane as suggested by the sewing ring. Alignment of the Doppler beam may be aided by observing the direction and orientation of the color flow jet.[41–44]

Using the peak instantaneous transvalvular flow velocities obtained with continuous wave Doppler, the peak and mean pressure gradients may be determined using the modified Bernoulli equation ($p = 4v^2$).[45] Excellent correlation has been obtained between gradients obtained by Doppler methods and catheterization pressure measurements of prosthetic valves, despite the possibilities that the assumptions made by using the Bernoulli formula may not have been fully validated for artificial valves.[46–49] Various reports[17,50–68] have defined the normal gradients obtained with individual cardiac prosthetic valve in relation to the position and size of the valve as obtained with echocardiography, cardiac catheterization and in-vitro testing, as summarized in the Appendix.

Similar to normal native cardiac valves, higher velocities may be obtained with the Doppler peak instantaneous gradients across prosthetic valves, compared with the peak-to-peak pressure gradients determined at catheterization, necessitating comparison of the mean gradients obtained with both methods. In any given prosthesis, high velocities may be recorded initially as the valve opens, which may give the erroneous impression of prosthetic valve obstruction.[69,70] Since higher velocities may be temporally related to forward blood flow due to valve dynamics, the mean gradient measurement is the most reliable gradient measurement in clinical practice.

Artificially high peak gradients may be obtained due to the effect of pressure recovery related to the geometry of the prosthetic valve.[71,72] This phenomenon is principally noted with high flow velocities recorded from the central orifice of bi-leaflet mechanical valves in the aortic position, but can occur with any prosthesis. It is noteworthy that these velocities are recorded on the initial postimplant echocardiogram and remain unchanged on subsequent follow-up echocardiographic studies. In such patients, transesophageal echocardiography demonstrates normal valve structure and mechanics despite the high mean and peak transvalve gradients. It is important to recognize increasing gradients on serial studies, though, since this finding is usually related to valve stenosis and not to pressure recovery. Baumgartner et al have shown that in patients who show high-localized Doppler gradients due to the pressure-recovery phenomenon, if the valve truly becomes pathologically stenotic, the high-pressure gradients tend to disappear,[73] emphasizing the importance of routine serial echocardiographic follow-up.

In addition to prosthetic valve gradients, Doppler sampling using the continuity principle or the vena contracta jet method provides an accurate assessment of prosthetic valve effective orifice area. Using the continuity principle, blood flow is calculated in one area of the heart and compared to the flow through the prosthetic valve, similar to quantification of native valve orifice areas. The continuity principle is valid provided that there is no significant regurgitation of the corresponding valve used for calculation of the forward flow. The pressure half-time method for measuring prosthetic valve obstruction has not been as successful as the continuity principle and therefore should not be routinely used for comparison with catheterization methods. However, the pressure-half-time method is valid for serial measurements in the same patient over time for the assessment of prosthetic valve obstruction.[41,44,73–76]

Doppler interrogation: physiological, transvalvular and paravalvular regurgitation

Due to the intrinsic design characteristics of prosthetic valves it is common to detect small regurgitant jet with transesophageal echocardiography.[77–86] This regurgitation is similar to native valves and has been labeled as physiological regurgitation. Physiological regurgitation is most prominent with mechanical valves and is produced by the backward motion of the occluder device or leaflet. Additionally when the valve is closed, there are small gaps that remain between the occluder or leaflets and the sewing rings which allow the backward flow of small amounts of blood. Each valve has an inherent forward flow dynamic velocity profile, and there is also a specific profile for physiological regurgitation. The amount of regurgitant flow is usually small, depending on the specific prosthetic valve type, and may only be present during part of the cardiac cycle. Color flow Doppler imaging demonstrates that the physiological regurgitant jet appears confluent in color without significant variance, resembling a 'flame-like' jet that flickers in and out of view.

The size of the color flow jet with physiological prosthetic regurgitation is often larger than in physiological regurgitation of a native valve. An important observation is that physiological regurgitant jets usually remain the same size and appearance on serial echocardiographic studies. Physiological regurgitation with mitral prostheses yield regurgitant jet areas of less than 2 cm^2 and jet lengths of less than 2.5 cm. In the aortic prosthetic, physiological jet areas are less than 1 cm^2 and jet length is less than 1.5 cm.[79] Bioprosthetic valves leak less frequently than mechanical valves. Bioprosthetic valve physiological regurgitant jets are usually small and usually do not occur over the entire duration of valve closure. One of the quality control issues for pericardial bioprosthesis is the in-vitro testing and recognition of valvular regurgitation for each valve during the manufacturing process.

Pathological prosthetic regurgitation results from valve malfunction, and may occur primarily as leakage through the valve (transvalvular regurgitation) as a result of leaflet or occluder damage, or as a result of paravalvular regurgitation due to blood flow between the valve-sewing ring and the native valve annulus. Pathological valvular regurgitation may be underestimated and falsely labeled as physiological or mild due to attenuation of the conventional or color Doppler signal by the prosthetic valve. Transesophageal echocardiography is extremely helpful for assessing true regurgitation either through the prosthesis or around the prosthesis. Color flow Doppler usually demonstrates a significant regurgitant jet with marked flow variance, producing a mosaic color display.

The echocardiographic techniques for identifying transvalvular regurgitation are identical to those for native valvular regurgitation. Transvalvular prosthetic regurgitation may appear similar to physiological regurgitation, but the transvalvular regurgitant jet is usually larger, and is associated with hemodynamic abnormalities that are readily demonstrated during the echocardiographic study. Pathological transvalvular regurgitation is usually associated with prosthetic valve malfunction, especially with mechanical type prostheses. In distinguishing pathological from physiological transvalvular regurgitation, it is vital to use conventional as well as color flow Doppler since the timing of regurgitant flow signals may be better described with pulsed or continuous wave techniques. Once the exact origin of the regurgitant flow jet is identified with color flow Doppler, conventional Doppler may assist in determining the severity of regurgitation. Color flow Doppler enables the jet area to be determined for mitral

prostheses, with areas less than 4 cm^2 consistent with mild, 4 to 8 cm^2 moderate and greater than 8 cm^2 signifying severe regurgitation, provided that the jet is not eccentric and impinging on the atrial surface. For aortic prostheses, the ratio of the width of the regurgitant jet at its origin to the left ventricular outflow tract diameter can be used to grade the regurgitation with ratios less than 38% as mild, 39 to 75% moderate, and greater than 75% consistent with severe regurgitation.[78]

Continuous wave Doppler with a higher signal-to-noise ratio may be more accurate for detecting abnormal flows by identifying weaker flow signals. Pulsed Doppler is limited by the Nyquist limit, since many prosthetic valves intrinsically produce flow with higher signals then can be accurately recorded with this technique. If the flows are accurately detected with pulse Doppler, this technique may be most helpful in determining the timing of the abnormal flow which helps in determining the severity of regurgitation.

Structural failure of a bioprosthetic valve due to deterioration of the valve leaflets most commonly produces transvalvular regurgitation.[87–90] Degeneration of the valve leaflets results in thickened and stiff leaflets that can produce ruptures or tears in the leaflet surface due to the wear and tear of motion during the cardiac cycle. Leaflet rupture may produce prolapse of the leaflet with significant regurgitation. In addition to leaflet rupture, the leaflet may tear completely away from the strut or sewing ring producing a flail leaflet appearance with acute severe regurgitation. With severely abnormal leaflet deformities, banding of the Doppler spectral display has been noted as a result of the high-velocity fluttering of the flail leaflet segment.

Transesophageal echocardiography is pivotal for distinguishing transvalvular regurgitation from paraprosthetic regurgitation, especially for prostheses in the mitral position. In paraprosthetic regurgitation, the actual defect producing the leak is frequently visualized with careful observation during rotation of the transducer from 0 to 180 degrees. The addition of color Doppler allows flow to be readily visualized emanating from the defect directed toward the left atrium. In patients with large paraprosthetic leaks, color flow Doppler may demonstrate antegrade and retrograde flow (to and fro flow) through the defect. Small paraprosthetic leaks are frequently detected immediately after implant, and have been reported to decrease or disappear over time. Transesophageal echocardiography plays a critical role at the time of surgical valve replacement defining severe paraprosthetic leaks and allowing the surgeon to correct them immediately, thus reducing early morbidity and mortality.

The early development of paraprosthetic leaks not present immediately after implant are usually the result of suture and/or annulus failure and must be monitored echocardiographically for acute or progressive worsening. Late developing paraprosthetic leaks may be the earliest signs of prosthetic valve endocarditis and coexistent annular abscess, which may result in valve dehiscence.[16,91–93] Large regurgitant jets are detected by color flow Doppler, in addition to rocking of the sewing ring during the cardiac cycle adjacent to the defect. Valve dehiscence is usually an ominous sign associated with severe regurgitation, requiring surgical correction and valve re-implantation.

Prosthetic valve endocarditis

Insertion of any foreign material such as a prosthetic valve introduces the risk of infection at the implant site during episodes of bacteremia. The risk of infection decreases once the prosthesis has endothelialized. Mechanical and bioprosthetic valves have a similar incidence for endocarditis. When patients with valvular prostheses develop signs of systemic infection such as fever, it is imperative to rule out prosthetic valve endocarditis.

The hallmark of endocarditis echocardiographically is the detection of valvular vegetations. Traditionally transthoracic echocardiography has been the technique of choice to visualize vegetations even though the sensitivity in prosthetic valve endocarditis is less than for native valve endocarditis.[95–99] Echocardiographic artifacts such as reverberations and shadowing from the prosthetic valve frequently obscure vegetations. New abnormalities such as valve instability, abnormal sewing ring motion, development of paraprosthetic regurgitation, and increased transvalve gradient with or without abnormal motion of the valve poppet or leaflet are suggestive of infected prosthetic valve endocarditis. Destruction of bioprosthetic leaflets with worsening hemodynamics may be detected even when vegetations are not visualized. Annular abscess is a known complication of endocarditis and may be the first evidence of infection.

Numerous studies have demonstrated a higher sensitivity for detecting prosthetic valve endocarditis, especially small vegetations with biplane and multiplane transesophageal echocardiography as compared with transthoracic echocardiography.[100–115] When the transthoracic echocardiogram is negative in patients with suspected prosthetic valve endocarditis, transesophageal echocardiography should be recommended. Vegetations appear echocardiographically as small irregular masses attached to some part of the valve structure, often indistinguishable from thrombus. Small vegetations may appear as small discrete masses, without significant mobility.[101] Larger vegetations usually appear mobile with chaotic motion. Occasionally vegetations impair valve poppet or leaflet motion, and produce obstruction and/or regurgitation.

Spread of infection to the annulus ring results in paravalvular abscess, pseudoaneurysms and fistulas, and is associated with a higher complication rate and poor clinical outcome.[105–111] Paravalvular abscess usually appears as an echo-free space adjacent to the prosthetic sewing ring, more common in the aortic position than the mitral, with an equal propensity in mechanical and bioprosthetic valves. In the aortic position an abscess may only appear as a thickening of the aortic root, with a heterogeneous echo texture. When a clear space is present within an area of thickening, an abscess is easier to diagnose, and represents rupture of the abscess and communication with the blood pool. In both the mitral and aortic position an abscess can be missed due to the surrounding echo artifact from the prosthesis, therefore identification of the abscess requires a meticulous search. Occasionally, the diagnosis of abscess can be made by visualizing exaggerated motion of the valve and sewing ring, with new paravalvular regurgitation and partial dehiscence of the prosthesis. The importance of serial follow-up echocardiographic studies cannot be over emphasized with prosthetic valves since we have frequently diagnosed abscesses by recognizing new abnormalities that were not present on previous studies and valve abscess is an indication for repeat valve replacement.

Pseudoaneurysm and/or fistulas are easier to identify due to their more uniform appearance with color flow Doppler, since the abnormal flow into the aneurysm and through the fistula is usually readily identified. Pseudoaneurysms appear echocardiographically as an echo-free perivalvular cavity with flow communicating with the adjacent cardiac chamber. Fistulus communications are generally narrow tracts that allow communication of flow between the aorta or left ventricular outflow tract to adjacent cardiac chambers (right atrium, left atrium, or right ventricle).

Transesophageal echocardiography has greatly enhanced the ability for detecting paravalvular abscess. Daniel et al, obtained a sensitivity of 87% and specificity of 95% for the diagnosis of abscesses for prosthetic and native valve endocarditis with transesophageal echocardiography.[108] San Roman et al studied only patients with prosthetic valve endocarditis and were able to identify 90% of paravalvular abscesses that were confirmed at the time of surgery.[110] The same group was able to identify 100% of pseudoaneurysms and fistulas with transesophageal echocardiography in the setting of prosthetic valve endocarditis.[110]

Prosthetic valve thrombosis

Prosthetic heart valve thrombosis is a rare but potentially fatal complication that invariably involves mechanical prostheses.[116–119] Prosthetic valve thrombi can run the

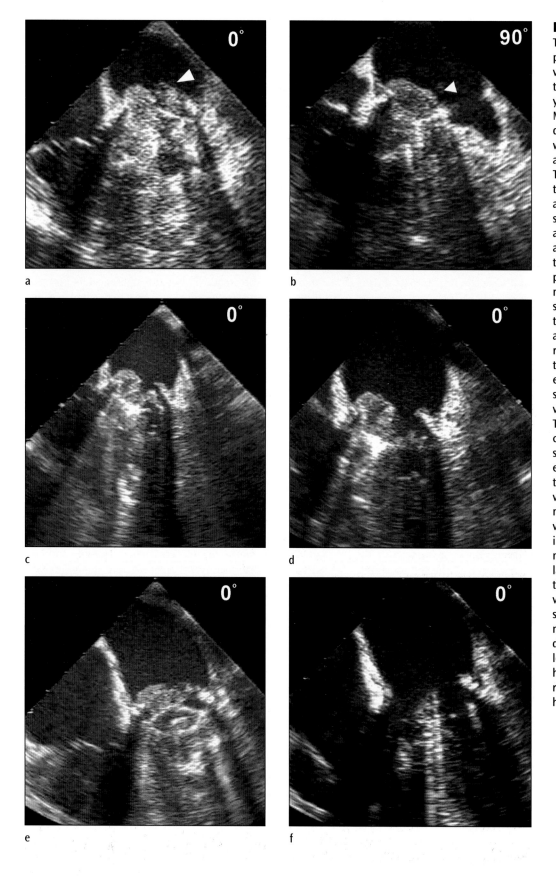

a

b

c

d

e

f

Figure 7.6
Thrombosed mitral prosthesis. A–F. Serial views of a thrombosed three year old St. Jude Mitral prosthesis during thrombolysis with the administration of TPA. The valve became thrombosed following an emergent bowel surgery and in-adequate anticoagulation. In the late postoperative period that was marred with post-surgical complications the patient arrested and following resuscitation a transthoracic echocardiogram suggested prosthetic valve malfunction. The patient was not a candidate for cardiac surgery and it was elected to attempt thrombolysis of the valve. Initially, the medial leaflet of the valve was found to be immobile with limited motion noted in the lateral leaflet. During thrombolysis the valve gradually started to move normally with debulking of the clot load and hemodynamics were restored within two hours.

gamut from small thrombi that may slightly interfere with valve function, to thrombi that may totally prevent poppet or leaflet motion leaving the valve partially open or partially closed, resulting in significant obstruction to antegrade flow or massive regurgitation. Prosthetic valve thrombosis may cause only intermittent sticking of the occluder device. Thrombi may occur in the setting of altered or insufficient anticoagulation, or may form in adequately anticoagulated patients when a structural abnormally associated with mechanical failure of the prosthetic valve components exists. Clinically, thrombosis should be suspected in any patient with a prosthetic valve who suddenly presents with florid heart failure.

Transthoracic or transesophageal echocardiography can be life-saving in establishing the diagnosis of a thrombosed valve in time to allow appropriate treatment.[116–123] Thrombus should be suspected when there is an increased echodensity within the valve structure and poppet or leaflet motion is either abnormal or undetectable. Doppler examination usually demonstrates an increased transvalvular gradient, indicating partial obstruction or new significant regurgitation. It is important to realize that when the valve is fixed in the open position, regurgitation may exhibit low velocities so that the severity of regurgitation may be underestimated. Transesophageal echocardiography has demonstrated a mass or thrombus, and a degree of hemodynamic impairment resulting from restricted poppet or leaflet motion, or an occluder fixed either in the open or closed position.[120–123]

Numerous reports have described the diagnosis of prosthetic valve thrombosis with cine-fluoroscopy, transthoracic and transesophageal echocardiographic imaging. Urgent transesophageal imaging is essential for diagnosing prosthetic malfunction in a hemodynamically unstable patient, when the findings with cine-fluoroscopy or transthoracic imaging are equivocal. Transesophageal echocardiography has a clear advantage over other techniques in evaluating patients with mitral prosthesis, atrial fibrillation and systemic embolic events.[123] Prosthetic valve thrombi appear as distinct masses, attached to the valve components and are visualized throughout the entire cardiac cycle. Pannus formation tends to be associated with the sewing ring, extends to the other valve structure and appears more echo-dense than thrombi. Ultrasound video intensity ratios of the mass as compared to the prosthesis have corroborated these findings. Differentiation of thrombus from pannus may still be difficult, especially since pathological studies have shown that thrombus may be adhered to pannus formation. Barbetseas et al reported the clinical and echocardiographic parameters that may help differentiate thrombus from pannus formation in prosthetic valve obstruction.[123] Factors that favor thrombus are short duration from time of valve insertion to malfunction, inadequate anticoagulation and shorter duration of

symptoms, and no change in NYHA class from the time of surgery. Thrombi tended to be larger, and extended to the left atrium surface of the valves in the mitral position, and always produced abnormal valve motion, in contrast to pannus formation where abnormal motion was only detected in 60%. Pannus formation tends to occur more common in the aortic position than does thrombus. In addition, the documentation of a soft mass on transesophageal echocardiography and a history of inadequate anticoagulation was similar to ultrasound video intensity alone in differentiating thrombus from pannus formation.

Numerous reports have described the role of transesophageal echocardiography in monitoring thrombolytic therapy in the treatment of thrombosed valves as depicted in Figure 7.6.[124–133]

Specific prosthetic valves
Starr-Edwards valve

The Starr-Edwards prosthesis[134–147] is a ball-cage valve and was one of the first prosthetic valves to be successfully implanted in humans (Figures 7.7 and 7.8). The Starr-Edwards valve is still used in the United States and abroad. The valve has gone through several modifications throughout the years, mirroring the developmental history of all prosthetic valves, but still maintains most of the original design. It is very important when examining a Starr-Edwards valve to know the model number, since specific valve malfunctions or problems may occur with a particular model. The major drawback of the Starr-Edwards valve is in its high profile produced by the ball and cage design. The central ball occluder is larger than the valve orifice of the sewing ring, and freely floats within the metallic cage during opening and closure. The large design profile of the Starr-Edwards valve limits the effective valve orifice area, which has a major impact in its hemodynamic profile. In addition the large profile of the valve fills the aorta when in the aortic position, often interfering with normal diastolic flow.

Modifications of the valve have occurred with change of composition of the ball, modifications of the struts and the sewing ring to enhance hemodynamic performance, and permanent fixation of the valve. There have been relatively few changes in the current models since 1968. Current models of the Starr-Edwards valve consist of an alloy cage with no welds and a silastic ball (poppet) with a circular sewing ring. The currently available aortic valve is model 1260 (Figure 7.7) and the mitral valve is model 6120 (Figure 7.8).

Previous models of the Starr-Edwards valve have been associated with specific abnormalities. Previous models employed various composition of the ball poppet, ranging

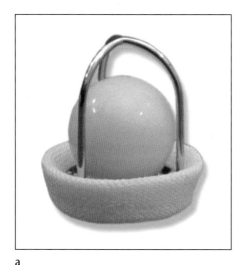

a

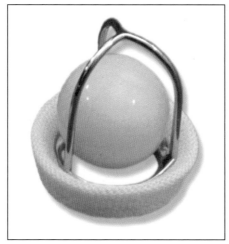

b

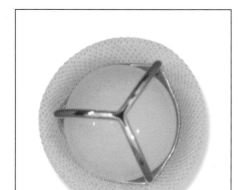

c

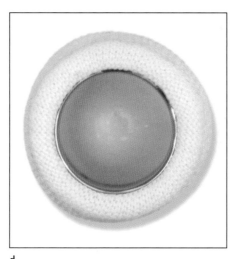

d

Figure 7.7
Starr-Edwards aortic silastic ball valve prosthesis (model 1260). The Starr-Edwards valve is constructed of an alloy cage with a rounded closed apex, free of welds which provides increased structural strength since there are no bends or hinges. Introduced in 1966, the valve is still implanted today in many parts of the world.

from silicone rubber (model 6000), and metal stellite (models 2310, 6300) to the modern silastic composition. The earlier poppet compositions resulted in stuck poppets within the cage due to ball variance from swelling or grooving, or escape of the poppet from the valve resulting in sudden catastrophic valve failure (Figure 7.9). These abnormalities are more of historical interest, and are not encountered today.

A few of the earlier manufactured valves (models 2300, 2320, 6300, 6320) were covered with cloth. This was abandoned because cloth disruption and disintegration occurred over time due to continual 'hammering' from the poppet during closure. Excessive turbulence produced by cloth disruption resulted in excessive hemolysis and/or embolic events greater than when the struts were left bare. Cloth disruption, especially of the struts, may be recognized by transesophageal echocardiography.[136,146–148]

With currently available models, the major risk of the Starr-Edwards prosthesis is for thromboembolic compli-

cations, similar to the other mechanical valves currently available. There is a low rate of thrombotic occlusion, mechanical sticking and encasement. The high valve profile and hemodynamic characteristics distinguish the Starr-Edwards valve from other available mechanical valves. Satisfactory hemodynamics are usually produced with prostheses in the mitral position, but significant gradients with hemolysis may occur in the aortic position.

Doppler color flow imaging defines two parallel lines of flow around the ball profile that converge downstream after the apex of the cage. An area of stagnant or vortical flow is produced behind the ball. To obtain the highest velocities of forward flow through the valve, the conventional Doppler must be directed to the lateral margins of the ball. Physiological regurgitation of the valve is limited to backflow produced by the ball movement during closure and results in a 'puff of smoke' appearance on color flow Doppler.

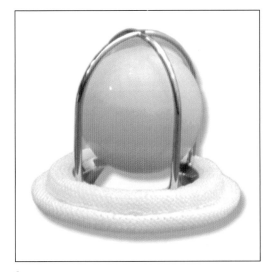

a

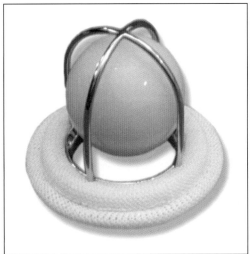

b

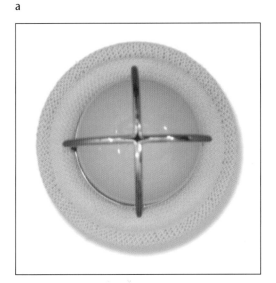

c

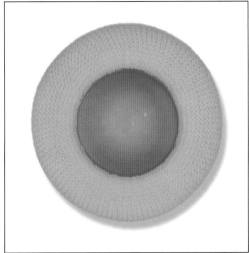

d

Figure 7.8
Starr-Edwards mitral silastic ball valve prosthesis (model 6120). The mitral prosthesis resembles the aortic prosthesis with differences in size and the sewing ring. The major risk of the Starr-Edwards prosthesis is for thromboembolic complications, similar to the other currently available mechanical valves. There is a reported low rate of thrombotic occlusion, mechanical sticking and encasement. The high valve profile and hemodynamic characteristics distinguishes the Starr-Edwards valve from the other available mechanical valves. Satisfactory hemodynamics are usually produced with prostheses in the mitral position. However significant gradients with hemolysis frequently occur in the aortic position.

Thrombosis of a Starr-Edwards valve with echocardiography is depicted as lack of excursion of ball, especially not reaching the top of the cage, producing a 'bouncing' effect of the ball. Tissue ingrowth or pannus formation impinging on the sewing ring orifice results in poor seating of the ball during closure, often presenting with significant regurgitation.

Beall-Surgitool valve

The Beall-Surgitool valve[149–164] is a low profile, central occluder disk valve, introduced in 1967, and is not currently available. The initial Beall-Surgitool valve, model 102, consisted of a flat extruded Teflon disk and titanium struts arranged in a guiding cage mechanism,

with an orifice completely covered with Dacron velour. Dacron velour was used as a thrombo-resistant lining and employed in other implantable cardiac devices designed in the mid-1960s. The Beall-Surgitool valve was prone to disk edge wear, and produced regurgitation, stenosis, hemolysis and disk embolization (Figure 7.9). The model 103 valve had a thicker compression-molded Teflon disk. The model 104 Beall-Surgitool valve incorporated an increase in the primary and secondary orifice of the smaller sized valves. The model 105 valve had a graphite disk, and the disk and wire struts were coated with a pyrolytic carbon-silicone alloy instead of Teflon. The model 106 valve, introduced in 1974, increased the diameter of the strut wire from 0.030 to 0.045 inches to prevent strut fracture, and modified the sewing ring to include both a standard sewing ring and a turtleneck ring (Figure 7.10).

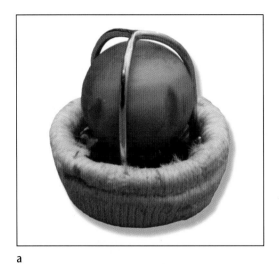

a

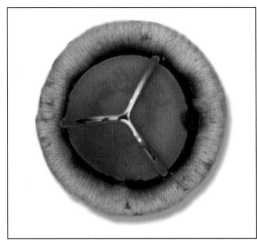

b

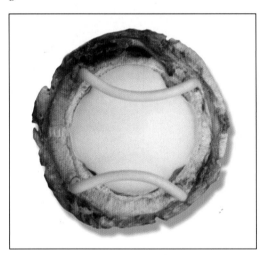

c

Figure 7.9
Variance. A, B. Grooved poppet of a Björk-Shiley aortic valve. The grooves are represented by the dark grooves in the ball and tend to cause abnormal poppet motion with opening and closing. In severe cases the ball may be embolized. C. Early clinical model of a Beall-Surgitool prosthesis exhibiting disk erosion. With severe erosion the Teflon coating may erode from the struts and the disk is expelled.

Normal echocardiographic visualization demonstrates brisk disk opening approximating the struts and closing promptly. It may be possible to still see a Beall-Surgitool valve, with the presentation cloth disintegration of the sewing ring and/or thrombosis producing delayed opening of the occluder (Figure 7.11).

Lillehei-Kaster valve

The Lillehei-Kaster valve[165–171] is a low profile, tilting disk valve, which was introduced in 1970 and is currently discontinued. The design served as the prototype for many currently available tilting disk valves. The valve consists of a free-floating, pivoting, pyrolytic carbon disk suspended in a titanium cage, and a Teflon sewing ring. The struts and the primary valve orifice are not covered with cloth. The disk opens to 80 degrees and when closed

is still tilted to 18 degrees. Both aortic and mitral valves were manufactured. The Lillehei Kaster valve was prone to prong perforation of the myocardium, which produced catastrophic thrombosis of the valve.

Omniscience valve I and II

The Omniscience (Lillehei-Medical) valve is a 'modified Lillehei-Kaster tilting disk valve' introduced in 1978, and currently manufactured by Medical Inc.[172–180] The valve consists of a curvilinear, pyrolytic carbon disk suspended in a one-piece titanium cage, supported by a Dacron covered sewing ring. The disk is inclined to 12 degrees when closed and opens to a maximum of 80 degrees in a shorter time period than the Lillehei-Kaster valve. The initial major modification distinguishing it from the Lillehei-Kaster valve are rounded, fin-like struts, which produce an additional

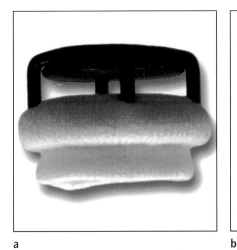

a

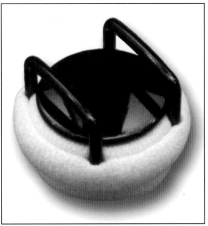

b

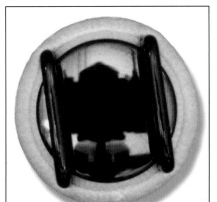

c

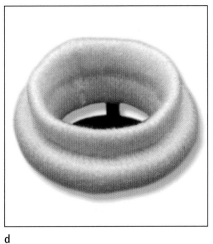

d

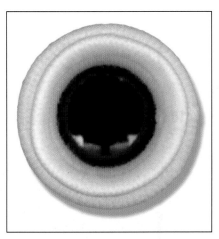

e

Figure 7.10
Beall-Surgitool valve (model 106). Turtle-neck model sewing ring incorporating pyrolytic carbon-coated struts and a pyrolytic carbon disk. The early models of the Beall-Surgitool valve were plagued with disk edge wear, producing regurgitation, stenosis, hemolysis and disk embolization. The model 106 valve, introduced in 1974, increased the diameter of the strut wire from 0.030 to 0.045 inches to prevent strut fracture, and modified the sewing ring to include both a standard sewing ring and a turtleneck ring.

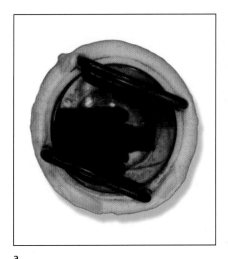

a

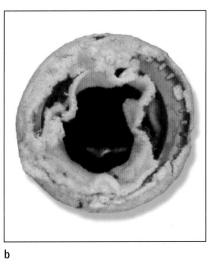

b

Figure 7.11
Explanted Beall-Surgitool sewing ring, cloth disintegration. Various materials have been used to construct the sewing ring and cover various valve parts. Many of the earliest materials would disintegrate and tear, producing thrombus formation and embolization.

advantage of a lower profile, replacing the longer prongs that were associated with myocardial perforation. The base of the valve is thinner to increase the inner-to-outer diameter ratio similar to that seen with a Bjork-Shiley valve. An additional modification of the Omniscience valve was changing to a Teflon sewing ring to avoid valve dehiscence. The newest design, the OmniCarbon valve, is constructed totally of pyrolytic carbon.

Doppler echocardiographic examination of the Omniscience valve exhibits one major inflow jet and usually two jets of minimal mitral regurgitation, which converge. The Omniscience valve occasionally demonstrates paraprosthetic valve regurgitation attributed to the sewing ring design.

Bjork-Shiley valve

The Bjork-Shiley valve is a low profile, tilting-disk valve that was introduced in 1969.[181-193] Three types of Bjork-Shiley valves were manufactured; the standard, spherical disk valve (R/S), the 60-degree and 70-degree convexo-concave disk valve (CC) (Figure 7.12) and the currently available monostrut valve (Alliance) (Figure 7.13).

The spherical disk prosthesis was composed of Delrin originally which was replaced by a flat pyrolytic carbon disk with a radio-opaque marker, suspended in a stellite metal cage. The disk is free-floating between two eccentrically situated support struts (inflow and outflow struts). The metal struts are heat-fused in place and then bent to allow insertion of the poppet. The disk is held in place by fitting the outflow strut into a central depression. The struts are then returned to their correct position. The sewing rings are thin and vertically oriented in the aortic valve and thicker and more horizontal in the mitral model. The disk opens to 60 degrees, creating a major and minor orifice, and when closed the disk rests on the valve ring. The R/S valve inherently leaks due to its design. Regurgitation of the valve is calculated to be about 2 to 5 percent of the stroke volume.

The spherical R/S valve is particularly vulnerable to accumulation of thrombus on the bare metal orifice and struts. Developing thrombus extends over the prosthesis margins and over the struts to occlude the lesser orifice. Clinically this produces a valve failure, typically producing fixation of the disk at an opening angle of 20 degrees, requiring emergency re-operation. Structural failure of the R/S valve was rare and resulted from inlet strut fracture attributed to the weld of the strut, which once identified was fixed.

In order to improve upon the hemodynamic characteristics of the R/S valve, the occluder disk was changed to a pyrolytic carbon disk with a convexo-concave shape

resembling an airplane wing, and the inlet and outlet struts were modified to accommodate the new disk. The Bjork-Shiley convexo-concave (C/C) valve replaced the R/S valve in 1976 and became one of the most popular prosthetic valves worldwide over the next 10 years. The C/C valve initially was manufactured with a 60-degree opening angle and then a later model was made with a 70-degree opening which was never available in the United States. With the 60 degree convexo-concave disk valve, the pivot point was moved 2.5 mm downstream to reduce obstruction by creating a larger minor orifice and a 12 degrees greater opening angle. The C/C valve, despite improved hemodynamics, was plagued with design fatigue of the outlet strut, due to the unique motion of the convexo-concave disk, which resulted in strut fracture and many deaths due to expulsion of the occluder disk. Repeated modification in the welding technique and improved design of the outlet strut remedied this problem, but the valve was subsequently withdrawn.

The monostrut Bjork-Shiley valve (Alliance) replaced the C/C model in 1982 and is available today, although not in the United States. The monostrut valve construction includes struts and ring formed by electromechanical machining from a single bar of cobalt base alloy, thus eliminating the strut welds. The monostrut valve incorporates the very good hemodynamics of the C/C valve without the history of valve structural failure, but has not enjoyed the success of the Bjork-Shiley C/C valve.

Color Doppler flow mapping is similar in all models and demonstrates two similar sized flow jets through the relatively equal flow diameters of the major and minor orifice created by the tilting disk, which converge downstream. Differences between flow jets or decreases in both jets have been shown to be associated with pannus ingrowth or valve thrombosis, and may result in reduction in occluder motion. Minimal physiological regurgitant jets are recorded with normal valves, thus significant regurgitation suggests valve malfunction.

Complications of the Bjork-Shiley valve other than mechanical failure include thrombosis and thromboembolic events. Obstruction of the valve may occur due to ingrowth or clot formation as illustrated in Figure 7.14, and is demonstrated echocardiographically with reduced amplitude of the disk opening, with dense echoes near the suture ring.

Medtronic-Hall valve (Hall-Kaster)

The Medtronic-Hall valve[194-211] is a pivoting disk valve introduced in 1977, and is a descendant of the Lillehei-Kaster valve design, with a lower valve profile (Figure 7.15). The valve consists of a pyrolytic carbon covered

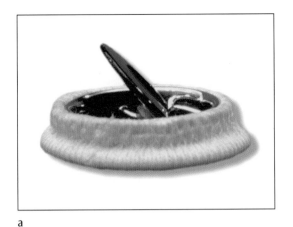

a

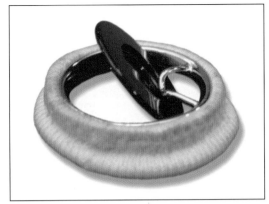

b

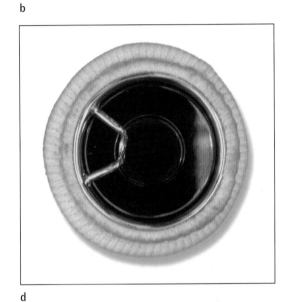

c

d

e

Figure 7.12

Björk-Shiley mitral valve. The Björk-Shiley valve is a low profile, tilting-disk valve and was introduced in 1969. Three types of Björk-Shiley valves were manufactured; the standard, spherical disk valve (R/S), the 60-degree and 70 degree convexo-concave disk valve (CC). The Björk-Shiley convexo-concave (C/C) valve replaced the R/S valve around 1976 and became one of the most popular prosthetic valves in the world for the next 10 years. The C/C valve initially was manufactured with a 60-degree opening angle and then a later model was made with a 70-degree opening which was never available in the United States. With the 60-degree convexo-concave disk valve the pivot point was moved 2.5 mm downstream to reduce obstruction by creating a larger minor orifice and a 12 degrees greater opening angle. The C/C valve, despite improved hemodynamics, was plagued with design fatigue of the outlet strut, due to the unique motion of the convexo-concave disk, which resulted in strut fracture and hemodynamic catastrophe due to expulsion of the occluder disk. Repeated modification in the welding technique and later improved design of the outlet strut remedied the problem, but the valve was still removed from the market.

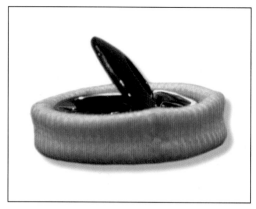

a

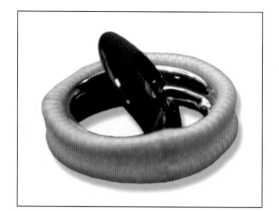

b

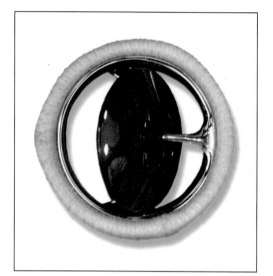

c

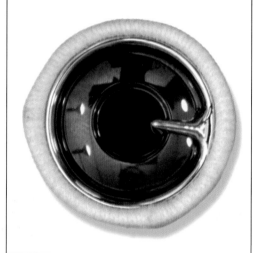

d

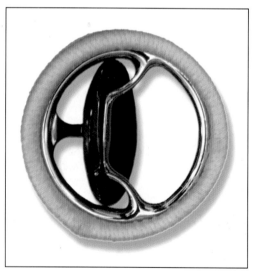

e

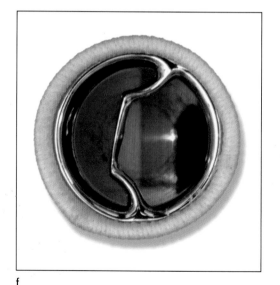

f

Figure 7.13
Björk-Shiley aortic valve. The monostrut Björk-Shiley valve (Alliance) replaced the C/C model in 1982 and is available today (manufactured by a different company) but is not available in the United States. The monostrut valve construction includes struts and ring formed by electromechanical machining process manufactured from a single bar stock of Haynes 25, cobalt base alloy, which eliminate the strut welds. The monostrut valve incorporates the same very good hemodynamics of the C/C valve without the experience of valve structural failure; however, the monostrut valve has not enjoyed the success of its predecessor the Björk-Shiley C/C valve.

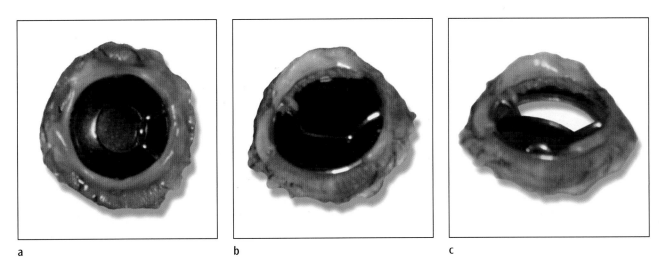

a   b   c

Figure 7.14
Explanted Björk-Shiley valve with pannus formation which covered the sewing ring and encroached on the valve orifice and interfered with leaflet motion. Sticking was produced with opening which was visualized with echocardiography by demonstrating the characteristic motion on m-mode.

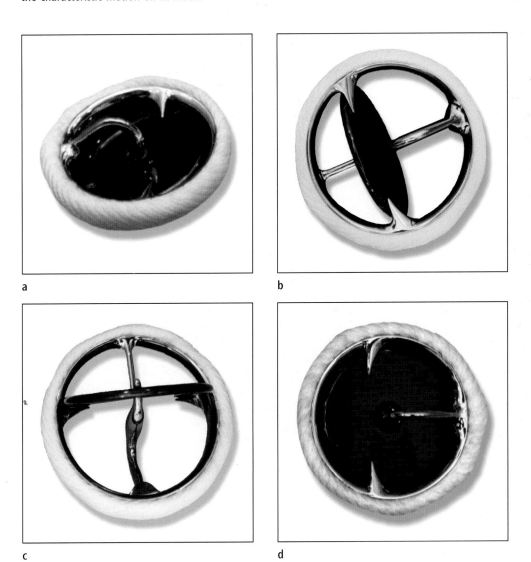

a   b

c   d

Figure 7.15
Medtronic-Hall tilting disk mechanical valve. The valve consists of a pyrolytic carbon covered disk that is suspended in a titanium cage and supported with a S-shaped central strut without welds, mounted to a Teflon sewing ring. The disk is guided during opening and closing by a rod guide strut projecting through a central disk perforation. The disk opens to a maximum of 75 degrees. The valve is available in aortic and mitral valve models. The valve can be rotated to allow for a disk parallel to flow orientation to produce an eccentric flow profile and provide good hemodynamics.

disk suspended in a titanium cage and supported with a S-shaped central strut without welds, mounted to a Teflon sewing ring. The disk is guided during opening and closing by a rod guide strut projecting through a central disk perforation. The disk opens to a maximum of 75 degrees. The valve is available in aortic and mitral valve types. Initially there were no reported cases of structural failure, although three cases of disk fracture have been reported.

Hemodynamically, flow occurs on both sides of the disk through a major and minor orifice, limiting the amount of flow stagnation behind the disk. Physiological regurgitation may be detected through the central perforation as well as around the disk periphery between the sewing ring. The central jet is frequently misinterpreted as pathological due to its large jet length. Careful evaluation of the central jet yields a thin jet without significant turbulence despite its long length.

St. Jude valve

The St. Jude valve introduced in 1977 was the first commercially available, low profile, bileaflet prosthesis.[212–228] The St.

Jude Standard valve is composed entirely of a pyrolytic carbon-coated graphite frame with two pyrolytic carbon leaflets impregnated with tungsten to make them radio-opaque, with a Dacron sewing ring (Figure 7.16). The leaflets open from an angle of 30 degrees to a maximum of 85 degrees from a central hinge point, which provides two lateral and one central orifice, with rapid opening which is not position-sensitive. Since the valve was introduced, there has only been one mechanical failure, after the first 50 valves were manufactured. The St. Jude valve is also available in an expanded cuff model that contains 25% more cuff material for the aortic model and 10% more cuff material for the mitral model than the standard cuff (Figure 7.17).

The St. Jude Hemodynamic Plus (HP) series include both aortic and mitral models for small annuli from 17 to 21 mm. The sewing ring is designed for a supra-annular position permitting a larger diameter orifice ring, which reduces the projection of the pivot guards into the left ventricular outflow tract.

The SJM Masters series allows the pivot guards to be rotated, after the valve has been sutured in place. The SJM Master's aortic model has a Hemodynamic Plus cuff and the

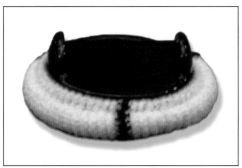
a

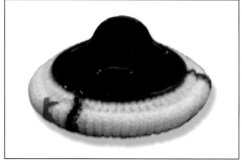
b

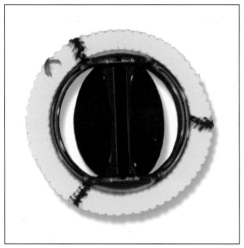
c

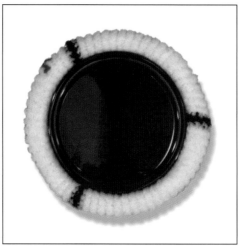
d

Figure 7.16

St. Jude bileaflet mitral prosthesis. The St. Jude valve was the first commercially available, low profile, bileaflet prosthesis and was introduced in 1977. The St. Jude Standard bileaflet valve is composed entirely of a pyrolytic carbon-coated graphite frame, two pyrolytic carbon leaflets impregnated with tungsten to make them radiopaque, and a Dacron sewing ring. The leaflets open from an angle of 30 degrees to a maximum of 85 degrees from a central hinge point, which provides two larger lateral and one smaller central orifice, with rapid opening which is not position-sensitive.

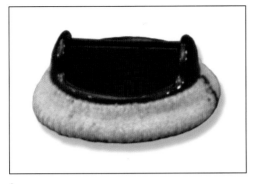

a

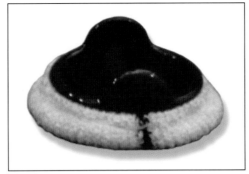

b

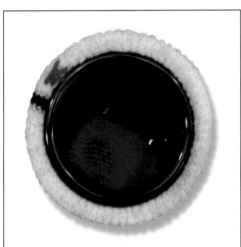

c

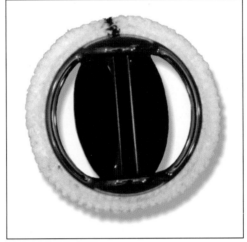

d

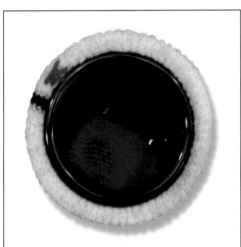

e

Figure 7.17

St. Jude bileaflet aortic prosthesis. The St. Jude aortic prosthesis is similar to the mitral model with a different sewing cuff. The St. Jude valve is also available in an expanded cuff model that contains 25% more cuff material for the aortic model and 10% more cuff material for the mitral model than the standard cuff. In addition to the standard and expanded cuff models the aortic prosthesis is also available in a Hemodynamic Plus (HP) series cuff to provide improved hemodynamics in patients with small aortic roots allowing the valve sewing cuff to be implanted on top of the annulus allowing a larger valve prosthesis and providing a larger effective orifice than would normally occur with a standard valve replacement. The SJM® Masters Series consists of mitral and aortic valves which have been modified to include rotatable leaflets which provide a mechanism (controlled torque rotation) for adjusting the orientation of the valve leaflets and pivot guards during implantation so there is no subvalvular tissue or foreign material that would interfere with leaflet motion. The valves also have improved radiopacity and extra suture markers on the sewing cuffs.

mitral model has a standard cuff. In the aortic model, the pivot guards should be rotated towards the left ventricular septum or towards residual sub-annular calcium that may interfere with the leaflets. In the mitral model, the leaflets are oriented in a plane perpendicular to the natural commissures to decrease the incidence of asynchronous leaflet closure.

A recent modification of the St. Jude valve was the addition of silver modified polyester, Silzone™ sewing ring (Figure 7.18). Although in-vitro studies showed lower bacterial counts on direct contact of the sewing ring, animal studies indicated that pannus organized more quickly but was thinner overall on the silver-coated versus

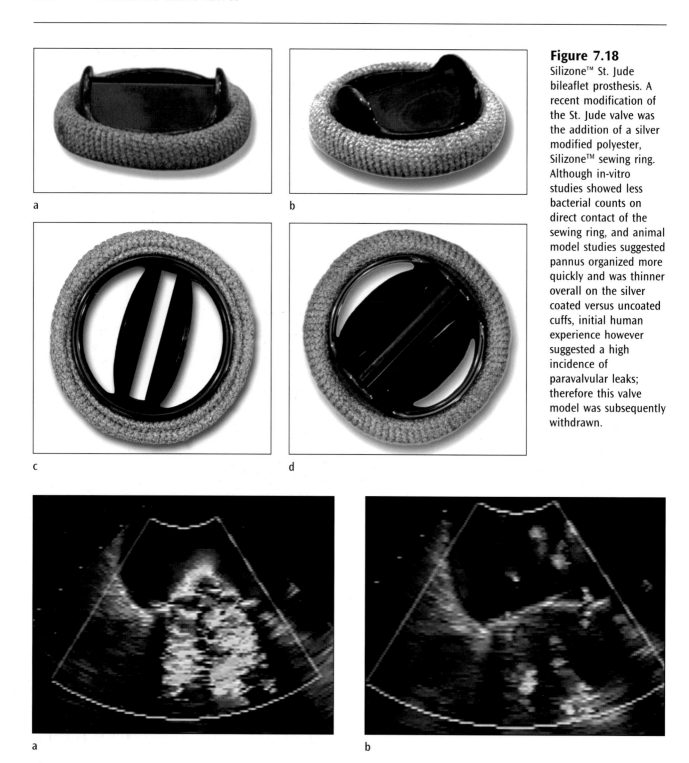

Figure 7.18
Silizone™ St. Jude bileaflet prosthesis. A recent modification of the St. Jude valve was the addition of a silver modified polyester, Silizone™ sewing ring. Although in-vitro studies showed less bacterial counts on direct contact of the sewing ring, and animal model studies suggested pannus organized more quickly and was thinner overall on the silver coated versus uncoated cuffs, initial human experience however suggested a high incidence of paravalvular leaks; therefore this valve model was subsequently withdrawn.

Figure 7.19
Normal color-flow doppler with a St. Jude bileaflet prosthesis. A. Flow through the bileaflet valve usually occurs through three orifices created by the valve leaflet arrangement creating two major and one minor central orifice exhibited by three areas of flow convergence on the opening surface of the valve ring. B. Transesophageal echocardiography provides an excellent assessment of the regurgitant jets to determine normal versus abnormal flows. Typically normal regurgitation of the St. Jude prosthesis consists of three small jets, two from the lateral portions of the leaflets and the sewing ring and one central jet representing a small amount of regurgitation during the valve's closing phase as demonstrated by systolic flow reversal on conventional doppler. In the aortic position there is usually little or no aortic regurgitation. Color flow doppler readily demonstrates abnormal regurgitation associated with bileaflet mechanical valves. Characteristics of abnormal transvalvular or paravalvular leaks in the mitral position are regurgitant jets that are asymmetric and cross the valve midline, are jets of long duration (pansystolic), or jets that exhibit a mosaic or turbulent flow pattern often along the atrial wall.

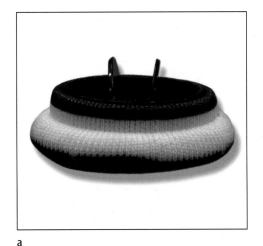

a

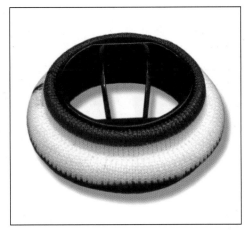

b

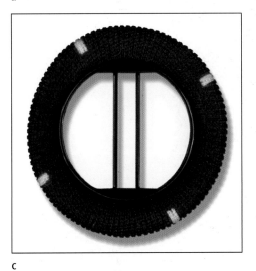

c

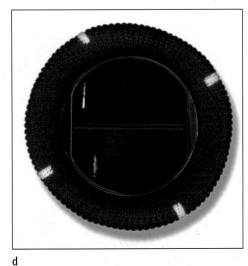

d

Figure 7.20
CPHV standard mitral valve. The Carbomedics prosthetic heart valve is a bileaflet mechanical valve and was introduced in 1986 and manufactured by Sulzer Carbomedics, Inc. The CPHV standard series has pyrolytic carbon leaflets designed for an intra-annular position and rotatable for optimum orientation. The valve design includes a recessed pivot mechanism, which promotes 'washing' of the mechanism as blood flows through the valve orifice. The sewing cuff is made of knitted polyester and is contoured which aids in seating the valve during implantation, with a few models composed of sewing rings coated with Biolite Carbon to reduce pannus growth. The Orbis Universal model, as its name implies, incorporates a sewing ring that may be implanted in either the aortic or mitral position.

uncoated cuffs. Initial human experience suggested a high incidence of paravalvular leaks, and the valve was subsequently withdrawn.

Echocardiographically, the St. Jude valve leaflets appear as two parallel lines during opening in both the long and short axis views. During valve closure the leaflets form a 'v' in long axis imaging, and disappear from view in short axis images. The valve leaflets are almost always visualized by transesophageal echocardiography despite the varying alignment of the leaflets.

Physiological regurgitation is usually demonstrated with color flow Doppler as three small jets (Figure 7.19). Two lateral jets originate for the edges of the valve leaflets and the sewing rings and point upwards away from the valve. One small jet also originates from the central orifice. Physiological regurgitant jets are short in duration. Smaller jets may also be visualized, especially with transesophageal echocardiography at the top and bottom of the valve when closed, demonstrating normal flow through the valve pivots. Physiological regurgitant jets are usually much better demonstrated with valves

in the mitral position than in the aortic position. In the normal mitral anatomically-positioned St. Jude valve (leaflet rotational axis parallel to the native commissure) the normal three jets are visualized at 0 degrees in the four-chamber view obtained in the mid to lower esophagus. With the mitral anti-anatomically-positioned valve (leaflet rotational axis pointed toward the aorta), a semicircular flare with color flow Doppler is seen with closure.

Carbomedics prosthetic heart valve

The Carbomedics prosthetic valve is a bileaflet mechanical valve introduced in 1986 and manufactured by Sulzer Carbomedics, Inc.[229–241] The CPHV standard series has pyrolytic carbon leaflets designed for an intra-annular position and rotatable for optimum orientation. The valve design includes a recessed pivot mechanism, which promotes washing of the leaflet by blood flow through the valve orifice (Figures 7.20 and 7.21). The sewing cuff is

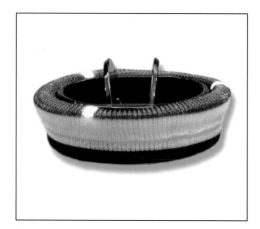

a

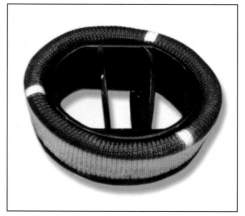

b

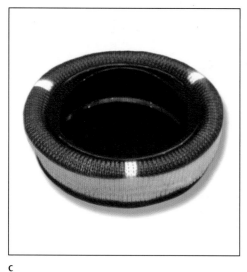

c

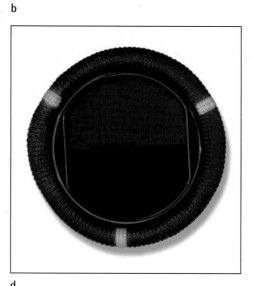

d

Figure 7.21
CPHV standard aortic valve and R series (reduced model) are designed for a narrow annulus and produce a larger sewing ring orifice to annulus ratio with no change in the internal orifice diameter. The Reduced valve model has a smaller, stiffer sewing ring (titanium) designed for narrow aortic roots.

made of knitted polyester and is contoured, with some models coated with Biolite Carbon to reduce pannus growth. Other available designs include the Top Hat valve, which is designed with a sewing ring for a supra-annular position (Figure 7.22). The Orbis Universal model, as its name implies, incorporates a sewing ring that may be implanted in either the aortic or mitral position. The Reduced valve model has a smaller, stiffer sewing ring made of titanium designed for narrow aortic roots.

On-X valve

The On-X valve is a bileaflet mechanical prosthesis currently under clinical investigation in Europe and the United States.[242–247] On-X valves are constructed of On-X carbon, which is the newest generation of pyrolytic carbon, manufactured without silicon. Pure pyrolytic carbon eliminates the imperfections found in silicon-alloyed carbon,

which results in increased strength, less blood trauma, and less thromboembolism. Other features of the On-X valve include a shaped orifice with flared inlet designed to reduce inlet turbulence, and an elongated orifice to organize flow and reduce exit losses. In addition, the leaflets are thinner and rotatable to be aligned with flow during implantation. The sewing ring is constructed of PTFE and fixed by titanium rings. The valve is available in aortic (Figure 7.23) and mitral (Figure 7.24) models, with a supra-annular sewing ring for small aortic valves ≤ 25 mm in size. The hinge mechanism provides a positive closing action due to a pivot design. Initial trial results have been promising, with low gradients even in the smaller size valves.

Edwards MIRA valve

The MIRA valve is a bileaflet mechanical prosthesis manufactured by Edwards Lifesciences. Four models are

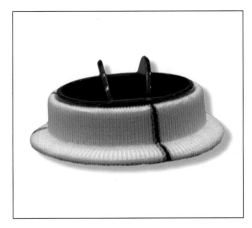

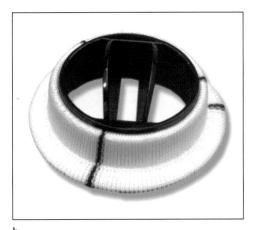

a

b

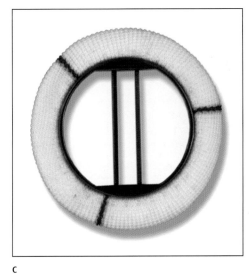

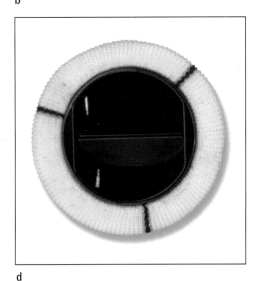

c

d

Figure 7.22
CPHV Top Hat aortic valve provides maximal blood flow with a 100% orifice-to-annulus ratio which is designed with a sewing ring for a supra-annular position to improve hemodynamics for a narrow aortic annulus.

available: the MIRA aortic mechanical valve; the MIRA Finesse aortic mechanical valve; the MIRA Ultra Finesse Aortic mechanical valve; and the MIRA Mitral mechanical valve. The MIRA valve leaflets have a curved leaflet profile and are mounted in a carbon coated titanium-alloy housing. The sewing rings contain a silicone sponge, which should provide stable anchoring of the valve and is unique for each model. The mitral sewing ring is hyperbolic in shape, with a gradual curvature to increase the sealing surface area.

ATS Medical Open Pivot™ valve

The ATS Medical Open Pivot™ heart valve is a bileaflet mechanical prosthesis, which is currently available outside the United States and as an investigational device in the US.[248–258] The leaflets are made from pyrolytic carbon impregnated with 20% tungsten. The open pivot design of

this bileaflet valve is unique and the traditional pivot cavities are replaced with smooth hemispheres, which may promote better open and closing of the leaflets. The sewing ring includes a titanium stiffening ring, which is rotatable. The ATS valve is available in two models. The standard valve is available in aortic and mitral models, and the advanced performance series for supra-annular placement with a reduced cuff size in both aortic and mitral models.

Ionescu-Shiley bioprosthesis

The Ionescu-Shiley bioprosthesis is a bovine pericardial xenograft.[259–281] Bovine pericardium is cut and a single strip of tissue sutured to the outside surfaces of rigid, symmetric titanium stents attached to a universal sewing ring or an aortic sewing ring, covered with Dacron. In smaller valves the stents are splayed outwards by 9 degrees to maximize hemodynamics. This design eliminated the asymmetric

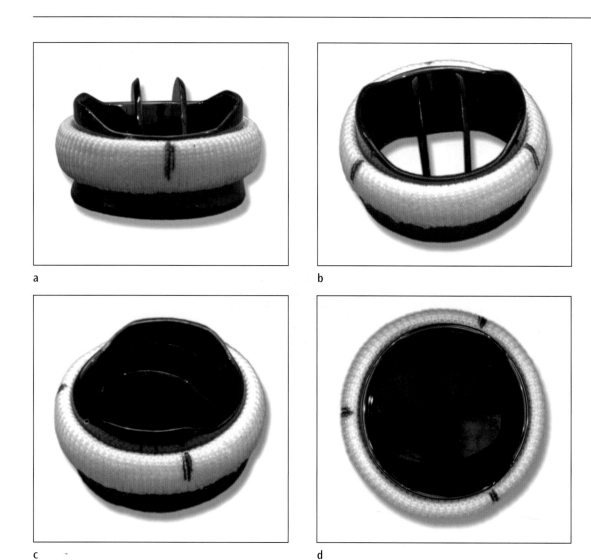

a

b

c

d

Figure 7.23
MCRI ON-X bileaflet aortic valve. The On-X valves are constructed of On-X carbon, which is the newest generation of pyrolytic carbon, manufactured without silicon that was used in previous pyrolytic valves. Pure pyrolytic carbon eliminates the imperfections found in silicon-alloyed carbon, which should result in less blood trauma with resultant thromboembolism, and increased strength. Other features of the On-X valve include a shaped orifice with flared inlet designed to reduce inlet turbulence, and an elongated orifice made to organize flow and reduce exit losses, with thinner leaflets that are rotatable to be aligned with flow during implantation. The sewing ring is constructed of PTFE and fixed by titanium rings. The valve is available in aortic and mitral models, with a supra-annular sewing ring for small aortic valves ≤25 mm in size. The hinge mechanism provides positive closing action due to an actuated pivot design. Initial trial results have been promising with low gradients in the smaller size valves.

opening of the valve leaflets, which occurs naturally with the normal porcine valve. Modifications of the Ionescu-Shiley valve included exchanging the rigid titanium stents with Delrin and the Dacron cloth with Microvel material to reduce valve leaflet abrasion and eliminate the outward stent placement and reduced stent profile height. Since the sewing ring is rather narrow, there is a high incidence of paravalvular regurgitation especially in the aortic position.

The greater back-pressure on the prosthesis in the mitral as compared to the aortic position usually causes abrasion of the pericardial tissue at the point of contact with the sewing ring and the stents, which facilitates calcification and restriction of the leaflets, resulting in valvular regurgitation. Restricted leaflet tissue is associated with perforations and tears sooner than observed with porcine valves. Calcification may also result in increased valvular gradients.

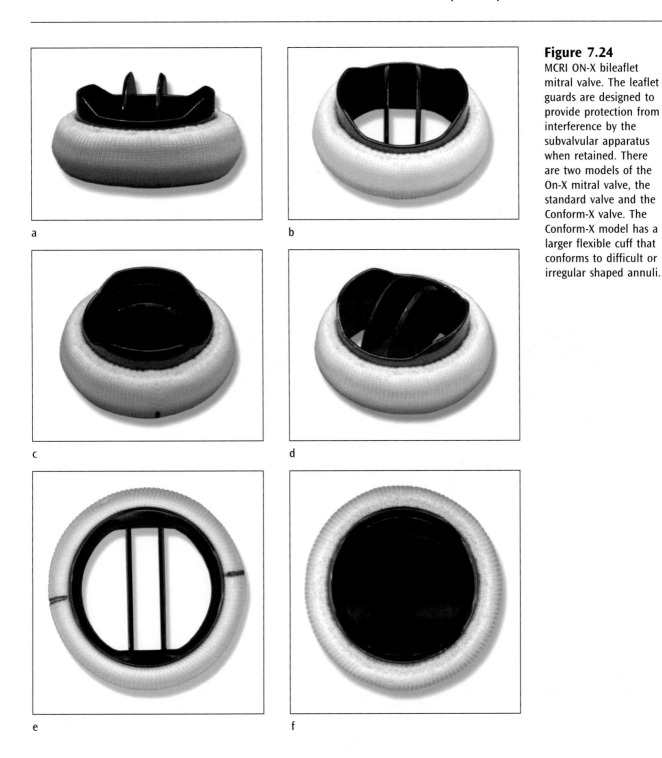

a

b

c

d

e

f

Figure 7.24
MCRI ON-X bileaflet mitral valve. The leaflet guards are designed to provide protection from interference by the subvalvular apparatus when retained. There are two models of the On-X mitral valve, the standard valve and the Conform-X valve. The Conform-X model has a larger flexible cuff that conforms to difficult or irregular shaped annuli.

Hancock bioprosthesis

The Hancock I valve was the first commercially available bioprosthetic valve.[282–291] The Hancock I valve consisted of a preserved whole porcine aortic valve mounted to a rigid metal stent and supported by a sewing ring. Rigid stents produced dehiscence of the valve tissue from its attachments to the stent posts.

In an effort to reduce the strain on the porcine valve and improve durability, the rigid frame was substituted for a flexible polyprolene frame reinforced with a rigid stellite orifice ring. The Hancock valve was continually modified to improve performance and durability. In an attempt to enlarge the effective valve orifice, the septal shelf of the porcine valve was eliminated by removing the right coronary cusp and substituting another

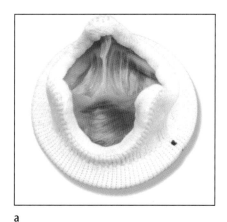
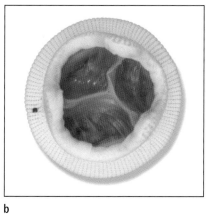
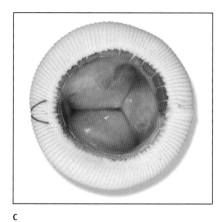

a   b   c

Figure 7.25
Hancock II. The Hancock valve has undergone many changes since it was first introduced to improve performance and durability. In an effort to reduce the strain on the porcine valve during closure promoting improved durability the rigid frame was substituted with a flexible polypropylene reinforced with a rigid stellite orifice ring. In an attempt to enlarge the effective valve orifice the septal shelf of the porcine valve was eliminated by removing the right coronary cusp and substituting another noncoronary cusp from a different valve in the mounting process. Further modifications of the Hancock prosthesis were changes in preservation from formalin fixation, to low-pressure glutaraldehyde and then to high-pressure fixation with glutaraldehyde. Improvements in flexibility lead to 'stent creep' or inward migration of the polyprolene stent post, producing valve obstruction and hemolysis. To prevent 'creep', the stent was replaced with Delrin, an acetyl resin that also allowed a shorter stent profile. The final flexible Hancock II valve, model 410, has a silastic core-sewing ring covered with Dacron material, and knitted polyester fabric stents. The aortic Hancock II valve is scalloped to conform to the natural aortic configuration, allowing the porcine valve leaflets to be mounted above the sewing ring, allowing for a larger orifice in smaller prostheses.

non-coronary cusp from a different valve in the mounting process.

Further modifications of the Hancock prosthesis included changes in preservation, from formalin fixation to low-pressure glutaraldehyde, and subsequently to high-pressure fixation with glutaraldehyde. Improvements in flexibility lead to 'stent creep' or inward migration of the polyprolene stent post, producing valve obstruction and hemolysis. To prevent 'creep', the stent was replaced with Delrin, an acetyl resin that also allowed a shorter stent profile.

The final flexible Hancock II valve, model 410, has a silastic core-sewing ring covered with Dacron material, and knitted polyester fabric stents (Figure 7.25). The aortic Hancock II valve is scalloped to conform to the natural aortic configuration, allowing the porcine valve leaflets to be mounted above the sewing ring and allowing for a larger orifice in smaller prostheses.

Carpentier-Edwards bioprosthesis

Carpentier-Edwards valves[292–299] are constructed from porcine valves preserved with glutaraldehyde and sterilized with formalin, surfactant and alcohol to prevent valve fungus. To minimize the septal bar in the Carpentier-

Edwards valve, it is incorporated into the annulus, making it asymmetric. The stent is constructed of an Elgiloy wire, a corrosion-resistant alloy of cobalt and nickel, which produces maximum flexibility and prevents stent 'creep'. In addition the stent posts of the Carpentier-Edwards valve are asymmetric, accommodating the natural shape of the aortic porcine valve. The sewing rings are composed of silicone rubber and covered with Teflon cloth specifically designed for the mitral or aortic position (Model 6625 or Model 2625, respectively), which further promotes flexibility. Care must be exercised during implantation of these valves since the increased flexibility of the stents and the sewing ring can be distorted, producing abnormal opening or closure of the valve and subsequent obstruction or regurgitation.

In addition to design characteristics, the Edward's laboratory was the first to recognize the inherent differences in each porcine valve, and specifically tested each valve for hydrodynamic standards prior to implant, including leak testing for regurgitation.

Carpentier-Edwards Perimount valve

The Carpentier-Edwards valve[300–305] is a bovine pericardial xenograft, model 2900, comparable in design to the

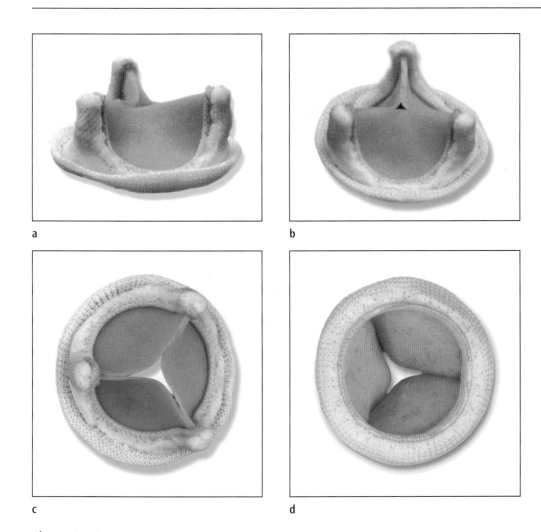

a   b

c   d

Figure 7.26

Carpentier-Edwards Perimount aortic bioprosthesis. The Carpentier-Edwards valve is a bovine pericardial xenograft, model 2900, comparable in design to the Ionescu-Shiley valve. Similar to the Carpentier-Edwards porcine valve, the Perimount valve incorporates an Elgiloy wire stent along with a silicone rubber insert, to promote flexibility as well as conformity to placement in the annulus. The valve is preserved with a buffered glutaraldehyde solution in the same fashion as the porcine valve. Unlike the Ionescu-Shiley valve the Perimount valve employs a novel and different attachment technique of pericardial tissue to stents, which appears to have eliminated the major problem associated with the Ionescu-Shiley valve of the separation of the leaflet from the supporting stent. The valve also comes in a SAV model for supra-annular placement.

Ionescu-Shiley valve. Similar to the Carpentier-Edwards porcine valve, the Perimount valve incorporates an Elgiloy wire stent with a silicone rubber insert, to promote flexibility as well as conform to placement in the annulus (Figures 7.26 and 7.27). The valve is preserved with a buffered glutaraldehyde solution in the same fashion as the porcine valve. Unlike the Ionescu-Shiley valve, the Perimount valve employs a novel and different attachment technique of pericardial tissue to stents, which may have eliminated the major problem associated with the Ionescu-Shiley valve.

Toronto SPV valve

The Toronto SPV valve is a stentless prosthesis created from a porcine aortic valve.[306–309] The porcine valve is cross-linked and sterilized in a glutaraldehyde solution. The sinuses of the Toronto SPV valve are scalloped and the whole valve is wrapped in a polyester fabric. The valve is sutured directly to the aortic root, which serves as the valve's stent, with the scalloped design allowing the preservation of the native sinuses (Figure 7.28).

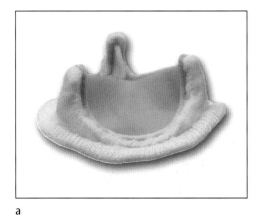

a

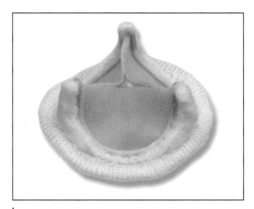

b

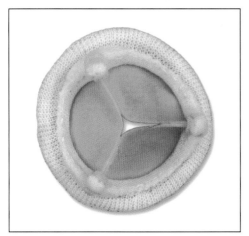

c

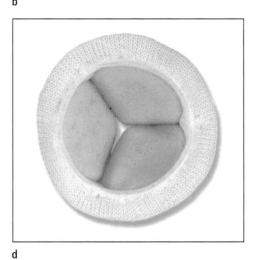

d

Figure 7.27
Carpentier-Edwards Duraflex Low Pressure Porcine Mitral bioprosthesis. The mitral and aortic valve is constructed with a XenoLogiX treatment which is thought to reduce phospholipids content to prevent calcification. The mitral valve receives a low pressure fixation to decrease the stress of the valve. The mitral model has an extended sewing ring to provide a larger surface area for attaching to the native annulus.

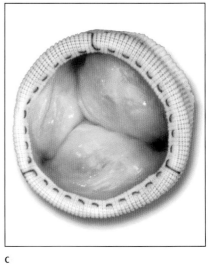

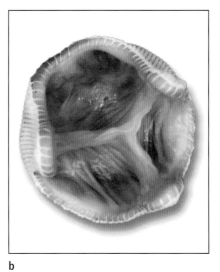

a   b   c

Figure 7.28
The St. Jude Toronto SPV® valve is a stentless prosthesis created from a porcine aortic valve. The porcine valve is cross-linked and sterilized in a glutaraldehyde solution. The sinuses of the Toronto SPV® valve are scalloped and the whole valve is wrapped in a polyester fabric to aid in suturing and securing the valve to the aorta. The valve is sutured directly to the aortic root, which serves as a substitute for the valve stents, with a scalloped design allowing for the preservation of the native sinuses.

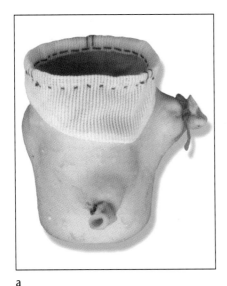
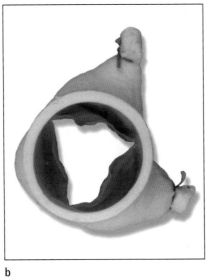
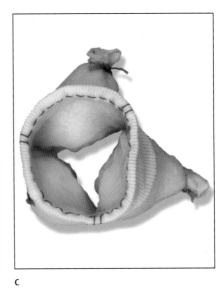

a   b   c

Figure 7.29
The Medtronic Freestyle valve uses the entire porcine aortic root with the valve. The total root design allows the surgeon to use the prosthesis for a full root replacement, tailor the prosthesis for the subcoronary technique where the valve is sculpted to fit around the coronaries or implanted as a root inclusion placing the prosthesis inside the native aorta. The porcine prosthesis is treated with an anti-mineralization process and fixed in glutaraldehyde rather than the typical pressure-fixed bioprosthesis. The total prosthesis is covered with polyester to strengthen and isolate the porcine myocardial tissue from the native aorta.

Transesophageal echocardiography is instrumental in determining the appropriate size of the valve prior to implant. Unlike homograft valves, where the size is determined in relationship to the aortic annulus, the Toronto SPV valve is sized through measurements of the sinotubular junction and the aortic annulus to allow the best spatial relationships of the three commissures. Pre-operative echocardiographic assessment includes measuring the dimensions of the aortic root as well as assessing the aortic root for excessive calcification, which could interfere with valve implantation or allow distortion of the prosthesis following implantation.

Post-bypass echocardiographic evaluation includes evaluation of the presence of regurgitation, and left ventricular size and function using the standard imaging views for the aortic valve. The Toronto SPV valve, once implanted, has the echocardiographical appearance of a normal native aortic valve. The valve prosthesis should be evaluated for normal leaflet motion with complete leaflet coaptation during closure. Immediately following surgery, the aortic root appears thickened, due to edema or hematoma that occurs with the trauma of surgical implantation. Occasionally this may influence the postoperative dimension of the left ventricular outflow tract. Serial assessment of the prosthesis has shown that thickening of the aortic root walls regress over time.

Color flow Doppler is helpful in determining transvalvular aortic regurgitation as well as near-normal antegrade flow through the prosthesis. Paravalvular leaks are rare.

Medtronic Freestyle aortic root bioprosthesis

The Freestyle valve uses the entire porcine aortic root with the valve (Figure 7.29).[310–313] The total root design allows the surgeon to use the prosthesis for a full root replacement, to tailor the prosthesis for the subcoronary placement where the valve is sculpted to fit around the coronaries, or implant it as a root inclusion, placing the prosthesis inside the native aorta. The porcine prosthesis is treated with an antimineralization process and fixed in glutaraldehyde rather than the typical pressure-fixed bioprosthesis. The total prosthesis is covered with polyester to strengthen and isolate the porcine myocardial tissue from the native aorta. Similar to homografts and other stentless prostheses, echocardiographically the Freestyle valve resembles the native aortic valve, irrespective of which surgical technique is employed. When these valves are implanted with the root inclusion technique and occasionally with the subcoronary approach, a double lumen may be visualized between the prosthesis and the native aortic wall. In the post-pump echocardiogram, minimal or mild aortic regurgitation is seen in approximately 50% of patients, which frequently resolves during early follow-up. Small paravalvular leaks may be seen in the post-pump echo, which also usually resolve over time.

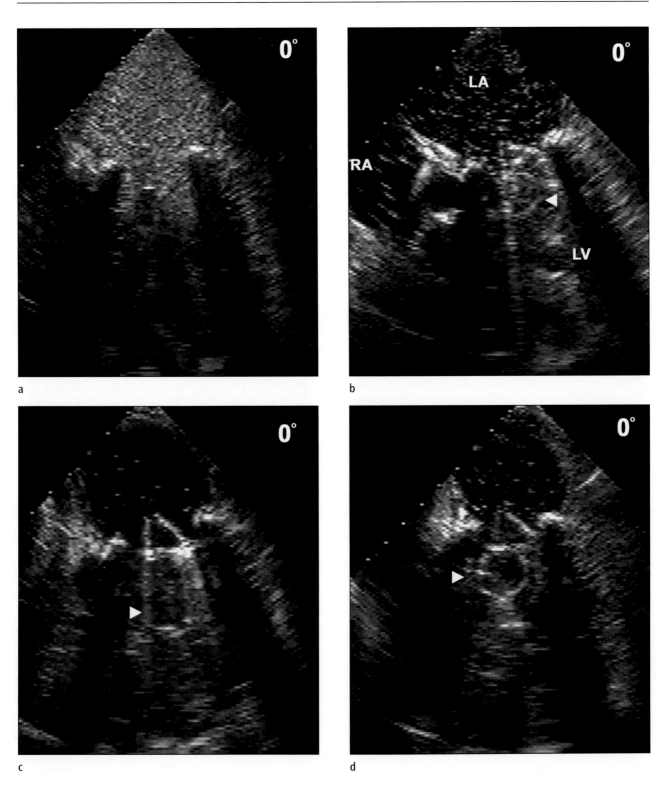

a

b

c

d

Case 7.1

Transesophageal echocardiography plays a major role in determining the success of valve replacement. A. Four-chamber view from the lower esophageal window immediately after closure of the left atrium and at the start of weaning from bypass. Contrast fills the left atrium demonstrating sluggish flow within the left atrium with the start of valve motion. B, C. With continuous observation the echocardiographic contrast clears with resumption of cardiac function. The two leaflets of the St. Jude mitral prosthesis opening and closing during the cardiac cycle. D. During the weaning process a left ventricular vent balloon catheter (arrow) is visualized across the mitral prosthesis which promotes the evacuation of retained air from the left ventricle and left atrium.

continued

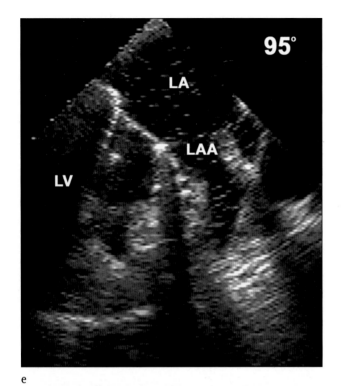

e

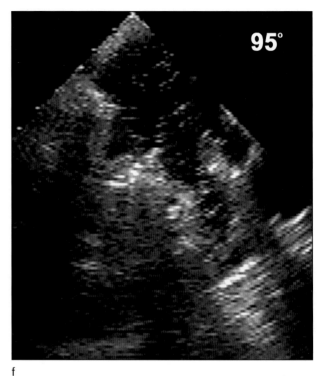

f

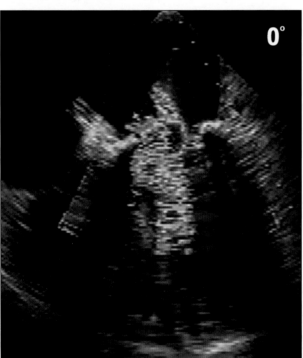

g

Case 7.1 *continued*

E, F. Two-chamber view demonstrating the St. Jude mitral prosthesis in a plane 90 degrees to the previous views. Only one leaflet is seen opening during the systolic frame (E) and closing during the diastolic frame (F) secondary to the vent crossing the valve. G. Color flow Doppler of the four-chamber view demonstrating diastolic flow across the valve before removal of the left ventricular vent catheter. LA, left atrium; LV, left ventricle; LAA, left atrial appendage; RA, right atrium.

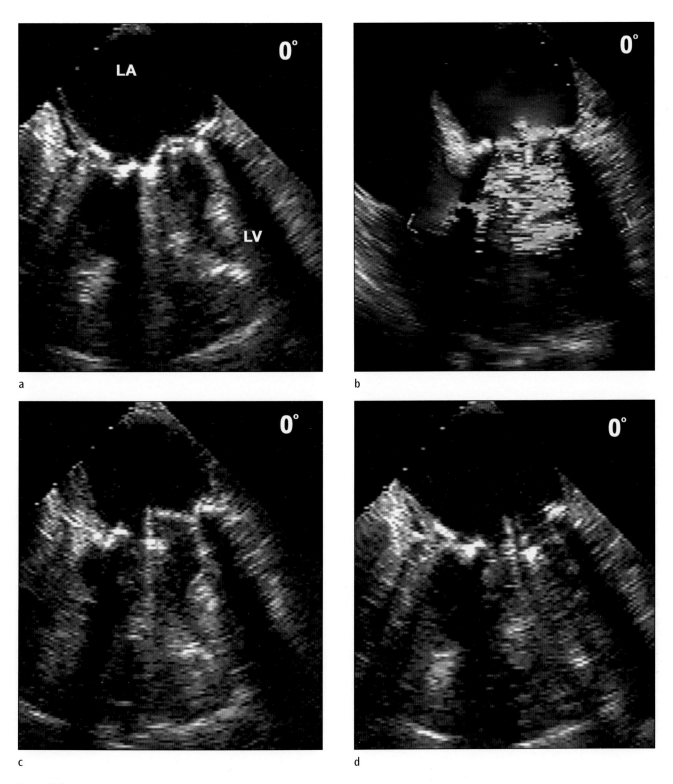

Case 7.2

Post-operative evaluation of a St. Jude bileaflet mitral prosthesis. A. Four-chamber view demonstrating the normal leaflet closure configuration following weaning from bypass. The valve leaflets, sewing ring and native annulus are easily visualized with transesophageal echocardiography in this view. B. Four-chamber view with color Doppler demonstrating forward flow through the prosthetic orifices. Forward flow demonstrates a mosaic pattern as flow mixes in the left ventricle. Flow convergence is noted on the left atrial side of the valve demonstrating the three orifices of the bileaflet valve. C–D. Only one leaflet is opening and closing normally with the other leaflet demonstrating delayed motion in reference to the normally moving leaflet. This is a frequent finding immediately following weaning which is due to low atrial pressure upon weaning of cardiopulmonary bypass.

continued

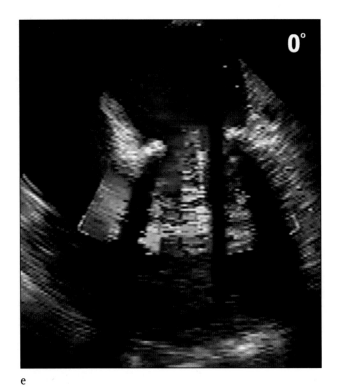

e

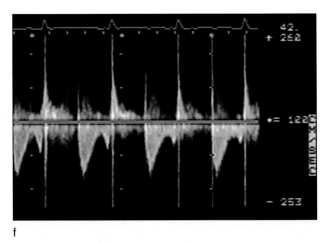

f

Case 7.2 *continued*

E. Color flow Doppler through the mitral prosthesis with only one leaflet opening demonstrating most of the flow through the side of the normally moving leaflet. F. Continuous wave Doppler interrogation in the same view. Note the regurgitant jet with lower velocity forward flow than is expected that is recorded through the valve orifice. LA, left atrium; LV, left ventricle.

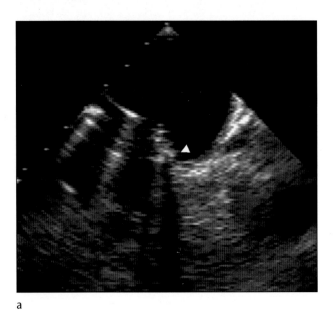

a

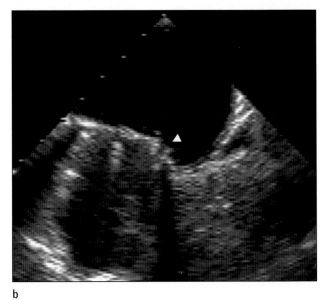

b

Case 7.3

St. Jude periprosthetic leak. Small periprosthetic leak which occurs between the native annulus and outer surface of the prosthetic valve sewing ring are frequently detected post-op. Many disappear with the endothelialization process that occurs with the valve ring. In mitral valve replacements periprosthetic leaks frequently occur in the posterior portion of the annulus and this is frequently associated with the loss of the normal oval orifice caused by annular calcification. A distorted annulus due to calcification may present a problem technically in approximating the sewing ring and may promote stress and breakage of the suture ring. A. Normal opening of a bileaflet valve. B. Normal closure of the valve, note the area of separation (dehiscence) between the sewing ring and the native annulus.

continued

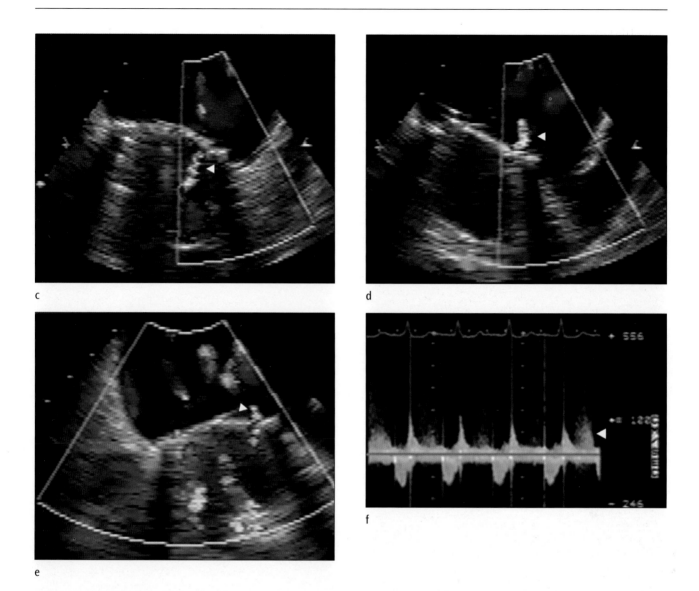

c

d

e

f

Case 7.3 *continued*

C. Color flow Doppler demonstrates the defect as a real communication between the left atrium and ventricle. D, E. Color flow Doppler demonstrating regurgitant flow from the defect which is distinct from the physiological regurgitation expected with a bileaflet valve in two planes 90 degrees apart. E. Small colour Doppler flow disturbances are seen on both leaflet surfaces of the bileaflet valve ring. Note the small transvalvular jets in the left atrium originating from each orifice of the bileaflet valve in distinction to the paravalvular leak. F. Continuous wave Doppler through the defect demonstrating a small paravalvular leak in the first and last beats.

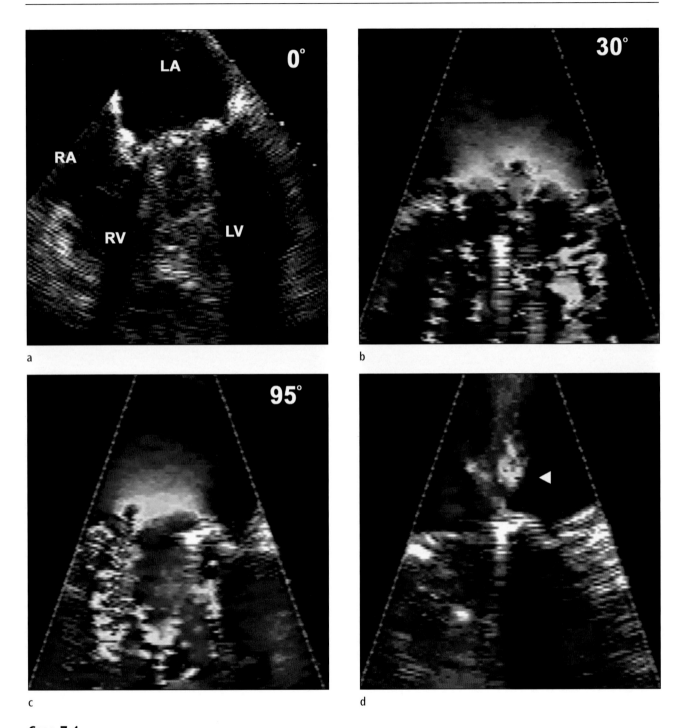

Case 7.4

St. Jude mitral prosthesis with pannus formation and a paravalvular leak. A. Four-chamber view demonstrating a St. Jude prosthesis in the mitral position. B. Normal color flow Doppler from the four-chamber view demonstrating flow convergence through the three orifices and (C) lateral view at 95 degrees during diastole. D. Systolic flow in the lateral portion demonstrating small transvalvular jets.

continued

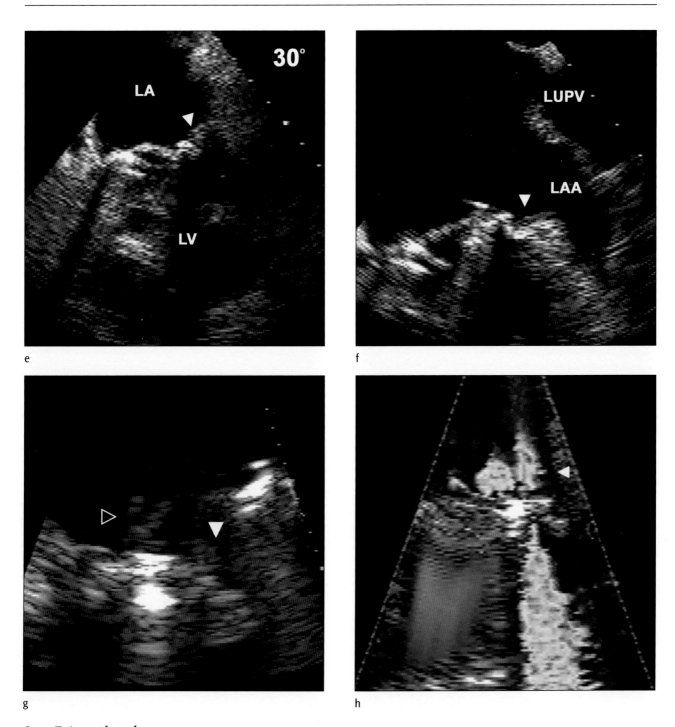

e   f

g   h

Case 7.4 *continued*

E. At 30 degrees a small defect (arrow) is noted near the lateral portion of the sewing ring. F. Magnified view demonstrating a defect (arrow) between the sewing ring and the native annulus in the approximate area of the atrial appendage. Noting specific cardiac landmarks and the vicinity of the defect aids the cardiac surgeon if repair is contemplated. G. With further magnification a shaggy hypodense echogenicity is noted around the sewing ring representing pannus formation. Pannus formation may not be readily distinguishable from vegetation with transesophageal echocardiography. H. Color flow Doppler demonstrates a high velocity forward flow jet through the defect which was responsible for significant hemolysis which initially led to the transesophageal echocardiography evaluation. LA, left atrium; RA, right atrium; LV, left ventricle; RV, right ventricle; LAA, left atrial appendage; LUPV, left upper pulmonary vein.

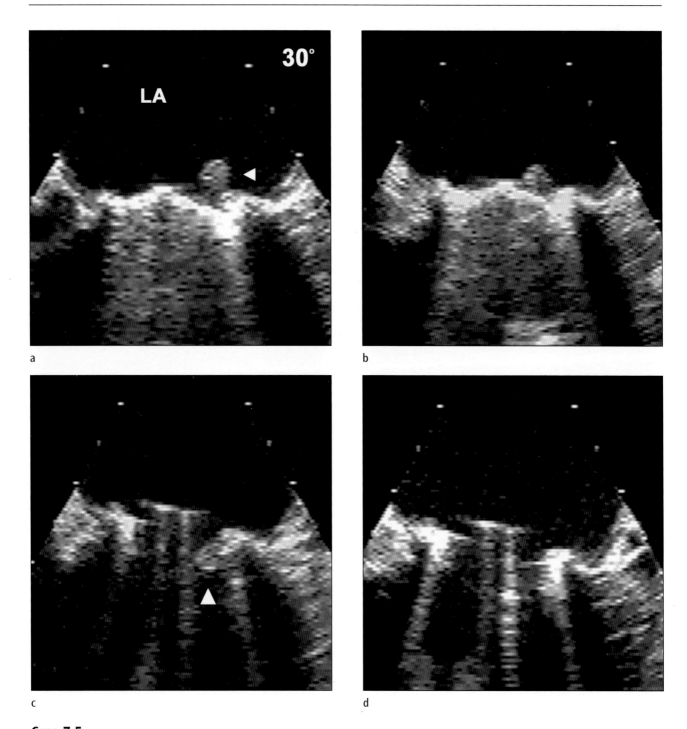

Case 7.5

Bileaflet prosthetic valve vegetation. Vegetations tend to demonstrate more motion, have a denser echogenicity and are usually better defined than pannus formation. These characteristics may be easily identified with transesophageal echocardiography especially in magnified images. A–D. A small oval mass (arrow) is demonstrated on the leaflet surface of the bileaflet valve which prolapsed back and forth through the valve orifice during the cardiac cycle consistent with vegetation. This diagnosis was confirmed at the time of surgery. LA, left atrium.

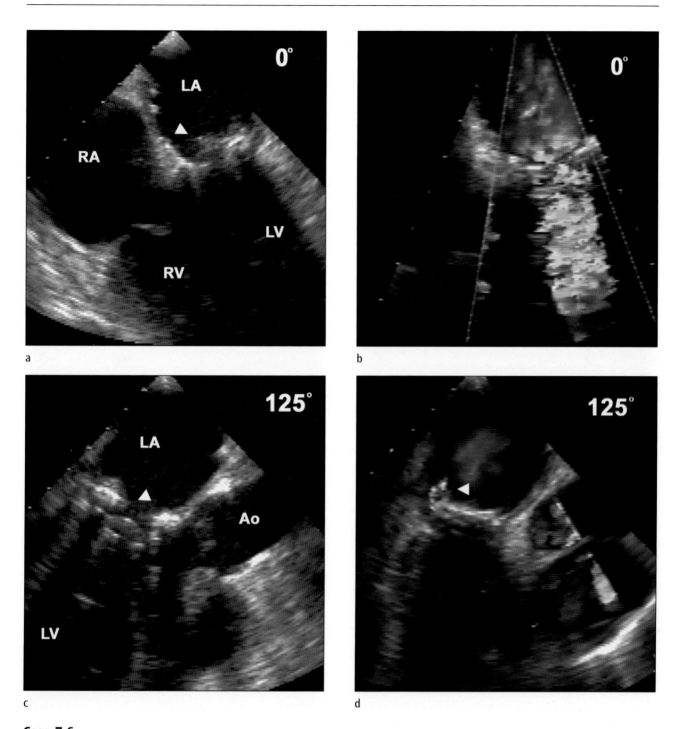

a

b

c

d

Case 7.6

Prosthetic disk valve pannus. A. Large shaggy, hypoechoic mass on the atrial surface of a bileaflet prosthesis in a four-chamber view at 0 degrees consistent with pannus in-growth and deterioration of the sewing ring. B. Color flow Doppler demonstrates a high velocity turbulent jet denoting obstruction of the valve orifice produced by the mass. C. Two-chamber view demonstrating pannus (arrow) narrowing of the orifice. D. Color flow Doppler demonstrates a small defect (arrow) in the posterior region of the annulus consistent with a small paravalvular leak (arrow). LA, left atrium; RA, right atrium; LV, left ventricle; RV, right ventricle; Ao, aorta.

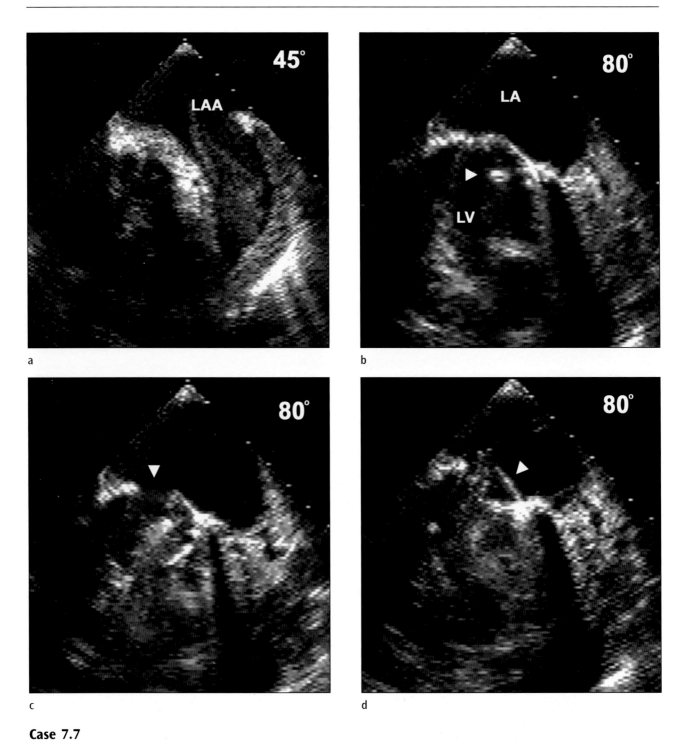

a

b

c

d

Case 7.7

St. Jude mitral prosthesis with a fixed leaflet. A. Spontaneous echocardiographic contrast filling the left atrial appendage denoting sluggish flow in the atrium. B. Echogenic mass (arrow) noted in the inflow area of the prosthesis with the valve in the closed position. C. During diastole only one leaflet (arrow) is noted to be opening. D. The other leaflet (arrow) was stuck in the closed position due to interference from the subvalvular apparatus.

continued

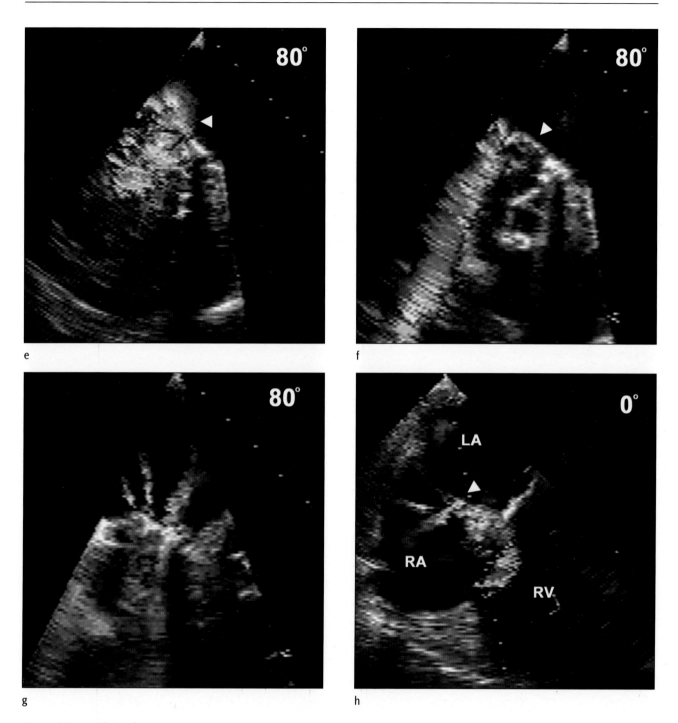

e   f

g   h

Case 7.7 *continued*

E. Color flow Doppler demonstrating only two areas of flow convergent (arrow) on the valve atrial surface, (F) with absence of flow through the fixed leaflet (arrow). G. During systole the valve demonstrated two normal physiological jets with a wide disturbed jet emanating from the fixed leaflet suggesting the leaflet was stuck in a semi closed position. H. A small continuous left-to-right shunt (arrow) was demonstrated through a patent foramen ovale and related to the high left atrial pressure created from the obstruction produced from the fixed leaflet. LAA, left atrial appendage; LA, left atrium; LV, left ventricle; RA, right atrium; RV, right ventricle.

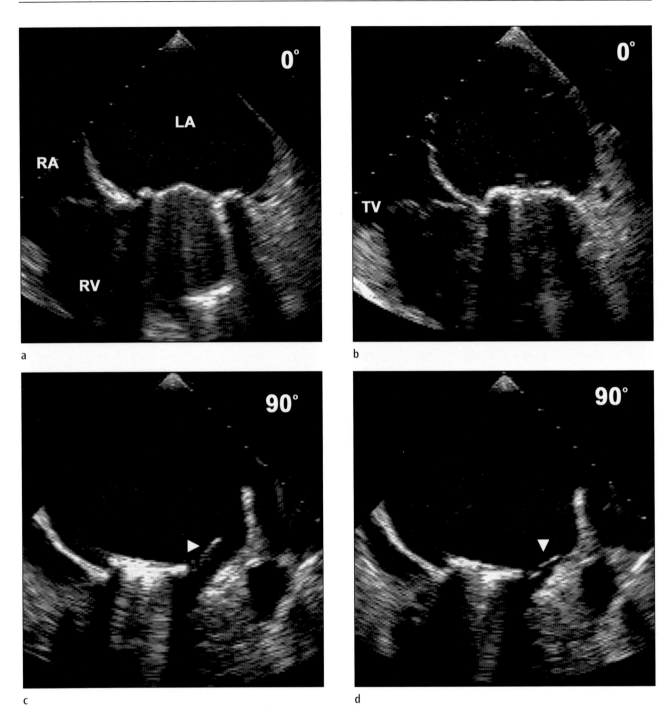

Case 7.8

Bileaflet mitral prosthesis with fibrous strands. A–D. Four-chamber view of a bileaflet mitral prosthesis during systole. Concentrating on the sewing ring and with rotation of the transducer multiple small linear fibrous strands (arrow) which exhibit chaotic motion are detected emanating on the atrial surface of the valve. Fibrous strands may represent pannus formation, or loose suture material, and need to be differentiated from vegetation. LA, left atrium; RA, right atrium; RV, right ventricle.

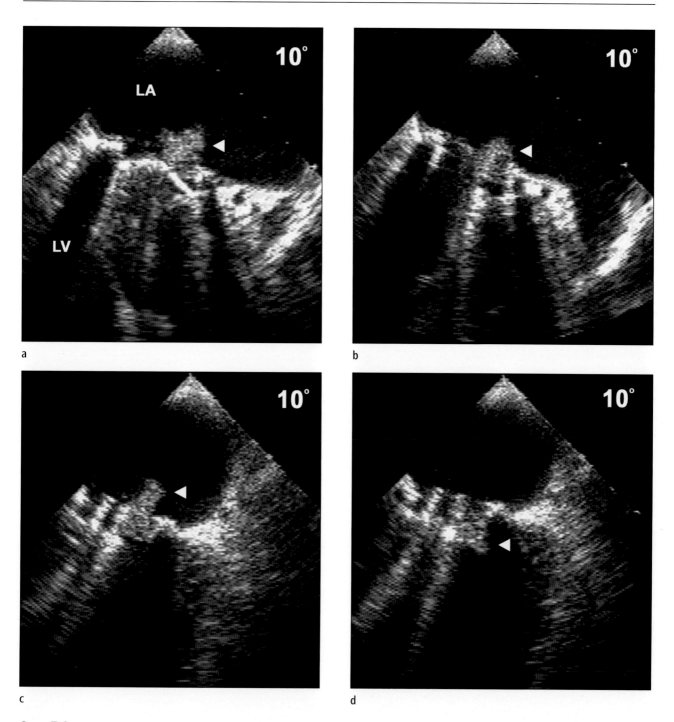

a

b

c

d

Case 7.9

Bileaflet mitral prosthesis with vegetation. Large echogenic mass (arrow) adherent to the atrial surface of bileaflet valve during systole. B–D. The mass (arrow) prolapses back and forth through the valve orifice during the cardiac cycle.

continued

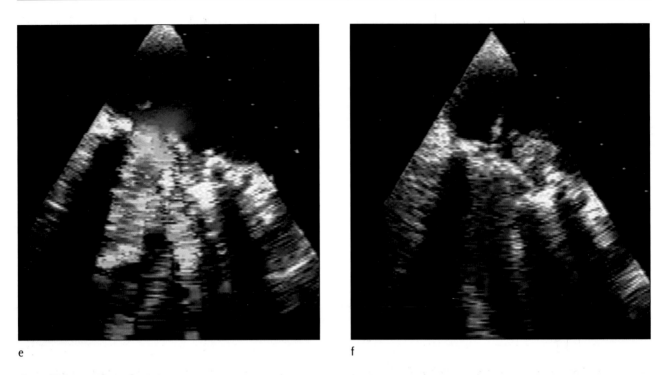

e

f

Case 7.9 *continued*

E. Color flow Doppler demonstrates a high velocity turbulent jet during diastole. Note color flow outlines and highlights the mass within the valve orifice. F. Color flow Doppler during systole demonstrating a lack of normal transvalvular regurgitation through the valve due to the mass. At the time of surgery the mass was consistent with a staphylococcus vegetation. LA, left atrium; LV, left ventricle.

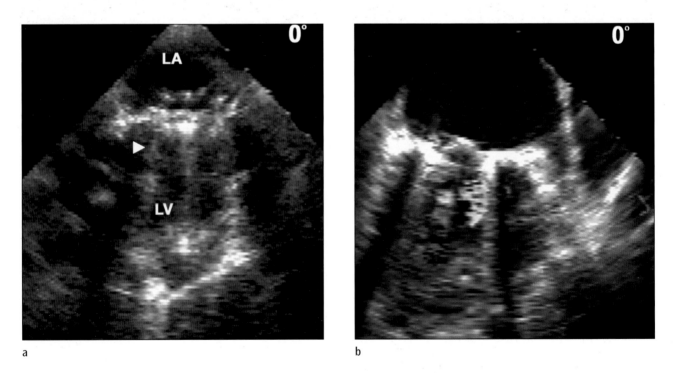

a

b

Case 7.10

Tilting disk valve with obstructing mass. A. Modified four-chamber view produced by retroflexion of the probe at 0 degrees which obliquely visualizes the sewing ring of a Medtronic-Hall valve. The normal artifact produced by the occluding disk is distorted (arrow). B. With color flow Doppler an obstructing mass is demonstrated in the minor orifice.

continued

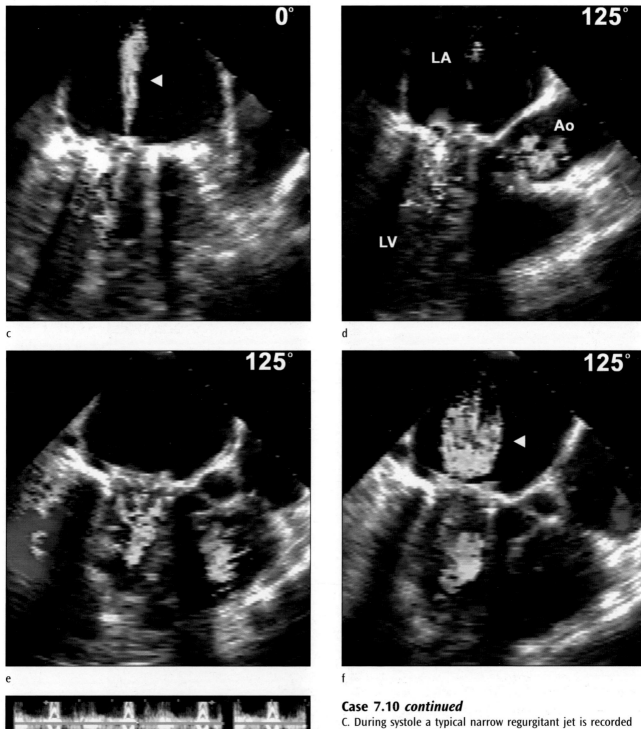

Case 7.10 *continued*
C. During systole a typical narrow regurgitant jet is recorded through the central hole in the disk. D, E. High velocity forward flow jet is recorded through the prosthetic valve. F. An abnormal regurgitant jet (arrow) emanates from the minor valve orifice demonstrating lack of closure of the disk due to the mass. G. Continuous-wave interrogation through the prosthetic valve demonstrates a delayed peaking, high velocity jet at 4 m/sec during diastole. LA, left atrium; LV, left ventricle; Ao, aorta.

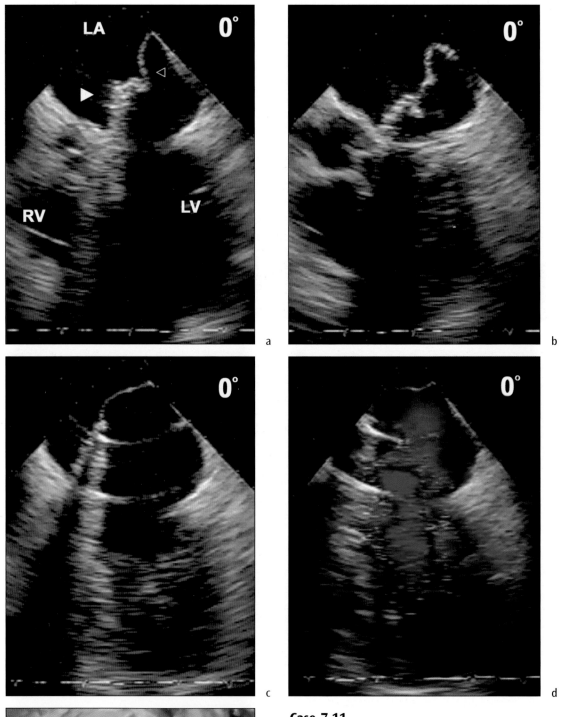

Case 7.11

AV groove dehiscence. Disruption of the atrial or ventricular wall may occur with prosthetic valve implantation. This occurs more frequently with high profile prostheses. Dehiscence with a St. Jude mitral prosthesis, on the fifth post-operative day presenting with hemodynamic collapse. A–C. Four-chamber view demonstrating the St. Jude mitral sewing ring (closed arrow) elevated from the native annular position (open arrow) swinging with the cardiac cycle. D. Color flow Doppler demonstrating flow in the area of the atrial wall disruption. E. Post-mortem anatomical preparation demonstrating the pocket (star) formed between the prosthesis sewing ring and the annular attachment producing a dissecting plane in the atrial wall. LA, left atrium; LV, left ventricle; RV, right ventricle.

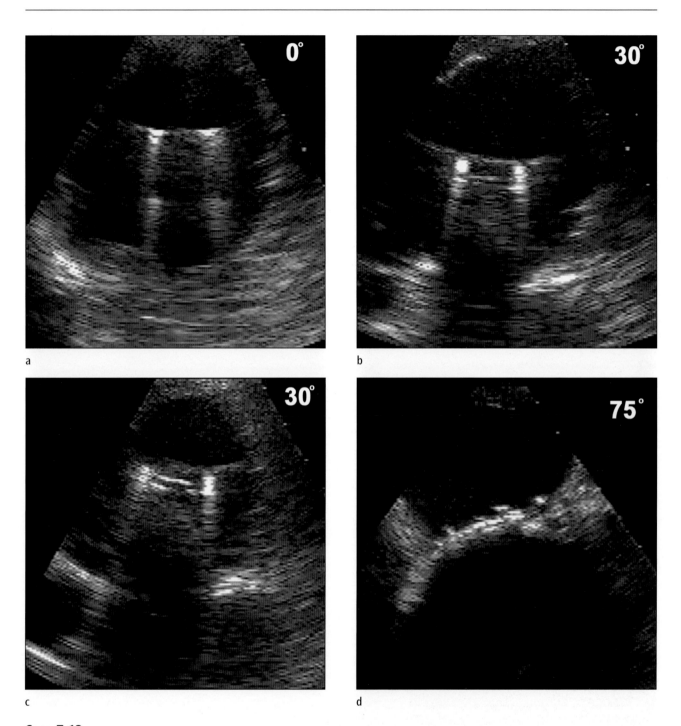

a

b

c

d

Case 7.12

Starr-Edwards mitral ball valve. Normal echocardiographic demonstration of a ball cage valve in the mitral position. A–C. Normal appearance of the valve struts in longitudinal views. Note the poppet movement (circular artifact of the superior portion of the ball) during the cardiac cycle. D. Magnification of the sewing ring. Doppler color flow imaging defines two parallel lines of flow around the ball profile that converge downstream after the apex of the cage. An area of stagnant or vertical flow is produced behind the ball. To obtain the highest velocities of forward flow through the valve the conventional Doppler must be directed to the lateral margins of the ball. Physiological regurgitation of the valve is limited to backflow produced by the ball movement during closure and results in a 'puff of smoke' appearance on color flow Doppler.

continued

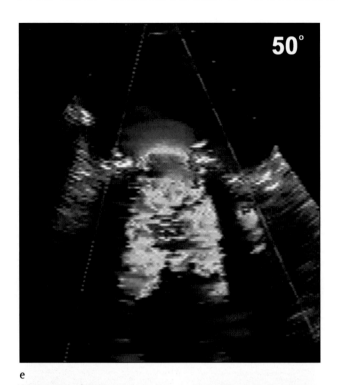

e

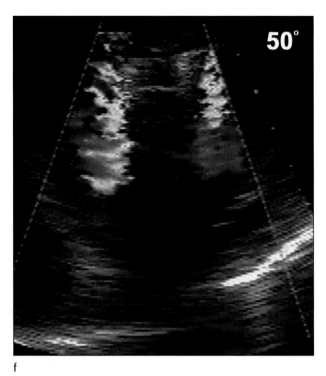

f

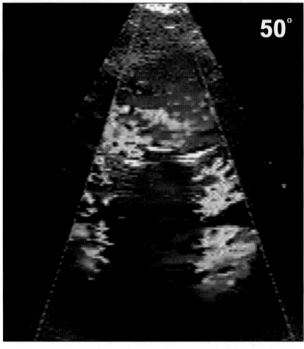

g

Case 7.12 *continued*

E–G. Normal diastolic color flow Doppler through the ball cage valve orifice. E. Initial diastolic frames demonstrate flow convergence at the valve orifice. F, G. Inflow produces the appearance of two jets that parallel the ball movement during opening.

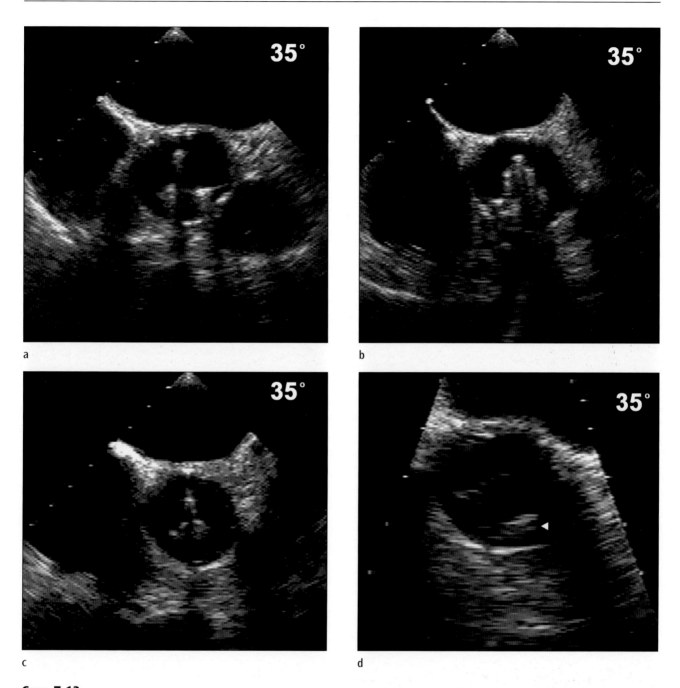

a

b

c

d

Case 7.13

Starr-Edwards aortic ball valve. Normal echocardiographic demonstration of a ball cage valve in short-axis from the basal view. A. Three struts are arranged in a triangular fashion in the center of the ascending aorta. B, C. During systole the ball artifact obscures the normal strut appearance. D. In another patient a large echodense mass (arrow) is depicted within the sewing ring in the short-axis basal view.

continued

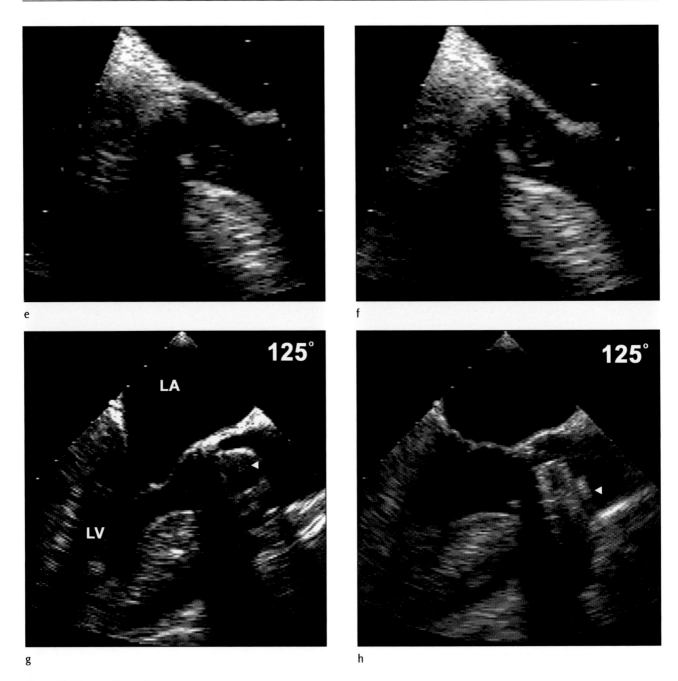

Case 7.13 *continued*

E, F. In a longitudinal projection at 0 degrees the mass is seen prolapsing into the left ventricular outflow tract. G–I. In a longitudinal view at 125 degrees the cage artifact is demonstrated with non-descript echogenicity (arrow) situated within the valve cage.

continued

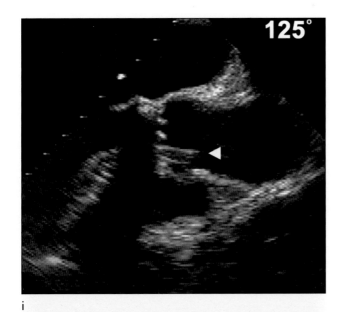

i

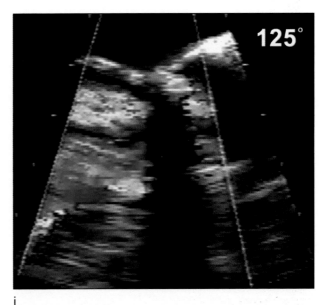

j

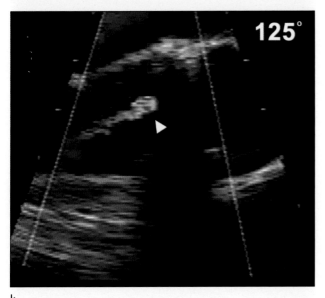

k

Case 7.13 *continued*

J, K. Color flow Doppler demonstrates aortic regurgitation. During replacement deterioration of the sewing ring and cloth was discovered which was covered with pannus and thrombus in a patient that did not receive anticoagulation. Despite the lack of anticoagulation the valve was implanted for 15 years without apparent embolic event. LA, left atrium; LV, left ventricle.

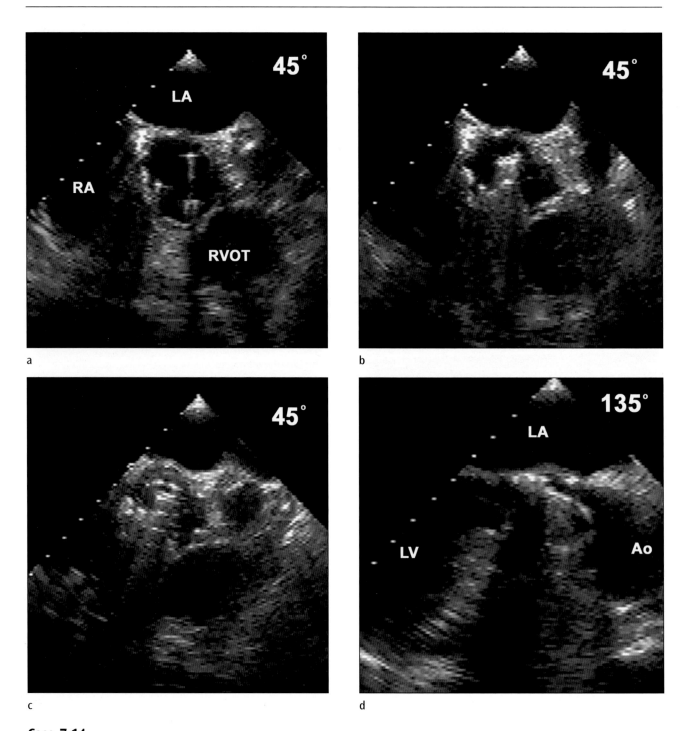

a

b

c

d

Case 7.14

Starr-Edwards aortic cloth covered ball valve. The model 2300 valve was totally cloth-covered (Dacron and Teflon) so there was no exposed metal on the base, orifice or cage. These valves exhibited suboptimal hemodynamics and strut cloth tears due to wear between the inner portion of the struts and a metal ball. The model 2400 valve had a single layer of loosely knit, thin polypropylene stretched over the struts except along the narrow inner track where the ball contacts only the Stellite cage. It is important to know the model number of the valve being examined in order to fully evaluate the valve's characteristics. A–C. Short-axis basal view of a model 2400 valve. D. Longitudinal views at 135 degrees.

continued

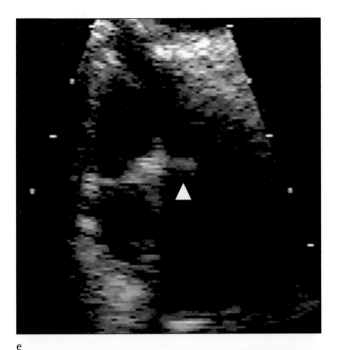

e

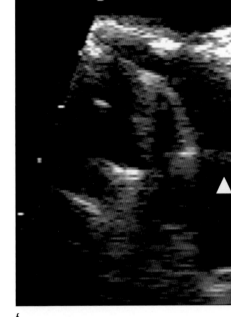

f

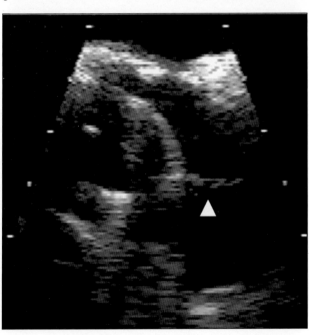

g

Case 7.14 *continued*

E–G. In zoom (magnification) mode and minor manipulation of the probe small chaotic projections (arrow) emanate from the valve cage struts demonstrating cloth wear. LA, left atrium; RA, right atrium; RVOT, right ventricular output tract.

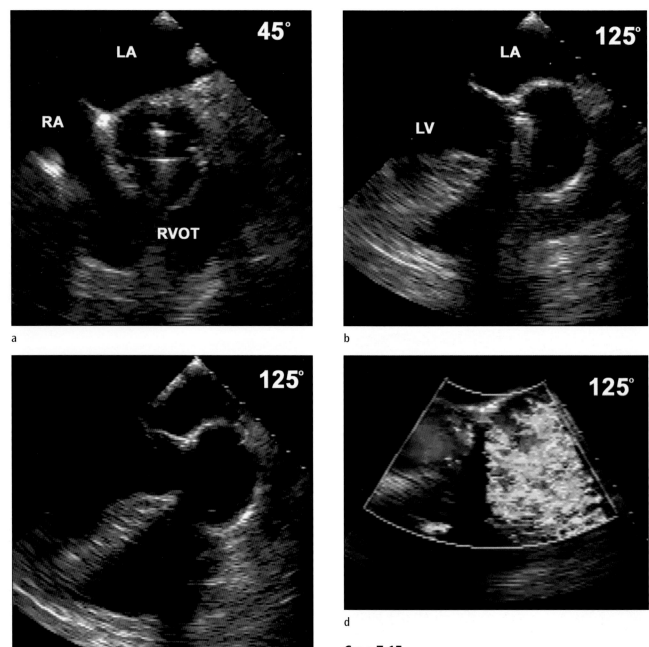

a

b

c

d

Case 7.15
Björk-Shiley aortic and mitral prosthesis. A. Short-axis view at the aortic valve level 45 degrees. Normal appearance of a Björk-Shiley aortic valve. B. Longitudinal diastolic and (C) systolic frames at 125 degrees demonstrating a normal Björk-Shiley valve. D. Color flow Doppler of a normal Björk-Shiley valve during systole demonstrating turbulent forward flow through the valve during systole filling the aortic root.

continued

Case 7.15 *continued*

E. M-mode taken through the aortic valve plane. F. Two-chamber view of a mitral Björk-Shiley valve during diastole and (G) during systole. H. Color flow Doppler demonstrating two forward flow jets through the major and minor orifice of the Björk-Shiley valve.

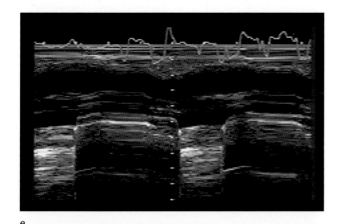

e

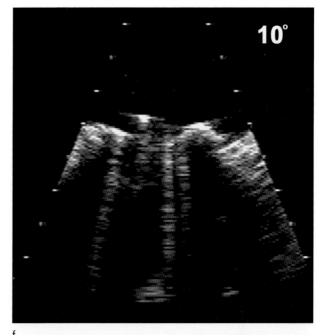

f

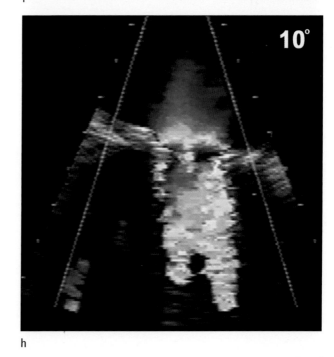

g

h

continued

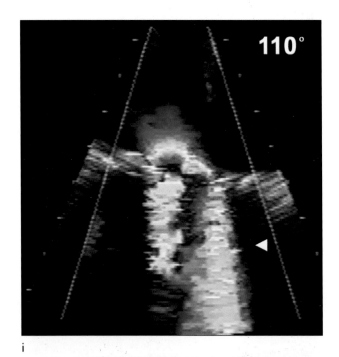

i

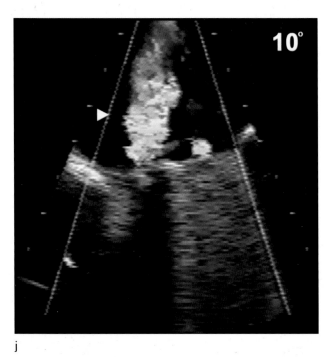

j

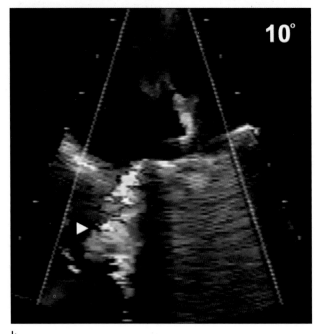

k

Case 7.15 *continued*

I. Color flow Doppler through the mitral prosthesis demonstrating flow convergence during early systole and a small periprosthetic leak (arrow) at 110 degrees. J. Normal regurgitation from the mitral prosthesis emanating from the minor and major orifice. K. At 10 degrees a small periprosthetic leak is also detected in addition to the normal leak. LA, left atrium; RA, right atrium; RVOT, right ventricular outflow tract; AV, aortic valve prosthesis.

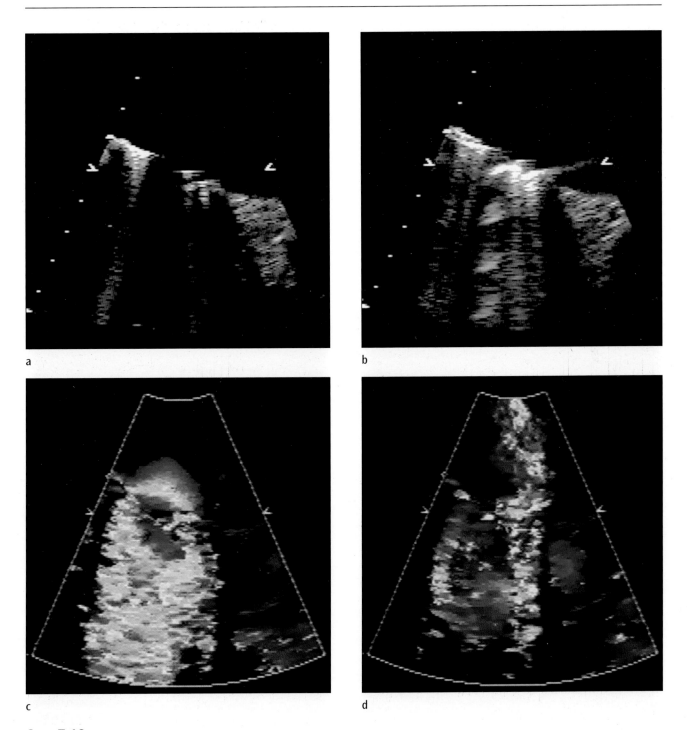

a

b

c

d

Case 7.16

Björk-Shiley mitral valve with pannus formation. A, B. Opening and closing of the valve. C. Color-flow Doppler during diastole demonstrating an accentuated disturbed turbulent flow jet. D. Severe regurgitation is created during systole as the valve does not close properly due to the pannus in-growth.

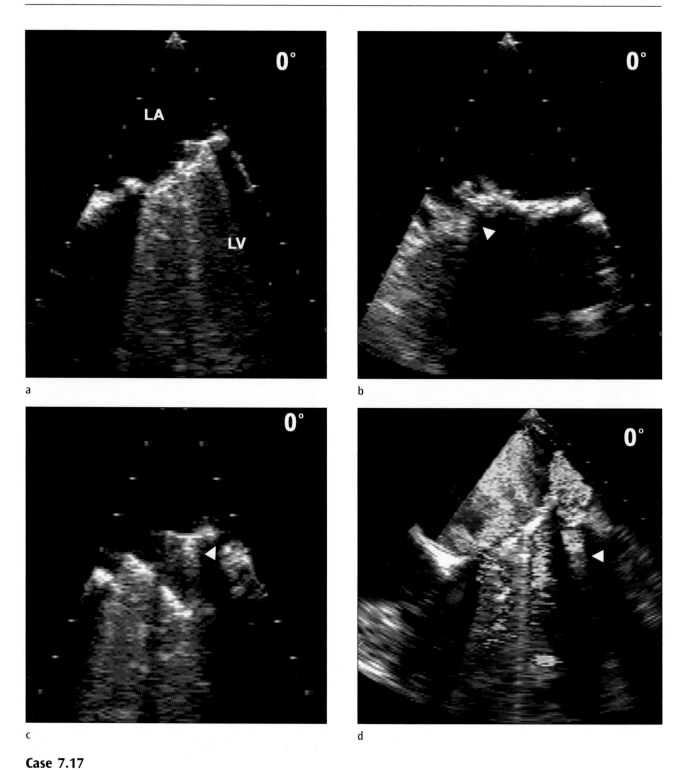

Case 7.17

Mitral tilting disk prosthesis with paravalvular regurgitation. A. Closed mitral tilting disk prosthesis in four-chamber view at 0 degrees. B, C. Defects with shaggy echo masses are detected in the lateral portion of the sewing ring between the natural annulus and the sewing ring. D. Color flow Doppler documents a paravalvular leak in the area of one of the defects.

continued

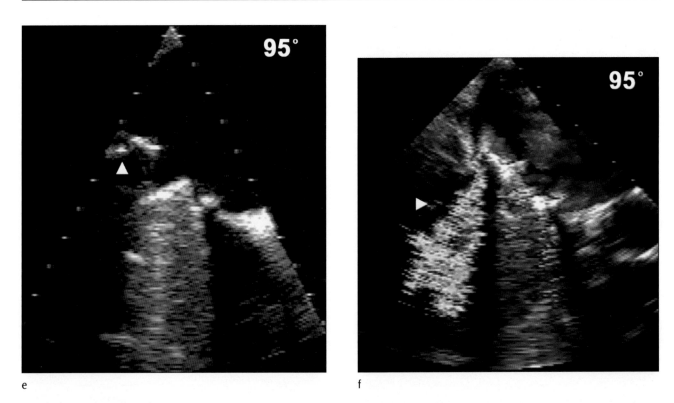

e   f

Case 7.17 *continued*

E. Rotation of the transducer to 95 degrees demonstrates the defect from a different plane and (F) color flow Doppler demonstrates high velocity, turbulent forward flow trough the defect which was associated with hemolysis. LA, left atrium; LV, left ventricle.

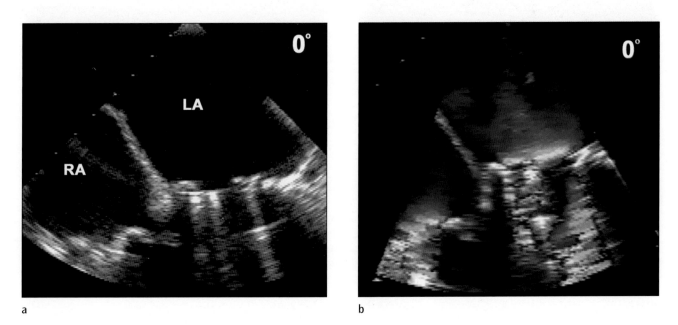

a   b

Case 7.18

Björk-Shiley mitral (tilting disk) prosthesis and a tricuspid prosthesis associated with a severely calcified mitral and tricuspid annulus. A. Four-chamber view of the tilting mitral prosthesis and a tricuspid prosthesis with heavy calcification of the native annulus of both valves. B. Color flow Doppler demonstrating forward flow through the prosthesis and tricuspid ring. Note two areas of flow convergence through the mitral prosthesis and one area through the tricuspid orifice.

continued

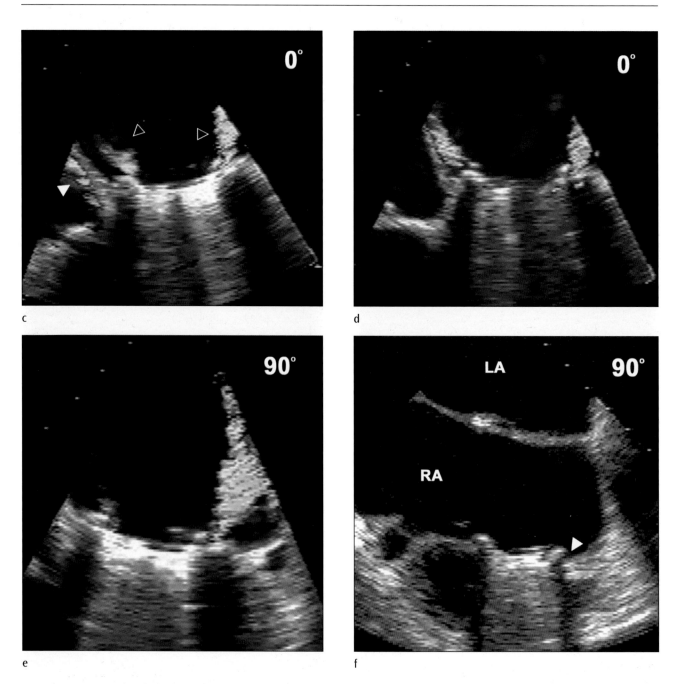

Case 7.18 *continued*

C. Small regurgitant jets (open arrows) associated with the mitral prosthesis and an eccentric tricuspid prosthetic regurgitant jet (closed arrow). D. Mild rotation of the probe demonstrates one of the jets as a small paraprosthetic leak. E. Rotation of the transducer to 90 degrees illustrates the full perspective of the periprosthetic leak. F. Bicaval atrial view concentrating on the tricuspid valve visualizing a defect between the sewing ring and the native annulus.

continued

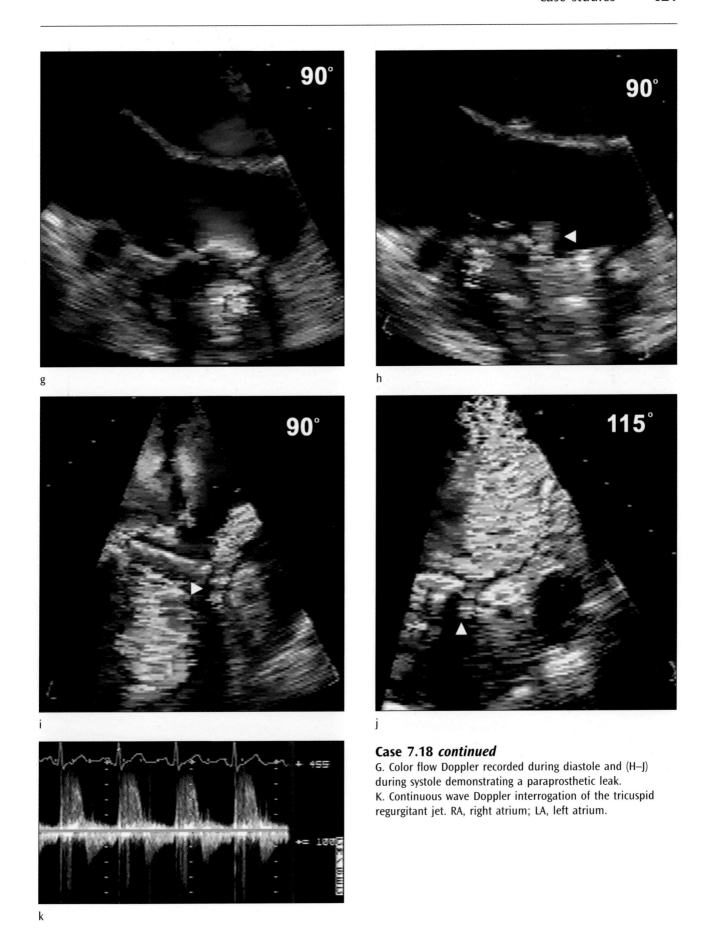

Case 7.18 *continued*
G. Color flow Doppler recorded during diastole and (H–J)
during systole demonstrating a paraprosthetic leak.
K. Continuous wave Doppler interrogation of the tricuspid
regurgitant jet. RA, right atrium; LA, left atrium.

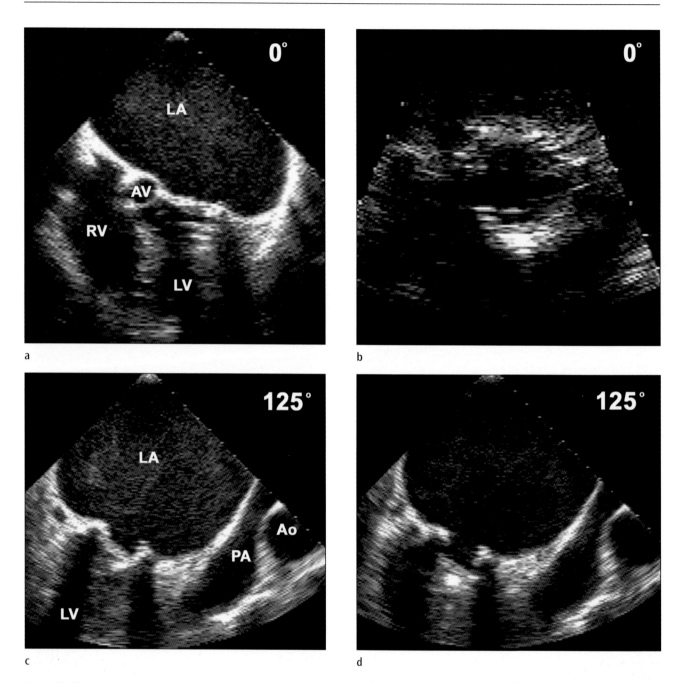

Case 7.19

Tilting disk mitral mechanical prosthesis. A. Four-chamber view demonstrating a closed mitral prosthesis. B. Modified short-axis view demonstrating the sewing ring enface. C, D. Two-chamber view at 125 degrees demonstrates dense echocardiographic smoke in the left atrium during systole with the valve closed which clears during diastole.

continued

Case 7.19 *continued*

E. M-mode through the mitral valve prosthesis. F–J. Magnified view at 125 degrees demonstrating flow convergence through the valve during diastole and a small degree of valvular regurgitation through the valve. LA, left atrium; RV, right ventricle; LV, left ventricle; AV, aortic valve prosthesis; Ao, aorta; PA, pulmonary artery.

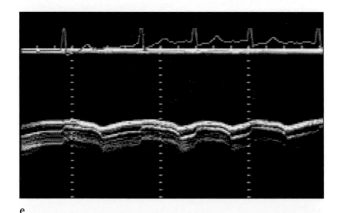

e

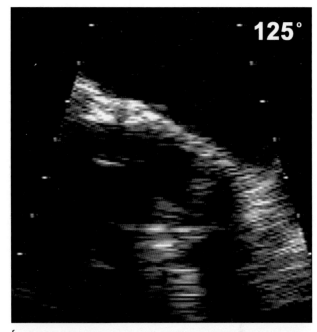

f

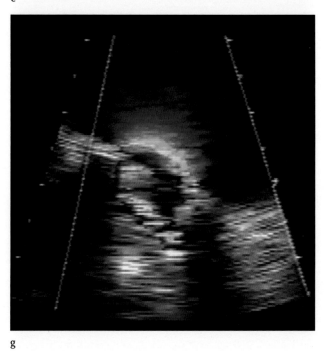

g

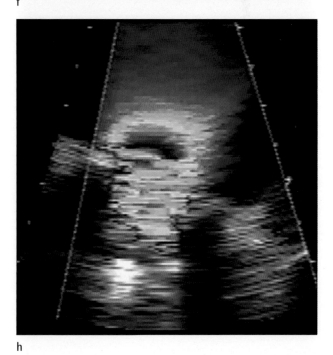

h

continued

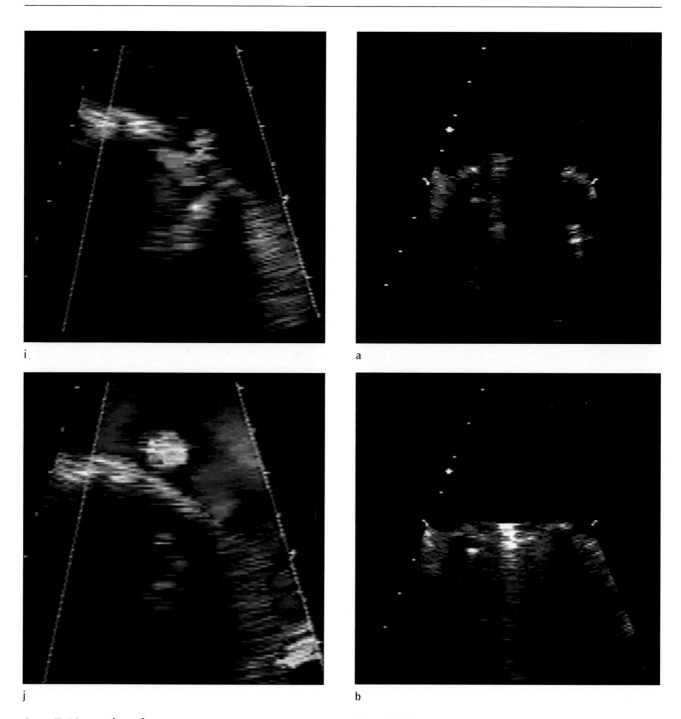

i

a

j

b

Case 7.19 *continued*

Case 7.20
Beal mitral prosthetic valve. A. Open valve during diastole
and (B) closed valve during systole.

continued

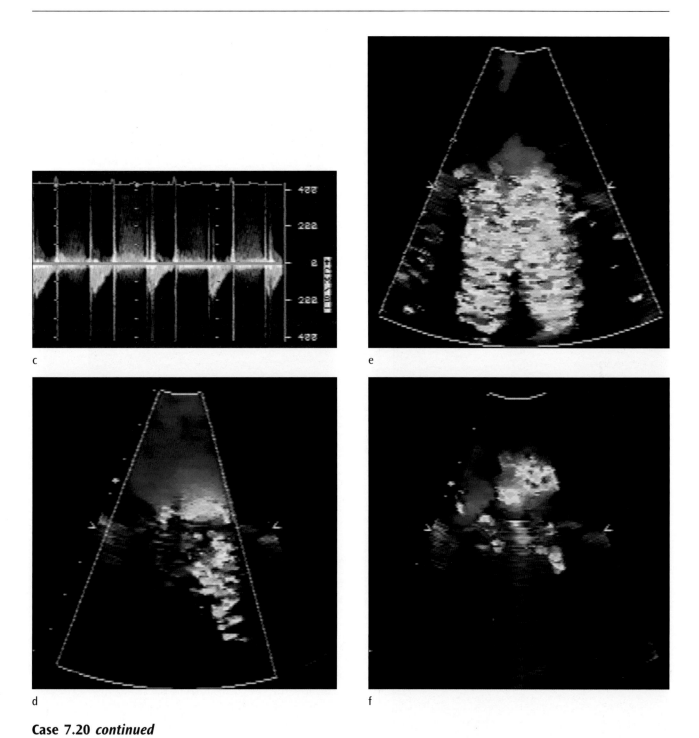

c

e

d

f

Case 7.20 *continued*
C. Continuous wave Doppler through the prosthesis. D, E. Color flow Doppler forward flow through the prosthesis. F. Normal regurgitation from a Star-Edwards valve.

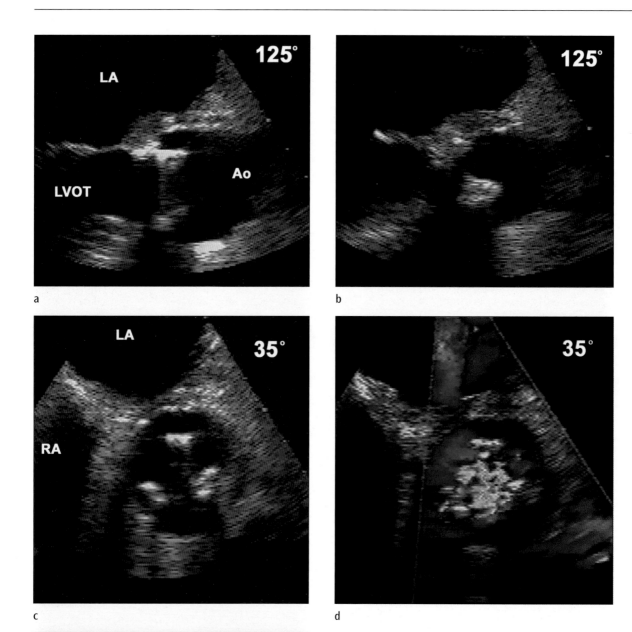

Case 7.21

Normal Carpentier-Edwards Perimount aortic valve.
A. Longitudinal view of the aortic root and a bioprosthetic aortic valve demonstrating the sewing ring bordered by two of the struts along the superior and inferior aortic walls. B. Mild angulation of the probe demonstrates a strut in longitudinal axis. C. Short-axis view at the aortic annulus level. The sewing ring is visualized within the aortic root and all three struts are visualized in a triangular orientation within the sewing ring. The valve leaflets are not well visualized at this level. D, E. Normal systolic flow with color flow Doppler recorded in early and late systole. LA, left atrium; RA, right atrium; Ao, aorta; LVOT, left ventricular output tract.

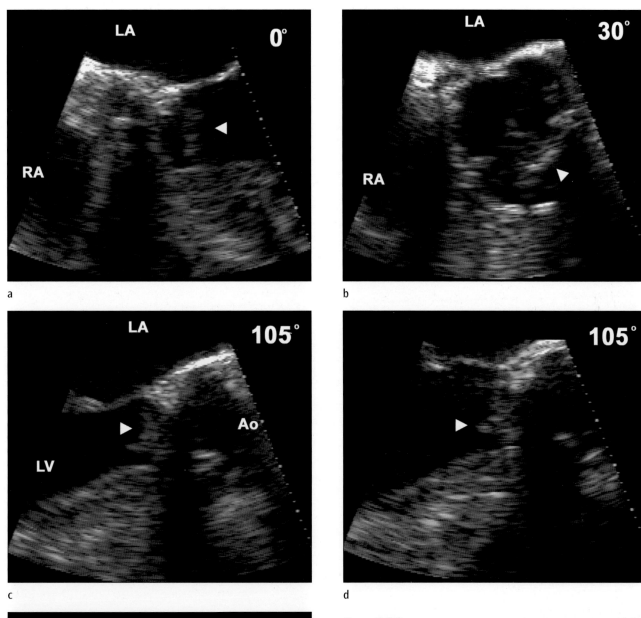

a

b

c

d

e

Case 7.22

Carpentier-Edwards porcine aortic valve with vegetation.
A. Modified four-chamber view demonstrating a soft, shaggy
mass (arrow) in the left ventricular outflow tract associated
with a aortic bioprosthesis. B. Short-axis view of the aortic
bioprosthesis at 30 degrees demonstrating a thickened leaflet
and increased echogenicity (arrow) in the cusp area suggesting
a mass. C–E. Longitudinal axis at 105 degrees demonstrating
the mass (arrow) prolapsing back and forth through the valve
with the cardiac cycle. LA, left atrium; RA, right atrium;
LV, left ventricle; Ao, aorta.

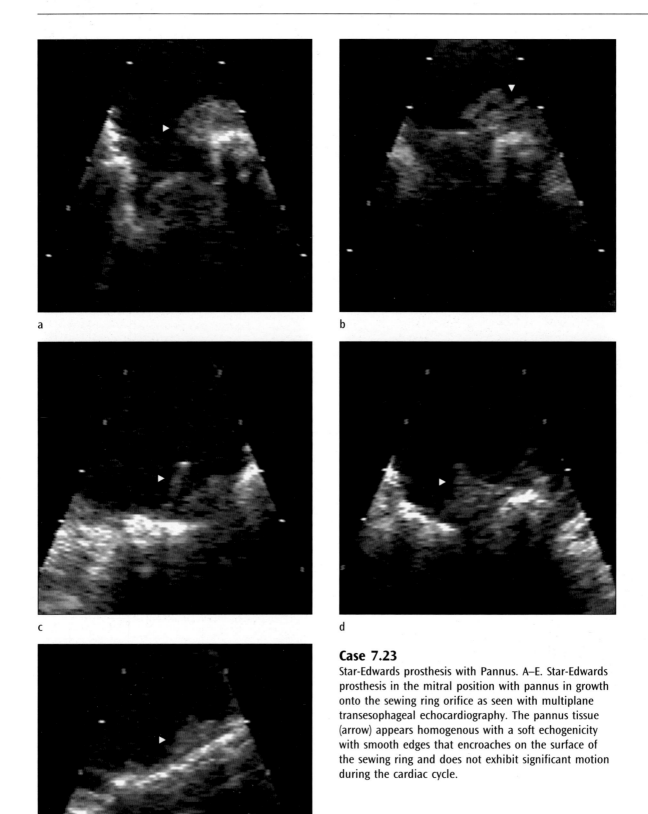

a

b

c

d

Case 7.23

Star-Edwards prosthesis with Pannus. A–E. Star-Edwards prosthesis in the mitral position with pannus in growth onto the sewing ring orifice as seen with multiplane transesophageal echocardiography. The pannus tissue (arrow) appears homogenous with a soft echogenicity with smooth edges that encroaches on the surface of the sewing ring and does not exhibit significant motion during the cardiac cycle.

e

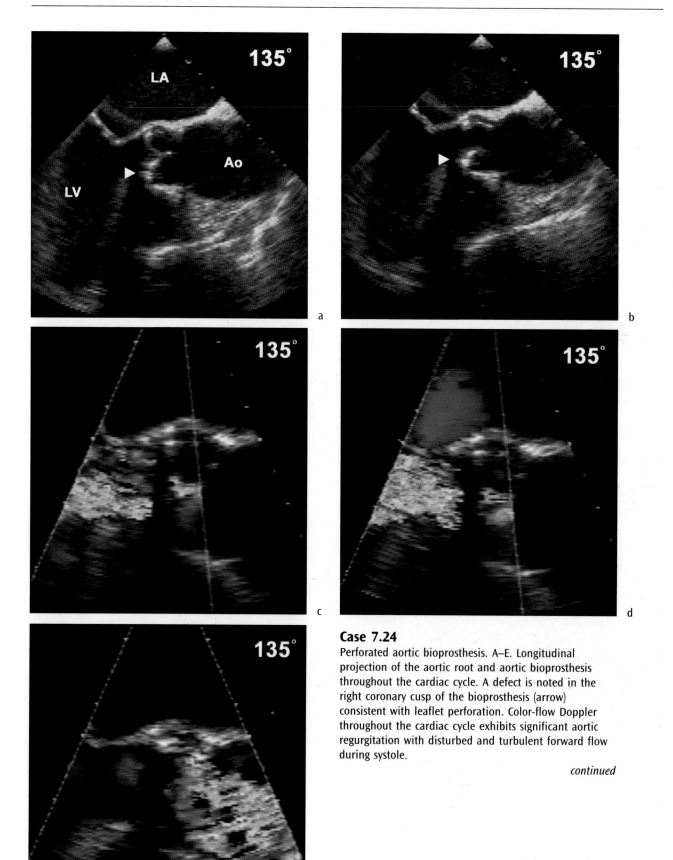

Case 7.24

Perforated aortic bioprosthesis. A–E. Longitudinal projection of the aortic root and aortic bioprosthesis throughout the cardiac cycle. A defect is noted in the right coronary cusp of the bioprosthesis (arrow) consistent with leaflet perforation. Color-flow Doppler throughout the cardiac cycle exhibits significant aortic regurgitation with disturbed and turbulent forward flow during systole.

continued

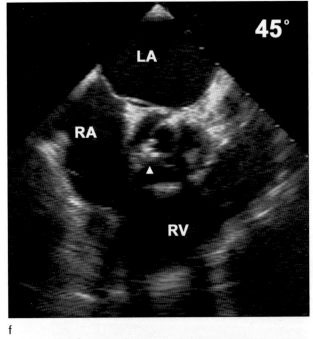

f

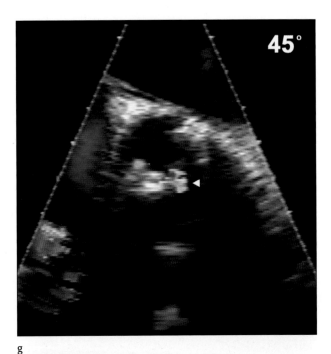

g

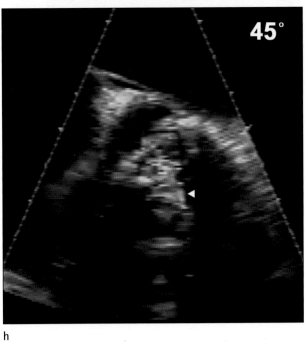

h

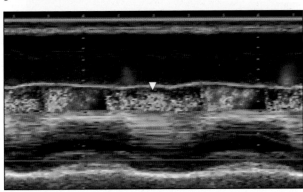

i

Case 7.24 *continued*

F. Short-axis view obtained at the aortic valve level demonstrates thickening and calcification of the bioprosthetic leaflets. G, H. Color-flow Doppler exhibits a prominent aortic regurgitant jet during diastole. I. Color m-mode Doppler demonstrating severe aortic regurgitation (arrow). LA, left atrium; Ao, aorta; LV, left ventricle; RV, right ventricle; right atrium.

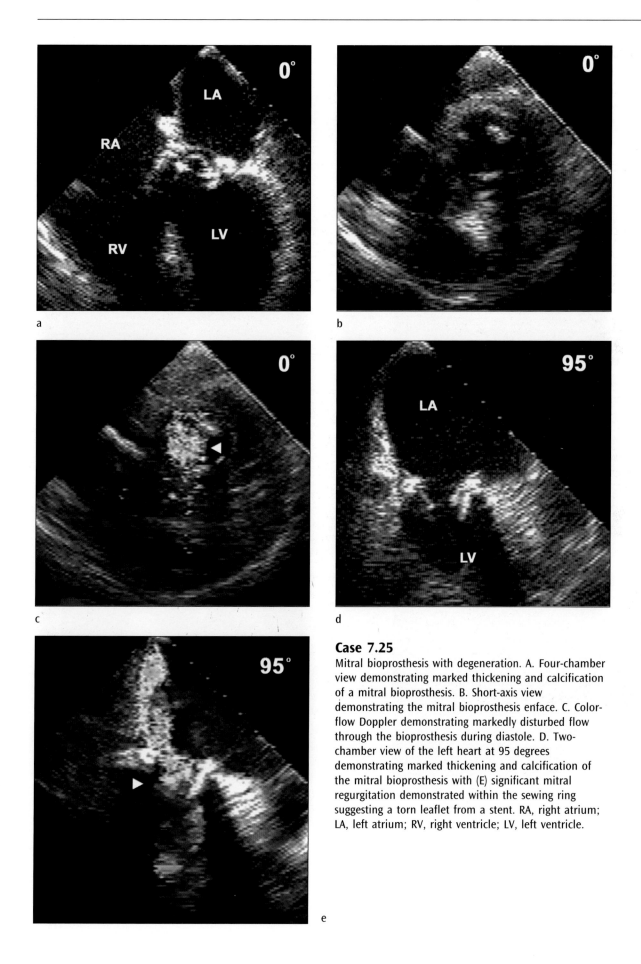

Case 7.25

Mitral bioprosthesis with degeneration. A. Four-chamber view demonstrating marked thickening and calcification of a mitral bioprosthesis. B. Short-axis view demonstrating the mitral bioprosthesis enface. C. Color-flow Doppler demonstrating markedly disturbed flow through the bioprosthesis during diastole. D. Two-chamber view of the left heart at 95 degrees demonstrating marked thickening and calcification of the mitral bioprosthesis with (E) significant mitral regurgitation demonstrated within the sewing ring suggesting a torn leaflet from a stent. RA, right atrium; LA, left atrium; RV, right ventricle; LV, left ventricle.

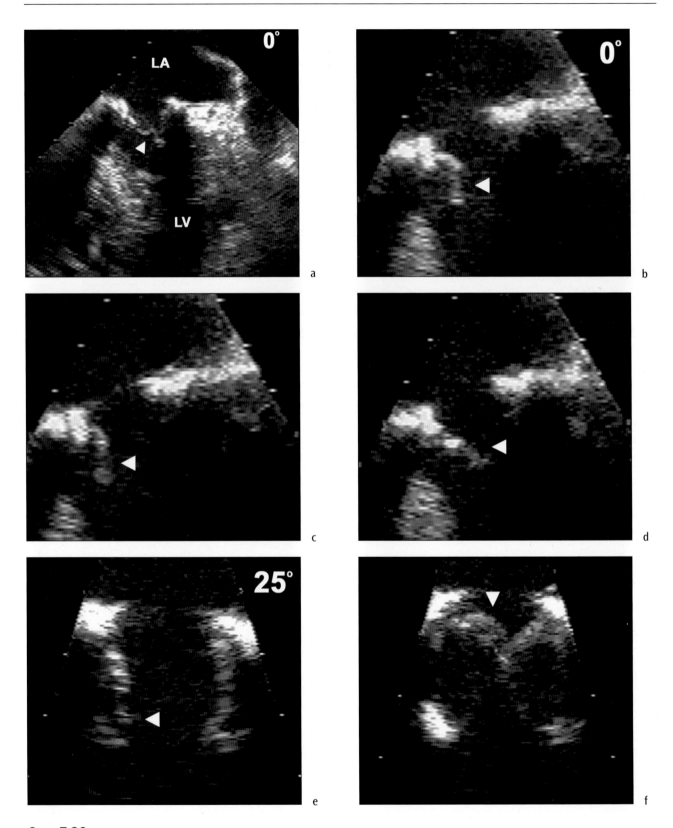

Case 7.26

Mitral bioprosthesis with degeneration. A. Modified four-chamber view at 0 degrees demonstrating a mitral bioprosthesis with thickening and a flail leafleted (arrow). B–G. Magnified views at 0 and 25 degrees demonstrating the flail bioprosthetic leaflet (arrow). At 25 degrees there is marked prolapse of the leaflet (arrow).

continued

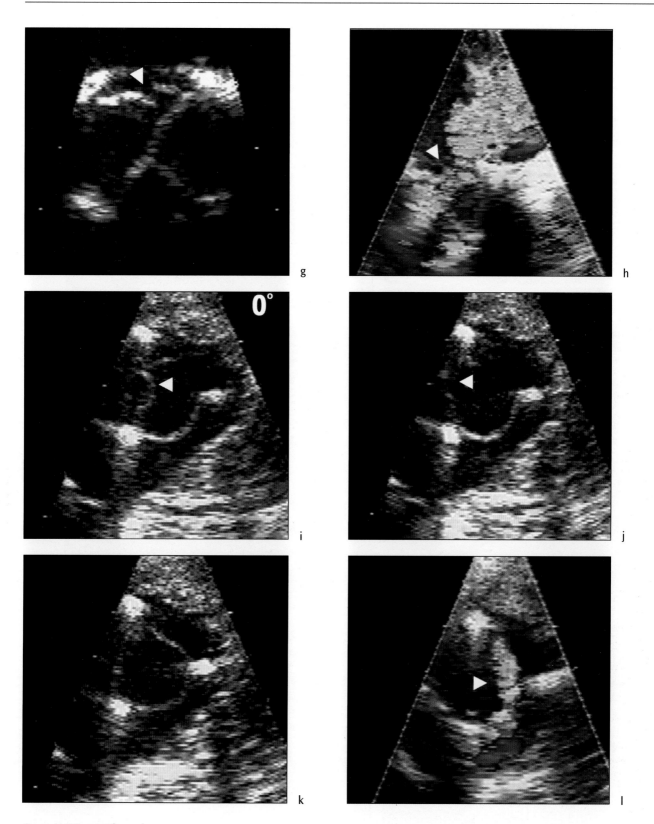

g

h

i

j

k

l

Case 7.26 *continued*

Color-flow Doppler demonstrates severe mitral regurgitation due to the flail and prolapsing bioprosthetic leaflet. I–K. Short-axis view at 0 degrees demonstrating the mitral bioprosthesis enface. The leaflets are thickened and therefore well visualized in-between the supporting stents of the valve. Chaotic motion (arrow) is noted in one leaflet (arrow). L. Color-flow Doppler demonstrating mitral regurgitation emanating from the flail leaflet. LA, left atrium; LV, left ventricle.

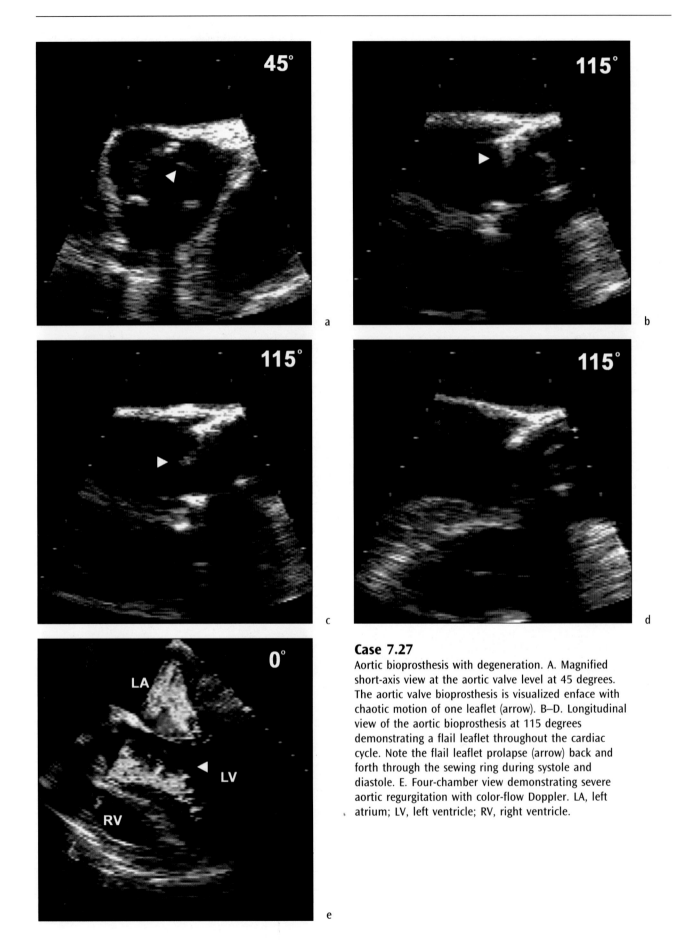

Case 7.27
Aortic bioprosthesis with degeneration. A. Magnified short-axis view at the aortic valve level at 45 degrees. The aortic valve bioprosthesis is visualized enface with chaotic motion of one leaflet (arrow). B–D. Longitudinal view of the aortic bioprosthesis at 115 degrees demonstrating a flail leaflet throughout the cardiac cycle. Note the flail leaflet prolapse (arrow) back and forth through the sewing ring during systole and diastole. E. Four-chamber view demonstrating severe aortic regurgitation with color-flow Doppler. LA, left atrium; LV, left ventricle; RV, right ventricle.

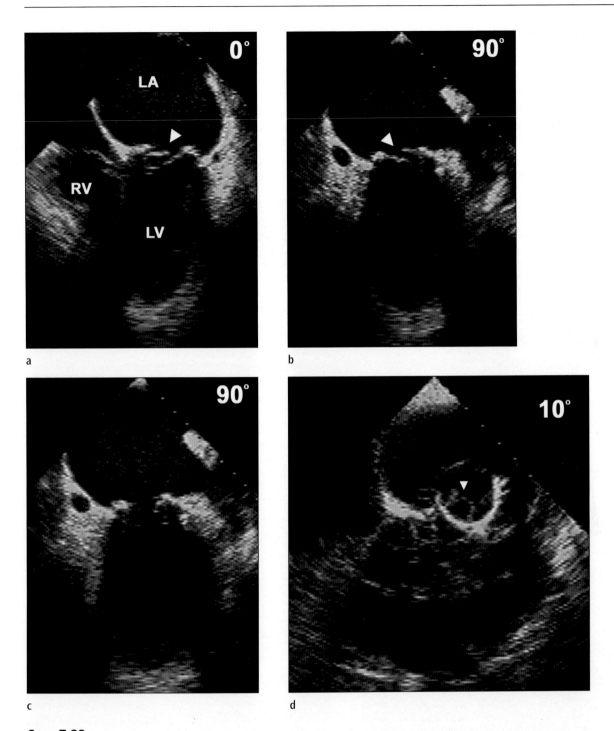

Case 7.28
Mitral bioprosthesis with degeneration and a torn leaflet. A. Four-chamber view at 0 degrees demonstrating marked left atrial enlargement with a flail and torn mitral bioprosthetic leaflet (arrow). B, C. Two-chamber view obtained at 90 degrees demonstrating a flail leaflet prolapsing beyond the sewing ring into the left atrium during systolic closure.

continued

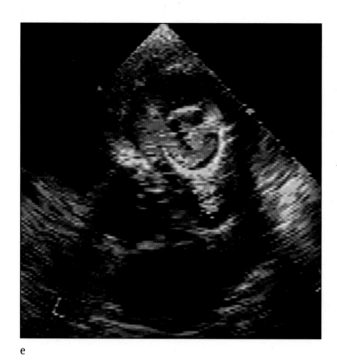

e

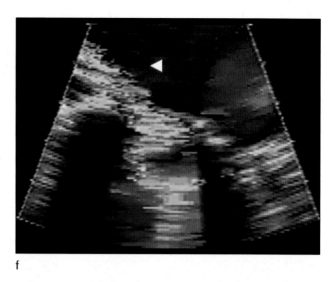

f

Case 7.28 continued

D, E. Short-axis view of the mitral bioprosthesis demonstrating the sewing ring and marked thickening and degeneration of the mitral bioprosthesis with a torn leaflet (arrow) with mitral regurgitation demonstrated with color-flow Doppler. F. Two-chamber view at 90 degrees demonstrating flow convergence and significant mitral regurgitation (arrow) in magnification mode. LA, left atrium; LV, left ventricle; RV, right ventricle.

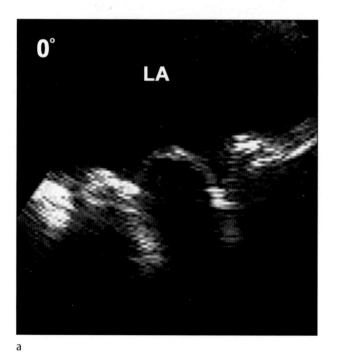

a

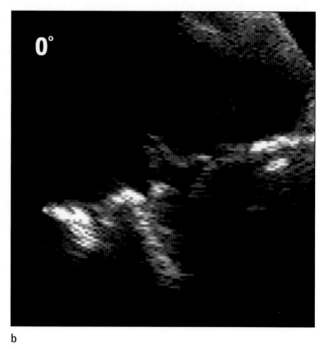

b

Case 7.29

Mitral bioprosthesis vegetation. A–D. Magnified mode of a mitral bioprosthesis at 0 and 25 degrees demonstrating a flail leaflet (arrow) secondary to infectious endocarditis. The flail leaflet is seen prolapsing into the left atrium during systole.

continued

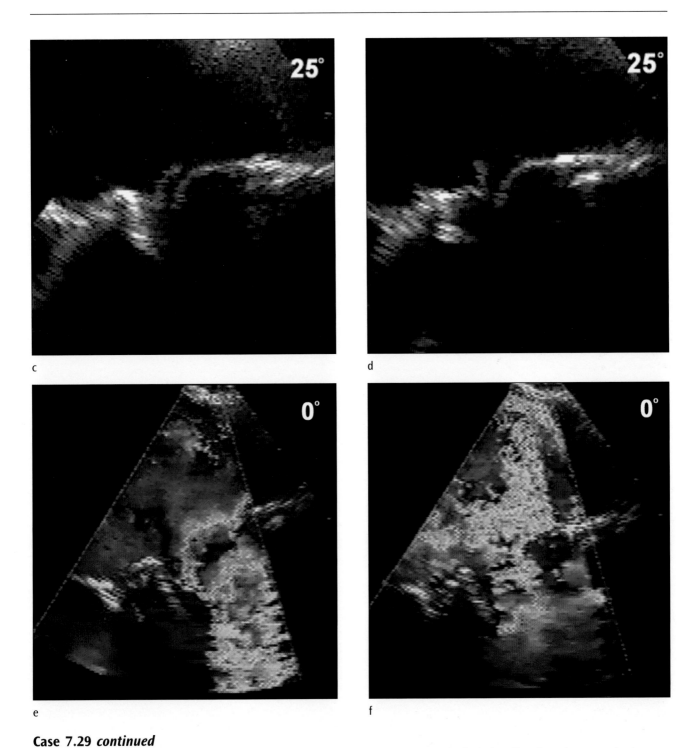

c

d

e

f

Case 7.29 *continued*
E, F. Color-flow Doppler at 0 degrees demonstrating turbulent flow through the prosthesis during diastole and severe mitral regurgitation during systole. LA, left atrium.

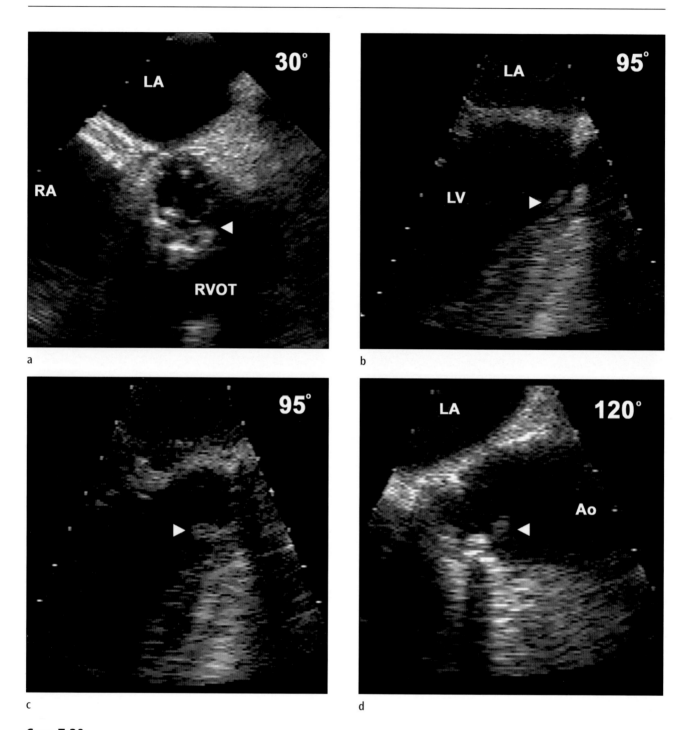

Case 7.30

Aortic bioprosthesis with vegetation. A. Short-axis view at the aortic valve level at 30 degrees with the aortic bioprosthesis viewed enface. The aortic sewing ring is visualized with an aortic valve abscess noted in the inferior portion of the annulus. There are multiple small areas of echolucency representing an unruptured abscess (arrow). B–D. Longitudinal views of the left ventricular outflow tract and 95 and 125 degrees demonstrating a soft echogenic mass which was a vegetation (arrow) that prolapsed between the left ventricular outflow tract and the aortic root during the cardiac cycle. LA, left atrium; RA, right atrium; RVOT, right ventricular outflow tract; LV, left ventricle; Ao, aorta.

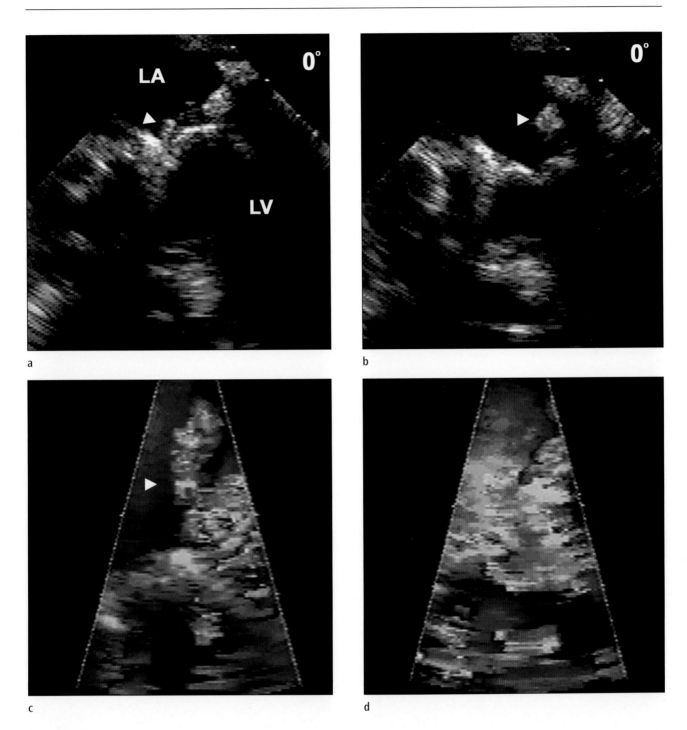

a

b

c

d

Case 7.31

Mitral bioprosthesis with vegetation. A, B. Four-chamber view at 0 degrees demonstrating a mitral bioprosthesis with marked thickening and degeneration of the valve. Pannus in growth has occurred surrounding the sewing ring with a small vegetation (arrow) noted on the aortic side of the sewing ring. C, D. Color-flow Doppler demonstrates mitral regurgitant jet (arrow) emanating from a small defect in-between the sewing ring and the native annulus representing a paraprosthetic leak due to a small dehiscence secondary to infection. Mild obstructive flow (star) is noted through the prosthesis during diastole (D).

continued

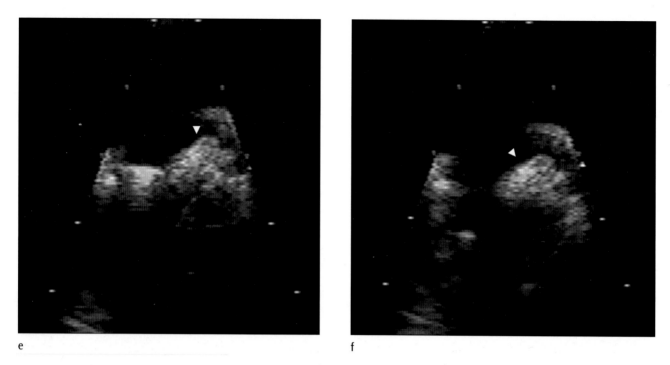

e

f

Case 7.31 *continued*

E, F. Short-axis view of the mitral prosthesis demonstrating marked degeneration of the valve leaflets enface with a large area of increased echogenic globular mass (arrow) representing pannus in-growth and thrombus formation. LA, left atrium; LV, left ventricle.

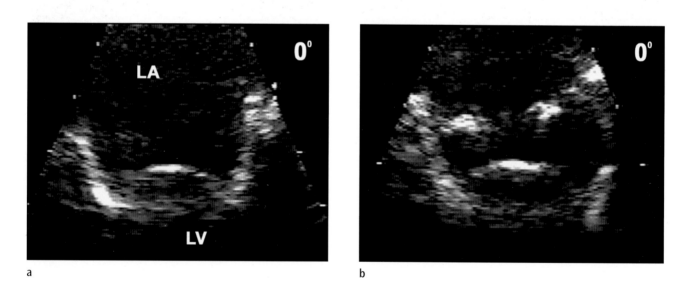

a

b

Case 7.32

Mitral bioprosthesis with small perforation. A, B. Magnified view at 0 degrees demonstrating a mitral bioprosthesis and small degree of degeneration.

continued

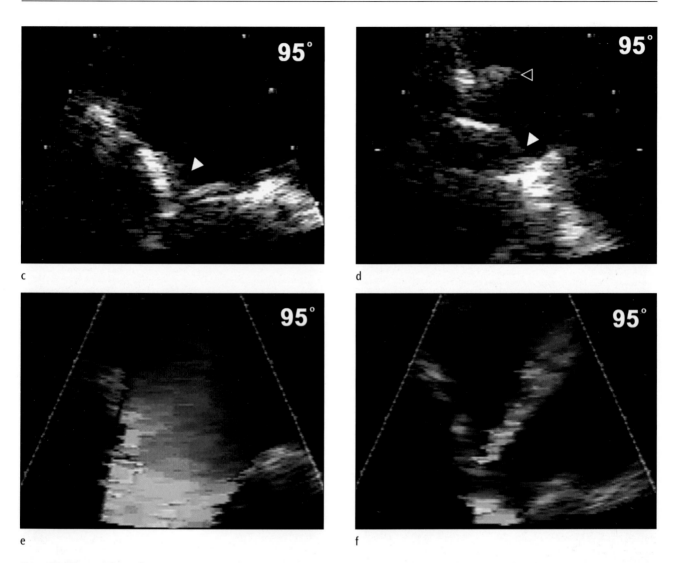

c

d

e

f

Case 7.32 *continued*

C, D. Magnified view at 95 degrees demonstrating thickened and calcified leaflets with separation of the leaflet from the sewing ring (arrow) demonstrating a torn leaflet. E, F. Color-flow Doppler demonstrates normal diastolic flow with a small regurgitant jet in the region of the torn leaflet. LA, left atrium; LV, left ventricle.

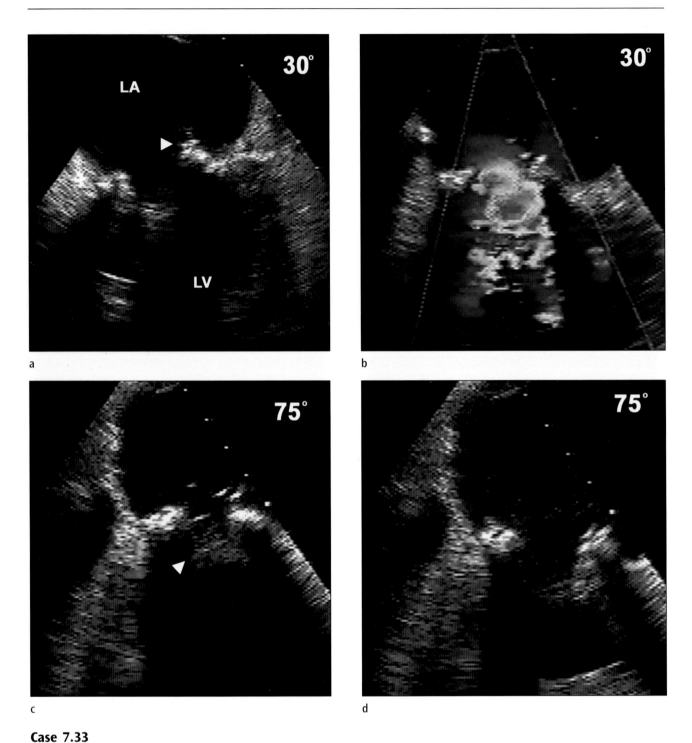

a

b

c

d

Case 7.33
Mitral bioprosthesis with vegetation. A. Two-chamber view at 30 degree demonstrating a large shaggy bright echogenic mass (arrow) prolapsing into the left atrium attached to the lateral aspect of the sewing ring. B. Color-flow Doppler demonstrating disturbed flow through the prosthesis during diastole near the area of the mass. C, D. Two-chambered view at 75 degrees demonstrating the vegetation prolapsing into the left ventricle. LA, left atrium; LV, left ventricle.

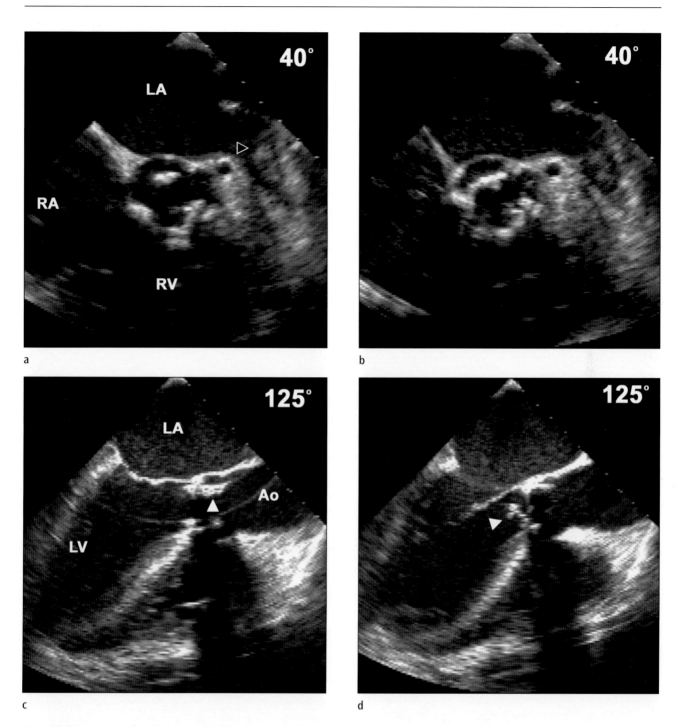

a

b

c

d

Case 7.34

Aortic bioprosthesis abscess. A. Short-axis view at the aortic valve level at 40 degrees demonstrating an aortic bioprosthesis with an echolucent area below the level of the left main coronary artery. B. In the same view echolucency and jagged areas are noted suggesting vegetation and abscess formation. The echolucency of the abscess suggests rupture. C–E. Longitudinal view of the aortic root demonstrating marked echogenicity of the sewing ring with a discreet vegetation noted near the area of the right coronary cusp that prolapses with the cardiac cycle.

continued

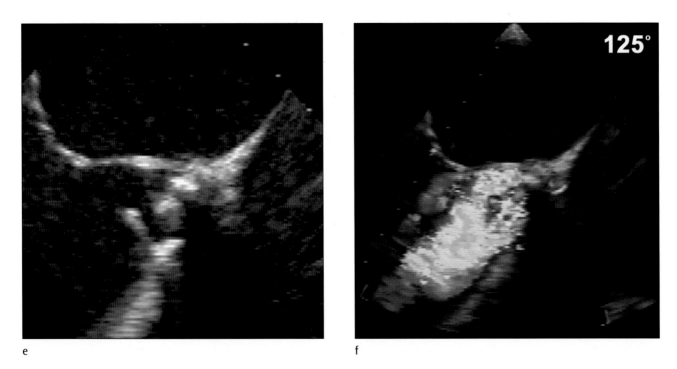

e

f

Case 7.34 *continued*
E. Magnified view demonstrating the vegetation. F. Color-flow Doppler demonstrating aortic regurgitation and disturbed flow in the outflow tract emanating from the abscess. LA, left atrium; RA, right atrium; RV, right ventricle; LV, left ventricle; Ao, aorta.

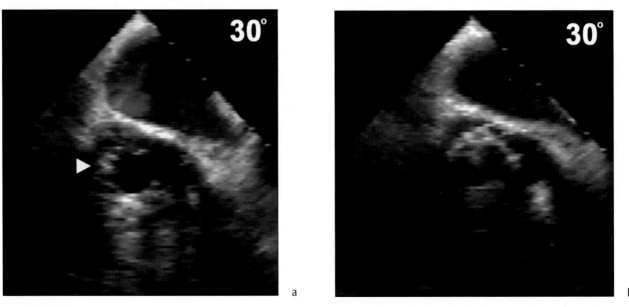

a

b

Case 7.35
Aortic bioprosthesis with dehiscence. A–D. Short-axis view of the aortic valve level at 30 degrees demonstrating the sewing ring of an aortic mechanical prosthesis. An echolucency is noted around the sewing ring consistent with abscess formation. Color-flow Doppler helps outline the area of the echo-free space in conjunction with imaging. Note the sewing ring moves throughout the cardiac cycle consistent with dehiscence. E–H. Longitudinal view during the cardiac cycle demonstrating rocking of the prosthetic sewing ring. I. Color-flow Doppler demonstrating aortic regurgitation.

continued

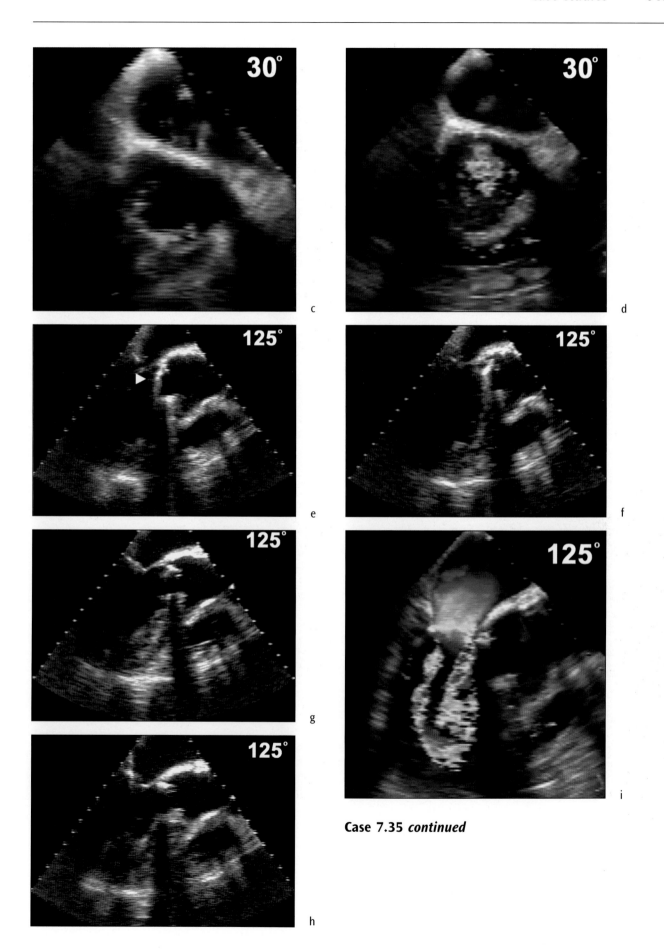

Case 7.35 *continued*

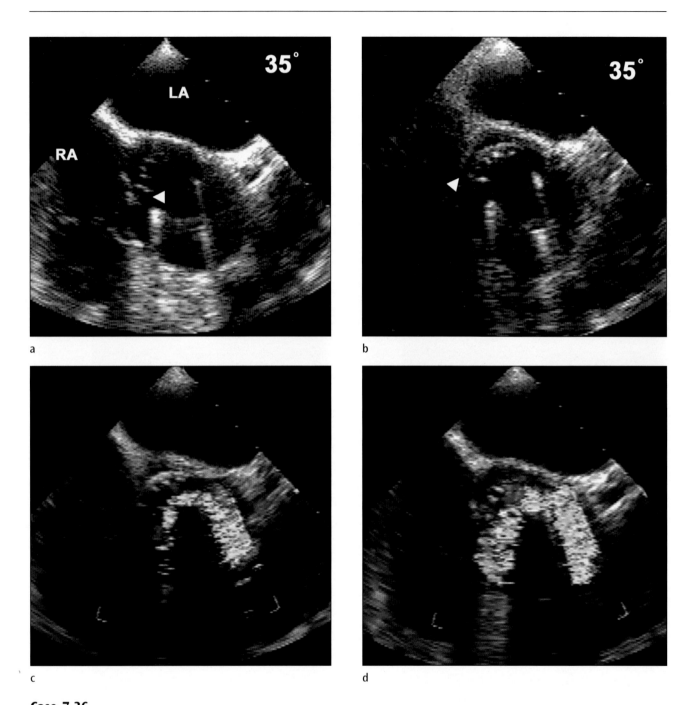

Case 7.36

Aortic prosthetic valve with abscess. A. Short-axis view of a ball-cage valve in the aortic position obtained at 35 degrees. Note the area of increased echogenicity of the lateral aspect of the sewing ring near the left atrial border. Multiple small linear echogenicities are noted in that area which exhibit chaotic motion during the cardiac cycle. Note the highly reflective struts of the cage, and the prominent echocardiography artifact of the ball. C, D. Color-flow Doppler demonstrate forward flow thorough the valve. These findings suggest degeneration of the sewing ring material and thrombus formation. LA, left atrium; RA, right atrium.

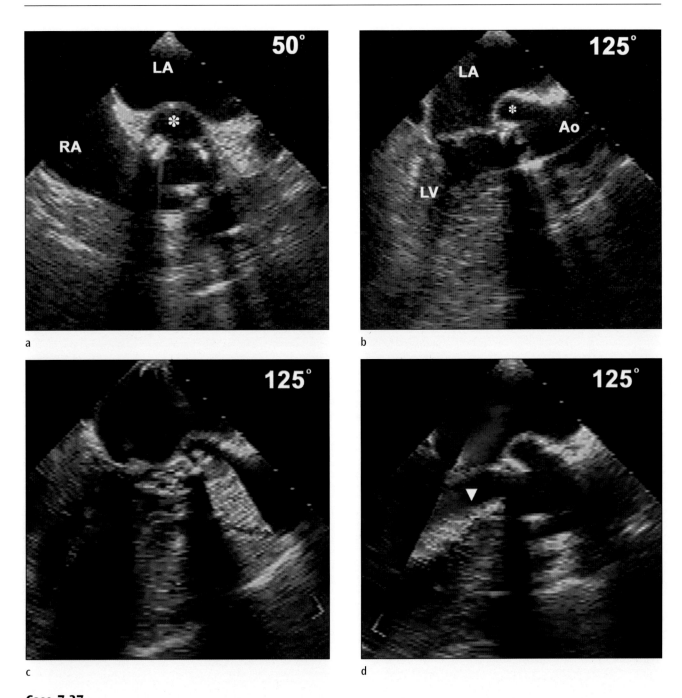

Case 7.37

Aortic bioprosthesis with abscess. A. Short-axis view at the aortic level obtained at 50 degrees. Note the area of increased echogenicity near the superior portion of the sewing ring protruding towards the left atrium (arrow). B. Longitudinal view demonstrating marked distortion of the left coronary cusp above the superior portion of the sewing ring (star). C, D. Color flow Doppler demonstrating systolic and diastolic flow with a small aortic regurgitant jet (arrow) in the left ventricular outflow tract.

continued

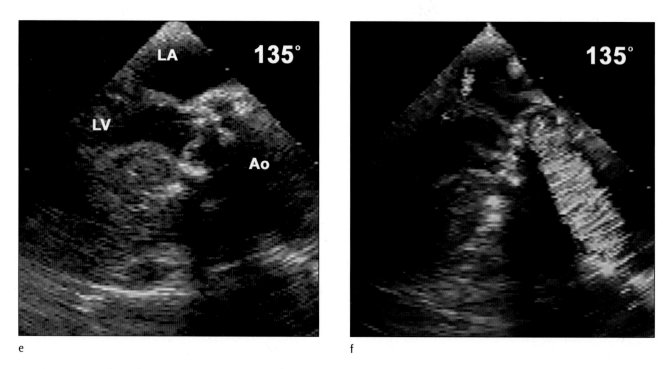

e

f

Case 7.37 *continued*

E, F. With rotation of the transducer to 135 degrees the area of protuberance of the sinus appears to be outlined by a jagged area which represented a true abscess that ruptured. Multiplane transesophageal echocardiography is extremely helpful in evaluating this area and differentiating abscess formation from a small sinus of Valsalva aneurysm which may occur during implantation of an aortic bioprosthesis. LA, left atrium; RA, right atrium; Ao, aorta; LV, left ventricle.

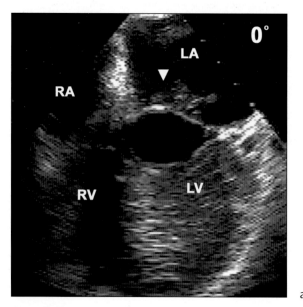

a

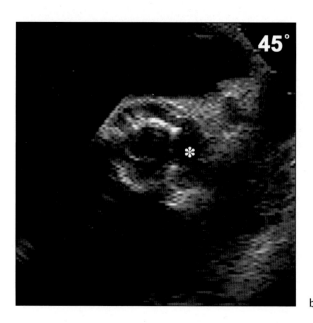

b

Case 7.38

Aortic prosthesis with abscess formation. A. Modified four-chamber view demonstrating a shaggy soft echogenic mass (arrow) appearing in the mitro-aortic curtain area. This area represents the fibrosa in-between the mitral and aortic valve. B. Short-axis view at the aortic valve level at 45 degrees demonstrating a large area of echolucency (star) surrounding the sewing ring which represents abscess formation.

continued

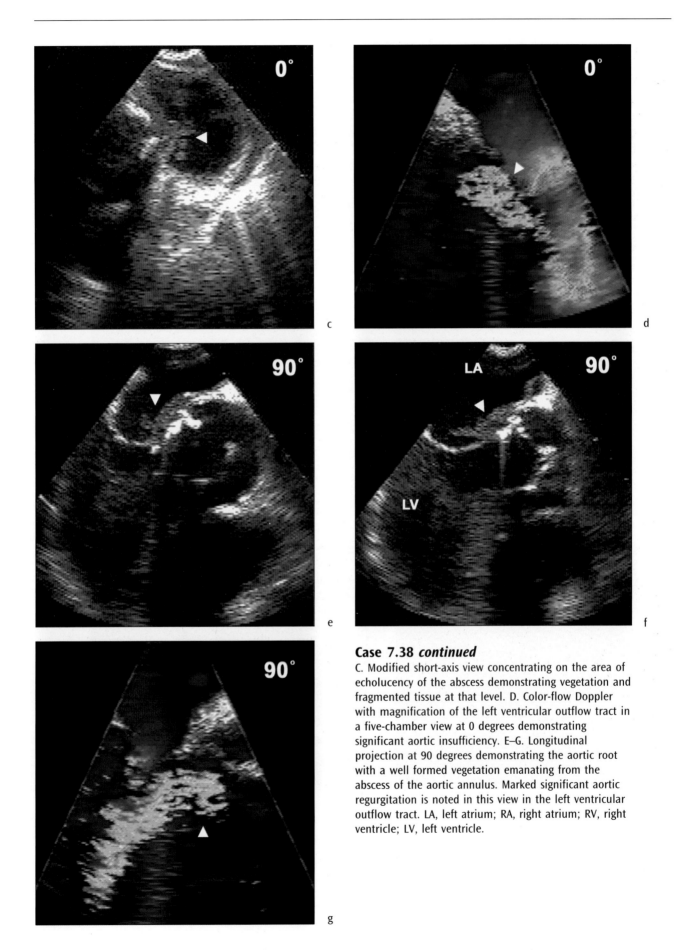

Case 7.38 *continued*

C. Modified short-axis view concentrating on the area of echolucency of the abscess demonstrating vegetation and fragmented tissue at that level. D. Color-flow Doppler with magnification of the left ventricular outflow tract in a five-chamber view at 0 degrees demonstrating significant aortic insufficiency. E–G. Longitudinal projection at 90 degrees demonstrating the aortic root with a well formed vegetation emanating from the abscess of the aortic annulus. Marked significant aortic regurgitation is noted in this view in the left ventricular outflow tract. LA, left atrium; RA, right atrium; RV, right ventricle; LV, left ventricle.

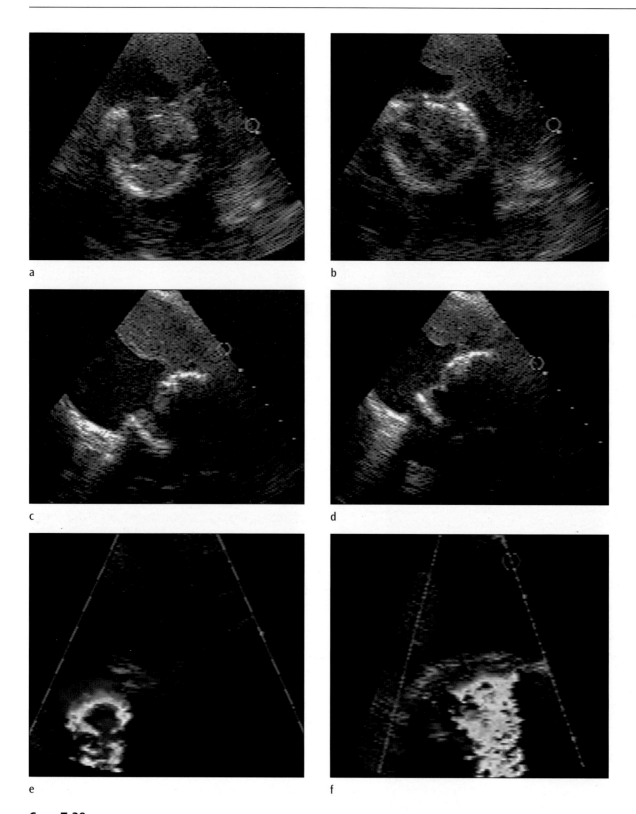

a

b

c

d

e

f

Case 7.39

Thrombosed mitral bioprosthesis. All prosthetic valves may be prone to thrombosis and obstruction, particularly mechanical prostheses. A. Mitral bioprosthesis viewed enface in a modified short-axis view. There is a soft echogenic mass (arrow) within the sewing ring of the prosthesis consistent with a thrombus. Oblique views of the left atrium demonstrate a large atrial thrombus in close proximity to the superior aspect of the sewing ring. E, F. Color flow Doppler during diastole demonstrates marked flow disturbance through the mitral prosthesis suggesting obstruction of the valve.

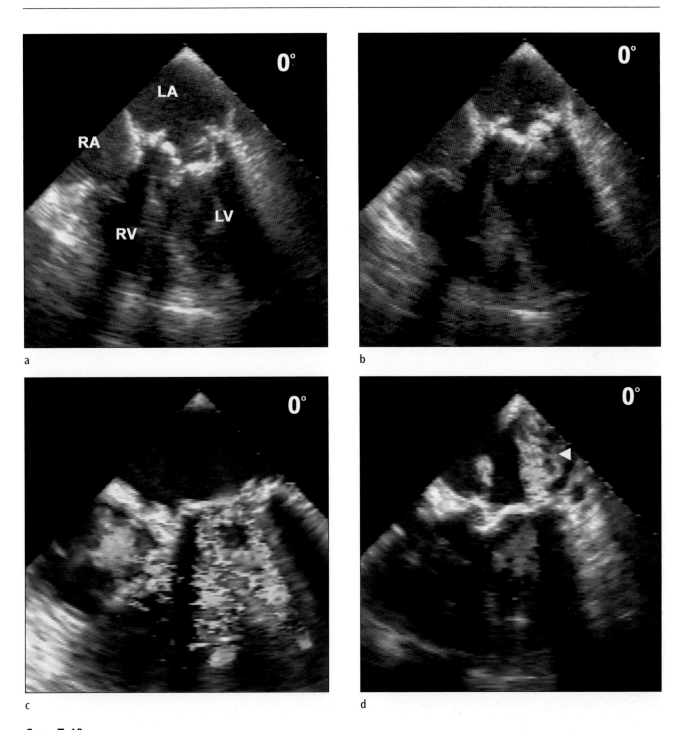

a

b

c

d

Case 7.40

Mitral bioprosthesis with stenosis. Marked degeneration consistent with calcification and thickening of the leaflets produced restrictive motion and obstruction of a mitral bioprosthesis. A. Four-chamber view obtained at 0 degrees demonstrating markedly increased echogenicity of the mitral bioprosthetic leaflets. B. There is marked restriction in opening motion of the valve leaflets during diastole. D. Color flow Doppler demonstrates severe disturbance of forward flow through the valve during diastole as well as mitral regurgitation (D) as a result of the fixed position of the leaflets due to restriction limiting valve opening and closing.

continued

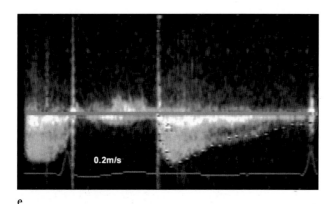

e

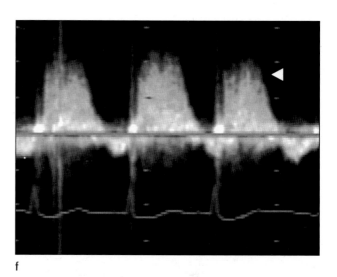

f

Case 7.40 *continued*

E. Continuous-wave Doppler through the prosthesis demonstrating increased velocity of 2 m/sec through the valve and a prolonged pressure half-time suggesting obstruction of forward flow. F. Continuous-wave Doppler during systole demonstrates mitral regurgitation (arrow). LA, left atrium; RA, right atrium; RV, right ventricle; LV, left ventricle.

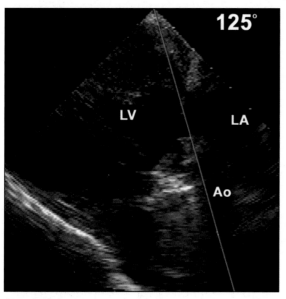

a

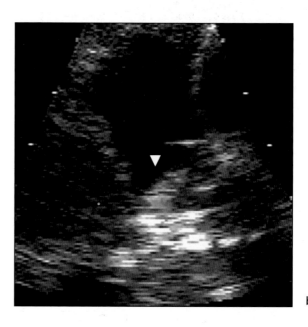

b

Case 7.41

Aortic mechanical prosthesis with thrombotic obstruction. A. Longitudinal view from the gastric window at 125 degrees demonstrating a soft echogenic mass on the ventricular surface of the aortic prosthesis obscuring the prosthetic leaflets from view. Note significant left ventricular hypertrophy. This is a good view for conventional Doppler interrogation of the aortic prosthesis. B–D. Magnified mode of the aortic prosthesis demonstrating numerous shaggy echoes with chaotic motion and marked turbulent flow through the aortic prosthesis with color Doppler. E. Continuous wave Doppler through the aortic prosthesis demonstrating increased flow at greater than 5 m/sec during systole. F–H. Longitudinal view at 115 to 135 degrees demonstrating thrombus associated with the aortic prosthesis with marked flow disturbance during systole in the aortic root. LA, left atrium; LV, left ventricle; Ao, aorta.

continued

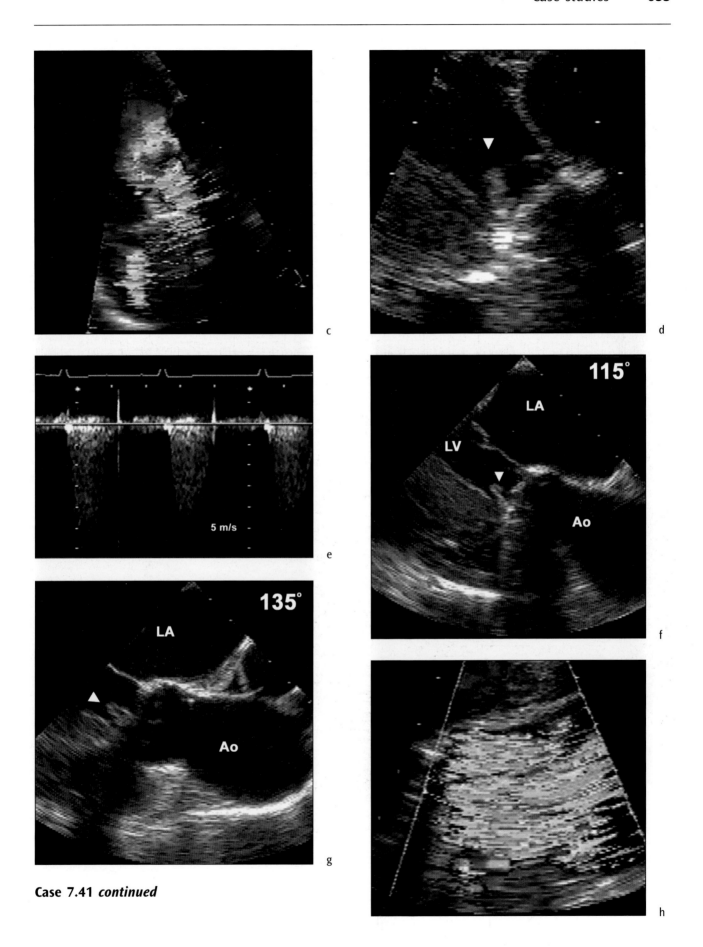

Case 7.41 *continued*

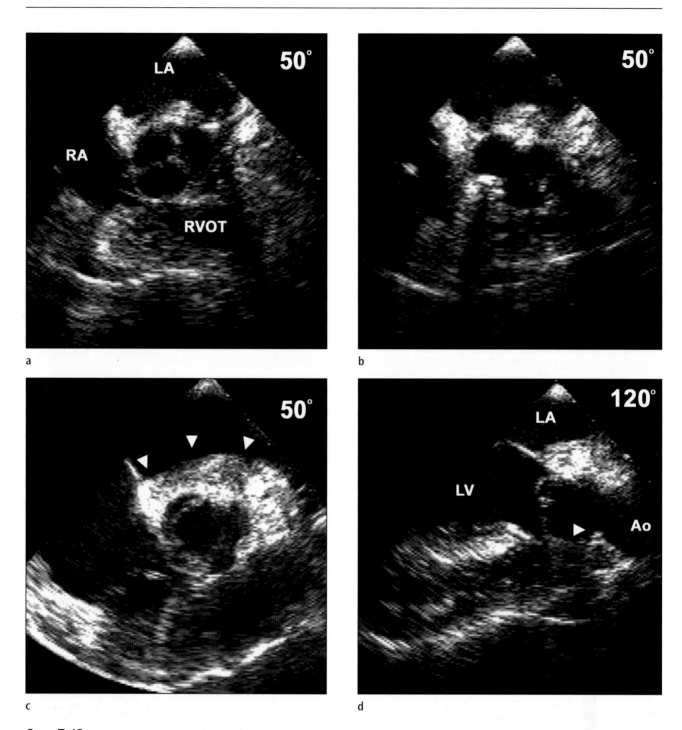

Case 7.42

Aortic valve homograft. Postoperative evaluation. A–C. Short-axis view at the aortic valve level. Increased echogenicity noted surrounding the aortic annulus which is consistent with edematous and swollen tissue produced during implantation of the homograft. The aortic valve appears similar to a native aortic valve. D–F. Longitudinal view of the aortic root at 125 degrees demonstrating the aortic valve homograft with imaging and color flow Doppler. Other than a slightly increased turbulence in forward flow during systole the color flow jets resemble a normal aortic valve pattern. LA, left atrium; RA, right atrium; RVOT, right ventricular outflow tract; LV, left ventricle; Ao, aorta.

continued

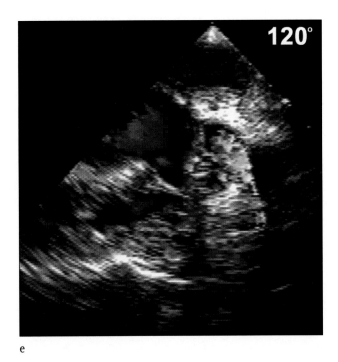

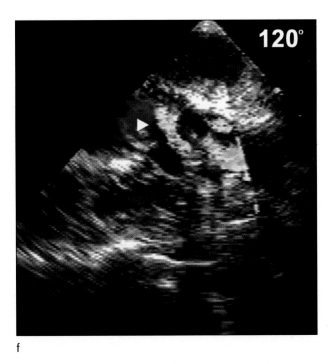

e

f

Case 7.42 *continued*

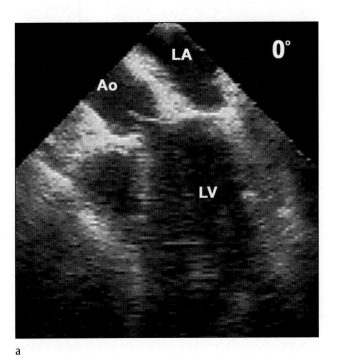

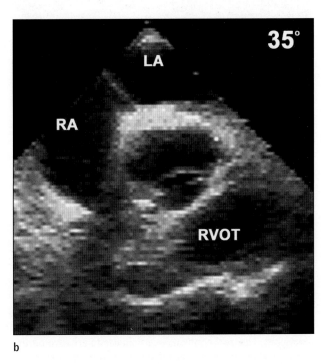

a

b

Case 7.43

Aortic valve homograft. Postoperative evaluation. A. Five-chamber view of the left ventricular outflow tract. B–D. Short-axis view at the level of the aortic valve at 35 degrees demonstrating the aortic homograft post-implantation. The aortic homograft appears similar to a native aortic valve. Color-flow Doppler demonstrates mild aortic regurgitation (arrow).

continued

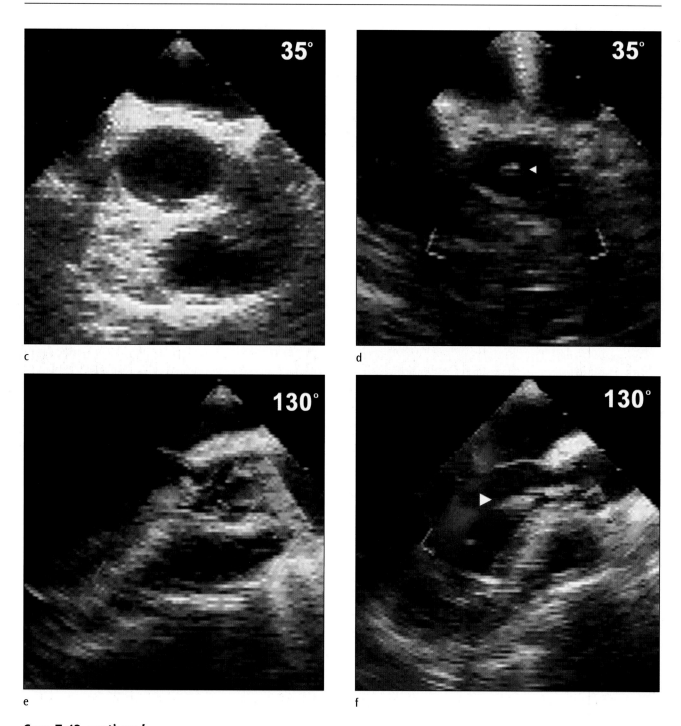

c

d

e

f

Case 7.43 *continued*

E, F. Color-flow Doppler of the aortic homograft in a longitudinal view at 130 degrees of the aortic root. E. Normal systolic forward flow with mild flow disturbance through the homograft. F. Mild aortic regurgitation (arrow) during diastole. Mild aortic regurgitation is frequently detected following implantation of the homograft and usually resolves in the early postoperative period. Increases in aortic regurgitation in the postoperative period should be followed closely. LA, left atrium; Ao, aorta; LV, left ventricle; RA, right atrium; RVOT, right ventricular outflow tract.

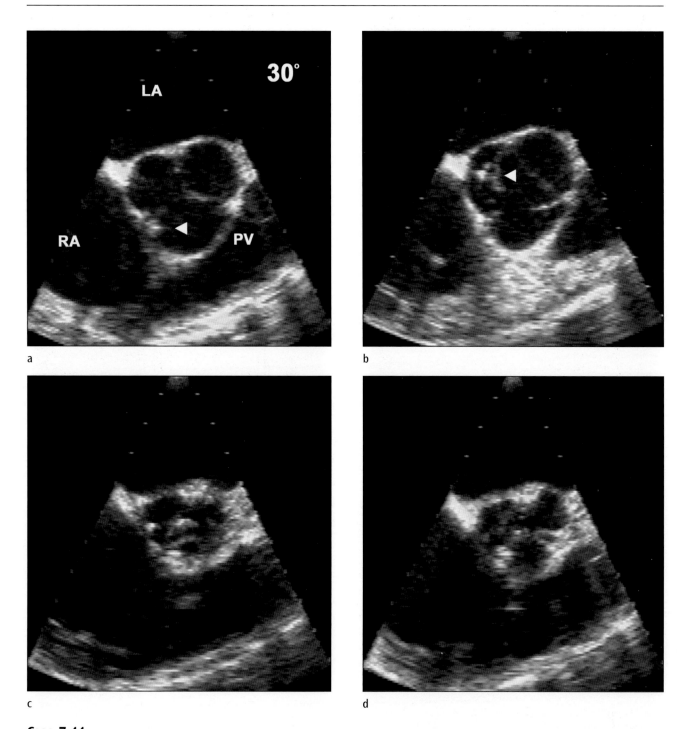

Case 7.44

Aortic St. Jude Toronto valve with vegetation. A. Aortic valve visualized enface with a mass noted in the commissure in the short-axis view at 30 degrees. B. Dense echogenic mass (arrow) associated with aortic valve leaflet during systole and (C) during early diastole. D. Short-axis view superior to the leaflet plane demonstrating mild narrowing of the aorta with imaging of the valve struts.

continued

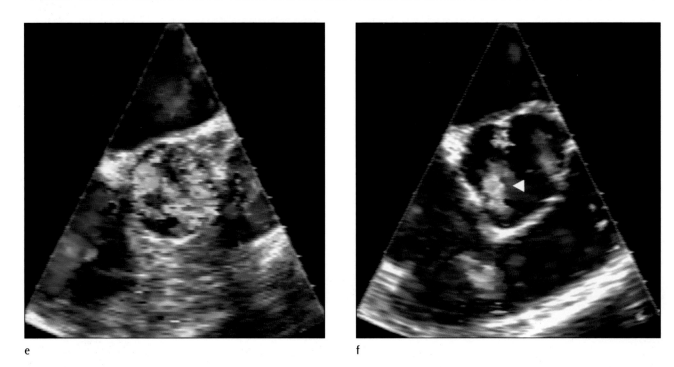

e   f

Case 7.44 *continued*
E. Color-flow Doppler in the short-axis view demonstrating systolic flow. F. During diastole a small aortic regurgitant jet (arrow) is visualized emanating from the area of the vegetation. LA, left atrium; RA, right atrium; PV, pulmonary valve.

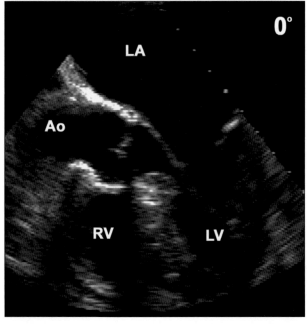

a

Case 7.45
Medtronic Freestyle. A. Five chamber view of the aortic root and left ventricular outflow tract visualizing the prosthesis in an oblique longitudinal projection. The prosthesis and leaflets are thickened suggesting degeneration. Normally the prosthesis is not as easily visualized and resembles a normal native valve.

continued

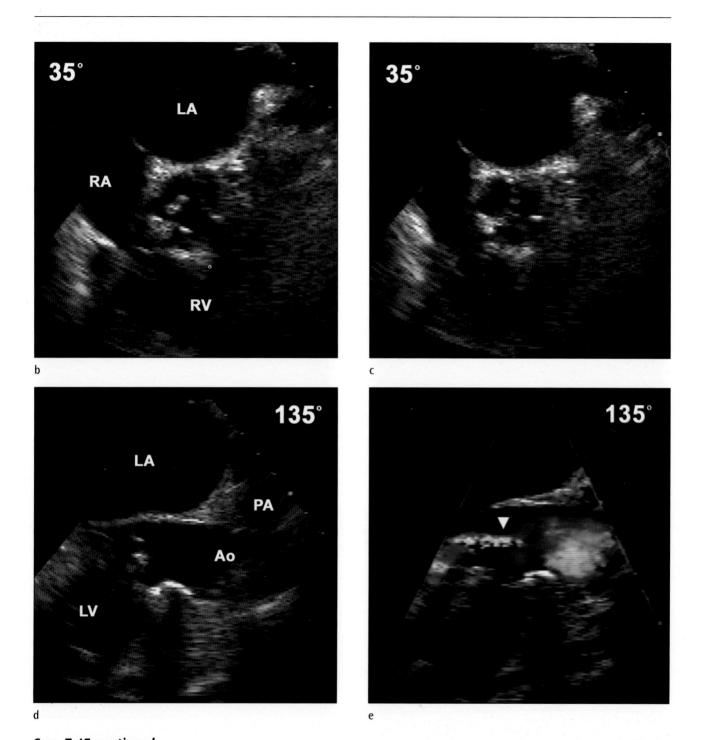

Case 7.45 *continued*

B, C. Short-axis view at the level of the leaflets at 35 degrees. Thickening and mild calcification of the valve is noted during systole and (E) diastole. D. Longitudinal view at 135 degrees of the aortic root demonstrating increased echogenicity of the prosthesis and valve leaflets. E. Color-flow Doppler demonstrating aortic regurgitation (arrow) associated with valve degeneration. LA, left atrium; Ao, aorta; RV, right ventricle; LV, left ventricle; RA, right atrium; PA, pulmonary artery.

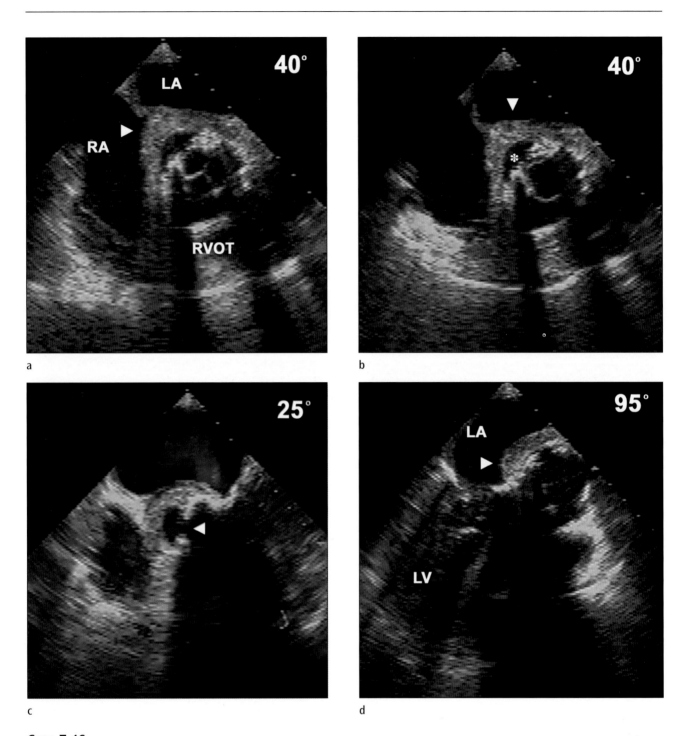

Case 7.46
Aortic valve homograft with abscess. A. Aortic valve homograft visualized enface in short-axis at 40 degrees. There is a well formed thickening (arrow) with homogenous echogenicity of the aortic root wall. B, C. With minor manipulation of the probe an abscess (arrow) is noted and at 25 degrees an abscess pocket (star) is also visualized. D. At 95 degrees color-flow Doppler highlights the area of the abscess pocket and flow is demonstrated within the pocket suggesting it has ruptured locally. LA, left atrium; RA, right atrium; RVOT, right ventricular outflow tract; LV, left ventricle.

References

1. Harken DE, Soroff HS, Taylor WJ, et al. Partial and complete prosthesis in aortic insufficiency. *J Thorac Cardiovasc Surg* 1960;40:744–62.

2. Starr A, Edwards ML. Mitral replacement: clinical experience with a ball valve prosthesis. *Ann Surg* 1961;154:726.

3. Roberts WC. Complications of cardiac valve replacement: characteristic abnormalities of prostheses pertaining to any or specific site. *Am J Cardiol* 1982;103:113–22.

4. Kotler MN, Segal BL, Parry WR. Echocardiographic and phonocardiographic evaluation of prosthetic heart valves. *Cardiovasc Clin* 1978;9:187–207.

5. Kotler MN, Mintz GS, Panidis I, et al. Non-invasive evaluation of normal and abnormal prosthetic valve function. *J Am Coll Cardiol* 1983;2:151–73.

6. Vongpatanasin W, Hillis LD, Lange RA. Prosthetic heart valves. *N Engl J Med* 1996;335:407–16.

7. Pandian NG, Hsu Tl, Schwartz SL, et al. Multiplane transesophageal echocardiography. *Echocardiography* 1992;9:649–66.

8. Daniel WG, Pearlman AS, Hausmann D, et al. Initial experience and potential applications of multiplane transesophageal echocardiography. *Am J Cardiol* 1993;71:358–61.

9. Zabalgoitia M. Echocardiographic assessment of prosthetic heart valves. *Curr Probl Cardiol* 1992;17:269–325.

10. Daniel WG, Mügge A, Grote J, et al. Comparison of transthoracic and transesophageal echocardiography for detection of abnormalities of prosthetic and bioprosthetic valves in the mitral and aortic positions. *Am J Cardiol* 1993;71:210–15.

11. Felner JM, Miller DD. Echocardiographic characteristics of mechanical prosthetic heart valves. *Echocardiography* 1984;1:261–310.

12. Horowitz MS, Goodman DJ, Fogarty TJ, et al. Mitral valve replacement with the glutaraldehyde-preserved porcine heterograft. *J Thorac Cardiovasc Surg* 1974;67:885–95.

13. Thomson FJ, Barrett-Boyes BG. The glutaraldehyde treated heterograft valve. Some engineering observations. *J Thorac Cardiovasc Surg* 1977;74:317.

14. Scharmm D, Baldauf W, Meisner H. Flow pattern and velocity field distal to human aortic and artificial heart valves as measured simultaneously by ultramicroscope anemometry in cylindrical glass tubes. *Thorac Cardiovasc Surg* 1980;28:133–40.

15. Yoganathan AP, et al. Bileaflet, tilting disk and porcine aortic valve substitutes: in vitro hydrodynamic characteristics. *J Am Coll Cardiol* 1984;3:313–20.

16. Chambers J, Monaghan M. Jackson G. Colour flow Doppler mapping in the assessment of prosthetic valve regurgitation. *Br Heart J* 1989;62:1–8.

17. Reisner SA, Meltzer RS. Normal values of prosthetic valve Doppler echocardiographic parameters: a review. *J Am Soc Echocardiogr* 1988;1:201–10.

18. Ross DN. Homograft replacement of the aortic valve. *Lancet* 1962;2:487.

19. Barrett-Boyes BG, et al. Homograft aortic valve replacement in aortic incompetence and stenosis. *Thorax* 1964;19:131.

20. Zabalgoita M. Echocardiographic assessment of prosthetic heart valves. *Curr Probl Cardiol* 1992;17:265–325.

21. Seward JB, Khandeheria BK, Freeman WK, et al. Multiplane transesophageal echocardiography: image orientation, examination technique, anatomic correlations, and clinical applications. *Mayo Clin Proc* 1993;68:523–51.

22. Feigenbaum H. Acquired valvular heart disease. In Feigenbaum H, *Echocardiography*. 5th Ed. Philadelphia, Lea & Febiger, 1994, 239–349.

23. Kotler MN, Jacobs LE, Movsowitz HD, et al. Noninvasive evaluation of normal and abnormal prosthetic valve function. In St John Sutton MG, Oldershaw PJ, Kottler MN (eds.) *Textbook of Echocardiography and Doppler in Adults and Children.* 2nd Ed. Oxford, Blackwell Science, Ltd. 1996, 277–322.

24. Wilkins GT, Flachskampf FA, Weyman AE. Echo-Doppler assessment of prosthetic heart valves. In Weyman AE (ed). *Principles and Practice of Echocardiography.* 2nd Ed. Philadelphia, Lea & Febiger, 1994, 1198–230.

25. Nottestad SY, Zabalgoitia M. Echocardiographic recognition and quantitation of prosthetic valve dysfunction. In Otto CM (ed). *The Practice of Clinical Echocardiography.* Philadelphia, WB Saunders, 1997, pp. 797–820.

26. Oh CC, Click Rl, Orszulak TA, et al. The role of intraoperative transesophageal echocardiography in determining aortic annulus diameter in homograft insertion. *J Am Soc Echocardiogr* 1998;11:638–42.

27. Bach DS, LeMire MS, Eberhart D, et al. Impact of intraoperative post-pump aortic regurgitation with stentless aortic bioprostheses. *Semin Thorac Cardiovasc Surg* 1999;11(Suppl 1):88–92.

28. Guarracino F, Zussa C, Polesel E, et al. Influence of transesophageal echocardiography on intraoperative decision making for Toronto stentless prosthetic valve implantation. *J Heart Valve Dis* 2001;10:31–4.

29. Greve HH, Farah I, Everlien M. Comparison of three different types of stentless valves: full root or subcoronary. *Ann Thorac Surg* 2001;71(5 Suppl):S293–6.

30. Baur LH, Peels K, Braun J. et al. Echocardiographic imaging of stentless aortic valve prostheses. *Echocardiography* 2000;17:625–9.

31. Del Rizzo DF, Abdoh A. Clinical and hemodynamic comparison of the Medtronic Freestyle and Toronto SPV stentless valves. *J Card Surg* 1998;13:398–407.

32. Pepper JR, Chir M. The stentless porcine valve. *J Card Surg* 1998;13:352–9.

33. Weinert L, Karp R, Vignon P, et al. Feasibility of aortic diameter for preoperative selection and preparation of homograft aortic valves. *J Thorac Cardiovasc Surg* 1996;112:954–61.

34. Andrade A, Vargas-Baron J, Romero-Cardenas A, et al. Transthoracic and transesophageal echocardiographic study of pulmonary autograft valve in aortic position. *Echocardiography* 1994;11:221–6.

35. Brown BM, Karalis DG, Ross JR, et al. Limited value of single plane transesophageal echocardiography in prosthetic aortic valve malfunction. *J Am Soc Echocardiogr* 1991;4:284.

36. Nanda NC, Pinheiro L, Sanyal RS, Storey O. Transesophageal biplane echocardiographic imaging: technique planes and clinical usefulness. *Echocardiography* 1990;7:771–88.

37. Bansal RC, Shakudo M, Shah PM, Shah PM, Biplane transesophageal echocardiography: technique, image orientation and preliminary experience in 131 patients. *J Am Soc Echocardiogr* 1990;3:348–66.

38. Khandheria BK, Seward JB, Oh JK, et al. Value and limitations of transesophageal echocardiography in assessment of mitral valve prostheses. *Circulation* 1991;83:1956–68.

39. Herrera CJ, Chaudhry FA, DeFrino PF, et al. Value and limitations of transesophageal echocardiography in evaluating prosthetic or bioprosthetic valve dysfunction. *Am J Cardiol* 1992;69:697–9.

40. Van den Brink R, et al. Comparison of transthoracic and transesophageal color Doppler flow imaging in patients with mechanical prostheses in the mitral valve position. *Am J Cardiol* 1989;63:1471–4.

41. Kapur KK, et al. Doppler color flow mapping in the evaluation of prosthetic mitral and aortic valve function. *J Am Cardiol* 1989;13:1561–71.

42. Holen J, Nitter-Hauge S. Evaluation of obstructive characteristics of mitral disk valve implants with ultrasound Doppler techniques. *Acta Med Scand* 1977;201:429–34.

43. Omoto R, Matsumura M, Asano H et al. Doppler ultrasound examination of prosthetic function and ventricular blood flow after mitral valve replacement. *Herz* 1986;11:346–50.

44. Ryan T, Armstrong WF, Dillion JC, Feigenbaum H. Doppler echocardiographic evaluation of patients with porcine mitral valves. *Am Heart J* 1986;111:237–44.

45. Hatle L, Angelsen BA, Tomsdal A. Non-invasive assessment of aortic stenosis by Doppler ultrasound. *Br Heart J* 1980;43:284–92.

46. Teirstein P, Yock PG, Popp RL. The accuracy of Doppler ultrasound measurement of pressure gradients across irregular dual, and tunnel-like obstruction to blood flow. *Circulation* 1985;72:577–84.

47. Simpson IA, Fisher J, Reece IJ, et al. Comparison of Doppler ultrasound velocity measurements with pressure differences across bioprosthetic valves in a pulsatile flow model. *Cardiovasc Res* 1986;20:317–21.

48. Wilkins GT, et al. Validation of continuous-wave Doppler echocardiographic measurements of mitral and tricuspid prosthetic valve gradients: a simultaneous Doppler-catheter study. *Circulation* 1986;74:786–95.

49. Burstow DJ, Nishimura RA, Bailey, et al. Continuous wave Doppler echocardiographic measurements of prosthetic valve gradients. *Circulation* 1989;80:504–14.

50. Panidis IP, Ross J, Mintz GS. Normal and abnormal prosthetic valve function as assessed by Doppler echocardiography. *J Am Coll Cardiol* 1986;8:317–26.

51. Williams GA, Labovitz AJ. Doppler hemodynamic evaluation of prosthetic (Starr-Edwards and Bjork-Shiley) and bioprosthetic (Hancock and Carpentier-Edwards) cardiac valves. *Am J Cardiol* 1985;56:325–32.

52. Curtius JM, Pawelzik H, Mittmann B, Breuer HW, Loogen F. Doppler echocardiography normal values in various types of mitral valve prostheses. *Z Radiol* 1987;76:25–9.

53. Cooper DM, Stewart WJ, Schiavone WA, et al. Evaluation of normal prosthetic valve function by Doppler echocardiography. *Am Heart J.* 1987;114:576–82.

54. Sagar KB, Wann S, Paulsen WHJ, Romhilt DW. Doppler echocardiographic evaluation of Hancock and Bjork-Shiley prosthetic valves. *J Am Coll Cardiol* 1986;7:681–7.

55. Ramirez ML, Wong M, Sadler N, Shah PM. Doppler evaluation of bioprosthetic and mechanical aortic valves: Data from four models in 107 stable, ambulatory patients. *Am Heart J* 1988;115:418–25.

56. Heldman D, Gardin JM. Evaluation of prosthetic valves by Doppler echocardiography. *Echocardiography* 1989;6:63.

57. Connolly HM, Miller FA, Taylor Cl, et al. Doppler hemodynamic profiles of eight-six normal tricuspid prostheses. *J Am Col Cardiol* 1991;14:69A.

58. Gray R, Chaux A, Matloff JM et al. Bileaflet, tilting disk and porcine aortic valve substitutes: In vivo hydrodynamic characteristic. *J Am Col Cardiol* 1984;3:321–7.

59. Lillehei, CW. The St. Jude cardiac valvular prosthesis: A clinical appraisal at two years. In St. Jude Medical, Inc. 1980 International Valve symposium. St. Paul, Minnesota: St. Jude Medical, Inc., 1980 pp 26–39.

60. Bach DS, David T, Yacoub M, et al. Hemodynamics and left ventricular mass regression following implantation of the Toronto SPV stentless porcine valve. *Am J Cardiol* 1998;82:1214–19.

61. Wang Z, Grainger N, Chambers J. Doppler echocardiography in normally functioning replacement heart valves: A literature review. *J Heart Valve Dis* 1995;4:591–614.

62. Dumesnil J, LeBlanc MH, Cartier P, et al. Hemodynamic features of the freestyle aortic bioprosthesis compared with stented bioprosthesis. *Ann Thorac Surg* 1998;66(Suppl 6):S130–3.

63. Gonzalez-Juanatey J, Garcia-Benoechea J, Garcia-Acuna J, et al. The influence of the design on medium to long-term hemodynamic behavior of the 19 mm pericardial aortic valve prostheses. *J Heart Valve Dis* 1996;5(Suppl 3):S317–23.

64. Freestyle aortic root bioprosthesis: Product performance report, data current to October, 1996, Medtronic (1997).

65. On-X PMA application to the U.S. Food and Drug Administration, August 2000.

66. Salomon NW, Okies JE, Krause AH et al. Serial follow-up of an experimental bovine pericardial aortic bioprosthesis. Usefulness of pulsed Doppler echocardiography. *Circulation* 1991;84(Suppl III)140–4.

67. Perier et al. Long term evaluation Carpentier-Edwards pericardial valve in the aortic position. *J Card Surg* 1991;6:589–94.

68. Aupart M, Neville P, Dreyfus X et al. The Carpentier-Edwards pericardial aortic valve: intermediate results in 420 patients. *Eur J Cardiothorac Surg* 1994;8:277–80.

69. Rothbart RM, Smucker ML, Gibson RS. Overestimation by Doppler echocardiography of pressure gradients across Starr-Edwards prosthetic valves in the aortic position. *Am J Cardiol* 1988;61:475–6.

70. Bhatia S, et al. Frequency of unusually high transvalvular Doppler velocities in patients with normal prosthetic valves. *J Am Coll Cardiol* 1987;9(Suppl.A):238A.

71. Levine RA, Jimoh A, Cape EG, et al. Pressure recovery distal to a stenosis: potential cause of gradient 'overestimation' by Doppler echocardiography. *J Am Coll Cardiol* 1989;13:706–15.

72. Baumgartner H, Kahn S, DeRobertis M et al. Discrepancies between Doppler and catheter gradients in aortic prosthetic valves in vitro. *Circulation* 1990;82:1467–75.

73. Baumgartner H, Schima H, Kuhn P. Effect of prosthetic valve malfunction on the Doppler-catheter gradient relation for bileaflet aortic valve prostheses. *Circulation* 1993;87:1320–7.

74. Hatle L, Angelson B, Tromsdal A. Noninvasive assessment of atrioventricular pressure half-time by Doppler ultrasound. *Circulation* 1979;60:1096–104.

75. Williams GA, Labovitz AJ. Doppler hemodynamic evaluation of prosthetic (Starr-Edwards and Bjork-Shiley) and bioprosthetic (Hancock and Carpentier-Edwards) cardiac valves. *Am J Cardiol* 1985;56:325–32.

76. Fawzy ME. Hemodynamic evaluation of porcine bioprostheses in the mitral position by Doppler echocardiography. *Am J Cardiol* 1987;59:643–6.

77. Hsiung MC, Ku CS, Wei J, et al. Transesophageal color Doppler flow imaging in the evaluation of prosthetic cardiac valves. *Echocardiography* 1992;9:583–8.

78. Nanda NC, Domanski MJ. Prosthetic valves and rings. In *Atlas of Transesophageal Echocardiography*. Baltimore, Williams & Wilkins, 1998 p 181.

79. Mohr-Kahaly S, Kupferwasser I, Erbel R, et al. Regurgitant flow in apparently normal valve prostheses: improved detection and semiquantitative analysis by transesophageal two-dimensional color-coded Doppler echocardiography. *J Am Soc Echocardiogr* 1990;3:187–95.

80. Khandheria BK. Transesophageal echocardiography in the evaluation of prosthetic valves. *Cardiol Clin* 1993:11:427–36.

81. Flachskampf FA, Hoffmann R, Franke A, et al. Does multiplane transesophageal echocardiography improve the assessment of prosthetic valve regurgitation? J Am Echocardiogr 1995;8:70–8.

82. Hixson CS, Smith MD, Mattson MD, et al. Comparison of transesophageal color flow Doppler imaging of normal mitral regurgitant jets in St. Jude Medical and Medtronic Hall cardiac prostheses. *J Am Soc Echocardiogr* 1992;5:57–62.

83. Nellessen U, Schnittger I, Appleton CP, et al. Transesophageal two-dimensional echocardiography and color Doppler flow velocity mapping in the evaluation of cardiac valve prostheses. *Circulation* 1988;78:848–55.

84. Taams MA, Gussenhoven EJ, Cahalan MK, et al. Transesophageal Doppler color flow imaging in the detection of native and Bjork-Shiley mitral valve regurgitation. *J Am Coll Cardiol* 1989;13:95–9.

85. Van den Brink RBA, Visser CA, Basart DCG, et al. Comparison of transthoracic and transesophageal color Doppler flow imaging in patients with mechanical prostheses in the mitral valve position. *Am J Cardiol* 1989;63:1471–4.

86. Gallet B, Berrebi A, Grinda JM, et al. Severe intermittent intraprosthetic regurgitation after mitral valve replacement with subvalvular preservation. *J Am Soc Echocardiogr* 2001;14:314–16.

87. Forman MB, Phelan BK, Robertson RM, Virmani R. Correlation of two-dimensional echocardiography and pathological findings in porcine valve dysfunction. *J Am Coll Cardiol* 1985;5:224–30.

88. Crupi G, Gibson D, Heard B, Lincoln C. Severe late failure of a porcine xenograft mitral valve: clinical, echocardiographic and pathological findings. *Thorax* 1980;35:210–12.

89. Nicholson WJ, Gracey JF, Martin CE. Echocardiographic identification of prolapsing leaflet of a malfunctioning aortic porcine xenograft. *Clin Cardiol* 1983;6:97.

90. Bansal RC, Morrison DL, Jacobson JG. Echocardiography of porcine aortic prosthesis with flail leaflets due to degeneration and calcification. *Am Heart J* 1984;107:591–3.

91. Jaggers J, Chetham PM, Kinnard TL, Fullerton DA. Intraoperative prosthetic valve dysfunction: detection by transesophageal echocardiography. *Ann Thorac Surg* 1995;59:755–7.

92. Schapira JN. Two-dimensional echocardiographic assessment of patients with bioprosthetic valves. *Am J Cardiol* 1979;43:510–19.

93. Kotler MN. Noninvasive evaluation of normal and abnormal prosthetic valve function. *J Am Coll Cardiol* 1983;2:151–73.

94. Mehta A. Two-dimensional echocardiographic observations in major detachment of a prosthetic aortic valve. *Am Heart J* 1981;101:231–3.

95. Effron MK, Popp RL. Two-dimensional assessment of bioprosthetic valve dysfunction and infective endocarditis. *J Am Coll Cardiol* 1983;2:597–606.

96. Alam M, et al. Echocardiography evaluation of porcine bioprosthetic valves: experience with 309 normal and 59 dysfunctional valves. *Am J Cardiol* 1983;52:309–15.

97. Arnett EN, Roberts WC. Prosthetic valve endocarditis: clinicopathologic analysis of 22 necropsy patients with comparison of observations in 74 patients with active infective endocarditis involving natural left-sided cardiac valves. *Am J Cardiol* 1976;38:281–92.

98. Rossiter SJ, Stimson EB, Oyer PE, et al. Prosthetic valve endocarditis: comparison of heterograft tissue valves and mechanical valves. *J Thorac Cardiovasc Surg* 1978;76:795–803.

99. Magilligan DJ Jr, Lewis JW Jr, Java FM et al. Spontaneous degeneration of porcine bioprosthetic valves. *Ann Thorac Surg* 1980;30:259–66.

100. Karalis DG, Bansal RC, Hauck AJ, et al. Transesophageal echocardiographic recognition of subaortic complications in aortic valve endocarditis: clinical and surgical implications. *Circulation* 1992;86:353–62.

101. Mugge A, Daniel WG, Frank G, et al. Echocardiography in infective endocarditis: reassessment of prognostic implications of vegetation size determined by transthoracic and transesophageal approach. *J Am Coll Cardiol* 1989;14:631–8.

102. Erbel R, Rohmann S, Drexler M, et al. Improved diagnostic value of echocardiography in patients with infective endocarditis by transesophageal approach: a prospective study. *Eur Heart J* 1988;1:43–53.

103. Daniel WG, Schroder E, Mugge A, et al. Transesophageal echocardiography in infective endocarditis. *Am J Cardiac Imag* 1988;2:78–85.

104. Taams MA, Gussenhoven EJ, Bose. Enhanced morphological diagnosis in infective endocarditis by transesophageal echocardiography. *Br Heart J* 1990;63:109–13.

105. Mardelli TJ, Ogawa S, Hubbard FE, et al. Cross-sectional echocardiographic detection of aortic ring abscess in bacterial endocarditis. *Chest* 1978;74:576–8.

106. Come PC, Riley MF. Echocardiographic recognition of perivalvular infection complicating aortic bacterial endocarditis. *Am Heart J* 1984;108:166.

107. Polak PE, Gussenhoven WJ, Roelandt JR. Transesophageal cross-sectional echocardiographic recognition of an aortic valve ring abscess and a subannular mycotic aneurysm. *Eur Heart J* 1987;8:664–6.

108. Daniel WG, Mugge A, Martin RP, et al. Improvement in the diagnosis of abscesses associated with endocarditis by transesophageal echocardiography. *N Engl J Med* 1991;324:795–800.

109. Kemp WE Jr, Citrin B, Byrd BF 3rd. Echocardiography in infective endocarditis. *South Med J* 1999;92:744–54.

110. San Roman JA, Vilacosta I, Sarria C, et al. Clinical course, microbiologic profile, and diagnosis of periannular complications in prosthetic valve endocarditis. *Am J Card* 1999;83:1075–9.

111. Shimomura T, Usui A, Watanabe T, Yasuura K. A case of aortic prosthetic valve endocarditis with aortic root aneurysm. *Jpn J Thorac Cardiovasc Surg* 1998;46:1354–7.

112. Liu F, Ge J, Kupferwasser I, et al. Has transesophageal echocardiography changed the approach to patients with suspected or known infective endocarditis? *Echocardiography* 1995;12:637–50.

113. Alam M, Rosman HS, Sun I. Transesophageal echocardiographic evaluation of St. Jude medical and bioprosthetic valve endocarditis. *Am Heart J* 1992;123:236–9.

114. Pedersen WR, Walker M, Olson JD, et al. Value of transesophageal echocardiography as an adjunct to transthoracic echocardiography in evaluation of native and prosthetic valve endocarditis. *Chest* 1991;100:351–6.

115. Vered Z, Mossinson D, Pelege E, et al. Echocardiographic assessment of prosthetic valve endocarditis. *Eur Heart J* 1995;16(Suppl B):63–7.

116. Boskovic D, Pechacek LW, Krajcer Z. Thrombosis of a Bjork-Shiley aortic valve prosthesis diagnosed by two-dimensional echocardiography. *J Clin Ultrasound* 1983;11:165–9.

117. Barzilai B, et al. detection of thrombotic obstruction of a Bjork-Shiley prosthesis by Doppler echocardiography. *Am Heart J* 1986;112:1088–90.

118. Morishita A, Shimakura T, Nonoyama M, et al. A case of thrombosed St. Jude Medical valve 16 years after initial mitral valve replacement. *Kyobu Geka* 2001;54:501–4.

119. Gonzalez-Santos JM, et al. Thrombosis of a mechanical valve prosthesis late in pregnancy. Case report and review of the literature. *Thorac Cardiovasc Surg* 1986;34:335–7.

120. Lin SS, Tiong IY, Asher CR, et al. Prediction of thrombus-related mechanical prosthetic valve dysfunction using transesophageal echocardiography. *Am J Card* 2000;86:1097–101.

121. Dzavik V, Cohen G, Chan KL. Role of transesophageal echocardiography in the diagnosis and management of prosthetic valve thrombosis. *J Am Coll Cardiol* 1991;18:1829–33.

122. Nakatani S, Andoh M, Okita Y, et al. Prosthetic valve obstruction with normal disk motion: usefulness of transesophageal echocardiography to define cause. *J Am Soc Echocardiogr* 1999;12:537–9.

123. Barbetseas J, Nagueh SF, Pitsavos C, et al. Differentiating thrombus from pannus formation in obstructed mechanical prosthetic valves: an evaluation of clinical, transthoracic and transesophageal echocardiographic parameters. *J Am Coll Cardiol* 1998;32:1410–17.

124. Lengyel M, Vegh G, Vandor L. Thrombolysis is superior to heparin for non-obstructive mitral mechanical valve thrombosis. *J Heart Valve Dis* 1999;8:167–73.

125. Ledain LD, et al. Acute thrombotic obstruction with disk valve prosthesis: diagnostic considerations and fibrinolytic treatment. *J Am Coll Cardiol* 1986;7:743–51.

126. Kumar S, Garg N, Tewari S, et al. Role of thrombolytic therapy for stuck prosthetic valves: a serial echocardiographic study. *Indian Heart J* 2001;53:451–7.

127. Vasan RS, Kaul U, Sanghvi S, et al. Thrombolytic therapy for prosthetic valve thrombosis: a study based on serial Doppler echocardiographic evaluation. *Am Heart J* 1992;123:1575–80.

128. Zoghbi WA, Desir RM, Rosen L, et al. Doppler echocardiography: application to the assessment of successful thrombolysis of prosthetic valve thrombosis. *J Am Soc Echocardiogr* 1989; 2:98–101.

129. Koblic M, Carey C, Webb-Peploe MM, Braimbridge MV. Streptokinase treatment of thrombosed mitral valve prosthesis monitored by Doppler ultrasound. *Thorac Cardiovasc Surg* 1986;34:333–4.

130. Lengyel M, Fuster V, Keltai M, et al. Guidelines for management of left-sided prosthetic valve thrombosis: a role for thrombolytic therapy. Consensus Conference on Prosthetic Valve Thrombosis. *J Am Coll Cardiol* 1997;30:1521–6.

131. Rittoo D, Buckley H, Cotter L. Recurrent prosthetic valve thrombosis: importance of prolonged Doppler echocardiography examination for diagnosis. *J Am Soc Echocardiogr* 1999;12:686–8.

132. Young E, Shapiro SM, French WJ, Ginzton LE. Use of transesophageal echocardiography during thrombolysis with tissue plasminogen activator of a thrombosed prosthetic mitral valve. *J Am Soc Echocardiogr* 1992;5:153–8.

133. Ozkan M, Kaymaz C, Kirma C, et al. Intravenous thrombolytic treatment of mechanical prosthetic valve thrombosis: a study using serial transesophageal echocardiography. *J Am Coll Cardiol* 2000;35:1881–9.

134. Akowuah EF, Onyeaka CV, Cooper GJ. A subtle sign of aortic outflow obstruction in an infected 29 year old Starr-Edward's valve. *Heart* 2001;85:384.

135. Moggio RA, Hammond GL, Stansel HC Jr, Glenn WW. Incidence of emboli with cloth-covered Starr-Edwards valve without anticoagulation and with varying forms of anticoagulation. Analysis of 183 patients followed for 3 1/2 years. *J Thorac Cardiovasc Surg* 1978;75:296–9.

136. Sakata K, Ishikawa S, Ohtaki A, et al. Malfunctioning Starr-Edwards mitral valve 21 years after installation. *J Cardiovasc Surg (Torino)* 1997;38:81–2.

137. Orszulak TA, Schaff HV, Puga FJ, et al. Event status of the Starr-Edwards aortic valve to 20 years: a benchmark for comparison. *Ann Thorac Surg* 1997;63:620–6.

138. Godje OL, Fischlein T, Adelhard K, et al. Thirty-year results of Starr-Edwards prostheses in the aortic and mitral position. *Ann Thorac Surg* 1997;63:613–19.

139. Pollock SG, Dent JM, Simek CL, et al. Starr-Edwards valve thrombosis detected preoperatively by transesophageal echocardiography. *Cathet Cardiovasc Diagn* 1994;31:156–7.

140. Alton ME, Pasierski TJ, Orsinelli DA, et al. Comparison of transthoracic and transesophageal echocardiography in evaluation of 47 Starr-Edwards prosthetic valves. *J Am Coll Cardiol* 1992;20:1503–11.

141. Schoevaerdts JC, Buche M, el Gariani A, et al. Twenty years' experience with the Model 6120 Starr-Edwards valve in the mitral position. *J Thorac Cardiovasc Surg* 1987;94:375–82.

142. Best JF, Hassanein KM, Pugh DM, Dunn M. Starr-Edwards aortic prosthesis: a 20-year retrospective study. *Am Heart J* 1986;111:136–42.

143. Jett GK, Jett MD, Barnhart GR, et al. Left ventricular outflow tract obstruction with mitral valve replacement in small ventricular cavities. *Ann Thorac Surg* 1986;41:70–4.

144. Starr A. The Starr-Edwards valve. *J Am Coll Cardiol* 1985;6:899–903.

145. Moggio RA, Hammond GL, Stansel HC, Glenn WW. Incidence of emboli with cloth-covered Starr-Edwards valve without anticoagulation and with varying forms of anticoagulation. Analysis of 183 patients followed for 3 1/2 years. *J Thorac Cardiovasc Surg* 1978;75:296–9.

146. Lamberti JJ, Gupta DS, Falicov R, Anagnostopoulos CE. An unusual form of late stenosis after aortic valve replacement with a cloth-covered Starr-Edwards prosthesis. *Chest* 1977;71:89–90.

147. Russell T 2nd, Kremkau EL, Kloster F, Starr A. Late hemodynamic function of cloth-covered Starr-Edwards valve prostheses. *Circulation* 1972;45(1 Suppl):I8–13.

148. Joob AW, Kron IL, Craddock GB, et al. A decade of experience with the Model 103 and 104 Beall valve prostheses. *J Thorac Cardiovasc Surg* 1985;89:444–7.

149. Ramsey HW, Williams JC Jr, Vernon CR, et al. Hemodynamic findings following replacement of the mitral valve with the Beall valve prosthesis. *J Thorac Cardiovasc Surg* 1971;62:624–30.

150. Linhart JW, Barold SS, Hildner FJ, et al. Clinical and hemodynamic findings following replacement of the mitral valve with a Beall valve prosthesis (Dacron Velour-covered Teflon-disk valve). *Circulation* 1969;39(5 Suppl 1):I127–34.

151. Vogel JH, Paton BC, Overy HR, et al. Advantages of the Beall valve prosthesis. *Chest* 1971;59:249–53.

152. Joob AW, Kron IL, Craddock GB, et al. A decade of experience with the Model 103 and 104 Beall valve prostheses. *J Thorac Cardiovasc Surg* 1985;89:444–7.

153. Ramsey HW, Williams JC, Vernon CR, et al. Hemodynamic findings following replacement of the mitral valve with the Beall valve prosthesis. *J Thorac Cardiovasc Surg* 1971;62:624–30.

154. Williams JC Jr, Vernon CR, Daicoff GR, et al. Hemolysis following mitral valve replacement with the Beall valve prosthesis. *J Thorac Cardiovasc Surg* 1971;61:393–6.

155. Hill RC, Sethi GK, Scott SM, et al. Disk embolization from a Beall mitral valve prosthesis. *J Cardiovasc Surg* 1989;30:384–7.

156. Coralli RJ, Dorney ER, Walter PF. Intermittent mitral regurgitation: an indicator of severe Beall valve dysfunction. *Clin Cardiol* 1987;10:419–22.

157. Conti VR, Nishimura A, Coughlin TR, Farrell RW. Indications for replacement of the Beall 103 and 104 disk valves. *Ann Thorac Surg* 1986;42:315–20.

158. Itzkoff JM, Curtiss EI, Reddy PS, Uretsky BF, Shaver JA. Intermittent mitral regurgitation due to Beall valve dysfunction: analysis of 13 patients with atrial fibrillation. *Am J Cardiol* 1984; 53:1071–4.

159. Ho KJ. Chronic systemic Dacron and Teflon embolization of a Beall model 103 mitral valve prosthesis. *J Thorac Cardiovasc Surg* 1979;77:875–9.

160. Montoya A, Sullivan HJ, Pifarre R. Disk variance: a potentially lethal complication of the Beall valve prosthesis. *J Thorac Cardiovasc Surg* 1976;71:904–6.

161. Salomon NW, Steele PP, Paton BC. Thromboembolism after Beall Valve replacement of the mitral valve. *Ann Thorac Surg* 1975;19:33–9.

162. Jost RG, McKnight RC, Roper CL. Failure of Beal mitral valve prosthesis. Clinical and radiographic features. *J Thorac Cardiovasc Surg* 1975;70:163–5.

163. Hildner FJ, Robinson MJ. Complications of Beall valve prosthesis. *Am J Cardiol* 1972;30:922.

164. Williams JC, Vernon CR, Daicoff GR, et al. Hemolysis following mitral valve replacement with the Beall valve prosthesis. *J Thorac Cardiovasc Surg* 1971;61:393–6.

165. Pyle RB, Mayer JE Jr, Lindsay WG, et al. Hemodynamic evaluation of Lillehei-Kaiser and Starr-Edwards prosthesis. *Ann Thorac Surg* 1978;26:336–43.

166. Mazzaro E, Bortolotti U, Milano A, et al. Long term survival without anticoagulation after aortic valve replacement with a Lillehei-Kaster prosthesis. A case report. *J Heart Valve Dis* 1993;2:420–2; discussion 423.

167. Olesen KH, Rygg IH, Wennevold A, Nyboe J. Aortic valve replacement with the Lillehei-Kaster prosthesis in 262 patients: an assessment after 9 to 17 years. *Eur Heart J* 1991;12:680–9.

168. Mikhail AA, Ellis R, Johnson S. Eighteen-year evolution from the Lillehei-Kaster valve to the Omni design. *Ann Thorac Surg* 1989;48(3 Suppl):S61–4.

169. Stewart S, Cianciotta D, Hicks GL, DeWeese JA. The Lillehei-Kaster aortic valve prosthesis. Long-term results in 273 patients with 1253 patient-years of follow-up. *J Thorac Cardiovasc Surg* 1988;95:1023–30.

170. Olesen KH, Rygg IH, Wennevold A, Nyboe J. Long-term follow-up in 54 patients after combined mitral and aortic valve replacement with the Lillehei-Kaster prosthesis. Overall results and prosthesis-related complications. *Eur Heart J* 1987;8:1090–8.

171. Thevenet A. Lillehei-Kaster prosthesis in the aortic position with and without anticoagulants. *J Cardiovasc Surg (Torino)* 1980;21:669–74.

172. Teijeira FJ. Long-term experience with the omniscience cardiac valve. *J Heart Valve Dis* 1998;7:540–7.

173. Mikhail AA. Omniscience valve evolution and literature. *Ann Thorac Surg* 1996;62:624–6.

174. Akalin H, Corapcioglu ET, Ozyurda U, et al. Clinical evaluation of the Omniscience cardiac valve prosthesis. Follow-up of up to 6 years. *J Thorac Cardiovasc Surg* 1992;103:259–66.

175. DeWall RA. Thrombotic complications with the Omniscience valve: a current review. *J Thorac Cardiovasc Surg* 1989;98:298–300.

176. Kazui T, Komatsu S, Inoue N. Clinical evaluation of the Omniscience aortic disk valve prosthesis. *Scand J Thorac Cardiovasc Surg* 1987;21:173–8.

177. Carrier M, Martineau JP, Bonan R, Pelletier LC. Clinical and hemodynamic assessment of the Omniscience prosthetic heart valve. *J Thorac Cardiovasc Surg* 1987;93:300–7.

178. Callaghan JC, Coles J, Damle A. Six year clinical study of use of the Omniscience valve prosthesis in 219 patients. *J Am Coll Cardiol* 1987;9:240–6.

179. Dewall R, Pelletier LC, Panebianco A, et al. Factors influencing thromboembolic complications in Omniscience cardiac valve patients. *Eur Heart J* 1984;5(Suppl D):53–7.

180. Fananapazir L, Clarke DB, Dark JF, et al. Results of valve replacement with the Omniscience prosthesis. *J Thorac Cardiovasc Surg* 1983;86:621–5.

181. Montero CG, Rufilanchas JJ, Juffe A, et al. Long-term results of cardiac valve replacement with the Delrin-disk model of the Bjork-Shiley valve prosthesis. *Ann Thorac Surg* 1984;37:328–36.

182. Sethia B, Turner MA, Lewis S, Rodger RA, Bain WH. Fourteen years' experience with the Bjork-Shiley tilting disk prosthesis. *J Thorac Cardiovasc Surg* 1986;91:350–61.

183. Bloomfield P, Wheatley DJ, Prescott RJ, Miller HC. Twelve-year comparison of a Bjork-Shiley mechanical heart valve with porcine bioprostheses. *N Engl J Med* 1991;324:573–9.

184. Febres-Roman PR, Bourg WC, Crone RA, et al. Chronic intravascular hemolysis after aortic valve replacement with Ionescu-Shiley xenograft: comparative study with Bjork-Shiley prosthesis. *Am J Cardiol* 1980;46:735–8.

185. Clements SD Jr, Perkins JV. Malfunction of a Bjork-Shiley prosthetic heart valve in the mitral position producing an abnormal echocardiographic pattern. *J Clin Ultrasound* 1978;6:334–6.

186. Lindower PD, Dellsperger KC, Johnson B, et al. Variability of regurgitation in Bjork-Shiley mitral valves and relationship to disk occluder design: an in vitro two-dimensional color-Doppler flow mapping study. *J Heart Valve Dis* 1996;5(Suppl 2):S178–83.

187. Lindblom D, Bjork VO, Semb BK. Mechanical failure of the Bjork-Shiley valve. Incidence, clinical presentation, and management. *J Thorac Cardiovasc Surg* 1986;92:894–907.

188. Wolfe SM, Greenberg A. Strut fractures with the Bjork-Shiley valve. *N Engl J Med* 1985;312:314–15.

189. Bjork VO, Lindblom D. The Monostrut Bjork-Shiley heart valve. *J Am Coll Card* 1985;6:1142–8.

190. Kenny A, Woods J, Fuller CA, et al. Hemodynamic evaluation of the Monostrut and spherical disk Bjork-Shiley aortic valve prosthesis with Doppler echocardiography. *J Thorac Cardiovasc Surg* 1992;104:1025–8.

191. Sava HP, McDonnell JT. Differences in spectral composition between monostrut Bjork-Shiley and Carbomedics valves implanted in the aortic position. *Med Bio Eng Comput* 1995;33:689–94.

192. Lindblom D. Long-term clinical results after aortic valve replacement with the Bjork-Shiley prosthesis. *J Thorac Cardiovasc Surg* 1988;95:658–67.

193. Lindblom D, Lindblom U, Henze A, Bjork VO, Semb BK. Three-year clinical results with the Monostrut Bjork-Shiley prosthesis. *J Thorac Cardiovasc Surg* 1987;94:34–43.

194. Butchart EG, Li HH, Payne N, et al. Twenty years' experience with the Medtronic Hall valve. *J Thorac Cardiovasc Surg* 2001;121:1090–100.

195. Hutchinson K, Hafeez F, Woods TD, et al. Recurrent ischemic strokes in a patient with Medtronic-Hall prosthetic aortic valve and valve strands. *J Am Soc Echocardiogr* 1998;11:755–7.

196. Nitter-Hauge S, Abdelnoor M, Svennevig JL. Fifteen-year experience with the Medtronic-Hall valve prosthesis. A follow-up study of 1104 consecutive patients. *Circulation* 1996;94(9 Suppl):II105–8.

197. Aris A, Ramirez I, Camara ML, et al. The 20 mm Medtronic Hall prosthesis in the small aortic root. *J Heart Valve Dis* 1996;5:459–62.

198. Rabago G, Corbi P, Tedy G, et al. Five-year experience with the Medtronic Hall prosthesis in isolated aortic valve replacement. *J Card Surg* 1993;8:85–8.

199. Hall KV. The Medtronic-Hall valve: a design in 1977 to improve the results of valve replacement. *Eur J Cardiothorac Surg* 1992;6(Suppl 1):S64–7.

200. Vallejo JL, Gonzalez-Santos JM, Albertos J, et al. Eight years' experience with the Medtronic-Hall valve prosthesis. *Ann Thorac Surg* 1990;50:429–36.

201. Keenan RJ, Armitage JM, Trento A, et al. Clinical experience with the Medtronic-Hall valve prosthesis. *Ann Thorac Surg* 1990;50:748–53.

202. Nitter-Hauge S, Abdelnoor M. Ten-year experience with the Medtronic Hall valvular prosthesis. A study of 1,104 patients. *Circulation* 1989;80(3 Pt 1):I43–8.

203. Butchart EG, Lewis PA, Grunkemeier GL, et al. Low risk of thrombosis and serious embolic events despite low-intensity anticoagulation. Experience with 1,004 Medtronic Hall valves. *Circulation* 1988;78(3 Pt 2):I66–77.

204. Antunes MJ, Wessels A, Sadowski RG, et al. Medtronic Hall valve replacement in a third-world population group. A review of the performance of 1000 prostheses. *J Thorac Cardiovasc Surg* 1988;95:980–93.

205. Beaudet RL, Poirier NL, Doyle D, et al. The Medtronic-Hall cardiac valve: 7 1/2 years' clinical experience. *Ann Thorac Surg* 1986;42:644–50.

206. Hall KV, Nitter-Hauge S, Abdelnoor M. Seven and one-half years' experience with the Medtronic-Hall valve. *J Am Coll Cardiol* 1985;6:1417–21.

207. Beaudet RL, Poirier NL, Guerraty AJ, Doyle D. Fifty-four months' experience with an improved tilting disk valve (Medtronic-Hall). *Thorac Cardiovasc Surg* 1983;31(Spec 2):89–93.

208. Butchart EG, Griffiths BE, Breckenridge IM. Clinical and echocardiographic assessment of the Medtronic-Hall valve: experience with 370 implanted valves. *Thorac Cardiovasc Surg* 1983;31(Spec 2):81–4.

209. Semb BK, Hall KV, Nitter-Hauge S, Abdelnoor M. A 5-year follow-up of the Medtronic-Hall valve: survival and thromboembolism. *Thorac Cardiovasc Surg* 1983;31(Spec 2):61–5.

210. Rabago G, Fraile J, Martinell J, et al. Early surgical results of the Medtronic-Hall valve. *Thorac Cardiovasc Surg* 1983;31(Spec 2):59–60.

211. Castro Farinas E, Ponce Rodriguez G. Medtronic-Hall valve: thromboembolic complications. *Thorac Cardiovasc Surg* 1983;31(Spec 2):94–6.

212. St John Sutton M, Roudaut R, Oldershaw P, Bricaud H. Echocardiographic assessment of left ventricular filling characteristics after mitral valve replacement with the St. Jude medical prosthesis. *Br Heart J* 1981;45:365–8.

213. Lund O, Nielsen SL, Arildsen H, et al. Standard aortic St. Jude valve at 18 years: performance profile and determinants of outcome. *Ann Thorac Surg* 2000;69:1459–65.

214. DiSesa VJ, Collins JJ Jr, Cohn LH. Hematological complications with the St. Jude valve and reduced-dose Coumadin. *Ann Thorac Surg* 1989;48:280–3.

215. Nair CK, Mohiuddin SM, Hilleman DE, et al. Ten-year results with the St. Jude Medical prosthesis. *Am J Cardiol* 1990;65:217–25.

216. Crawford FA Jr, Kratz JM, Sade RM, et al. Aortic and mitral valve replacement with the St. Jude Medical prosthesis. *Ann Surg* 1984;199:753–61.

217. Fisher J. Comparative study of the hydrodynamic function of the size 19mm and 21mm St. Jude Medical Hemodynamic Plus Bileaflet Heart valves. *J Heart Valve Dis* 1994;3:75–80.

218. Khan SS. Assessment of prosthetic valve hemodynamics by Doppler: lessons from in vitro studies of the St. Jude valve. *J Heart Valve Dis* 1993;2:183–93.

219. Eber B, Brussee H, Auer T, Rotman B. The St. Jude Valve: thrombolysis as the first line of therapy for cardiac valve thrombosis. *Circulation* 1993;88:809–10.

220. Nair CK, Mohiuddin SM, Hilleman DE, et al. Ten-year results with the St. Jude Medical prosthesis. *Am J Cardiol* 1990;65:217–25.

221. Myers ML, Lawrie GM, Crawford ES, et al. The St. Jude valve prosthesis: analysis of the clinical results in 815 implants and the need for systemic anticoagulation. *J Am Coll Cardiol* 1989;13:57–62.

222. Czer LS, Matloff JM, Chaux A, et al. The St. Jude valve: analysis of thromboembolism, warfarin-related hemorrhage, and survival. *Am Heart J* 1987;114:389–97.

223. Jones TW, Thomas GI, Stavney LS, Manhas DR. The St. Jude experience. *Am J Surg* 1984;147:593–7.

224. Panidis IP, Ren JF, Kotler MN, et al. Clinical and echocardiographic evaluation of the St. Jude cardiac valve prosthesis: follow-up of 126 patients. *J Am Coll Cardiol* 1984;4:454–62.

225. St John Sutton M, Roudaut R, Oldershaw P, Bricaud H. Echocardiographic assessment of left ventricular filling characteristics after mitral valve replacement with the St. Jude medical prosthesis. *Br Heart J* 1981;45:365–8.

226. Lange HW, Olson JD, Pederson WR, et al. Transesophageal color Doppler echocardiography of the normal St. Jude medical mitral valve prosthesis. *Am Heart J* 1991;122:489–94.

227. Seipelt RG, Vazquez-Jimenez JF, Seipelt IM, et al. The St. Jude "Silzone" valve: midterm results in treatment of active endocarditis. *Ann Thorac Surg* 2001;72:758–62.

228. Kjaergard HK, Tingleff J, Abildgaard U, Pettersson G. Recurrent endocarditis in silver-coated heart valve prosthesis. *J Heart Valve Dis* 1999;8:140–2.

229. Li HH, Hahn J, Urbanski P, et al. Intermediate-term results with 1,019 Carbomedics aortic valves. *Ann Thorac Surg* 2001;71:1181–7; discussion 1187–8.

230. Shapira Y, Nili M, Hirsch R, et al. Mid-term clinical and echocardiographic follow up of patients with CarboMedics valves in the tricuspid position. *J Heart Valve Dis* 2000;9:396–402.

231. Copeland JG 3rd, Sethi GK. Four-year experience with the CarboMedics valve: the North American experience. North American team of clinical investigators for the CarboMedics prosthetic heart valve. *Ann Thorac Surg* 1994;58:630–7; discussion 637–8.

232. Bernal JM, Rabasa JM, Gutierrez-Garcia F, et al. The CarboMedics valve: experience with 1,049 implants. *Ann Thorac Surg* 1998;65:137–43.

233. Rodler SM, Moritz A, Schreiner W, et al. Five-year follow-up after heart valve replacement with the CarboMedics bileaflet prosthesis. *Ann Thorac Surg* 1997;63:1018–25.

234. Copeland JG. The CarboMedics prosthetic heart valve: a second generation bileaflet prosthesis. *Semin Thorac Cardiovasc Surg* 1996;8:237–41.

235. Nistal JF, Hurle A, Revuelta JM, Gandarillas M. Clinical experience with the CarboMedics valve: early results with a new bileaflet mechanical prosthesis. *J Thorac Cardiovasc Surg* 1996;112:59–68.

236. Abe T, Kamata K, Kuwaki K, Komatsu K, Komatsu S. Ten years' experience of aortic valve replacement with the Omnicarbon valve prosthesis. *Ann Thorac Surg* 1996;61:1182–7.

237. Fiane AE, Saatvedt K, Svennevig JL, et al. The CarboMedics valve: midterm follow-up with analysis of risk factors. *Ann Thorac Surg* 1995;60:1053–8.

238. Copeland JG. An international experience with the CarboMedics prosthetic heart valve. *J Heart Valve Dis* 1995;4:56–62.

239. Copeland JG, Sethi GK. Four-year experience with the CarboMedics valve: the North American experience. North American team of clinical investigators for the CarboMedics prosthetic heart valve. *Ann Thorac Surg* 1994;58:630–7; discussion 637–8.

240. de Luca L, Vitale N, Giannolo B, et al. Mid-term follow-up after heart valve replacement with CarboMedics bileaflet prostheses. *J Thorac Cardiovasc Surg* 1993;106:1158–65.

241. Subotic S, Petrovic P, Boskovic D, et al. Clinical and functional evaluation of the Carbomedics Prosthetic Heart Valve in the mitral position. Preliminary results. *J Cardiovasc Surg* 1990;31:509–11.

242. Laczkovics A, Heidt M, Oelert H, et al. Early clinical experience with the On-X prosthetic heart valve. *J Heart Valve Dis* 2001;10:94–9.

243. Walther T, Falk V, Tigges R, et al. Comparison of On-X and SJM HP bileaflet aortic valves. *J Heart Valve Dis* 2000;9:403–7.

244. Birnbaum D, Laczkovics A, Heidt M, et al. Examination of hemolytic potential with the On-X(R) prosthetic heart valve. *J Heart Valve Dis* 2000;9:142–5.

245. Fraund S, Pethig K, Wahlers T, et al. ON-X bileaflet valve in aortic position—early experience shows an improved hemodynamic profile. *Thorac Cardiovasc Surg* 1998;46:293–7.

246. Chambers J, Ely JL. Early postoperative echocardiographic hemodynamic performance of the On-X prosthetic heart valve: a multicenter study. *J Heart Valve Dis* 1998;7:569–73.

247. Hwang NH, Reul H, Reinhard P. In vitro evaluation of the long-body On-X bileaflet heart valve. *J Heart Valve Dis* 1998;7:561–8.

248. Shiono M, Sezai Y, Sezai A, et al. Multi-institutional experience of the ATS open pivot bileaflet valve in Japan. *Ann Thorac Cardiovasc Surg* 1996;2:51–8.

249. Van Nooten G, Caes F, François K, et al. Clinical experience with the first 100 ATS heart valve implants. *Cardiovasc Surg* 1996;4:288–92.

250. Karpuz H, Jeanrenaud X, Hurni M, et al. Doppler echocardiographic assessment of the new ATS medical prosthetic valve in the aortic position. *Am J Card Imaging* 1996;10:254–60.

251. Westaby S, Van Nooten G, Sharif H, Pillai R, Caes F. Valve replacement with the ATS open pivot bileaflet prosthesis *Eur J Cardiothoracic Surg* 1996;10:660–5.

252. Aoyagi S, Kawara T, Fukunaga S, et al. Cineradiographic Evaluation of ATS Open Pivot Bileaflet Valves. *J Heart Valve Dis* 1997;6:258–63.

253. Van Nooten G, Van Belleghem Y, Caes F, et al. Anticoagulation revised for mechanical ATS heart valve implants. In: Krian A, Matloff JM, Nicoloff DM, eds. *Advancing the Technology of Bileaflet Mechanical Heart Valves* (Darmstadt: Steinkopff Verlag, 1998), pp. 23–36.

254. Kim HJ, Kim WJ, Jo WM, et al. Clinical evaluation of the ATS Medical valve. In: Krian A, Matloff J M, Nicoloff DM, eds *Advancing the Technology of Bileaflet Mechanical Heart Valves* (Darmstadt: Steinkopff Verlag, 1998), pp. 47–52.

255. Krian A. Clinical results of a large series of ATS valve implants. In: Krian A, Matloff JM, Nicoloff DM, eds. *Advancing the Technology of Bileaflet Mechanical Heart Valves* (Darmstadt: Steinkopff Verlag, 1998), pp. 53–72.

256. Tesar PJ, O'Brien MF, Mau TK, Pohlner PG. Queensland/Australian experience with the ATS mechanical valve November 1996. In: Krian A, Matloff JM, Nicoloff DM, eds. *Advancing the Technology of Bileaflet Mechanical Heart Valves*, (Darmstadt: Steinkopff Verlag, 1998), pp. 75–88.

257. Fraile J, Martinell J, Artiz V, et al. ATS Medical mechanical valve prosthesis in reoperations. In: Krian A, Matloff JM, Nicoloff DM, eds. *Advancing the Technology of Bileaflet Mechanical Heart Valves* (Darmstadt: Steinkopff Verlag, 1998), pp. 101–10.

258. Parravicini R, Barchetti M, Reggianini L, et al. ATS prosthetic valves AP series: echocardiographic evaluation. In: Krian A, Matloff JM, Nicoloff DM, eds. *Advancing the Technology of Bileaflet Mechanical Heart Valves* (Darmstadt: Steinkopff Verlag, 1998), pp. 111–16.

259. Revuelta JM, Garcia-Rinaldi R, Johnston RH Jr, et al. The Ionescu-Shiley valve: a solution for the small aortic root. *J Thorac Cardiovasc Surg* 1984;88:234–7.

260. Walker WE, Duncan JM, Frazier OH Jr, et al. Early experience with the Ionescu-Shiley pericardial xenograft valve. Accelerated calcification in children. *J Thorac Cardiovasc Surg* 1983;86:570–5.

261. Febres-Roman PR, Bourg WC, Crone RA, et al. Chronic intravascular hemolysis after aortic valve replacement with Ionescu-Shiley xenograft: comparative study with Bjork-Shiley prosthesis. *Am J Cardiol* 1980;46:735–8.

262. Masters RG, Walley VM, Pipe AL, Keon WJ. Long-term experience with the Ionescu-Shiley pericardial valve. *Ann Thorac Surg* 1995;60(2 Suppl):S288–91.

263. Walley VM. Ionescu-Shiley valve failures. *Ann Thorac Surg* 1993;55:1048–9.

264. Walley VM, Keon CA, Khalili M, et al. Ionescu-Shiley valve failure. II: Experience with 25 low-profile explants. *Ann Thorac Surg* 1992;54:117–22; discussion 122–3.

265. Walley VM, Keon CA, Khalili M, et al. Ionescu-Shiley valve failure. I: Experience with 125 standard-profile explants. *Ann Thorac Surg* 1992;54:111–16.

266. Eng J, Ravichandran PS, Kay PH, Murday AJ. Long-term results of Ionescu-Shiley valve in the tricuspid position. *Ann Thorac Surg* 1991;51:200–3.

267. Bojar RM, Diehl JT, Moten M, et al. Clinical and hemodynamic performance of the Ionescu-Shiley valve in the small aortic root. Results in 117 patients with 17 and 19 mm valves. *J Thorac Cardiovasc Surg* 1989;98:1087–95.

268. Jacobs LE, Parry WR, Kotler MN. Pulsed, continuous, and color flow Doppler echocardiographic assessment of normal and abnormal Ionescu-Shiley pericardial valves. *J Card Surg* 1988;3(3 Suppl):429–35.

269. Walley VM. The low-profile Ionescu-Shiley valve. *J Thorac Cardiovasc Surg* 1988;96:969–70.

270. Daenen W, Noyez L, Lesaffre E, et al. The Ionescu-Shiley pericardial valve: results in 473 patients. *Ann Thorac Surg* 1988;46:536–41.

271. Goldman B, Scully H, Tong C, et al. Clinical results of pericardial xenograft valves: the Ionescu-Shiley and Hancock valves. *Can J Cardiol* 1988;4:328–32.

272. Revuelta JM, Duran CM. Performance of the Ionescu-Shiley pericardial valve in the aortic position: 100 months clinical experience. *Thorac Cardiovasc Surg* 1986;34:247–51.

273. Gallo I, Nistal F, Revuelta JM, et al. Incidence of primary tissue valve failure with the Ionescu-Shiley pericardial valve. Preliminary results. *J Thorac Cardiovasc Surg* 1985;90:278–80.

274. Toon RS, Grooters RK, Soltanzadeh H. Ionescu-Shiley valve defect. *Ann Thorac Surg* 1984;37:180.

275. Revuelta JM, Garcia-Rinaldi R, Johnston RH, et al. The Ionescu-Shiley valve: a solution for the small aortic root. *J Thorac Cardiovasc Surg* 1984;88:234–7.

276. Revuelta JM, Duran D, Figueroa A, Vega JL, Duran CM. The Ionescu-Shiley pericardial bioprostheses in the aortic position. A 5-year perspective. *J Cardiovasc Surg* 1984;25:199–204.

277. Walker WE, Duncan JM, Frazier OH, et al. Early experience with the Ionescu-Shiley pericardial xenograft valve. Accelerated calcification in children. *J Thorac Cardiovasc Surg* 1983;86:570–5.

278. Szkopiec RL, Torstveit J, Desser KB, et al. M-Mode and 2–dimensional echocardiographic characteristics of the Ionescu-Shiley valve in the mitral and aortic positions. *Am J Cardiol* 1983;51:973–80.

279. Gabbay S, Factor SM, Strom J, et al. Sudden death due to cuspal dehiscence of the Ionescu-Shiley valve in the mitral position. *J Thorac Cardiovasc Surg* 1982;84:313–14.

280. Becker RM, Sandor L, Tindel M, Frater RW. Medium-term follow-up of the Ionescu-Shiley heterograft valve. *Ann Thorac Surg* 1981;32:120–6.

281. Febres-Roman PR, Bourg WC, Crone RA, et al. Chronic intravascular hemolysis after aortic valve replacement with Ionescu-Shiley xenograft: comparative study with Bjork-Shiley prosthesis. *Am J Cardiol* 1980;46:735–8.

282. Khan SS, Chaux A, Blanche C, et al. A 20–year experience with the Hancock porcine xenograft in the elderly. *Ann Thorac Surg* 1998;66(6 Suppl):S35–9.

283. Magilligan DJ Jr, Quinn EL, Davila JC. Bacteremia, endocarditis, and the Hancock valve. *Ann Thorac Surg* 1977;24:508–18.

284. Kawachi Y, Tominaga R, Hisahara M, et al. Excellent durability of the Hancock porcine bioprosthesis in the tricuspid position. A sixteen-year follow-up study. *J Thorac Cardiovasc Surg* 1992;104:1561–6.

285. Bortolotti U, Milano A, Thieve G, Mazzucco A. Original expectations of the Hancock valve and 20 years of clinical reality. *Eur J Cardiothorac Surg* 1992;6(Suppl 1):S75–8.

286. Khan SS, Mitchell RS, Derby GC, et al. Differences in Hancock and Carpentier-Edwards porcine xenograft aortic valve hemodynamics. Effect of valve size. *Circulation* 1990;82(5 Suppl):IV117–24.

287. Gallo JI, Ruiz B, Carrion MF, et al. Heart valve replacement with the Hancock bioprosthesis: a 6-year review. *Ann Thorac Surg* 1981;31:444–9.

288. Ubago JL, Figueroa A, Colman T, et al. Hemodynamic factors that affect calculated orifice areas in the mitral Hancock xenograft valve. *Circulation* 1980;61:388–94.

289. Broom ND, Thomson FJ. Influence of fixation conditions on the performance of glutaraldehyde-treated porcine aortic valves: towards a more scientific basis. *Thorax* 1979;34:166–76.

290. Bortolotti U, Gallucci V, Casarotto D, Thiene G. Fibrous tissue overgrowth on Hancock mitral xenografts: a cause of late prosthetic stenosis. *Thorac Cardiovasc Surg* 1979;27:316–18.

291. Buch WS, Pipkin RD, Hancock WD, Fogarty TJ. Mitral valve replacement with the Hancock stabilized glutaraldehyde valve. Clinical and laboratory evaluation. *Arch Surg* 1975;110:1408–15.

292. Le Tourneau T, Savoye C, McFadden EP, et al. Mid-term comparative follow-up after aortic valve replacement with Carpentier-Edwards and Pericarbon pericardial prostheses. *Circulation* 1999;100(19 Suppl):II11–16.

293. Bove EL, Marvasti MA, Potts JL, et al. Rest and exercise hemodynamics following aortic valve replacement. A comparison between 19 and 21 mm Ionescu-Shiley pericardial and Carpentier-Edwards porcine valves. *J Thorac Cardiovasc Surg* 1985;90:750–5.

294. Blair KL, Hatton AC, White WD, et al. Comparison of anticoagulation regimens after Carpentier-Edwards aortic or mitral valve replacement. *Circulation* 1994;90(5 Pt 2):II214–19.

295. Khan SS, Mitchell RS, Derby GC, et al. Differences in Hancock and Carpentier-Edwards porcine xenograft aortic valve hemodynamics. Effect of valve size. *Circulation* 1990;82(5 Suppl):IV117–24.

296. Nashef SA, Sethia B, Turner MA, et al. Bjork-Shiley and Carpentier-Edwards valves. A comparative analysis. *J Thorac Cardiovasc Surg* 1987;93:394–404.

297. Franzen SF, Nylander E, Olin CL. Aortic valve replacement with pericardial valves in patients with small aortic roots. Clinical results in a consecutive series of patients receiving 19 and 21 mm prostheses. *Scand Cardiovasc J* 2001;35:114–18.

298. Firstenberg MS, Morehead AJ, Thomas JD, et al. Short-term hemodynamic performance of the mitral Carpentier-Edwards PERIMOUNT pericardial valve. Carpentier-Edwards PERIMOUNT Investigators. *Ann Thorac Surg* 2001;71(5 Suppl):S285–8.

299. Jamieson WR, Janusz MT, MacNab J, Henderson C. Hemodynamic comparison of second- and third-generation stented bioprostheses in aortic valve replacement. *Ann Thorac Surg* 2001;71(5 Suppl):S282–4.

300. Marchand MA, Aupart MR, Norton R, et al. Fifteen-year experience with the mitral Carpentier-Edwards PERIMOUNT pericardial bioprosthesis. *Ann Thorac Surg* 2001;71(5 Suppl):S236–9.

301. Milano AD, Blanzola C, Mecozzi G, et al. Hemodynamic performance of stented and stentless aortic bioprostheses. *Ann Thorac Surg* 2001;72:33–8.

302. Eric Jamieson WR, Marchand MA, Pelletier CL, et al. Structural valve deterioration in mitral replacement surgery: comparison of Carpentier-Edwards supra-annular porcine and Perimount pericardial bioprostheses. *J Thorac Cardiovasc Surg* 1999;118:297–304.

303. Bortolotti U, Scioti G, Milano A, et al. Performance of 21-mm size Perimount aortic bioprosthesis in the elderly. *Ann Thorac Surg* 2000;69:47–50.

304. Marchand M, Aupart M, Norton R, et al. Twelve-year experience with Carpentier-Edwards PERIMOUNT pericardial valve in the mitral position: a multicenter study. *J Heart Valve Dis* 1998;7:292–8.

305. Frater RW, Furlong P, Cosgrove DM, et al. Long-term durability and patient functional status of the Carpentier-Edwards Perimount pericardial bioprosthesis in the aortic position. *J Heart Valve Dis* 1998;7:48–53.

306. Nagy ZL, Fisher J, Walker PG, Watterson KG. The effect of sizing on the in vitro hydrodynamic characteristics and leaflet motion of the Toronto SPV stentless valve. *J Thorac Cardiovasc Surg* 1999;117:92–8.

307. Bach DS, David T, Yacoub M, et al. Hemodynamics and left ventricular mass regression following implantation of the Toronto SPV stentless porcine valve. *Am J Cardiol* 1998;82:1214–19.

308. Del Rizzo DF, Goldman BS, David TE. Aortic valve replacement with a stentless porcine bioprosthesis: multicenter trial. Canadian Investigators of the Toronto SPV Valve Trial. *Can J Cardiol* 1995;11:597–603.

309. Del Rizzo DF, Goldman BS, Joyner CP, et al. Initial clinical experience with the Toronto Stentless Porcine Valve. *J Card Surg* 1994;9:379–85.

310. Nagy ZL, Fisher J, Walker PG, Watterson KG. The effect of sizing on the hydrodynamic parameters of the Medtronic freestyle valve in vitro. *Ann Thorac Surg* 2000;69:1408–13.

311. Melina G, Rubens MB, Birks EJ, et al. A quantitative study of calcium deposition in the aortic wall following Medtronic Freestyle compared with homograft aortic root replacement. A prospective randomized trial. *J Heart Valve Dis* 2000;9:97–103.

312. Katsumata T, Vaccari G, Westaby S. Stentless xenograft repair of excavating aortic root sepsis. *J Card Surg* 1998;13:440–4.

313. Sintek CF, Pfeffer TA, Kochamba GS, et al. Freestyle valve experience: technical considerations and mid-term results. *J Card Surg* 1998;13:360–8.

Appendix
Aortic valve prostheses

Valve	Size (mm)	V$_{max}$ (m/s)	Peak grad (mmHg)	Mean grad (mmHg)	Area (cm^2)
Starr Edwards		3.1 ± 0.5	40 ± 3.0	24 ± 4	
Bjork-Shiley	19			21.0 ± 7.0	
	21	2.76 ± 0.9	30.5 ± 19.9	16 ± 5	
	23	2.59 ± 0.42	27.3 ± 8.7	14.0 ± 5	
	25	2.14 ± 0.31	18.4 ± 5.3	13.3 ± 2.5	
	27	1.91 ± 0.2	14.6 ± 3.1	9.7 ± 2.5	
	29	1.87 ± 0.2	13.9 ± 2.5	7.0 ± 6	
St. Jude	19	3.0 (2.0–4.5)	29 ± 10	20 (10–30)	1.0
	21	2.7 (2.5–3.5)	27 ± 10	14 (10–30)	1.3
	23	2.5 (2.0–3.5)	25 ± 8	12 (10–30)	1.3
	25	2.4 (2.0–3.5)	22 ± 8	12 (5–30)	1.8
	27	2.2 (2.0–3.1)	22 ± 10	11 (5–20)	2.4
	29	2.0 (2.0–2.5)		10 (5–15)	2.7
	31	2.1 (1.5–2.5)		10 (5–15)	3.1
St. Jude HP	17				1.6
	19				2.1
	21				2.6
Medtronic-Hall	19	21 ± 7			
	21	2.8 ± 0.9	16		
	23	2.6 ± 0.4	14 ± 5		
	25	2.1 ± 0.3	13 ± 3		
	27	1.9 ± 0.2	10 ± 3		
	29	1.9 ± 0.2	7 ± 6		
ATS	16/19			20.2 ± 2.8	1.2 ± 0.3
	18/21			18.0 ± 1.6	1.5 ± 0.1
	20/23			13.1 ± 0.8	1.7 ± 0.1
	22/25			11.1 ± 0.8	2.1 ± 0.1
	24/27			8.0 ± 0.8	2.5 ± 0.2
	26/29			7.8 ± 1.1	3.1 ± 0.4
CarboMedics	19			21.7 ± 9.1	0.9 ± 0.3
	21			16.2 ± 7.9	1.3 ± 0.4
	23			9.9 ± 4.2	1.4 ± 0.4
	25			10.5 ± 2.8	1.5 ± 0.3
	27			7.2 ± 3.9	2.2 ± 0.7
	29/31			5.1 ± 2.8	3.2 ± 1.5
On-X	19		17.1 ± 5.3	8.9 ± 3.1	1.5 ± 0.34
	21		14.2 ± 5.4	7.7 ± 2.9	1.9 ± 0.5
	23		12.4 ± 6.2	6.7 ± 3.1	2.4 ± 0.7
	25		8.9 ± 4.6	4.3 ± 2.4	2.7 ± 0.7
	27/29		9.8 ± 5.3	5.6 ± 3.1	2.9 ± 0.7
Ionescu-Shiley		2.38 ± 0.35	23.0 ± 6.71	11.0 ± 2.29	
Carpentier-Edwards	19	2.8 ± 0.66	31.6 ± 14.9	14.4 ± 5.7	
	21		27.3 ± 9.9	14.5 ± 6	
	23	2.56 ± 0.44	26.6 ± 8.9	12.7 ± 5.7	
	25	2.54 ± 0.4	24.3 ± 7.9	10.4 ± 2.3	
	27	2.41 ± 0.37	23.6 ± 7.2	9.9 ± 1	
	29	2.38 ± 0.44	22.8 ± 8.4	11.6	
	31	2.36 ± 0.43	22.3 ± 8.1		
Hancock	21	3.5	49		
	23	2.37 ± 0.24	23.2 ± 8.7	12.0 ± 2	
	25	2.26 ± 0.25	20.7 ± 4.57	11.0 ± 2	
	27	2.12 ± 0.35	20.5 ± 5.69	10 ± 3	
	29	2.23 ± 0.4	31.6 ± 14.9	16.5 ± 1.4	*continued*

Valve	Size (mm)	V_{max} (m/s)	Peak grad (mmHg)	Mean grad (mmHg)	Area (cm²)
Toronto-SPV		2.2 ± 0.4		3 (2–20)	1.8 – 2.3
	21		18.4 ± 11.8	7.3 ± 4.4	1.3 ± 0.7
	23		15.1 ± 8.8	7.4 ± 4.5	1.5 ± 0.5
	25		11.6 ± 6.6	6.1 ± 3.1	1.7 ± 0.4
	27		9.6 ± 5.0	4.9 ± 2.4	2.0 ± 0.4
	29		7.2 ± 4.1	4.0 ± 2.1	2.4 ± 0.6
Freestyle	19			12.1 ± 4.9	1.26 ± 0.27
	21			9.6 ± 7.3	1.52 ± 0.54
	23			8.7 ± 7.8	1.77 ± 0.59
	25			5.9 ± 4.4	2.08 ± 0.62
	27			4.2 ± 3.0	2.54 ± 0.74
Aortic Homograft		1.8 ± 0.4		7 ± 3	2.2 (1.7–3.1)

Refs. 17, 50–68.

Mitral valve prostheses

Prosthesis	Size	V_{max} (m/s)	Peak grad (mmHg)	Mean grad (mmHg)	Half-time	Area (cm²)
Starr-Edwards		1.88 ± 0.42	14.6 ± 5.5	4.55 ± 2.4	109.5 ± 26.6	2.01 ± 0.49
Lillehei-Kaster		1.84	13.54	3.35	125 ± 29	1.88 ± 0.56
Beall-Surgitool		1.8 ± 0.2	13.4 ± 4.0	6.0 ± 2.0	129.4 ± 15.2	1.7 ± 0.2
Bjork-Shiley		1.61 ± 0.33	10.72 ± 2.74	2.90 ± 1.61	90.2 ± 22.4	2.44 ± 0.62
St. Jude	27	1.54 ± 0.2	9.69 ± 3.06	5.0 ± 2.0	137.5	1.6
	29	1.59 ± 0.27	10.11 ± 3.43	2.71 ± 1.36	78.0 ± 16	2.93 ± 0.6
	31	1.54 ± 0.36	9.90 ± 4.49	5.0 ± 3.0	57.9 ± 6.10	3.8 ± 0.4
	33					5.18
Medtronic-Hall	25	2.1 ± 0.3	13 ± 3			
	27	1.9 ± 0.2	10 ± 3			
	29	1.9 ± 0.2	7 ± 6			
ATS	22/25*			5.4 ± 4.7		1.8 ± 0.5
	24/27*			4.5 ± 0.9		2.9 ± 0.9
	26/29			3.7 ± 0.7		2.8 ± 0.3
	28/31/33			3.1 ± 0.2		2.9 ± 0.2
CarboMedics	25			4.3 ± 1.7		2.7 ± 0.8
	27			3.9 ± 1.0		2.9 ± 1.3
	29/31/33			4.6 ± 2.0		3.0 ± 0.8
On-X	25			3.5 ± 1.1		3.0 ± 0.8
	27/29			4.7 ± 2.0		2.7 ± 0.6
	31/33			4.5 ± 1.3		2.3 ± 0.6
Ionescu-Shiley		1.46 ± 0.27	8.53 ± 2.91	3.28 ± 1.19	93.3 ± 25	2.36 ± 0.75
Carpentier-Edwards		1.76 ± 0.24	12.5 + 3.64	6.5 ± 2.1	90 ± 25.4	2.45 ± 0.7
Hancock		1.5 ± 0.26	9.7 + 3.2	4.29 ± 2.1	129 ± 31	1.7 ± 0.4

Refs. 17, 50–68.

8

Evaluation of cardiac masses and tumors

Cardiac masses comprise thrombi and cardiac tumors, with thrombi occurring much more commonly. Cardiac tumors are rare, but, there is an increased frequency for the diagnosis of cardiac tumors with clinical imaging techniques. The signs and symptoms produced by cardiac masses are largely non-specific and resemble those produced by other forms of heart disease. The diagnosis of a cardiac mass is usually made as a coincidental finding on a standard imaging technique such as echocardiography during a general cardiac work-up, CT scanning, MRI, or rarely during cardiac catheterization. Except in rare cases, the diagnosis of a cardiac mass is not entertained unless the diagnosis of cancer has been established or when a cardiac source of embolus is suspected. In our laboratories, echocardiography is frequently requested to rule out cardiac source of embolus, and when transthoracic echocardiography does not yield a diagnosis, transesophageal echocardiography is undertaken as the next step, especially when the transthoracic imaging is not optimal.

Echocardiography is excellent for evaluating and diagnosing cardiac masses, due to its widespread availability. In most cases, transthoracic echocardiographic examinations are sufficient for diagnosis, especially when interpreted together with the clinical history and physical examination. In patients with recent myocardial infarction and an embolic event, in patients with a known malignancy and signs of pericardial effusion or embolic events, or valvular disease and embolic events, or in patients with hemodynamic alterations and no known cardiac disease, echocardiography frequently yields a diagnosis. Frequently, transesophageal echocardiography does not add incremental information to the diagnosis of cardiac masses over the transthoracic echocardiogram. The echocardiographic characteristics of cardiac masses are often subtle and are highly dependent upon the experience of the sonographer, as well as knowing the prevalence and natural history of cardiac masses. Ultrasonic tissue characterization may provide additional diagnostic information, but thus far has not equalled that of MRI scanning. Transesophageal-echocardiography-guided biopsy is extremely helpful in certain cases and is being used with increased frequency as physicians become familiar with the technique.

The treatment of cardiac masses is variable. Thrombi are usually treated with anticoagulation, and in rare cases where anticoagulation or thrombolysis are unsuccessful or prohibited in patients with multiple life-threatening embolic events, surgery may be indicated. Surgical resection is the treatment of choice for benign tumors, especially when they are well encapsulated. Malignant tumors have a dismal prognosis and are only occasionally surgically resectable, although debulking may provide relief from symptoms when hemodynamics are affected. Only in specific tumor types is adjuvant chemotherapy or radiation therapy helpful.

Cardiac thrombi

The most common cause of a cardiac mass is cardiac thrombus. Thrombi occur in the right heart chambers as the result of the peripheral embolization of venous thrombi from the legs or the pelvis, and also occur in association with indwelling catheters, in patients with or without associated heart disease. Left-sided cardiac thrombi occur in the left atrium in valvular disease, in the left ventricle after acute myocardial infarction, in dilated cardiomyopathy, and in the aorta in association with atherosclerotic debris. Recently, the frequency of cardiac thrombi in endomyocardial disease and diseases in association with anticardiolipin antibody type syndromes has been appreciated by transesophageal echocardiography. The diagnosis of cardiac thrombus is usually entertained to rule out pulmonary embolus, or to rule out cardiac source of thromboembolism in patients with stroke or peripheral systemic embolization. Transthoracic imaging is often adequate, and transesophageal echocardiography is necessary only for evaluating smaller thrombi in the left atrium or aorta. In patients with left ventricular thrombus, transthoracic imaging has a clear advantage over transesophageal echocardiography because the left ventricular apex is less well visualized even with multiplane transesophageal echocardiography, due to foreshortening of the ventricle in most views.

Left atrial thrombi

Transesophageal echocardiography is the optimal evaluation for left atrial thrombi. The close proximity of the left atrium to the esophagus allows for better evaluation of both atria by transesophageal echocardiography than by transthoracic echocardiography. Transesophageal echocardiography is most useful in two specific clinical circumstances, in patients undergoing elective cardioversion for atrial arrhythmias, and in patients before undergoing mitral balloon valvuloplasty to rule out atrial thrombi, and in patients with neurological or peripheral embolic events.

Transesophageal echocardiography has a major role in patients undergoing elective cardioversion and undergoing ablation in the electrophysiology lab. However, the role of transesophageal echocardiography in the electrophysiology lab is not as well defined as in electrical cardioversion.

Atrial fibrillation is frequently encountered in patients with or without heart disease, and accounts for a substantial number of hospital admissions yearly.[1] The prevalence of atrial fibrillation increases with age, occurs frequently in younger patients without structural heart disease, and can result in hemodynamic compromise in older patients with heart disease who require the atrial kick and a slow ventricular response to maintain

adequate cardiac output. In elderly patients over the age of 80, paroxysmal atrial fibrillation occurs in 9% of that population.[2] Alterations in atrial rhythm result in loss of normal atrial function, leading to blood stasis, which predisposes to thrombus formation especially in the left atrial appendage. Atrial flutter is less frequent, but also predisposes to systemic thromboembolism even though there is a preservation of atrial function. The role of echocardiography in general has been defined in atrial fibrillation.

Echocardiographic studies have shown that the atria slowly dilate in response to atrial fibrillation. M-mode echocardiographic measurements of atrial dimension have correlated with other imaging techniques and have shown that reversion to sinus rhythm from atrial fibrillation is associated with regression of atrial size. However, left atrial dimensions greater than 6 cm are less likely to maintain sinus rhythm and frequently revert to atrial fibrillation.[3] The likelihood of maintaining sinus rhythm after cardioversion is dependent on the duration of atrial fibrillation and left atrial size before cardioversion.

Cardioversion, either medical or electrical, has been associated with thromboembolic events, with a substantial yet reduced risk of 7% in patients with atrial fibrillation of less than 48 hours' duration.[4–8] In patients receiving warfarin for 3 to 4 weeks before cardioversion, the risk of thromboembolism is reduced to 1%.[4–10] In an effort to obviate the recommended 1-month period of oral anticoagulation, and to avoid the complications of anticoagulant therapy, studies have investigated the use of transesophageal echocardiography to assess the presence of atrial thrombi and the possibility of cardioverting patients safely without anticoagulation. Reducing the duration of atrial fibrillation increases the likelihood of maintaining sinus rhythm, after cardioversion and allows faster recovery of atrial mechanical function. Manning and colleagues[11] showed that in patients with atrial fibrillation for less than 2 weeks, atrial mechanical function was restored within 24 hours. When the duration of atrial fibrillation extended from 2 to 6 weeks, recovery of atrial function took 1 week, and when the duration was greater than 6 weeks, recovery often took up to 3 weeks if the patient did not revert to atrial fibrillation.

Most left atrial thrombi reside in the left atrial appendage (90%) in patients with atrial fibrillation, and therefore transthoracic echocardiographic imaging of these patients is insufficient.[12–14] Multiplane transesophageal echocardiography has a sensitivity of 93–100%, specificity of 93–100%, and a predictive accuracy of 99–100% for the diagnosis of left atrial thrombi.[15–20]

Although currently no large-scale results are available, a few small studies have addressed the safety of cardioversion

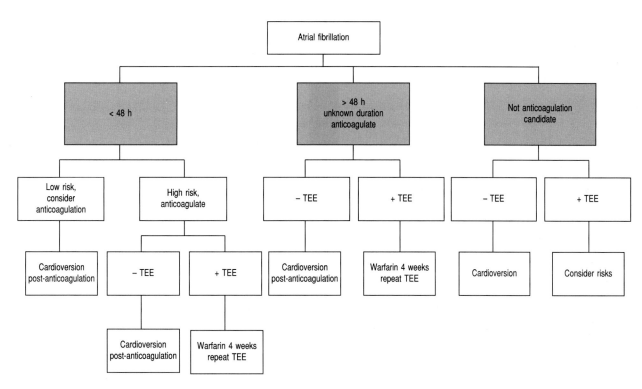

Figure 8.1
Pre-cardioversion transesophageal echocardiography (TEE) in atrial fibrillation.
Anticoagulate: heparin with partial thromboplastin time 2× control, initiate warfarin therapy.
High risk: patient with mitral stenosis, prosthetic mitral valve, significant mitral annular calcification, previous history of thromboembolism, patent foramen ovale.
TEE: no left atrial, left atrial appendage or right atrial thrombus.
Cardioversion: pharmacological or electrical cardioversion.
Post-anticoagulation: continue warfarin for 4 weeks, stop heparin when INR (international normalzied ratio) ≥ 2.0; if not a warfarin candidate continue heparin for at least 24 hours depending on risk or return of atrial mechanical function.
Consider risks: consider not cardioverting versus risk of atrial fibrillation, or using some form of anticoagulation.
Modified from Silverman and Manning.[27]

using prior transesophageal echocardiography without 4 weeks of warfarin before cardioversion. The ACUTE trial (Assessment of Cardioversion Using Transesophageal Echocardiography), which included over 3000 patients, should resolve these issues.[9] Preliminary, smaller trials of transesophageal echocardiography before cardioversion have shown that in patients with atrial fibrillation for more than 48 hours, the incidence of atrial thrombi is approximately 15%.[2,21–23] Atrial spontaneous echocardiographic contrast, reduced left ventricular systolic function, and the occurrence of embolic events are predictors for the presence of atrial thrombi.[2,21,22] Although a few reports have suggested that mitral regurgitation gives a protective effect against formation of atrial thrombus, by performing a mechanical washout of the areas for stagnant flow, atrial thrombi are frequently observed in that subset of patients.[9,18] Initial data from these studies suggest that

transesophageal-echocardiography-guided cardioversion is at least as safe as conventional warfarin treatment before cardioversion.[2,9,21,22] In our own institutions, systemic thromboembolic events have occurred after cardioversion even with negative transesophageal echocardiography evaluations before cardioversion.[24]

Current recommendations for transesophageal-echocardiography-guided cardioversion, as illustrated in Figure 8.1, include anticoagulation with heparin and/or warfarin with adequate laboratory anticoagulation levels before cardioversion irrespective of the transesophageal echocardiography results.[25] Transesophageal echocardiography should be done close to the time of cardioversion, and in our laboratories is done as a combined procedure.[26] The rationale for this strategy is that the time for thrombus formation is unknown. Since cardioversion requires general anesthesia, a better-tolerated transesophageal echocardiographic examination is assured. Adequate systemic anticoagulation should be maintained for 4 weeks after successful cardioversion. Prolonged anticoagulation should be protective until atrial mechanical function returns.[11,27,28]

Patients with positive transesophageal echocardiography findings for atrial thrombi, should be treated by conventional anticoagulation for 4 weeks. After 4 weeks of therapy a repeat transesophageal echocardiography shows resolution of thrombus in 50–80% of patients.[9,11,29–31] The highest resolution rates have been reported in non-rheumatic atrial fibrillation patients.[30] Whether patients with documented atrial thrombi on the first study should be restudied is controversial. Since this approach does not yield a 0% thromboembolism rate for cardioversion it is especially compelling to restudy patients with initially positive transesophageal echocardiograms, especially when thrombi are large and mobile. No good data exist on propagation of thrombi by cardioversion or the embolic potential of thrombi in regard to size or mobility. In addition, many embolic episodes are clinically silent, as illustrated by postmortem studies in which emboli to the spleen and other areas are found.

There is general agreement that patients with atrial fibrillation of less than 48 hour duration are at low risk for clinical thromboembolic events. Extrapolating data from patients who are observed to convert spontaneously or with medical therapy to sinus rhythm, the incidence of embolism is approximately 0.8%.[32,33] Patients at higher risk of embolic events, those with known valvular disease, reduced left ventricular function, and a previous history of atrial fibrillation or documented embolic events, should be screened with transesophageal echocardiography prior to cardioversion.

Left ventricular thrombi

Most studies of the characteristics of ventricular thrombi have used transthoracic echocardiography.[34,35] Transesophageal echocardiography is not a good technique for showing ventricular thrombi unless they are large and highly mobile. Multiplane transesophageal echocardiography often does not allow good visualization of the ventricular apex, so apical left ventricular thrombi may not be diagnosed. The best transesophageal echocardiographic views for visualizing apical ventricular thrombi are the deep transgastric views. Transesophageal echocardiography is especially helpful in the preoperative screening of patients with suspected thrombi, because the thrombi may be dislodged during manipulation of the heart during surgery.

The most common cause of left ventricular thrombus is acute myocardial infarction. Postmortem studies

suggest a greater than 50% prevalence after fatal acute myocardial infarction.[36–42] The incidence of systemic emboli determined by echocardiography after acute myocardial infarction approaches 12%, and was related to the cause of death in 12–33% in the pre-thrombolytic era, and usually occurs in anterior wall infarctions, with a higher frequency with apical aneurysmal formation.[40–42] The sensitivity and specificity of ventricular thrombus by echocardiographic techniques during myocardial infarction is 90%. Most large contemporary echocardiographic series have shown a 0 to 27% embolic rate within 4 months.[43–46] Ventricular mural thrombi appear as distinct masses, producing a disruption of the endocardial contour and increased echogenicity. A distinguishing characteristic of all thrombi is that they frequently have central areas of echolucency, suggesting clot liquefaction. Occasionally, ventricular thrombi appear as localized thickening in areas of regional wall motion defects adjacent to ventricular myocardial thinning, and these must be differentiated from myocardial trabeculations and hypertrophied papillary muscles. Myocardial trabeculations occur with ventricular hypertrophy, are usually more diffuse throughout the ventricle, do not exhibit greater echogenicity than the adjacent myocardium, and rarely have irregular margins. Transthoracic imaging is usually adequate for this differentiation, but transesophageal echocardiography may be helpful in some cases.

Echocardiographic predictors of thromboembolism include the degree of protrusion of the thrombus into the ventricular cavity (40% increase in embolization) and the degree of mobility of the thrombus (60% increase in embolic potential).[47–51] Ultrasonic tissue characterization may be useful to assess the tissue texture of thrombi, which may identify those with greater likelihood of embolization.

Left ventricular thrombus detected by echocardiography after myocardial infarction requires anticoagulant therapy for 3–6 months, irrespective of complete resolution of the thrombus.[52] Ventricular thrombi after infarction usually organize and shrink in size, and may completely disappear with time. Residual or chronic ventricular thrombi have increased echogenicity, are laminated usually sessile, and may be indistinguishable from ventricular trabeculations. Chronic thrombi may occasionally calcify. Thrombi may increase in size or recur after discontinuation of anticoagulant therapy, and warrant aggressive anticoagulant therapy.

The second most frequent cause of left ventricular thrombus is dilated cardiomyopathy, with a prevalence rate of 40% by echocardiography and in postmortem studies. Thrombus is most frequent in the left ventricular apex, but also occurs rarely in the right ventricular apex.[53] The incidence of embolic events for left ventricular thrombus approaches 10%, and thus patients with cardiomyopathy may require lifelong anticoagulant therapy.[54–59]

Ventricular thrombi are also associated with endomyocardial disease, anti-cardiolipin syndromes, and certain malignancies.

Right heart thrombi

Primary thrombus in the right atrium and ventricle are rare in comparison with left heart thrombi. Case reports have described right atrial appendage thrombi in patients with atrial fibrillation, and right ventricular thrombi after right ventricular infarction or in association with cardiomyopathies.[60–65] Primary right heart thrombi are usually sessile and appear more heterogeneous as layered masses on echocardiography.[65] Most right heart thrombi occur as a result of peripheral embolization, or in association with indwelling catheters or pacemaker leads. Recently, reports have illustrated right heart thrombi following tissue injury produced by electrophysiological catheter ablation.[66,67]

Embolization of thrombus from the systemic veins to the right heart may be visualized in the right heart chamber or proximal pulmonary arteries. They are usually extremely mobile and resemble venous casts, and may become caught on Eustachian valves, in a patent foramen ovale or pulmonary valve, or entangled in the tricuspid valve apparatus. Occasionally, thrombi may float freely within the cardiac chambers, unable to pass into the pulmonary artery because of their size. Although the incidence of thrombi in postmortem series is only 0.7%, it is as high as 9% in patients with documented deep venous thrombosis, although it is not unusual to visualize these thrombi on echocardiography.[68,69]

Cardiac tumors

Cardiac tumors occur rarely, but are usually easily recognized by echocardiography. The most common cardiac tumors are metastases from the heart, lung, colon, etc. Primary tumors of the heart are extremely rare, with a prevalence in postmortem studies of 0.0017–0.28%.[70–77] Benign tumors are more frequent than primary malignant cardiac tumors and are listed in Table 8.1. The clinical signs and symptoms of cardiac tumors are non-specific, and may cause chest pain, dyspnea, congestive heart failure, right heart failure, pericardial effusion, pulmonary hypertension, arrhythmias, cardiac syncope, or bacterial endocarditis (Table 8.2). Usually transthoracic echocardiography is sufficient for diagnoses of cardiac tumors, although transesophageal echocardiography is more sensitive when echocardiography is the only diagnostic test before surgery. Echocardiographic tissue signature is often

Table 8.1 Incidence and location of cardiac tumors

Cardiac tumors	Relativer frequency (%)	Site of distribution
Benign		
Myxoma	60.4	LA, RA, RV, LV, V
Papillary fibroelastoma	5.3	V, RA, LA, RV, LV
Rhabdomyoma	4.5	LV, RV, RA, LA
Lipoma	2.5	AS, AV-groove, P
Teratoma	1.4	Mediastinum, P
Fibroma		V, VS, LV and RV free-wall
Hemangioma	1.4	VS, RV, RA, LA
Mesothelioma	1.2	AV node
Angioma	0.9	AV node
Hamartoma	0.8	V myocardium
Neurofibroma	0.3	P, V myocardium
Granular cell tumor	0.3	LA, LV, RA, LV
Thyroid	0.2	P
Malignant		
Sarcoma	14.4	
Angiosarcoma	4.8	RA, VC, TV, P, LA
Rhabdomyosarcoma	3.5	RA, LA
Fibrosarcoma	2.2	RA, LA
Leiomyosarcoma	0.8	LA
Myosarcoma	0.6	LA, MV
Myxosarcoma	0.5	LA, RA, RV, P
Liposarcoma	0.5	P, RA
Osteosarcoma	0.5	LA wall, RA
Malignant mesothelioma	1.6	LA, P
Lymphoma	0.7	P, LV and RV wall
Malignant teratoma	0.3	P

RA = right atrium; RV = right ventricle; LA = left atrium; LV = left ventricle; AS = atrial septum; IVC = inferior vena cava; P = pericardium; PE = pericardial effusion; MV = mitral valve; AV = aortic valve; TV = tricuspid valve; V = valve. Modified from reference 70.

Table 8.2 Differential diagnosis of cardiac tumors by signs and symptoms

Pericarditis
Coronary artery disease
Dilated cardiomyopathy
Congestive heart failure
Pulmonary hypertension (primary or secondary)
Restrictive cardiomyopathy
Bacterial endocarditis
Autoimmune diseases
Rheumatic disease
Valvular heart disease

sufficient to differentiate tumor from thrombus. Transesophageal echocardiography can be used to direct and guide percutaneous biopsy for histological diagnosis.

Primary cardiac tumors are usually benign, with a reported prevalance of 80% of all cardiac tumors.[70,71] The distribution of benign cardiac tumors includes myxoma (70%), papillary fibroelastoma (7%), and lipoma (3%).[70,71] In the pediatric population transesophageal echocardiography is rarely needed. The most common type is rhabdomyoma, followed by fibromas, teratomas, and hemangioma.

Sarcomas are the most frequent primary malignant cardiac tumor, comprising 80% of all cases including angiosarcoma and osteosarcoma.[70,71,75] Mesothelioma is the second most common primary malignant cardiac tumor, occurring in 10% of cases.[70,71]

Metastatic tumors affect the heart through involvement of the pericardium, hematogenous or lymphatic spread, and less frequently by direct extension of the primary tumor. Metastatic tumors, such as carcinomas of the lung, breast, or esophagus, involve the heart by direct extension of the primary tumor, or by hematogenous or lymphatic spread with pericardial involvement. Malignant melanoma metastasize hematogenously while lymphoma involvement occurs by lymphatic extension. Lung and breast carcinoma often involve the pericardium by direct invasion, while melanoma and leukemia rarely involve the pericardium.

Myxoma

The most common cardiac tumor is the benign myxoma.[70,71] Myxomas are most commonly found in the left atrium, followed by the right atrium, right ventricle, and, very rarely, the left ventricle, or on the cardiac valves.[70,71,78–83] Rarely, myxomas may be multiple, with the most common presentation being bi-atrial myxomas.[79] In one report, myxomas occurred in all four cardiac chambers. Myxomas are generally adult cardiac tumors, and predominate in women. Myxomas are either sessile with a broad base or pedunculated on a stalk, both taking origin from the atrial septum around the foramen ovale.[71,78] Mobile myxomas usually present with findings of obstructive atrioventricular valvular disease, since they may produce obstruction when prolapsing through the valve during diastole. Myxomas may grow to sizes that nearly fill the whole atrial chamber. In one of our cases, the myxoma was so large that when the patient was in the supine position it prolapsed backwards and occluded the pulmonary veins, producing severe dyspnea. When mobile myxomas occur in the right atrium, they may frequently produce severe tricuspid insufficiency.[80,81]

Echocardiographically and pathologically, myxomas may appear firm and smooth with a broad base, or may appear gelatinous, with multiple finger-like projections. Occasionally, myxomas present with cystic areas of echolucency within the tumor, which histologically represent areas of hemorrhage or necrosis. Gelatinous myxomas frequently present with systemic embolus or sudden death.[70,71,75] In one case, a young nurse, previously evaluated for atypical chest pain, had sudden death with unsuccessful resuscitation. Transesophageal echocardiography performed during the resuscitation showed a small friable myxoma in the left atrium, and tumor fragments throughout the aorta, producing total obstruction of the abdominal aorta.

When myxomas are discovered they should be removed surgically. The role of transesophageal echocardiography is to define the site of attachment so the tumor can be removed with the least manipulation, to avoid fragmentation and embolization.

Lipomas

Lipomas comprise 3–6% of benign cardiac tumors.[70,71,75] Lipomas are encapsulated tumors that may occur anywhere within the heart or pericardium. They usually occur either in the atrial septum or the outer margins of fibrous skeleton near the atriovenous groove. Lipomas of the atrial septum are frequently confused with lipomatous hypertrophy or with amyloid infiltration of the atrial septum, and care must be taken to distinguish these entities. Most lipomas are sessile, with 50% originating from the subendocardial layer, 25% from the subepicardial layer, and 25% from the intramuscular layer.[84,85] Lipomas in the muscle layers are firmly attached to surrounding cardiac structures, and they therefore cannot be easily removed surgically.

Lipomas may grow to significant size, and although they are histologically benign, they may produce symptoms from obstruction or promote thrombus formation. In most cases lipomas are moderate in size and do not present with signs and symptoms of cardiac disease.

Lipomatous hypertrophy represents accumulation of non-encapsulated adipose tissue into the atrial septum contiguous with subendocardial fat. Lipomatous hypertrophy appears as brighter echogenic protuberances of the atrial septum usually above, below, and sometimes surrounding the foramen ovale. Transthoracic echocardiography descriptions of lipomatous hypertrophy have described a "dumb-bell" appearance of the atrial septum.[84,85]

Papillary fibroelastoma

Statistically, papillary fibroelastomas are the second most common cardiac tumor, occurring with a frequency of 7% in most postmortem series.[70,71] The true incidence of papillary fibroelastomas has probably been underestimated, since with the increased use of transesophageal echocardiography these small tumors are frequently recognized arising from valvular apparatus, in contrast to the infrequency of these tumors found on postmortem examinations.

Papillary fibroelastomas are small tumors usually 2–3 mm in dimension, attached to valve leaflet margins, the chordae tendinae, or papillary muscles, and are predominately associated with the left heart valves.[70,71] Papillary fibroelastomas are mobile and present with chaotic motion projecting towards the ventricular outflow tract or prolapse between cardiac chambers either the atrioventricular or semilunar valves. Multiplane transesophageal echocardiography is especially useful in detecting papillary fibroelastomas, since tumors are small and may only appear as linear thin projections, while when viewed in multiple planes these tumors may appear as small polyps. Multiple papillary fibroelastomas have been described but are rare.[86,87] Most papillary fibroelastomas are symptom-free, most commonly attached to the aortic valve and may result in systemic embolism, which have been implicated in neurological events and sudden cardiac death.[88–90]

Papillary fibroelastomas must be differentiated from normal anatomic variants such as Lambl's excrescences of the heart valves.[71,91,92] Two types of Lambl's excrescences are associated with the normal aortic valve on echocardiography.[71,91] In patients under 30 years old, lamellar excrescences are found along the lower border of the lunulas, often with thickening of the body of the cusp. In older patients, filiform excrescences emanate from the nodule of Arantes and along the free margin of the cusp. The connective tissue core of the filiform excrescences contain collagen fibrils arranged in opposing layers of elastic material, with a central zone devoid of identifiable connective tissue.[71,91] Similar, multiple excrescences are found on the mitral valve and apparatus, but they have not been reported to occur in the first year of life. Lamellar and sublunar excrescences may form because of the shear stress caused by the blood flow or because of friction of the valve surfaces during valve closure. The incidence of valve excrescences is not known, because they may be confused with degenerative changes described pathologically that occur on all valve margins, especially the left sided valves, producing "hair-like" projections.[91–94] Whether these entities represent a true cardiac source of embolus is unknown.[93,94]

Pediatric tumors

Rhabdomyomas are the most common cardiac tumors in newborns and infants.[95–97] These tumors may be very small, or large enough to fill the right or left ventricles producing heart failure. Rhabdomyomas are usually multiple involving the ventricular myocardium, with a strong association with tuberous sclerosis (50%).[96] Tumors may be pedunculated and mobile or project from the ventricular or septal wall. Since these tumors are slow growing, they may be surgically resectable.

Fibromas are usually solitary tumors, and are the second most common tumor in infants and children.[70,71]

Fibromas occur in the free wall of the left ventricle and tend to produce obstruction as they increase in size. Fibromas are located on the endocardial surface in 50% of cases. Complete surgical resection is not always possible, but debulking of the tumor is advantageous in some cases, with good long-term survival.

Hemangiomas are rare, with most reported cases found at autopsy. Complete resection has been accomplished when the tumor is diagnosed early.[70,71,95]

The other benign cardiac tumors are teratomas, mesotheliomas, angiomas, hamartomas, neurofibromas, granular cell tumors, and thyroid tumors. These tumors occur with much less frequency and possess the same echocardiographic characteristics of the benign tumors. They have been described in isolated reports, are generally diagnosed only by histology, and are usually discovered coincidentally at necropsy. Surgery is reserved for obstructive tumors.

Malignant tumors

Malignant cardiac tumors produce similar echocardiographic findings as benign tumors, with an increased prevalence in the right heart, especially the right atrium. Although malignant cardiac tumors carry a dismal prognosis, the proper histological diagnosis should be made, since occasional reports have described some success with chemotherapy (Table 8.3)[98] or radiation therapy.

Sarcomas represent the most common group of malignant primary cardiac tumors, and may occur in all age groups. Angiosarcoma is the most common tissue type and involves the right atrial cavity in 70% of cases.[70,71] One in four of all angiosarcomas are intracavitary, and produce valvular obstruction and right heart failure. Some are complicated by hemorrhagic pericardial effusion and subsequent tamponade. Angiosarcomas rapidly enlarge and spread to the myocardium and pericardium, and/or lung and mediastinum. These tumors are usually already metastatic at the time of diagnosis, precluding surgical resection.[99,100]

Table 8.3 Primary cardiac tumors sensitive to chemotherapy
Angiosarcoma
Undifferentiated sarcoma
Myxosarcoma
Rhabdomyosarcoma
Osteogenicsarcoma
Leiomyosarcoma
Liposarcoma

Loffler H, Grille W. Classification of malignant cardiac tumors with respect to oncological treatment. *Thorac Cardiovasc Surg* 1990;38:173–5.

Myxosarcomas have been called the malignant variety of the myxoma.[75] In one case report the tumor was removed at surgery, and was thought to be a benign myxoma. At the time of surgery, the atrial septum was not resected and the tumor recurred within 1 year.[75] Even when wide excision of the atrial septum is performed, the tumor may recur. Obstruction at the level of the atrioventricular valve is frequent.

Osteosarcoma, rhabdomyosarcoma, fibrosarcoma, and spindle cell sarcoma share similar echocardiographic characteristics with other sarcomas, except that they may occur more frequently in the left heart than the right heart.

Malignant mesothelioma is the second most common malignant cardiac tumor in the adult.[70,71] Malignant mesotheliomas are usually large tumors of the visceral or parietal pericardium, and frequently cause compression of the adjacent cardiac structure, rarely spreading to the myocardium.

Metastatic cardiac tumors

Metastatic cardiac tumors are found at necropsy in 10% of all metastatic malignancies.[75,76,101–103] Almost all malignant tumors have been reported to spread to the heart and pericardium, with lung cancer, breast cancer, malignant melanoma, leukemias, and lymphomas occurring most frequently. Cardiac involvement occurs in over 50% of malignant melanoma and leukemias.[103,104]

Metastatic cardiac tumors occur more frequently in the right heart and the pericardium.[101–107] Metastatic tumors may produce intracavitary or pericardial "filling" masses. Masses may extend into the right heart chambers via the vena cava. Cardiac metastases may occur as single or multiple intramyocardial masses, or purely extracardiac masses compressing cardiac structures. In many patients, computed tomographic scanning or magnetic resonance imaging is a useful adjunct to transesophageal echocardiography in further defining metastasis.

When metastatic malignancies spread to the heart via direct extension, pericardial involvement is the norm.[70,71] The echocardiographic characteristics of malignant pericardial involvement include pericardial effusion, which may be large, with or without dyspnea, and often with pericardial tamponade. Pericardial involvement commonly includes multiple or discrete visceral, epicardial nodules that may penetrate the myocardium.[108–113] Pericardial nodules may also occur in organizing inflammatory pericardial effusions that are not malignant.[111]

Echocardiographic pseudotumors

Various normal and abnormal structures may masquerade as cardiac masses. Lipomatous hypertrophy of the atrial septum may mimic lipomas of the heart. It is important to recognize these variants and not to misinterpret their presence as indicative of malignancy.

Lipomatous hypertrophy is rarely greater than 2–3 cm in diameter. Transesophageal echocardiography may be useful in distinguishing lipomatous hypertrophy when images are non-diagnostic with transthoracic echocardiography. Prominent accumulations of tissue may occur at the atrial septum primum, where the superior vena cava enters the right atrium and joins the right atrial appendage, and where the left pulmonary vein enters the left atrium near the superior margin of the left atrial appendage (Q-tip sign). Occasionally, prominent pectinate muscles in the atrium may be confused with thrombus. Hypertrophied trabeculations of the ventricles and large papillary muscles may occasionally resemble tumors, but may be recognized because they are sessile and have the same echocardiographic texture as surrounding cardiac structures.

Hiatal hernia may be detected echocardiographically as a thick walled retrocardiac mass with hypo-echoic centers. Usually, clinical history helps in delineating this diagnosis. Esophageal and gastric varicies are infrequently encountered during routine transesophageal echocardiographic examinations. The first evidence of esophageal varicies is poor cardiac image quality. Cardiac structures are usually displayed about 3 to 4 cm from the apex of the image sector. Varices appear as very prominent rugal folds, as seen in the stomach. The folds are different echocardiographically in that they are usually thicker and occasionally large, with the homogenicity of a hematoma that is well encapsulated. In addition there may be an echo-free interface noted between the transducer and esophagus and the cardiac image, representing ascites. The liver may be enlarged or small with prominent hepatic channels, and epigastric lobe may be seen floating in the ascitic fluid in the gastric or lower esophageal views in between the posterior wall of the heart and the esophagus.

Pericardial cysts are symptom-free congenital dilations of the pericardium.[109,110] Although pericardial cysts are rare, they may be seen with transesophageal echocardiography as thin walled, circular cystic structures with echo-free centers, resembling loculated pericardial effusion, usually located near the diaphragm at the cardiophrenic angle. In addition to cysts, epicardial fat accumulation can occasionally be confused with pericardial tumor studding. When an accurate diagnosis cannot be made with transthoracic echocardiographic imaging, transesophageal echocardiography is recommended. With transesophageal echocardiography, prominent adipose tissue accumulations may be identified along the atriovenous groove, on the anterior surface of the right ventricle and/or pulmonary artery, in the transverse sinus, or near the left atrial appendage. Adipose tissue is diagnosed with echocardiographically as homogenous, with echogenicity in direct continuity with the epicardial surface predominantly in obese patients.

Case studies

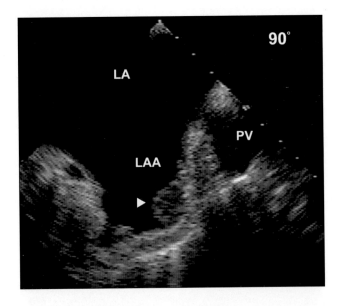

Case 8.1

Left atrial appendage thrombus. The left atrial appendage is a frequent site of thrombus formation in patients with atrial fibrillation. Multiplane TEE is well suited to evaluate the left atrial appendage. The left atrial appendage is visualized from the upper esophageal window to the left of the aortic valve plane. Antegrade flexion is useful in many cases to aid in visualizing the appendage at 0°. To evaluate the whole appendage the transducer is rotated through 90° in the zoom mode. LAA, left atrial appendage; LA, left atrium; PV, pulmonary vein.

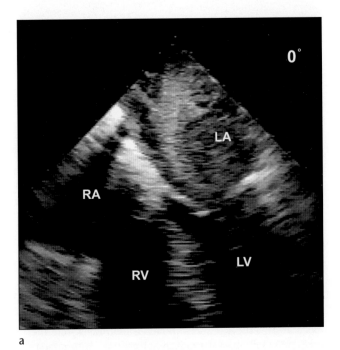

a

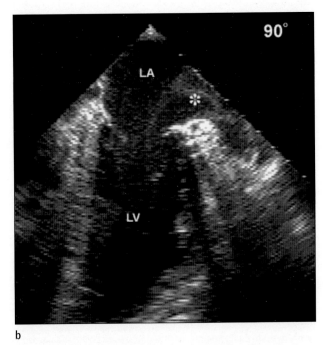

b

Case 8.2

Spontaneous contrast. Spontaneous contrast or echocardiographic smoke is a phenomenon frequently observed within the left atrium denoting stasis or sluggish flow implicated as a precursor for thrombus formation. (a) Spontaneous contrast filling the whole left atrium in a patient with mitral stenosis. Increasing the overall gain helps detect spontaneous contrast. (b) Spontaneous contrast (star) filling the left atrial appendage. Heavy echo smoke in the left atrial appendage may obscure small thrombi and may carry an increased risk associated with cardioversion. LA, left atrium; LV, left ventricular; RA, right atrium; RV, right ventricle.

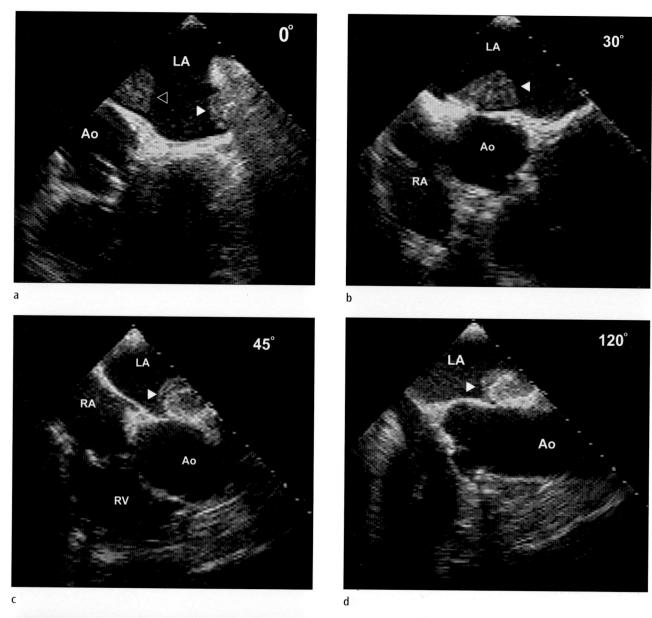

Case 8.3

Left atrial thrombi. Multiple atrial thrombi in a patient with severe mitral stenosis and a heavily calcified mitral annulus. (a) Left atrial cavity thrombus attached near the atrial septum (open arrow). There is also a thrombus protruding from the area of the left atrial appendage (solid arrow). With rotation of the transducer (b) 30°, (c) 45°, (d) 120° the thrombi in the left atrial cavity is better visualized. (e) Small freely mobile thrombus is noted exiting the SVC attached to a catheter (solid arrow). LA, left atrium; Ao, aorta; RA, right atrium; RV, right ventricle; LA, left atrium; SVC, superior vena cava.

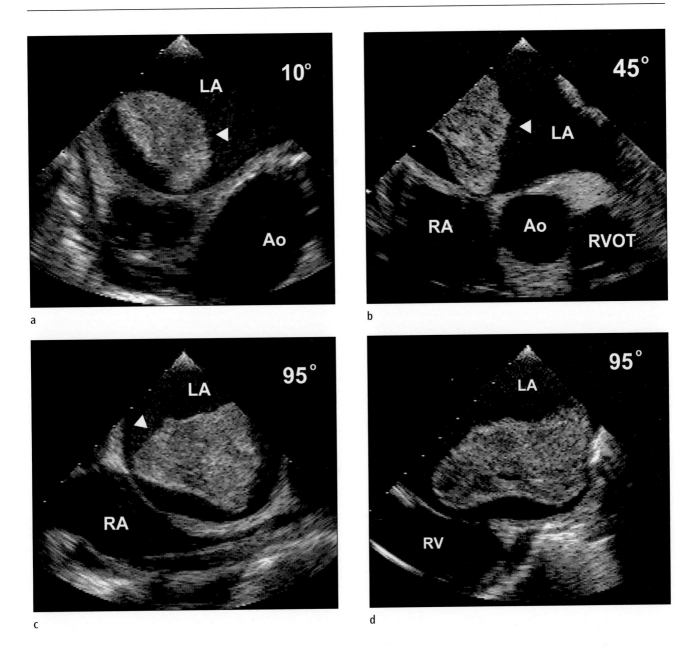

Case 8.4

A large left atrial cavity thrombus (arrow) attached to the posterior wall of the left atrium seen in multiple views (a–d). The thrombus was detected during a TEE to rule/out cardiac source of embolus. The thrombus was not well visualized on a transthoracic study due to poor acoustic windows secondary to lung disease. A pacemaker catheter is noted in the right atrium. LA, left atrium; Ao, aorta; RA, right atrium; RVOT, right ventricular outflow tract.

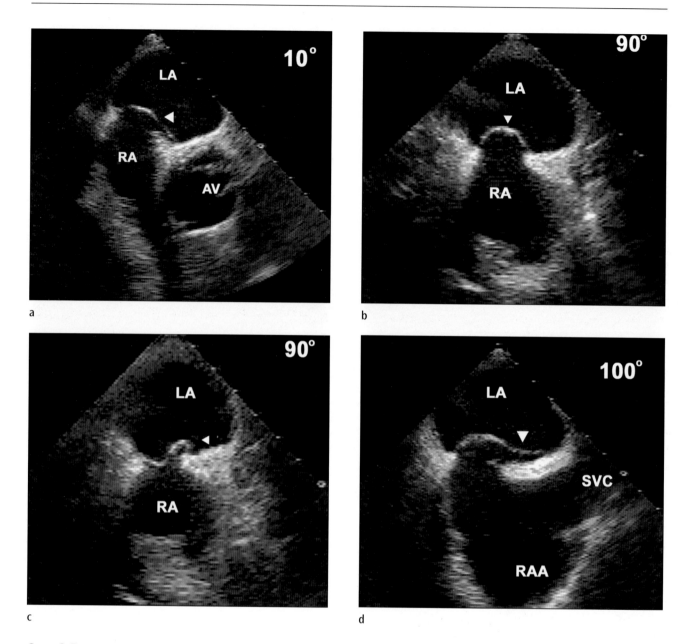

Case 8.5

Thrombus associated with an atrial septal aneurysm. Atrial septal aneurysms have been associated as a cardiac source of embolus. A defect or ridge is produced by the atrial septal aneurysm (arrows) on the left atrial surface, which allows for formation of a thrombus, which probably can embolize with excursion of the atrial septal aneurysm. Motion of the ASA is demonstrated in multiple views (a–d).

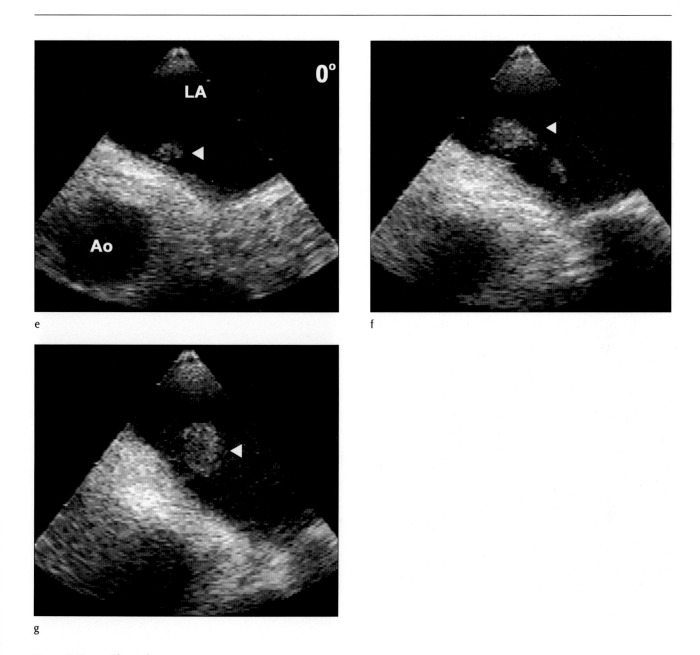

Case 8.5 *continued*

By providing multiple imaging planes, multiplane TEE the sensitivity for detecting small thrombi is dramatically improved. A small echo-dense mass is denoted in (e) near the ASA on the left atrial surface. With zooming in on that area (f, g), a thrombus is noted attached to the redundant septal tissue (arrow). LA, left atrium; Ao, aorta; RA, right atrium; AV, aortic valve; RAA, right atrial appendage; SVC, superior vena cava.

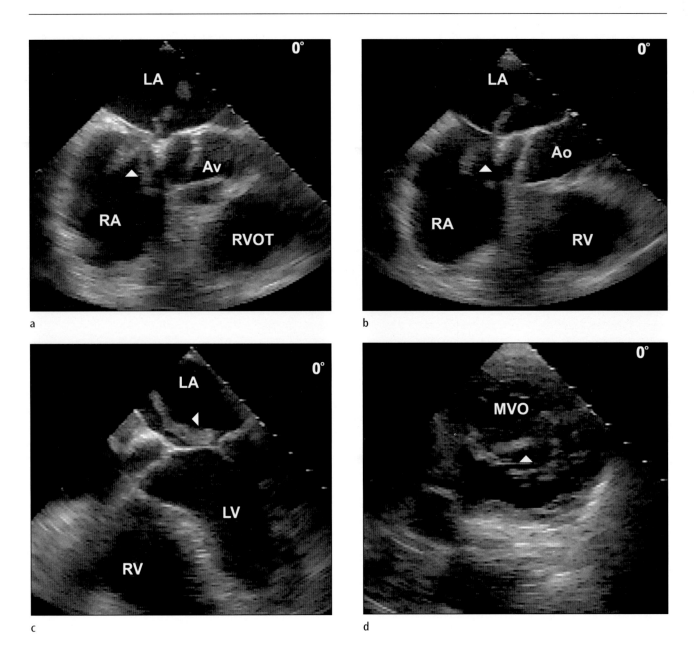

Case 8.6

Thrombus trapped within a patent foramen ovale. Venous casts that embolized from the systemic venous system enter the right atrium through the IVC. Due to the orientation of the ostia of the IVC, these casts may be directed toward and across a patent foramen ovale or atrial septal defect, resulting in left sided (paradoxical) embolism. Clot in the foramen (solid arrow) floating in the RA and LA (a, b). The clot resembling a linear thrombus seen next to the mitral valve (c). In a short axis projection of the mitral orifice the clot is seen moving in and out of the mitral orifice (solid arrow) (d). LA, left atrium; RA, right atrium; AV, aortic valve; RVOT, right ventricular outflow tract; RV, right ventricle; Ao, aorta; LV, left ventricle; MVO, mitral valve orifice.

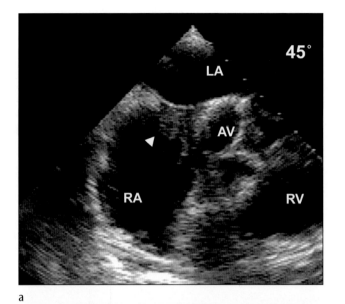

a

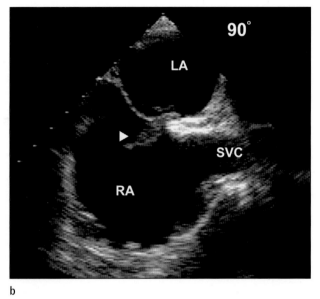

b

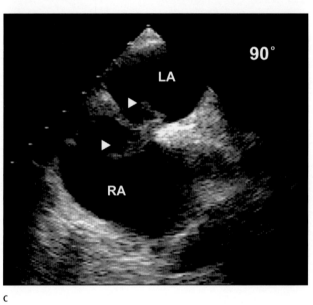

c

Case 8.7

Small thrombus visualized in a patent foramen ovale in a patient presenting with multiple transient ischemic attacks. A very mobile, shaggy thrombus is seen in multiple views (a–c). LA, left atrium; RA, right atrium; RV, right ventricle; AV, aortic valve; SVC, superior vena cava.

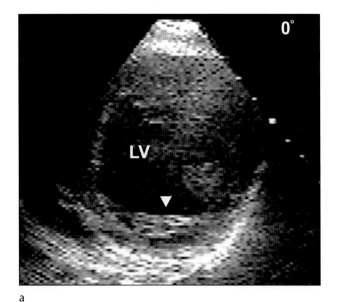 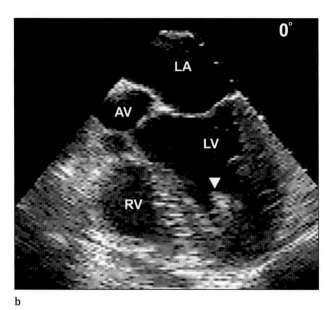

a   b

Case 8.8

Ventricular thrombus associated with an anterior wall myocardial infarction. Ventricular thrombi are usually better appreciated by the transthoracic approach since the ventricular apex is frequently foreshortened and difficult to visualize from the esophageal approach. (a) Thrombus demonstrated attached to the anterior wall in a short axis view of the left ventricle. The thrombus is defined as an area of increased echogenicity in comparison to the adjacent ventricular myocardium. (b) In the lower esophageal window the thrombus appears as a filling defect of the left ventricular apex. LV, left ventricle; LA, left atrium; RV, right ventricle; AV, aortic valve.

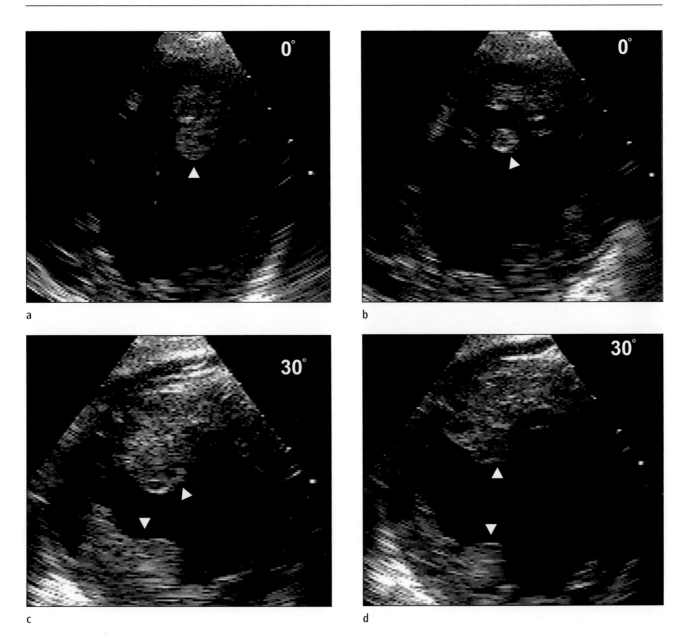

Case 8.9

Large mobile thrombi associated with a recent inferior apical infarction. The thrombus (arrows) is demonstrated in multiple views as a large mildly hyporeflective mass protruding into the ventricular cavity. (a–d) The thrombus can usually be differentiated from a papillary muscle due to it echogenicity and position in the left ventricle. In addition, the demonstration of chaotic motion in an area exhibiting a regional wall motion abnormality helps identify thrombus.

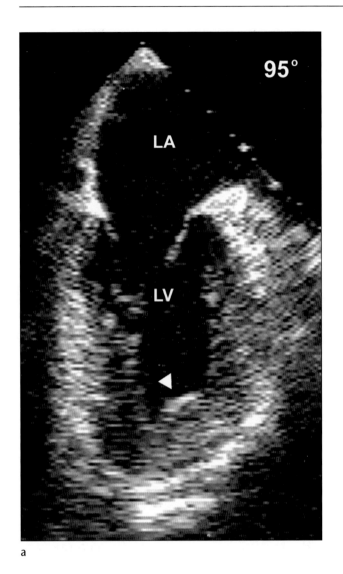

a

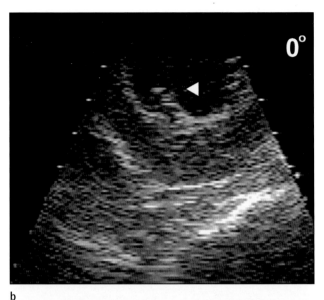

b

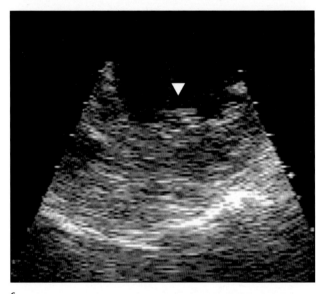

c

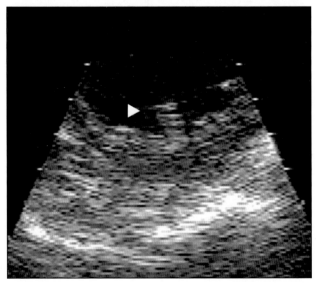

d

Case 8.10

Anterior apical thrombus in a patient with a recent anterior infarct. (a) Initially the thrombus appears sessile in a two chamber view at 90°, however due to the increased resolution available with TEE the thrombus exhibits a great deal of mobility during the cardiac cycle (b–d). LA, left atrium; LV, left ventricle.

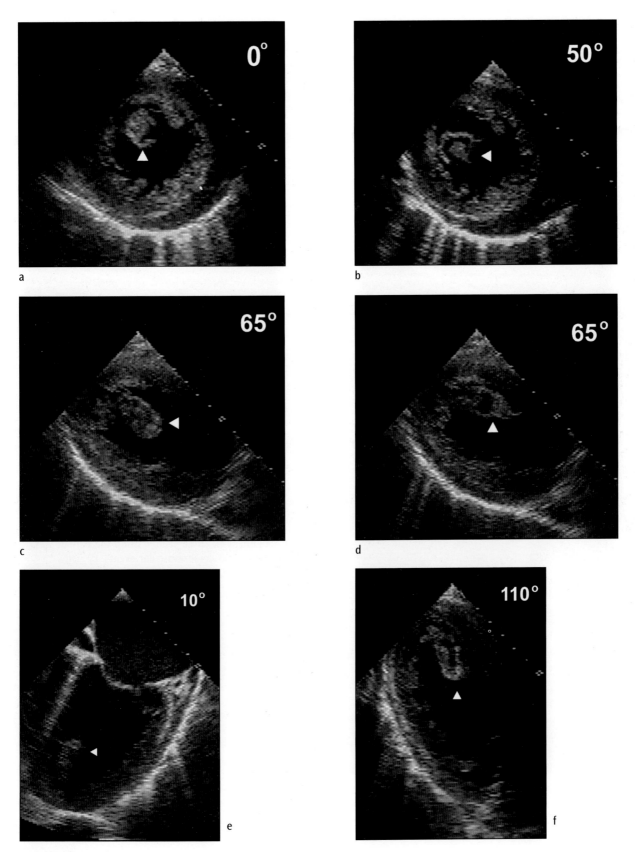

Case 8.11

Large apical thrombus associated with a dilated cardiomyopathy. (a–f) The thrombus appears polypoid, with an echolucent center. The thrombus emanated from the apex of the left ventricle with a great deal of motion with the cardiac cycle in a patient with multiple embolic events.

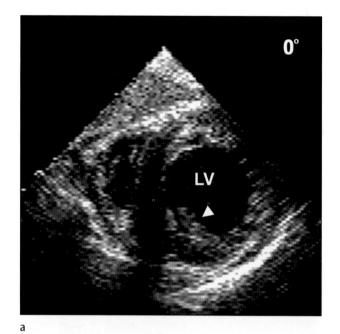

a

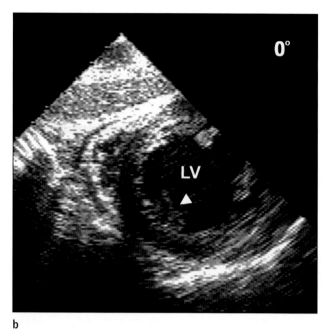

b

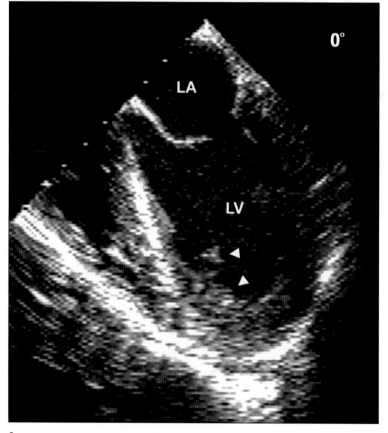

c

Case 8.12

Endomyocardial disease. Multiplane TEE was performed in a young female with a known history of systemic lupus with multiple cerebrovascular events. (a–f) TEE exhibited multiple areas with small masses and fronds exhibiting chaotic motion. The patient was taken to surgery and a "peel" was easily excised from the endocardial surface that covered approximately two-thirds of the ventricular endocardium. The ventricular apex and peel was best appreciated in the transgastric views at 90 to 110° (d–f). Three years post-op the patient was free from cerebrovascular events. LV, left ventricle; LA, left atrium.

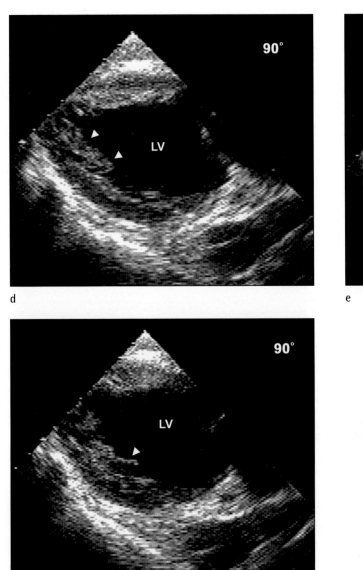

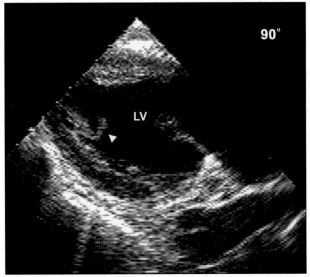

d

e

f

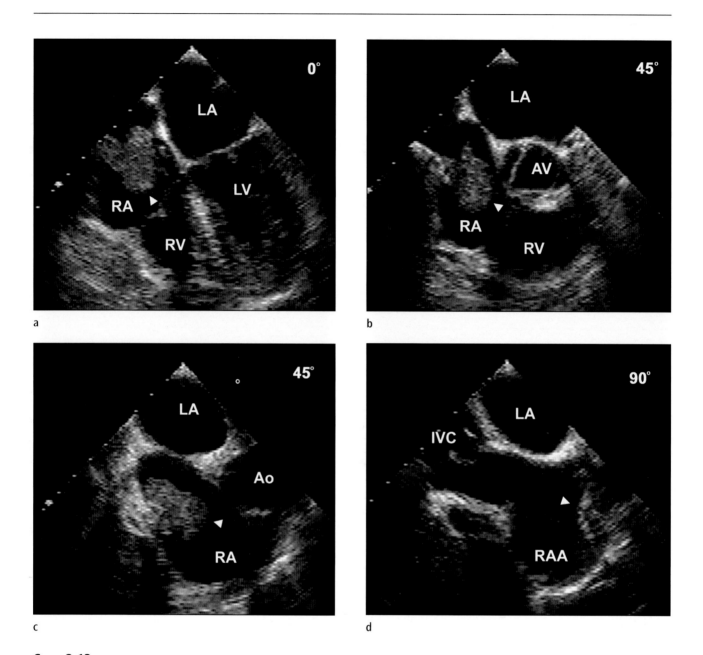

Case 8.13

Superior vena cava catheter thrombus. Thrombi frequently develop on and become attached to catheters. The origin and size of thrombi that are visualized in the right atrium can be readily determined with multiplane TEE. (a) Thrombus (arrow) seen filling the right atrium at 0° in the four chamber view. At the base of the heart the thrombus is seen near the orifice of the inferior vena cava, (b) at 0° and (c) at 45°. At 90° (d), the inferior vena cava demonstrates a prominent Eustachian valve. The thrombus is seen attached to a catheter situated in the superior vena cava. RA, right atrium; LA, left atrium; RV, right ventricle; LV, left ventricle; AV, aortic valve; Ao, aorta; RAA, right atrial appendage; IVC, inferior vena cava.

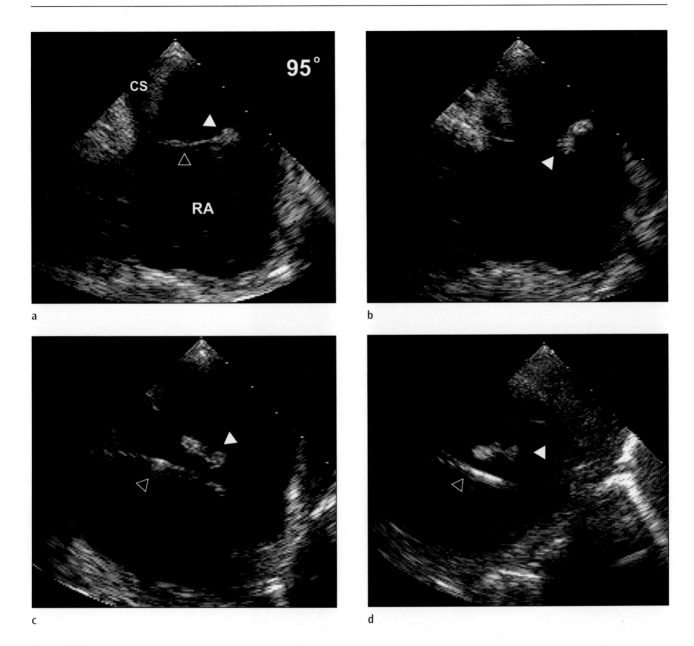

a

b

c

d

Case 8.14

Small thrombus attached to a Chiari Network. Modified bicaval views at 95° illustrate a Chiari Network (open arrow). A thrombus (probable small venous cast ruminant) is seen undulating during the cardiac cycle and firmly attached in the Chiari Network (a–d). RA, right atrium; CS, coronary sinus.

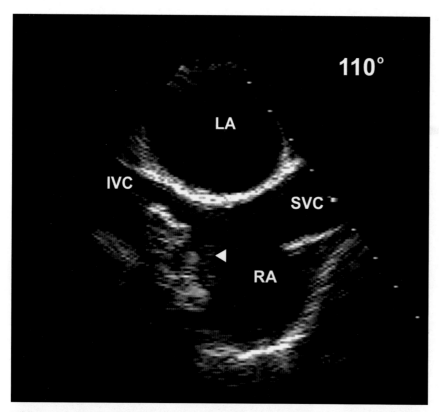

a

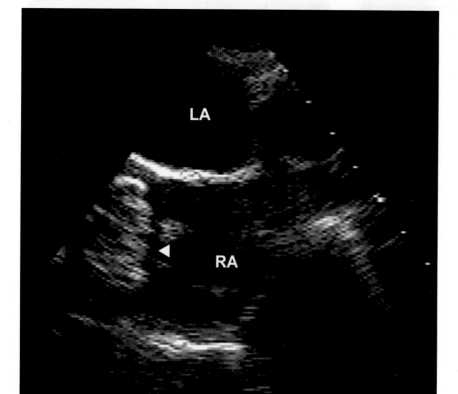

b

Case 8.15
Inferior vena cava thrombus. A large multilobed thrombus is seen protruding from the inferior vena cava orifice, entering the right atrium.
(a) Bicaval view at 110° demonstrating the thrombus (arrow). (b) Better appreciation of the size of the thrombus is demonstrated by rightward lateral flexion of the scope. A small mobile projection of the thrombus is also appreciated (arrow). RA, right atrium; LA, left atrium; IVC, inferior vena cava; SVC, superior vena cava.

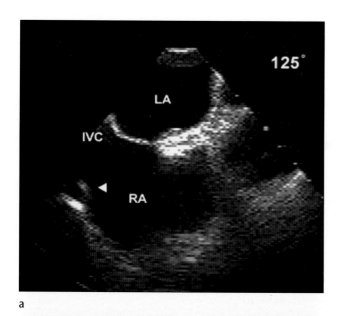

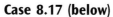

a

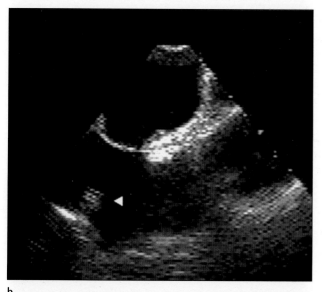

b

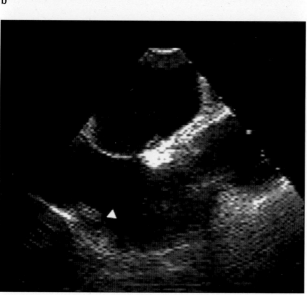

c

Case 8.16 (left)

Small mobile thrombus attached to the right atrial wall (a–c). This is a frequent sight of thrombus production when a superior venous catheter extends too far into the atrium. It has been suggested, that the thrombi are produced when the catheter abrade on the atrial endocardium. RA, right atrium; LA, left atrium; IVC, inferior vena cava.

Case 8.17 (below)

A large right atrial echodense mass consistent with a thrombus attached to the posterior wall of the right atrium (a) that prolapses across the tricuspid valve (b) during diastole. RA, right atrium; LA, left atrium; RV, right ventricle; LV, left ventricle.

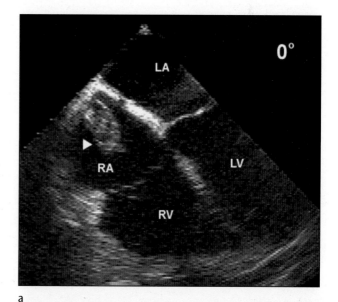

a

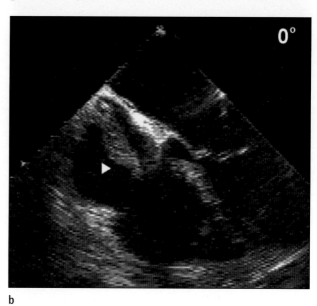

b

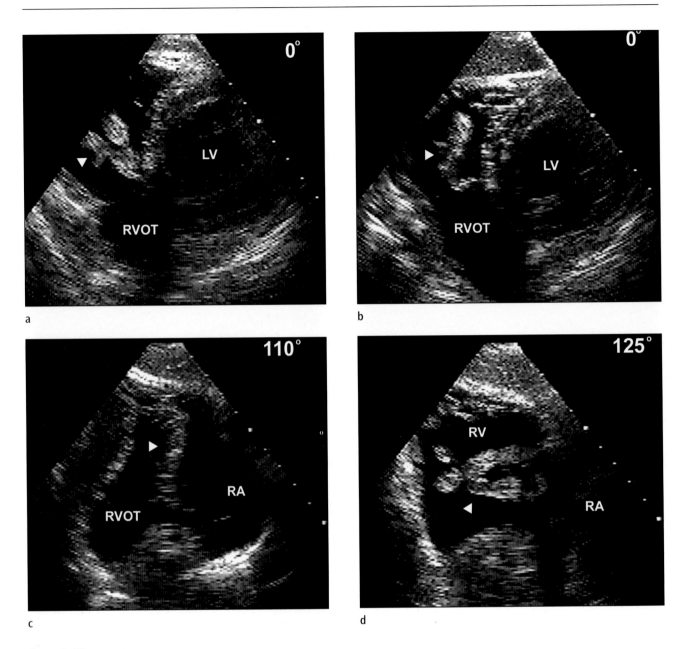

Case 8.18

Venous cast emanating from the inferior vena cava extending across the tricuspid valve and ending in the right ventricular outflow tract as viewed with multiplane TEE in multiple imaging planes. The patient studied had a history of multiple pulmonary emboli. Highly, mobile, thromboembolus (arrow) visualized in the right ventricle (a) and extending to the right ventricular outflow tract (b) obtained from the transgastric views at 0°. With rotation of the transducer to 110° (c) and 125° (d) the thromboembolic venous cast is seen folded on itself and moving freely within the right ventricular cavity.

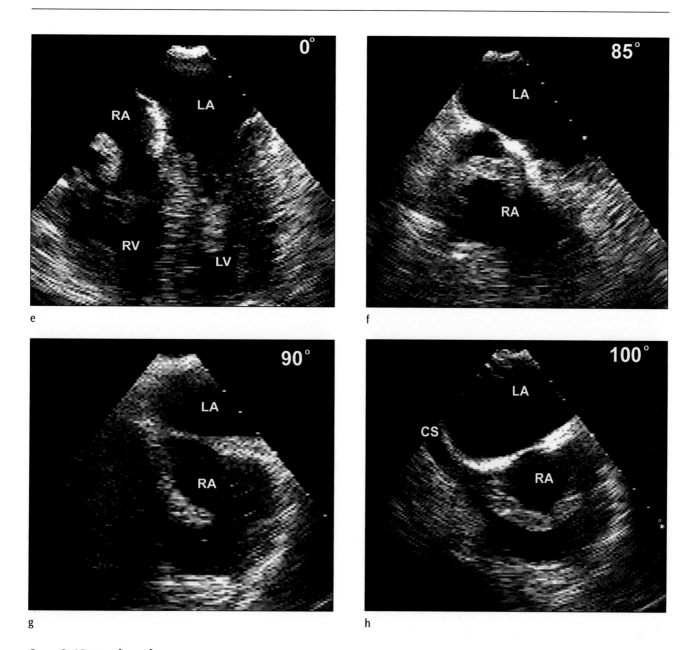

Case 8.18 continued

In the upper esophageal views the thrombus is appreciated in the right atrium (e–h) with its origin from the inferior vena cava (g). LV, left ventricle; RVOT, right ventricular outflow tract; RA, right atrium; RV, right ventricle; LA, left atrium; CS, coronary sinus.

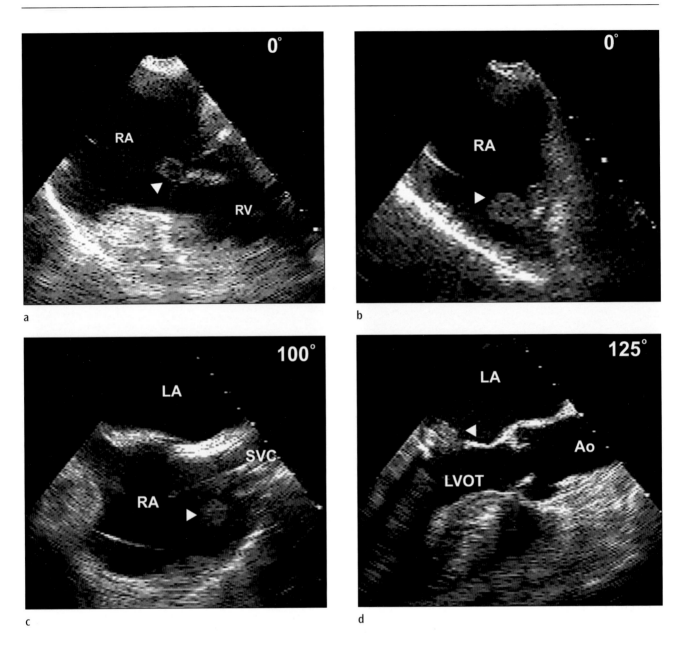

Case 8.19

Multiple small thrombi associated with a catheter in the right heart associated with a thrombus associated with the mitral annulus in a patient with protein S deficiency. Echodense mass caught at the tricuspid valve level (a) between the right atrium and ventricle. A curvilinear echo density representing the catheter is seen in the superior vena cava, right atrium (b, c) with multiple small echodense thrombi attached to the catheter. A small thrombus is seen (arrow) attached to the posterior annular portion of the posterior leaflet of the mitral valve (d). RA, right atrium; RV, right ventricle; SVC, superior vena cava; LA, left atrium; LVOT, left ventricular outflow tract; Ao, aorta.

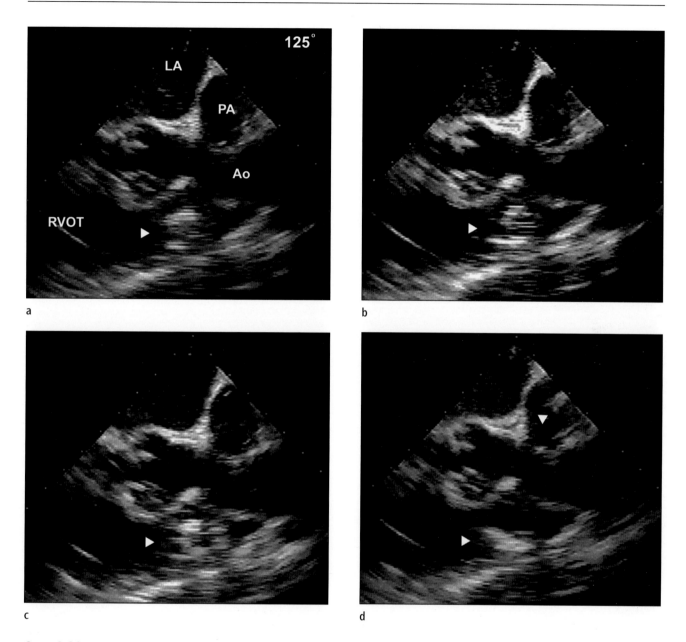

Case 8.20

Thrombus caught on the pulmonary valve leaflet. A highly, mobile thrombus (arrows) is seen in multiple positions (a–d) during the cardiac cycle and is attached to a Swan–Ganz catheter in a preoperative patient. It was postulated that the Swan–Ganz catheter, which was just inserted, carried the thrombus from the venous vessels during insertion. LA, left atrium; PA, pulmonary artery; RVOT, right ventricular outflow tract; Ao, aorta.

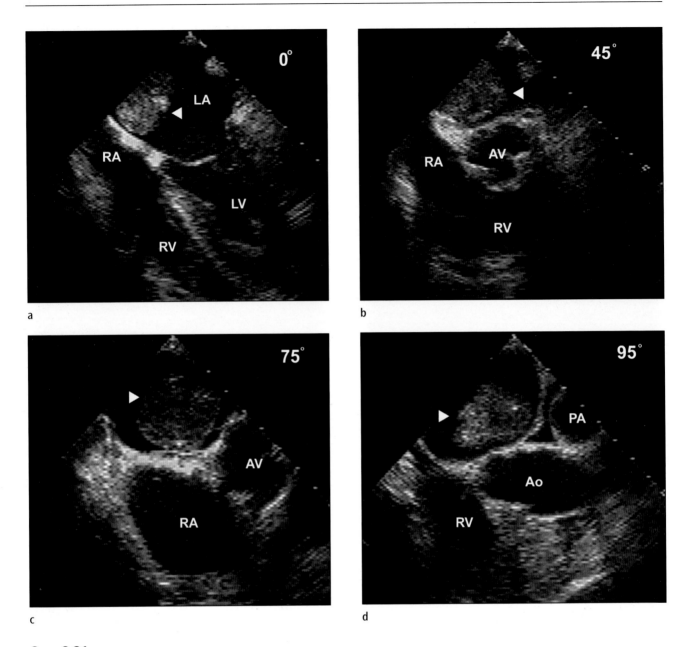

Case 8.21

Left atrial myxoma. The most common cardiac tumor is the benign myxoma, which is usually found in the left atrium. Myxomas may appear firm and smooth with a broad base or may appear gelatinous, with multiple finger-like projections. Multiplane TEE (a–d) demonstrating a left atrial myxoma from 0 to 95°. The tumor appears globular with an attachment site on the atrial septum at the foramen level (c). The advantage for TEE is in determining the site of attachment, the size and degree of mobility of the tumor. These features also assist in the certainty for diagnosis.

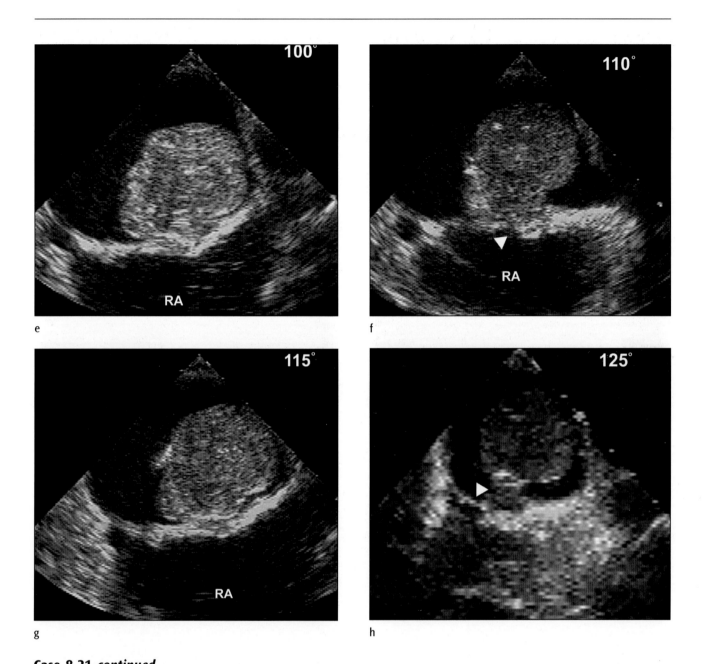

Case 8.21 *continued*
The stalk of the atrial myxoma is readily appreciated and demonstrated in zoom mode (e–h). RA, right atrium; LA, left atrium; RV, right ventricle; LV, left ventricle; AV, aortic valve; Ao, aorta; PA, pulmonary artery.

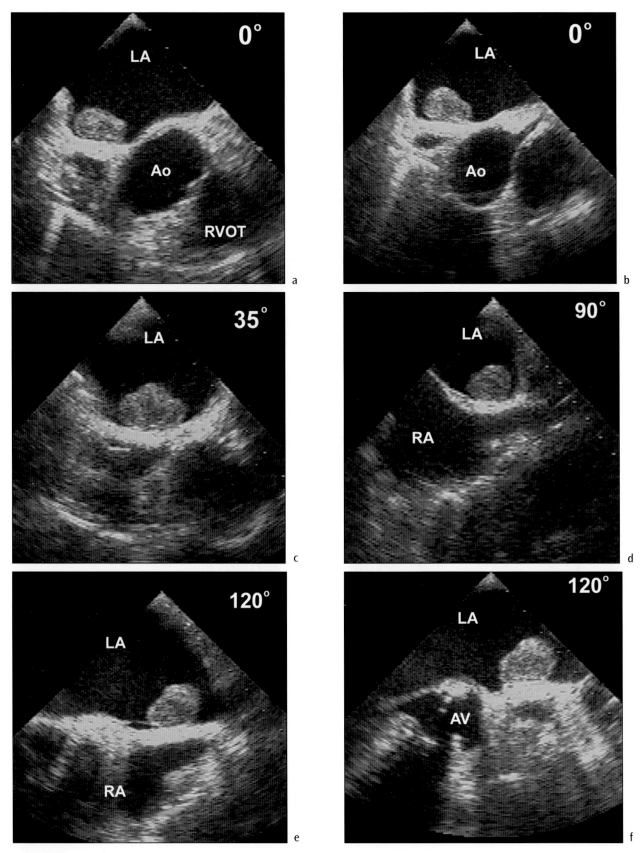

Case 8.22
Left atrial myxoma. A small left atrial myxoma not visualized with transthoracic echocardiography but diagnosed with multiplane TEE (a–f) The atrial myxoma appears firm and smooth with a broad base of attachment. The myxoma was an incidental finding. Ao, aorta; RVOT, right ventricular outflow tract; LA, left atrium; RA, right atrium.

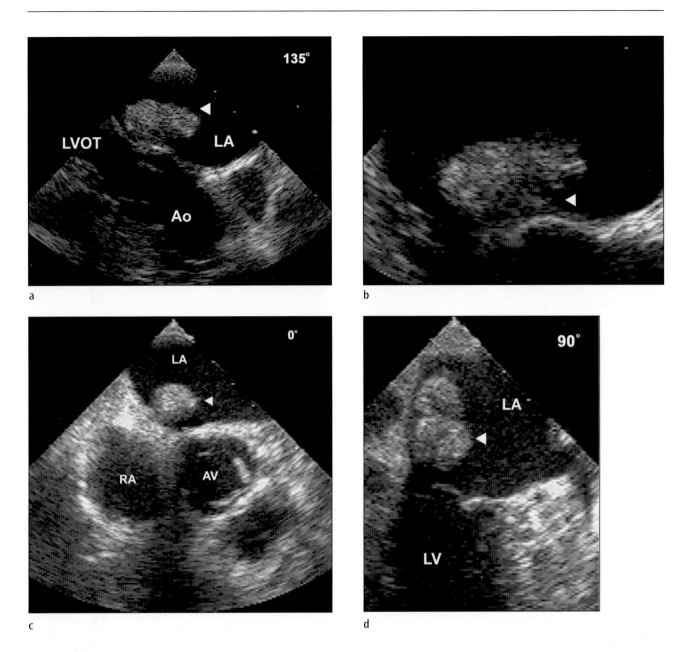

Case 8.23

Left atrial myxoma. Small left atrial myxoma attached to the atrial septum at the foramen level discovered during a rule/out cardiac source of embolus study in a patient with a stroke. The tumor was not well visualized in the left atrium but suspected on a transthoracic echocardiogram. With TEE the tumor appeared gelatinous and multilobular (a–d). LA, left atrium; LVOT, left ventricular outflow tract; Ao, aorta; RA, right atrium; AV, aortic valve; LV, left ventricle.

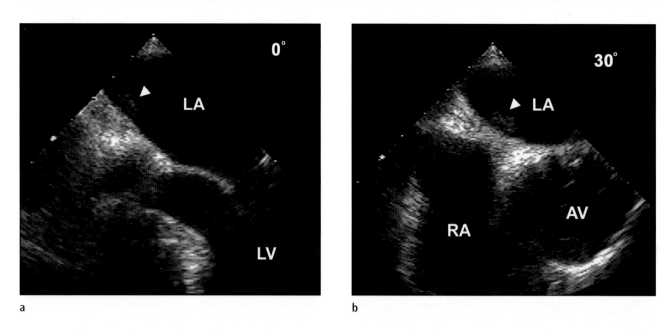

a
b

Case 8.24
Recurrent left atrial myxoma. Small left atrial myxoma attached to the atrial septum (a, b). The patient had surgical removal 3 years previous and was re-evaluated to rule/out thrombus on a pre-cardioversion study after developing atrial fibrillation. LA, left atrium; RA, right atrium; AV, aortic valve; LV, left ventricle.

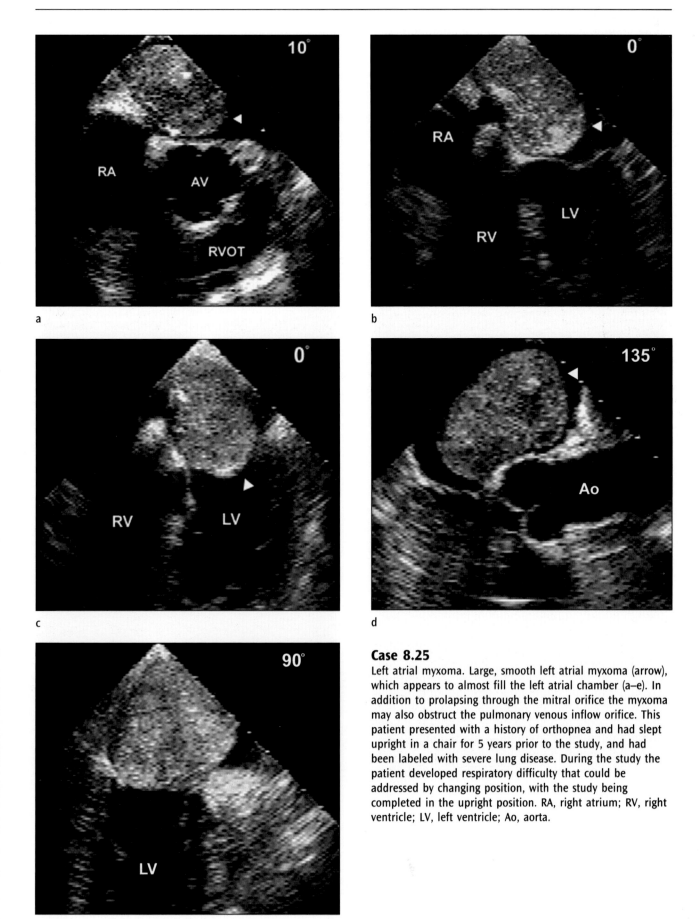

Case 8.25

Left atrial myxoma. Large, smooth left atrial myxoma (arrow), which appears to almost fill the left atrial chamber (a–e). In addition to prolapsing through the mitral orifice the myxoma may also obstruct the pulmonary venous inflow orifice. This patient presented with a history of orthopnea and had slept upright in a chair for 5 years prior to the study, and had been labeled with severe lung disease. During the study the patient developed respiratory difficulty that could be addressed by changing position, with the study being completed in the upright position. RA, right atrium; RV, right ventricle; LV, left ventricle; Ao, aorta.

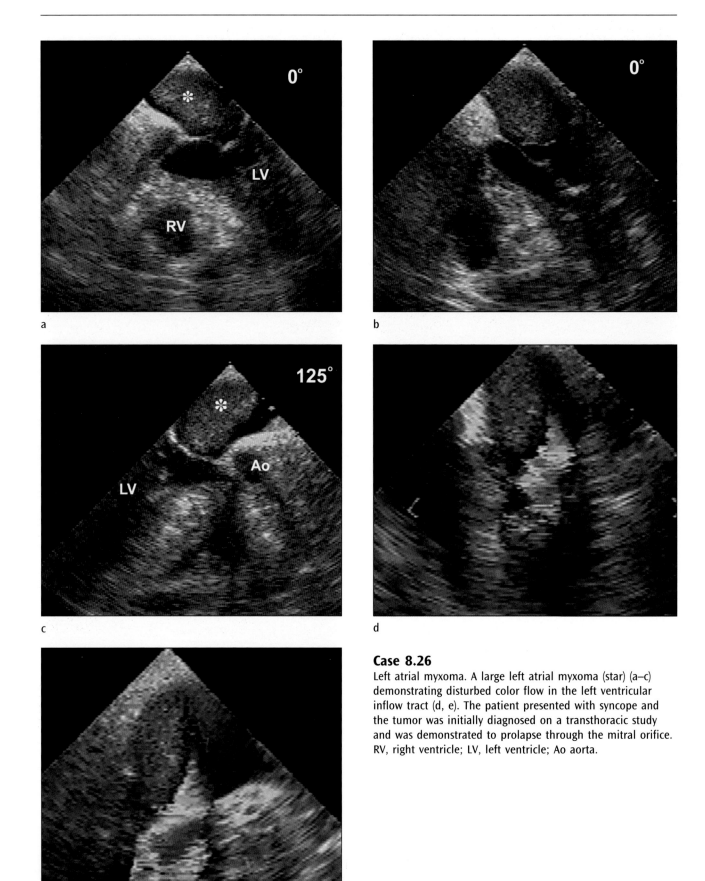

Case 8.26

Left atrial myxoma. A large left atrial myxoma (star) (a–c) demonstrating disturbed color flow in the left ventricular inflow tract (d, e). The patient presented with syncope and the tumor was initially diagnosed on a transthoracic study and was demonstrated to prolapse through the mitral orifice. RV, right ventricle; LV, left ventricle; Ao aorta.

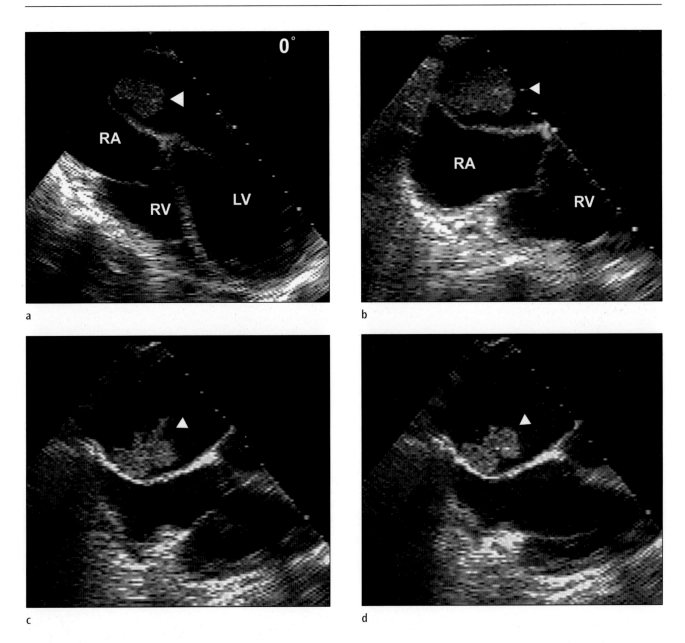

a

b

c

d

Case 8.27

Left atrial myxoma. A small, shaggy, fragmented, gelatinous myxoma discovered in a young nurse following an unexplained cardiac arrest. The patient was in the process of being worked up for chest pain and had a normal cardiac catheterization 2 months prior to the cardiac arrest. Immediately following the arrest the patient was pulseless in both lower extremities and right carotid despite adequate return of blood pressure. A post-arrest transthoracic study demonstrated a possible left atrial mass. Multiplane TEE demonstrated a gelatinous tumor with multiple finger-like projections in multiple planes (a–g).

continued overleaf

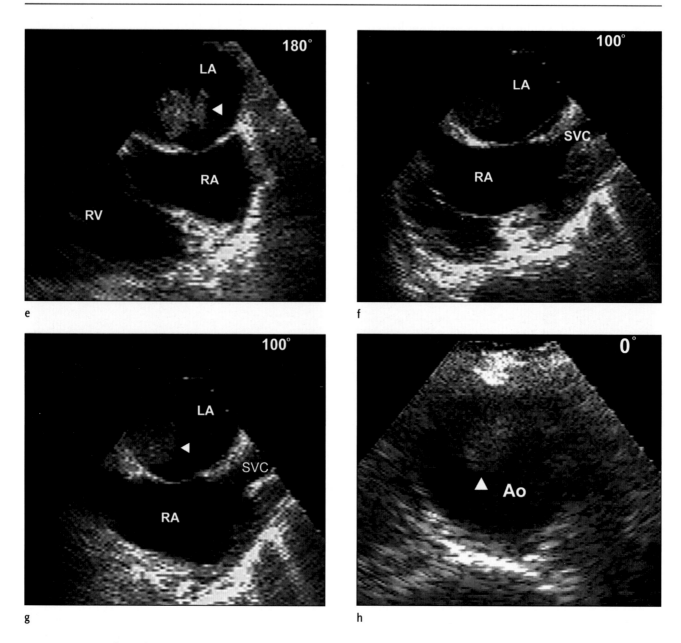

Case 8.27 *continued*
Visualization of the thoracic aorta in the mid chest level (h) demonstrated complete occlusion of the aorta. Embolectomy of the thoracic, abdominal aorta and femoral arteries yielded multiple myxoma tumor fragments. RA, right atrium; RV, right ventricle; LA, left atrium; Ao, aorta; Ao, aorta; LV, left ventricle; SVC, superior vena cava.

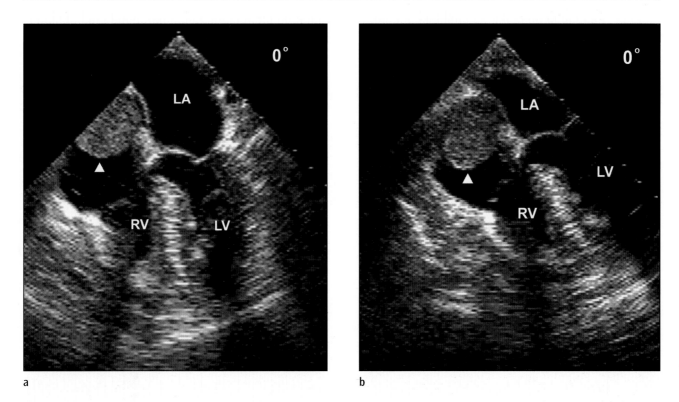

a   b

Case 8.28

Right atrial myxoma. A firm, smooth myxoma with a broad base of attachment to the atrial septum at the foramen level (a, b). Thickening of the atrial septum in (b) was in fact a second small myxoma lobe. RV, right ventricle; LA, left atrium; LV, left ventricle.

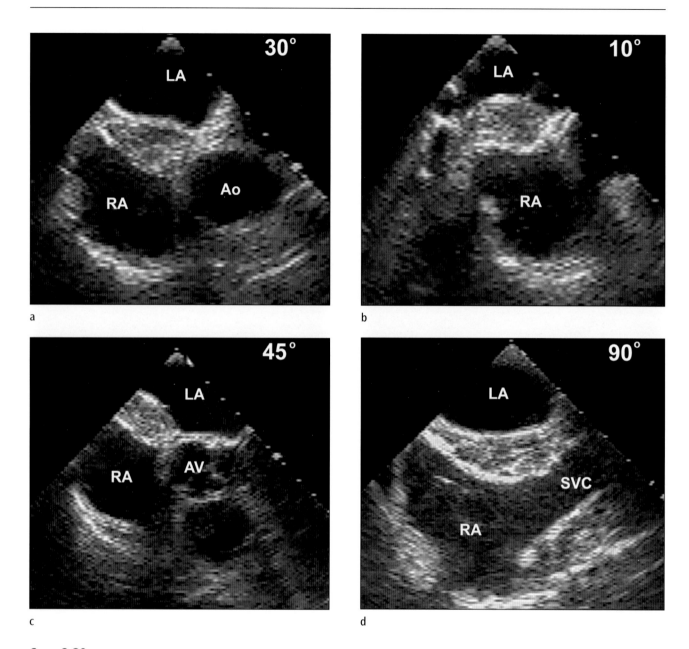

Case 8.29

Lipomatous hypertrophy. Plurality fatty deposits in the heart are virtually absent at birth, however they increase with advancing age. When fatty deposits accumulate in the atrial septum (a–d) they are referred to as lipomatous hypertrophy, as denoted as a septal cephalad thickness of greater than 2 cm. Patients usually exhibit fatty deposits elsewhere including the subepicardial adipose tissue. RA, right atrium; LA, left atrium; Ao, aorta; AV, aortic valve; SVC, superior vena cava.

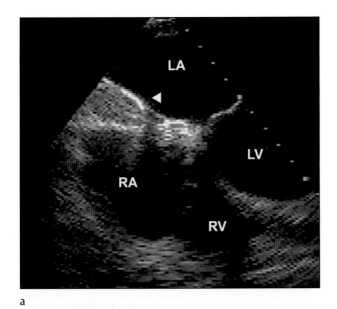

a

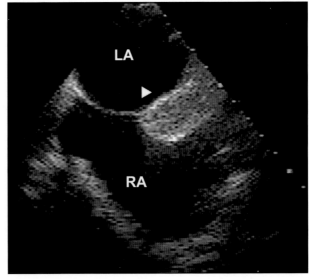

b

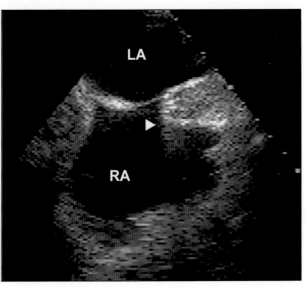

c

Case 8.30

Lipomatous hypertrophy. Lipomatous hypertrophy usually occurs in the cephalad portion of the atrial septum, but also may occur in the caudal portion, sparing the fossa ovalis, producing a characteristic dumbbell pattern to the atrial septal wall (a–c). RA, right atrium; LA, left atrium; RV, right ventricle; LV, left ventricle.

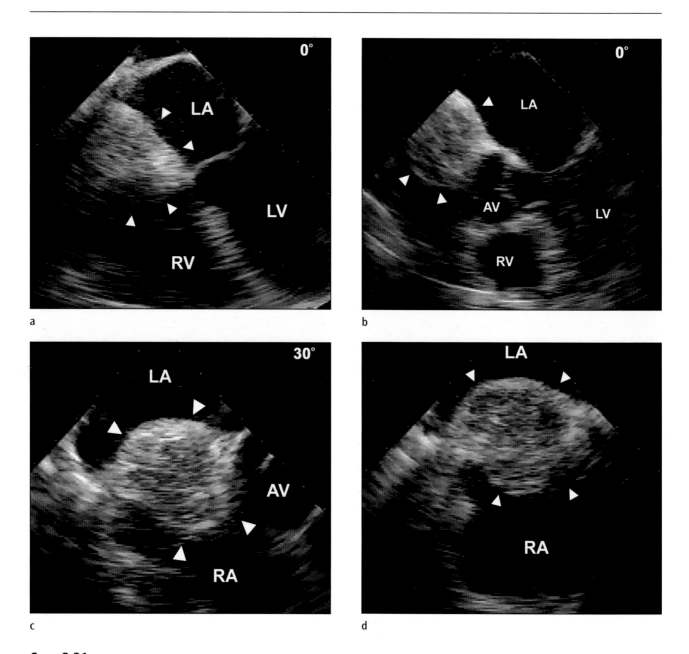

Case 8.31

Lipoma of the atrial septum. Large lipoma of the atrial septum visualized with multiplane TEE. Lipomas are common benign tumors found in adults. True lipomas of the atrial septum also occur and frequently are indistinguishable from lipomatous hypertrophy or fatty infiltration of the atrial septum. A lipoma (arrow) usually presents as a discreet mass (a–d) however with the appearance of a capsule on TEE, rather that a generalized thickening of the septal wall. RA, right atrium; LA, left atrium; RV, right ventricle; LV, left ventricle; AV, aortic valve.

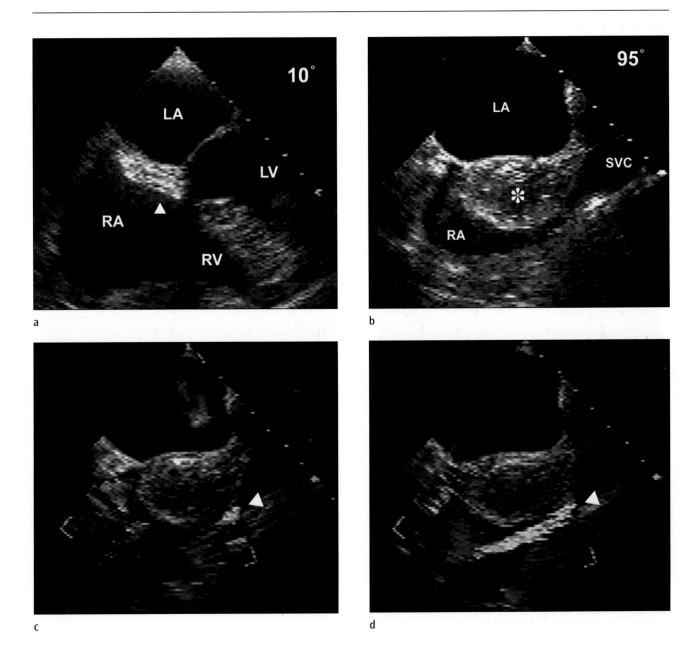

Case 8.32

Lipoma of the atrial septum. Discrete lipoma (star) of the upper atrial septum (a–c). Although generally benign the position of this lipoma caused narrowing and flow disturbance (d) at the orifice of the superior vena cava demonstrated with color flow Doppler. The functional consequence of this abnormality is not known however; various reports have suggested hemodynamic consequence. RA, right atrium; LA, left atrium; RV, right ventricle; LV, left ventricle; SVC, superior vena cava.

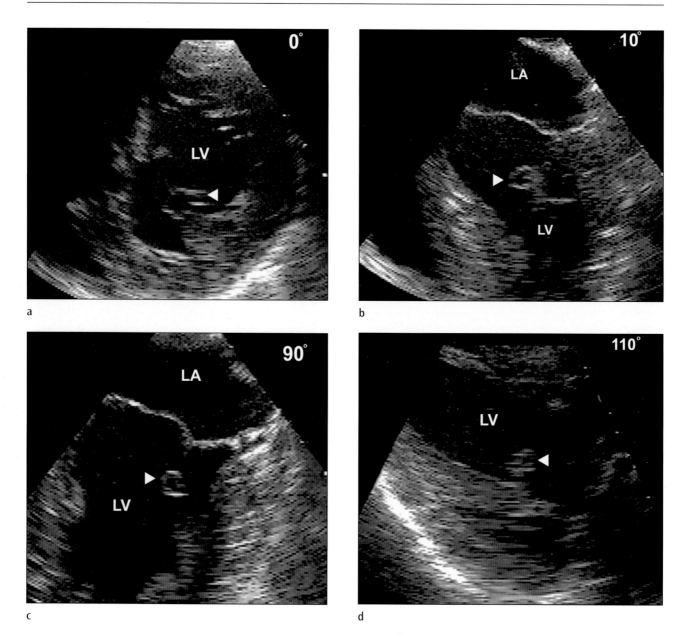

Case 8.33

Papillary fibroelastoma of the mitral valve. Cardiac tumors involving valves are rare. However, 87% are papillary fibroelastomas, and are associated with embolic events. Small papillary fibroelastoma (arrow) attached to the chordae tendinae as seen in multiple planes with TEE (a–d).

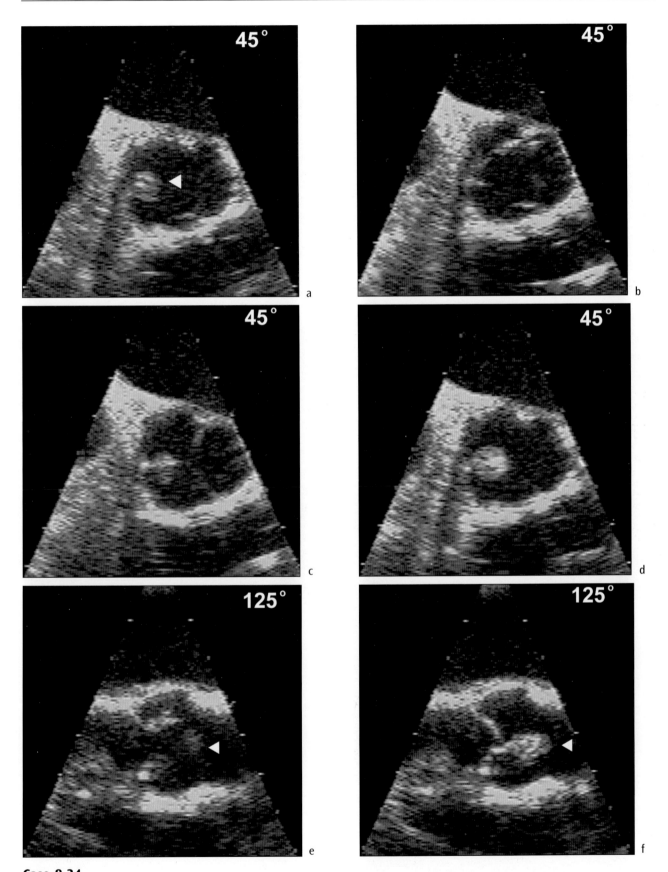

Case 8.34

Papillary fibroelastoma of the aortic valve. Papillary fibroelastomas are more frequently associated with the aortic valve in comparison to the other valves. Short axis views (a–d) of the aortic valve show a small round mass attached with a short stalk to the aortic valve cusp freely moving with the cardiac cycle. Long axis view of the aortic root illustrating the papillary fibroelastoma (e, f).

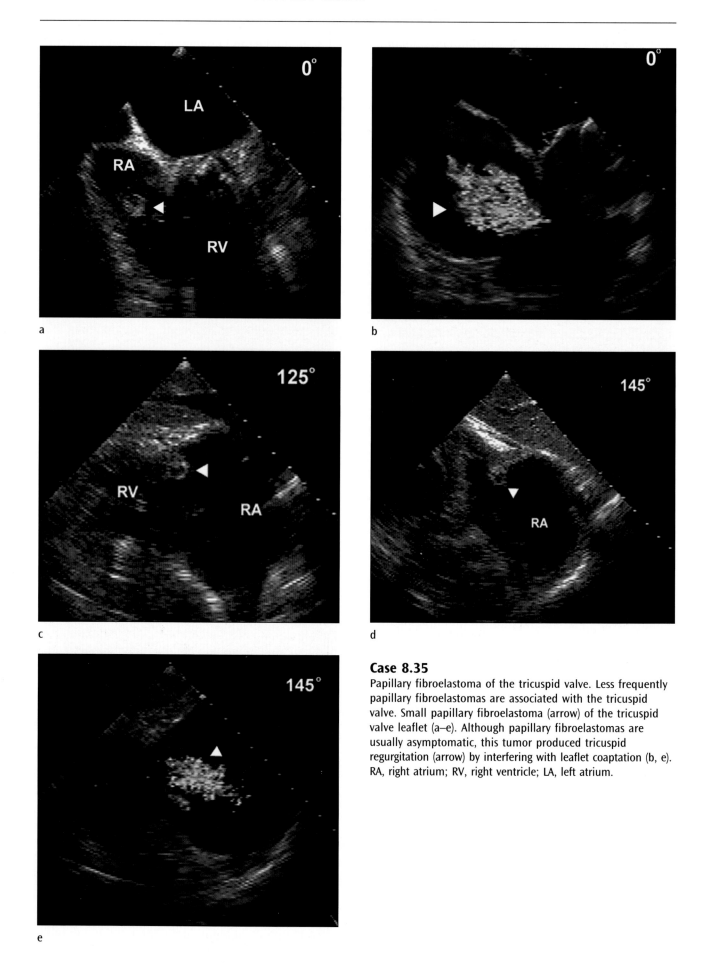

Case 8.35

Papillary fibroelastoma of the tricuspid valve. Less frequently papillary fibroelastomas are associated with the tricuspid valve. Small papillary fibroelastoma (arrow) of the tricuspid valve leaflet (a–e). Although papillary fibroelastomas are usually asymptomatic, this tumor produced tricuspid regurgitation (arrow) by interfering with leaflet coaptation (b, e). RA, right atrium; RV, right ventricle; LA, left atrium.

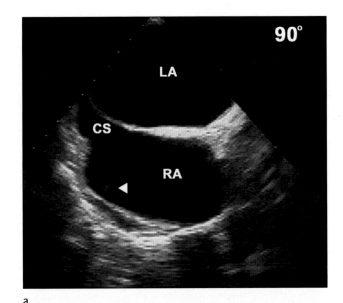

a

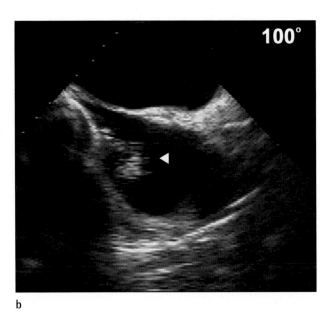

b

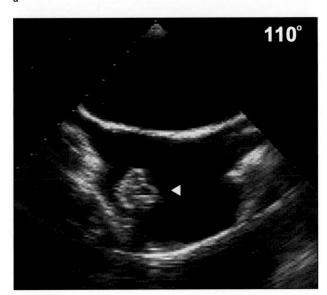

c

Case 8.36

Papillary fibroelastoma of the right atrium. Although papillary fibroelastomas are found frequently attached to the valves, they can be found anywhere in the heart. Small, biopsy proven papillary fibroelastoma (arrow) attached to the right atrial free wall (a–c). RA, right atrium, LA, left atrium; CS, coronary sinus.

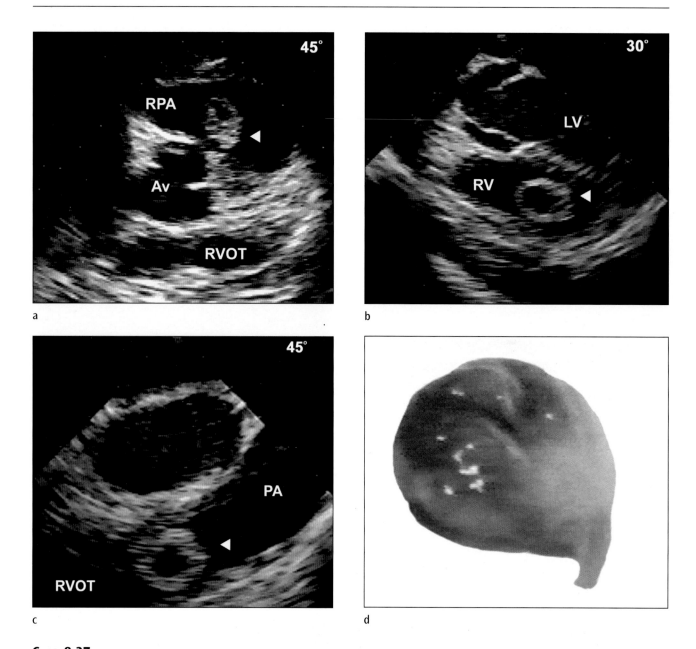

Case 8.37

Capillary hemangioma of the right ventricular outflow tract. Multiplane TEE was performed in a 14 y/o male who exhibited syncope on numerous occasions while playing basketball. A round mass (arrow) with an echogenic center was noted to be freely prolapsing in and out of the right ventricular outflow tract (a–c). The mass was noted to be frequently trapped in the pulmonary valve during systole. The mass was excised (d) and had no further syncopal events. RPA, right pulmonary artery; AV, aortic valve; RVOT, right ventricular outflow tract.

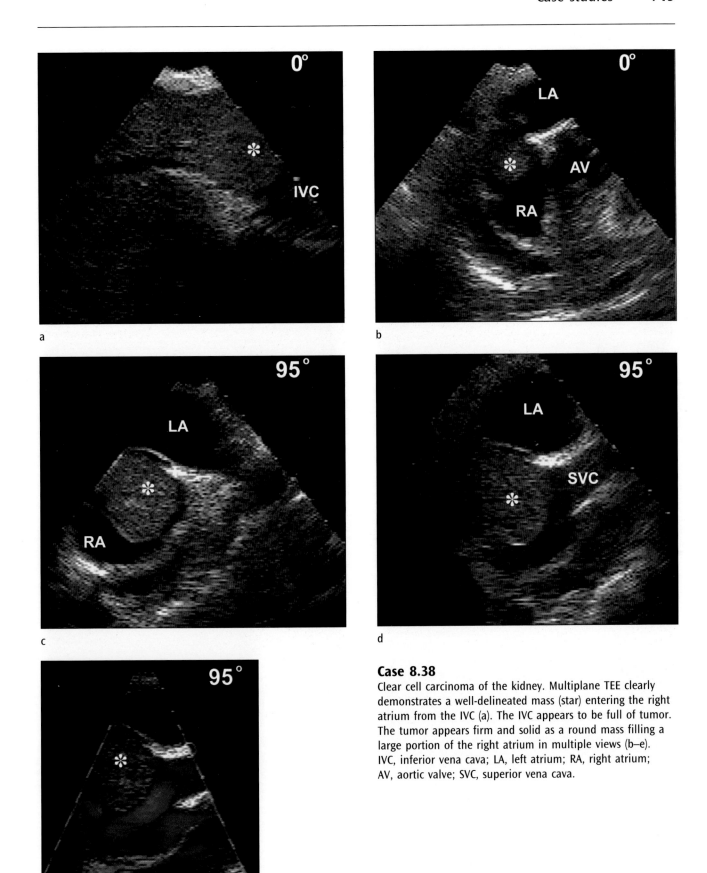

Case 8.38

Clear cell carcinoma of the kidney. Multiplane TEE clearly demonstrates a well-delineated mass (star) entering the right atrium from the IVC (a). The IVC appears to be full of tumor. The tumor appears firm and solid as a round mass filling a large portion of the right atrium in multiple views (b–e). IVC, inferior vena cava; LA, left atrium; RA, right atrium; AV, aortic valve; SVC, superior vena cava.

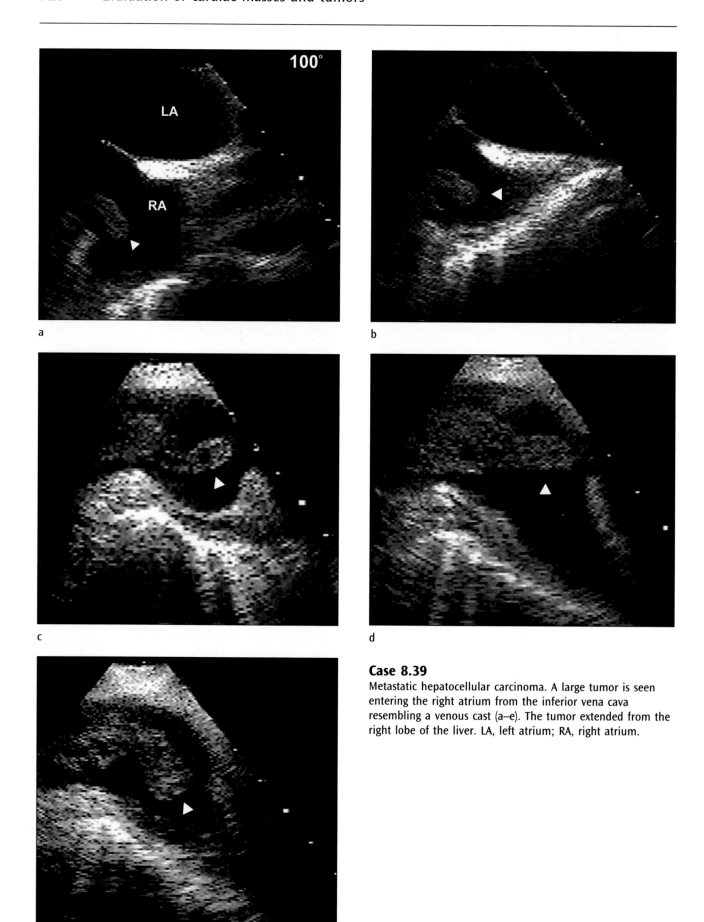

a

b

c

d

e

Case 8.39

Metastatic hepatocellular carcinoma. A large tumor is seen entering the right atrium from the inferior vena cava resembling a venous cast (a–e). The tumor extended from the right lobe of the liver. LA, left atrium; RA, right atrium.

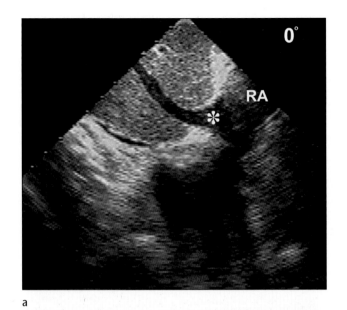

a

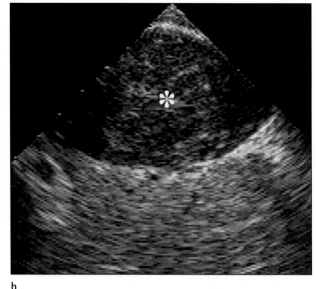

b

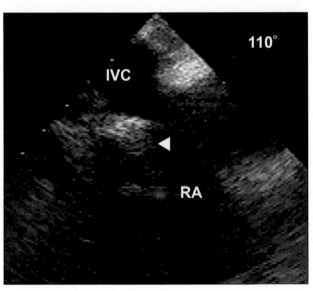

c

Case 8.40
Metastatic melanoma. Large right atrial tumor (star) associated with melanoma with extension to the inferior vena cava (a–c). RA, right atrium; IVC, inferior vena cava.

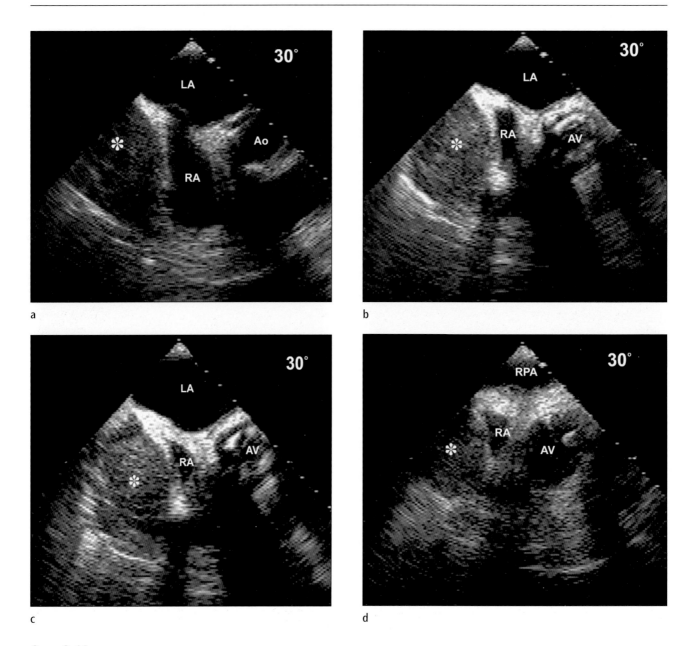

Case 8.41

Mesothelioma. The second most common type of malignant tumor is the mesothelioma, which arises from the visceral or parietal pericardium. A large mesothelioma (star), which caused extrinsic compression of the right atrium, as demonstrated in multiple levels with multiplane TEE. LA, left atrium, RA, right atrium; Ao, aorta; AV, prosthetic aortic valve; RPA, right pulmonary artery.

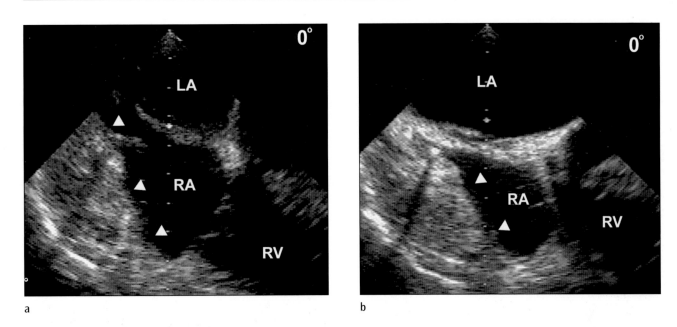

a   b

Case 8.42

Angiosarcoma of the right atrium. Sarcomas are the most common malignant primary tumor of the heart. Large cavity filling tumor (arrow) of the right atrium, which appears confluent with the atrial wall (a, b). Over 70% of sarcomas occur in the right atrium, which readily expand into the myocardium and pericardium and frequently metastasize to the lungs and mediastinal lymph nodes. LA, left atrium; RA, right atrium; RV, right ventricle.

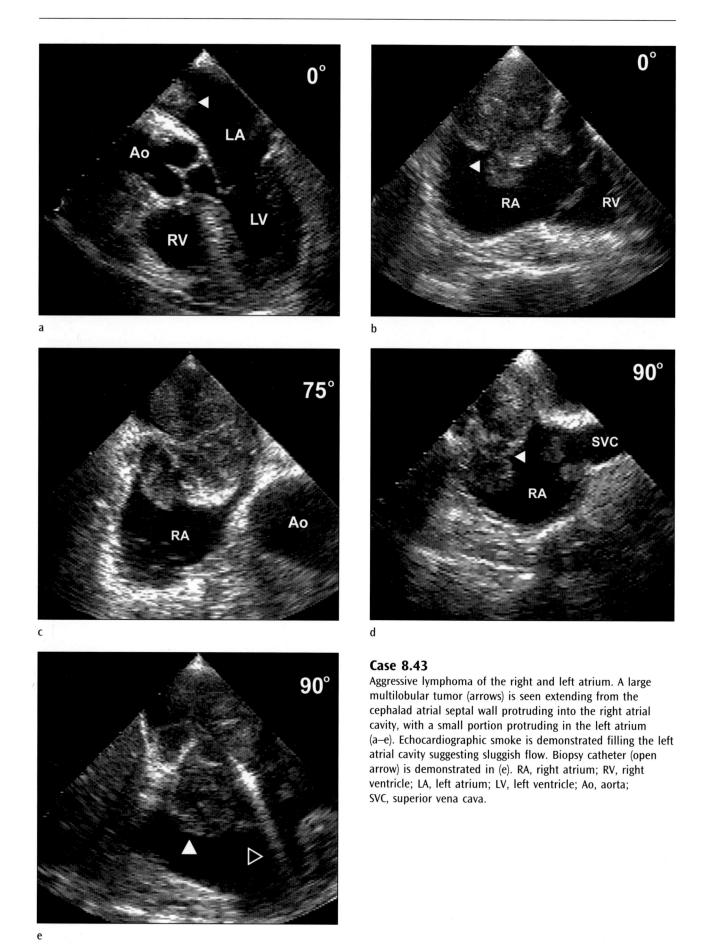

Case 8.43

Aggressive lymphoma of the right and left atrium. A large multilobular tumor (arrows) is seen extending from the cephalad atrial septal wall protruding into the right atrial cavity, with a small portion protruding in the left atrium (a–e). Echocardiographic smoke is demonstrated filling the left atrial cavity suggesting sluggish flow. Biopsy catheter (open arrow) is demonstrated in (e). RA, right atrium; RV, right ventricle; LA, left atrium; LV, left ventricle; Ao, aorta; SVC, superior vena cava.

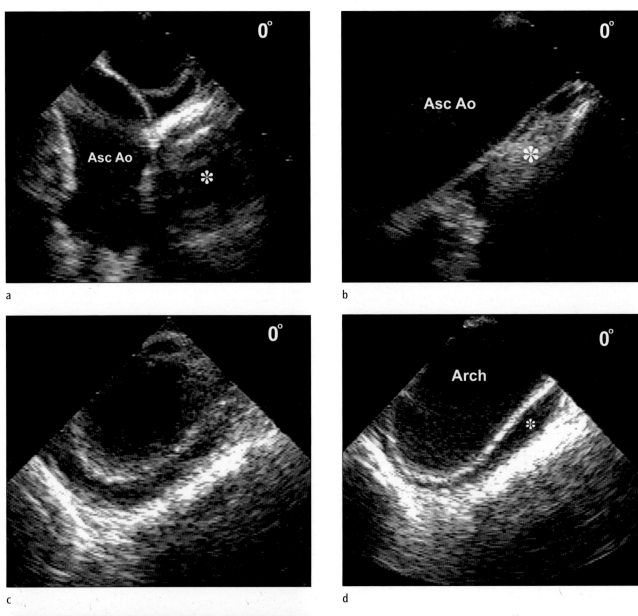

Case 8.44

Non-Hodgkin's lymphoma. Large mediastinal lymph nodes are visualized as large echodense masses (star) lying adjacent to the thoracic aorta (a–d). Echo-free space is seen outlining the great vessels representing fluid. In zoom mode (e) a lymph node is seen with excellent detail. ASC Ao, ascending aorta; Arch, aortic arch.

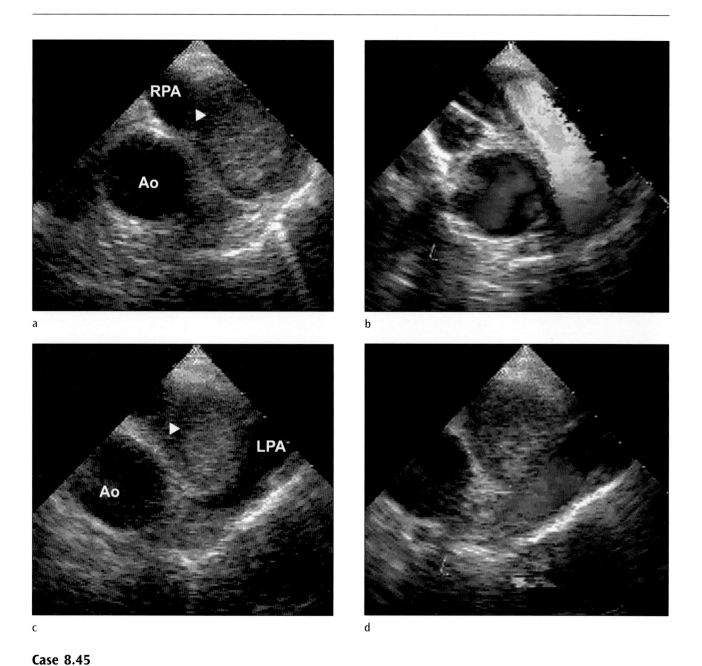

a

b

c

d

Case 8.45

Paraganglioma. Tumors, which arise from the chemoreceptor system, are called chemodectomas or nonchromaffin paraganglioma, and most represent benign indolent growths. A paraganglioma or aortic body tumor (arrow) is seen adjacent to the ascending aorta and main pulmonary artery (a–h). Extrinsic compression of the pulmonary artery is noted; with high velocity flow noted by color flow Doppler (d).

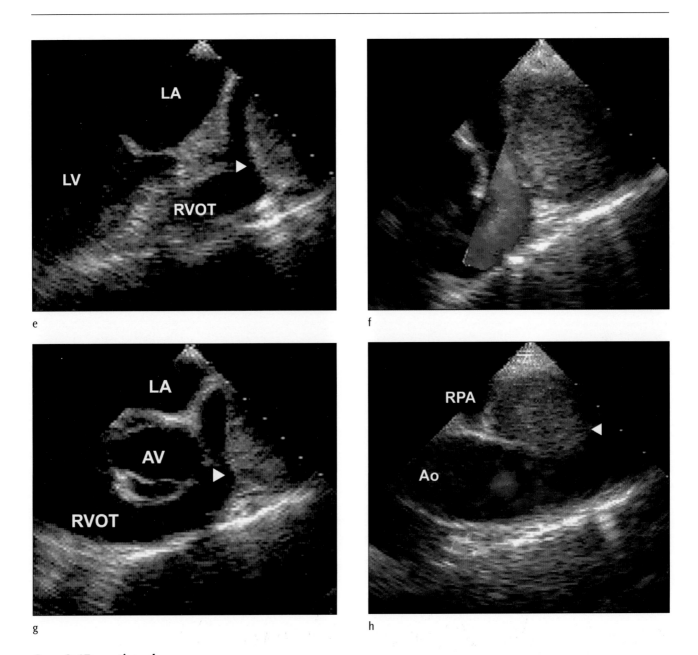

e

f

g

h

Case 8.45 *continued*

Occasionally these tumors are difficult to remove surgically, however this tumor was well encapsulated and was successfully excised. Ao, aorta; RPA, right pulmonary artery; LPA, left pulmonary artery; LA, left atrium; LV, left ventricle; RVOT, right ventricular outflow tract, AV, aortic valve.

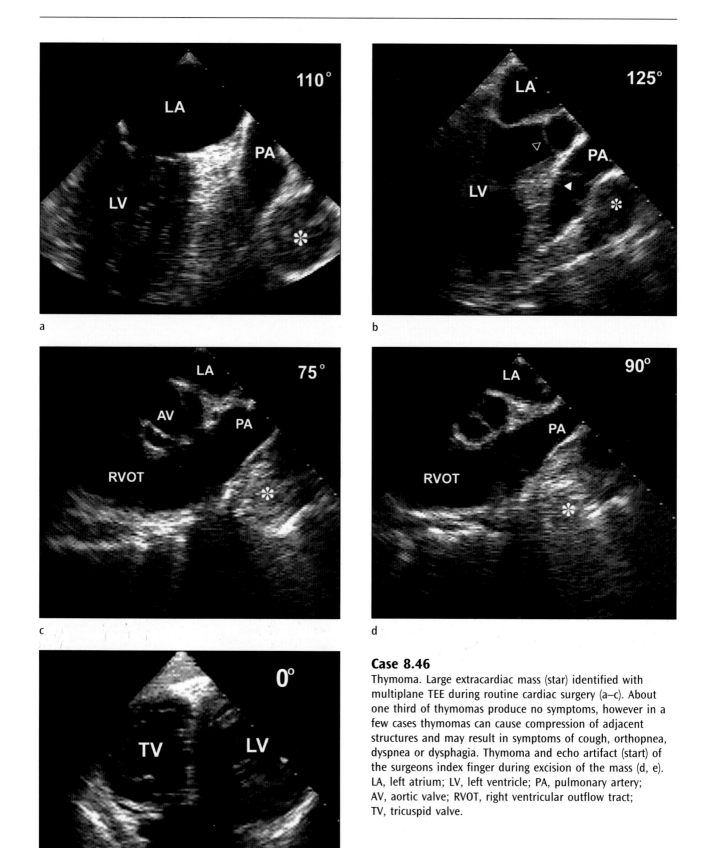

Case 8.46

Thymoma. Large extracardiac mass (star) identified with multiplane TEE during routine cardiac surgery (a–c). About one third of thymomas produce no symptoms, however in a few cases thymomas can cause compression of adjacent structures and may result in symptoms of cough, orthopnea, dyspnea or dysphagia. Thymoma and echo artifact (start) of the surgeons index finger during excision of the mass (d, e). LA, left atrium; LV, left ventricle; PA, pulmonary artery; AV, aortic valve; RVOT, right ventricular outflow tract; TV, tricuspid valve.

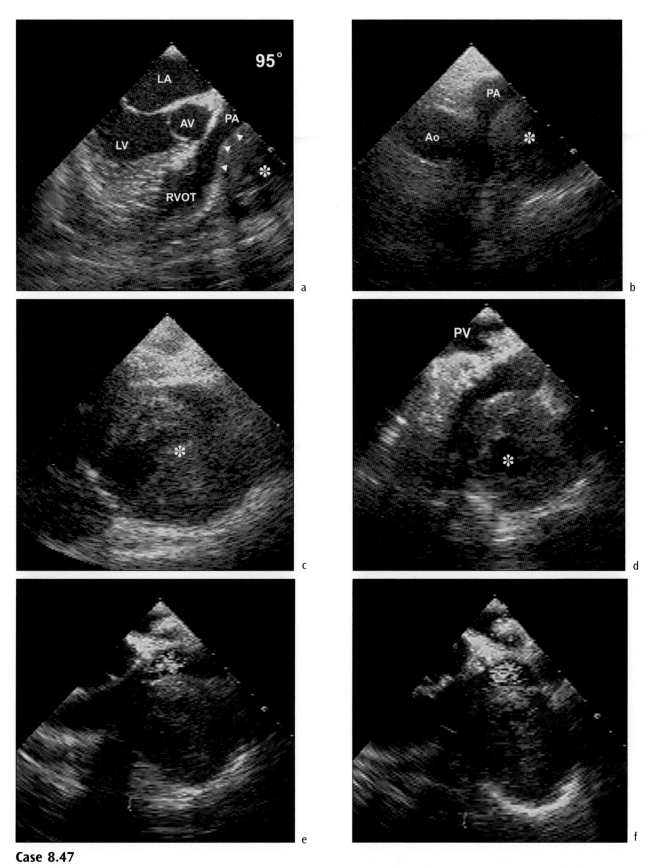

Case 8.47

Lung tumor. A large tumor mass (star) is demonstrated with multiplane TEE producing external compression of the right ventricular outflow tract and main pulmonary artery (a–f). Increased velocities are demonstrated in the pulmonary artery with color flow Doppler. In most cases of metastatic spread of lung carcinoma to the heart by hematogenous or lymphatic spread. LA, left atrium; LV, left ventricle; AV, aortic valve; RVOT, right ventricular outflow tract; PA, pulmonary artery.

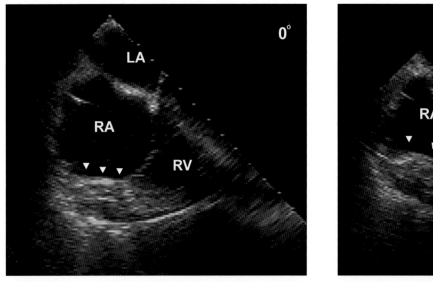
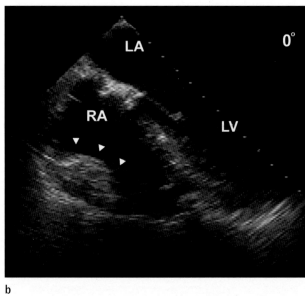

a   b

Case 8.48

Metastatic breast carcinoma. Large metastatic mass infiltrating the wall of the right atrium and pericardium by direct extension in a patient with aggressive breast carcinoma (a, b). Metastasis from breast carcinoma usually only involves the pericardium without infiltrating the myocardium. RA, right atrium; LA, left atrium; LV, left ventricle.

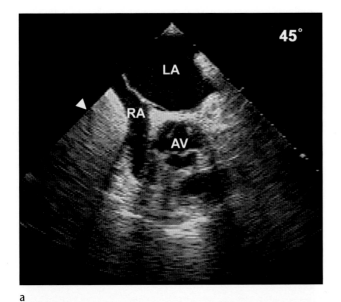

a

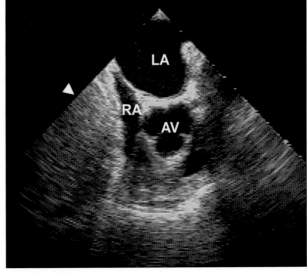

b

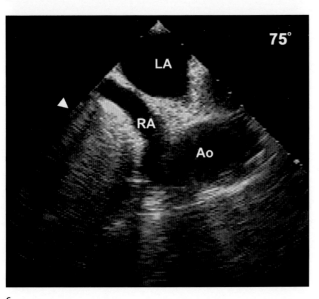

c

Case 8.49

Malignant lymphoma. Large intrapericardial mass (arrow) compressing the right atrium in a patient with malignant lymphoma (a–c). Other views demonstrated pericardial effusion. RA, right atrium; LA, left atrium; AV, aortic valve, Ao, aorta.

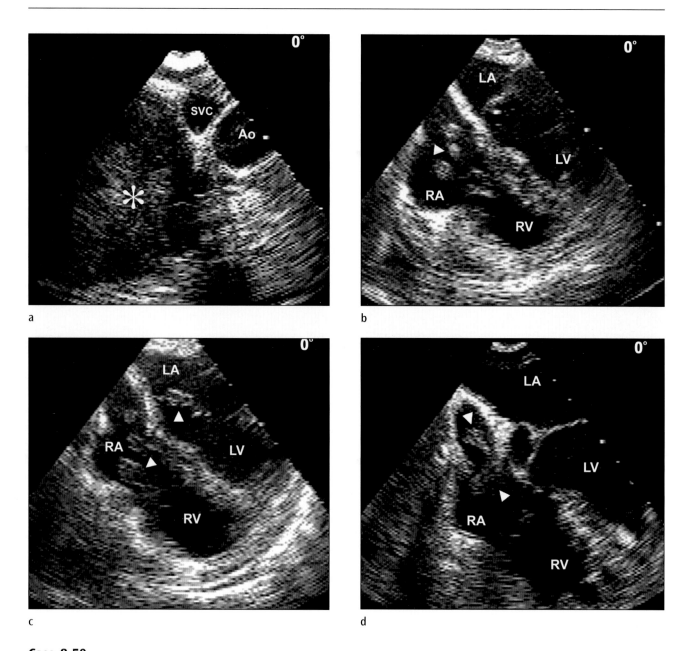

Case 8.50

Lung tumor and thrombus. Large lung carcinoma (star) with multiple small mobile masses (arrows) thought to be thrombi, identified in the right and left atrial cavities, in a patient with a hypercoaguable state (a–d).

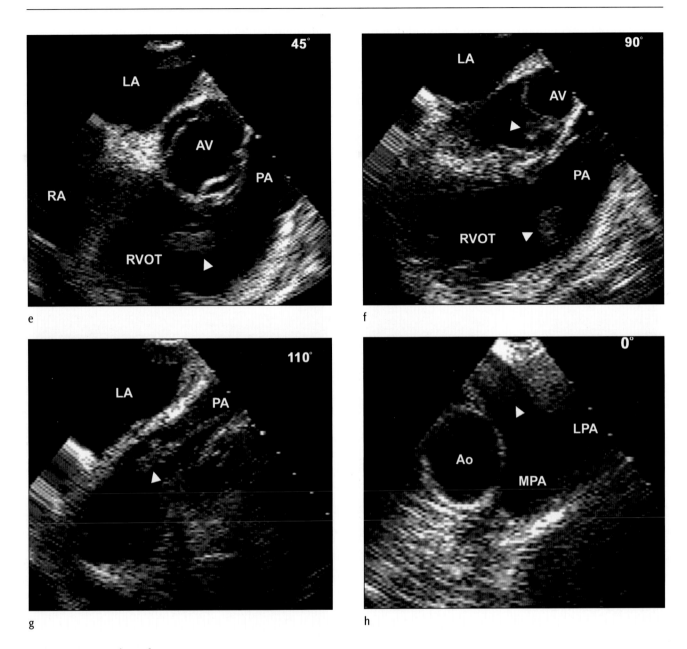

Case 8.50 *continued*
RA, right atrium; RV, right ventricle; LA, left atrium; LV, left ventricle; SVC, superior vena cava; Ao, aorta.

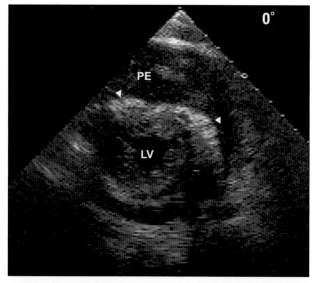

a

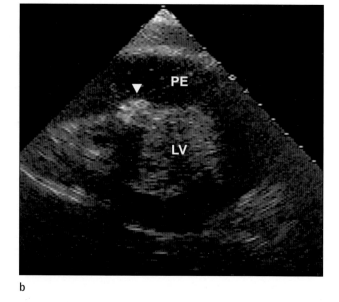

b

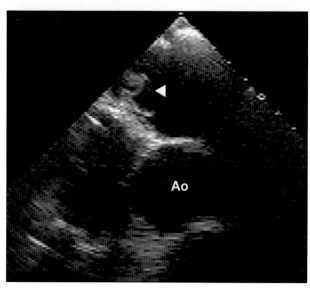

c

Case 8.51

Malignant pericardial effusion and pericardial metastasis.
Malignant pericardial effusion is usually produced with
lymphatic spread of a malignant tumor. Breast and lung
carcinomas are frequently associated with just an effusion,
however melanoma and leukemia commonly involve the
heart and pericardium. Pericardial metastasis is suggested by
the demonstration of discrete masses or nodules attached to
the visceral or parietal pericardium associated with thickening
of the pericardium and usually pericardial fluid. Multiplane
TEE was performed in a patient with symptoms of pericarditis
with a history of leukemia. A pericardial effusion was noted
in all views (a–f) with small nodular masses and areas of
pericardial thickening denoted as the echo dense areas of the
parietal pericardium (arrows) in a young patient with
leukemia.

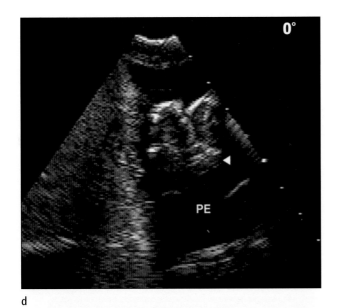

d

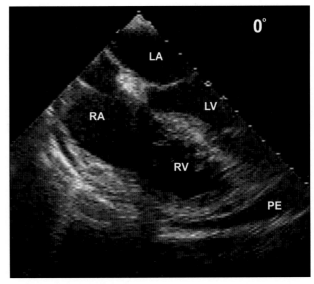

e

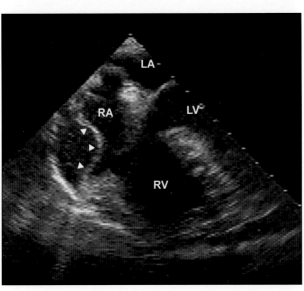

f

Case 8.51 *continued*
Although demonstrated by transthoracic echocardiography, the identification of metastatic nodules are better appreciated with TEE. PE, pericardial effusion; LV, left ventricle; Ao, aorta; RA, right atrium; LA, left atrium; RV, right ventricle; LV, left ventricle.

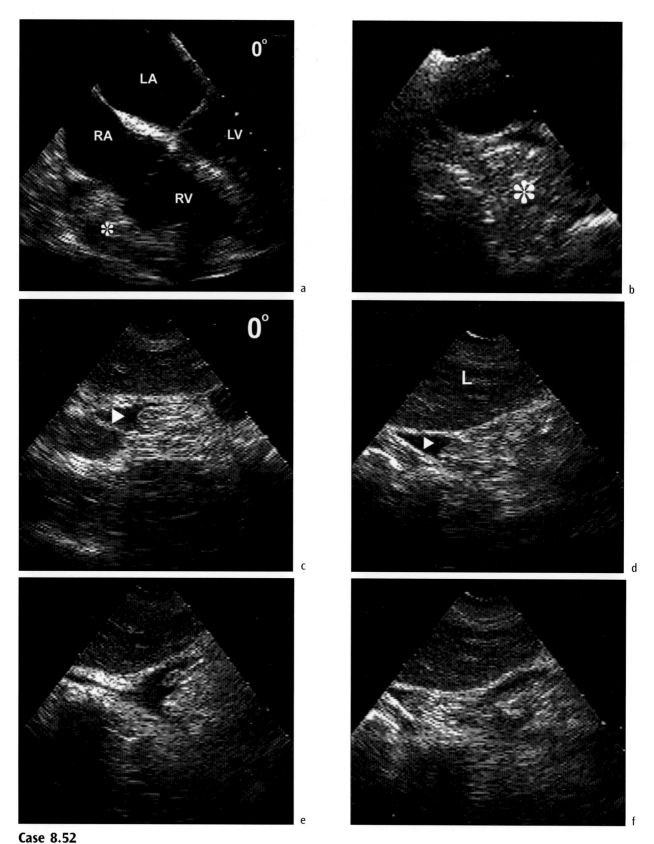

Case 8.52
Pericardial metastasis. Discrete masses noted attached to the pericardium in a patient with adenocarcinoma of the colon (a–f), thought to be cured. Pericardial metastatic lesions usually do not exhibit chaotic motion in comparison to pericardial debris or fibrous bands that occur with inflammatory disease of the pericardium. This patient also demonstrated multiple discrete smaller lesions (arrow) and a rather large pericardial mass (star) and a small pericardial effusion along the roof of the right atrium.
RA, right atrium; LA, left atrium; RV, right ventricle; LV, left ventricle; L, liver.

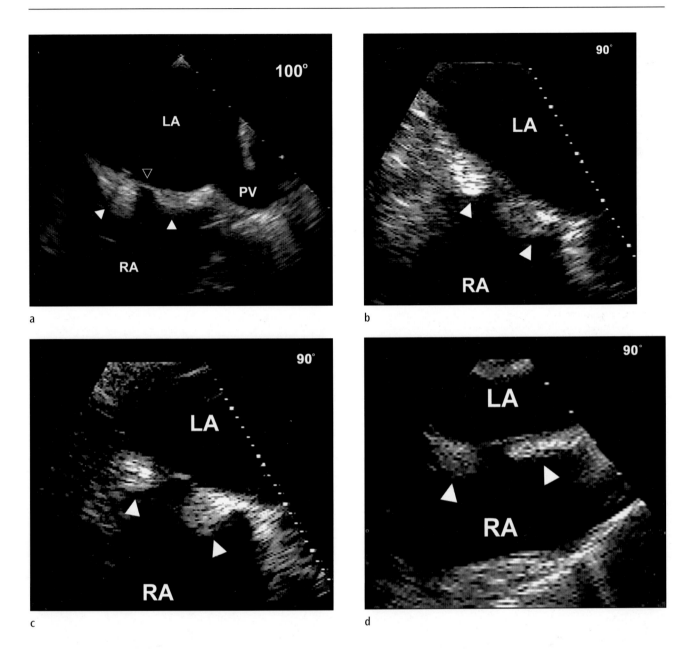

a

b

c

d

Case 8.53

Pseudotumors. Lipomatous hypertrophy of the atrial septum may appear as globular polyps, which may be confused with tumors especially with transthoracic echocardiography. The dumbbell appearance (a–d) produced by cephalad and caudal thickening (solid arrow) of the atrial septum bordering a spared foramen area (open arrow) suggest the diagnosis of lipomatous hypertrophy, which is often better appreciated with TEE. LA, left atrium; RA, right atrium; PV, pulmonary vein.

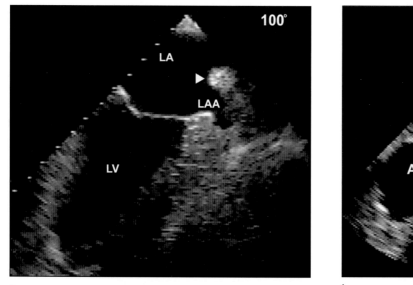

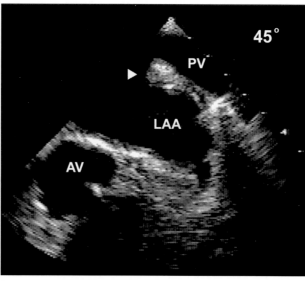

a

b

Case 8.54

Pseudotumors. "Q-tip sign". Prominent accumulations of tissue (arrow) may be created with ultrasound, especially in the region where the left pulmonary vein enters the left atrium near the superior margin of the left atrial appendage (a, b), and must not be confused with thrombus or tumor. LA, left atrium; LAA, left atrial appendage; LV, left ventricle; PV, pulmonary vein.

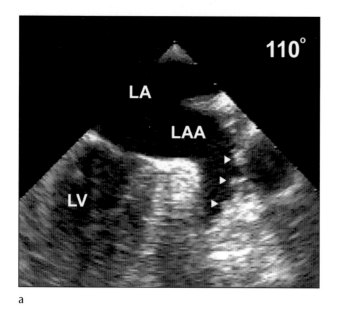

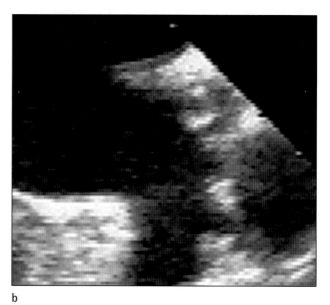

a

b

Case 8.55

Left atrial appendage pectinate muscle. Prominent pectinate muscles (a) often produce folds that protrude from the atrial wall that appear on two-dimensional imaging as small masses (arrows). Careful attention in zoom mode (b) helps to differentiate these from thrombi by denoting the echogenicity of the structure in comparison to the atrial wall and the lack of mobility of the mass. LA, left atrium; LAA, left atrial appendage; LV, left ventricle.

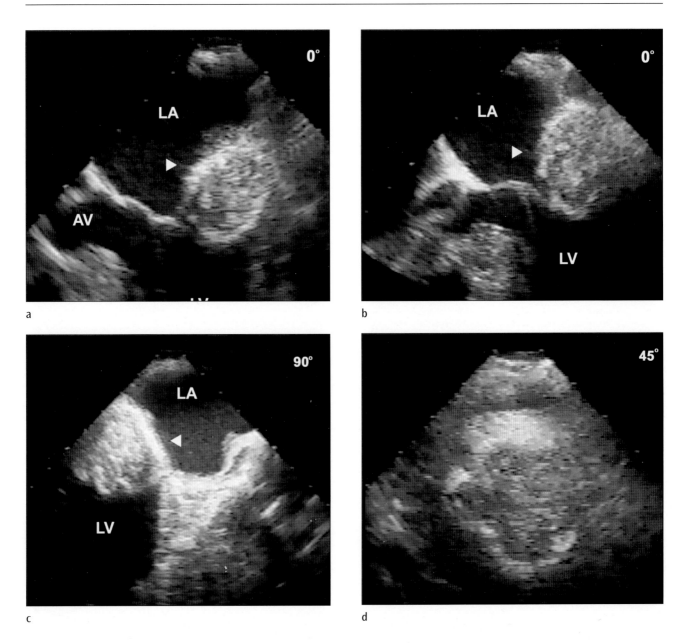

a

b

c

d

Case 8.56

Extensive mitral annular calcification. Multiplane TEE examination (a–d) was performed to investigate a possible left atrial mass (arrow) seen on a transthoracic study, in a patient with hyperparathyroidism. The mass is high reflective and shadowing is seen suggesting calcification in the region around the mitral annulus. LA, left atrium; LV, left ventricle; AV, aortic valve.

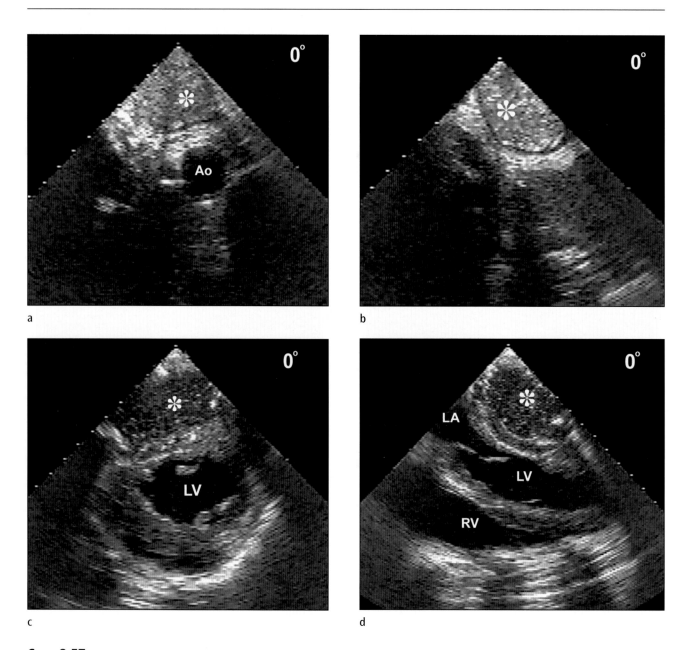

Case 8.57

Mediastinal abscess. A large mass (star) with a course hyper-refractile granular appearance is seen compressing the posterior cardiac structures in-between the heart and the esophagus. The patient underwent a pericardial stripping 10 years earlier for tuberculosis. The abscess encased the anterior portion of the heart and eroded through the anterior chest wall with a small fistulous tract. The abscess is demonstrated as a hyperechoic mass (a, b). The large abscess appears to be compressing the posterior borders of the right and left ventricle (c, d). With posterior rotation of the probe toward the left chest a pleural effusion is demonstrated with pleural debris noted (e, f). With further rotation of the probe a large cystic area of the mass (star) is noted, with clear margins and septae within the mass (g–j). LA, left atrium; LV, left ventricle; Ao, aorta; RV, right ventricle.

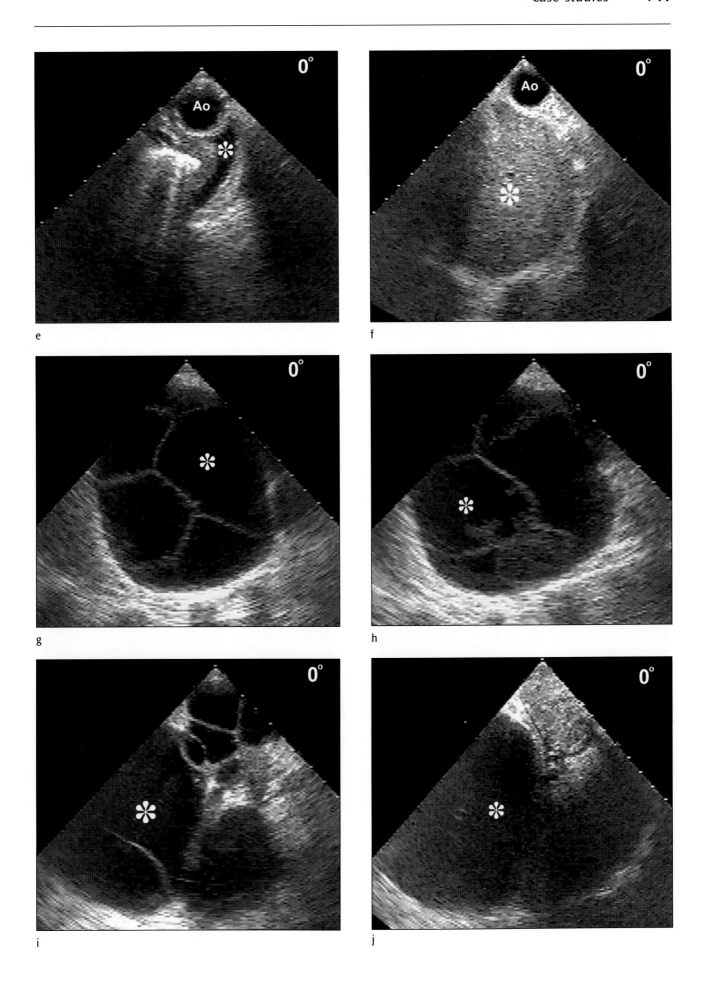

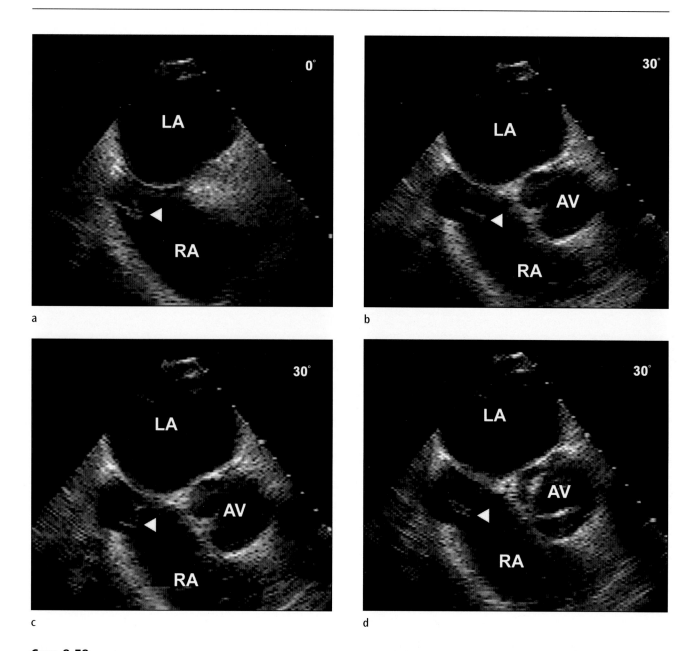

Case 8.58

Prominent Eustachian valve. A prominent, floppy Eustachian valve is frequently seen on echocardiographic studies and may be misinterpreted as a mass or thrombus especially with transthoracic echocardiography. On TEE they are identified by their position at the inferior vena cava and thin linear echo produced (arrow) that undulate during the cardiac cycle. LA, left atrium; RA, right atrium; AV, aortic valve.

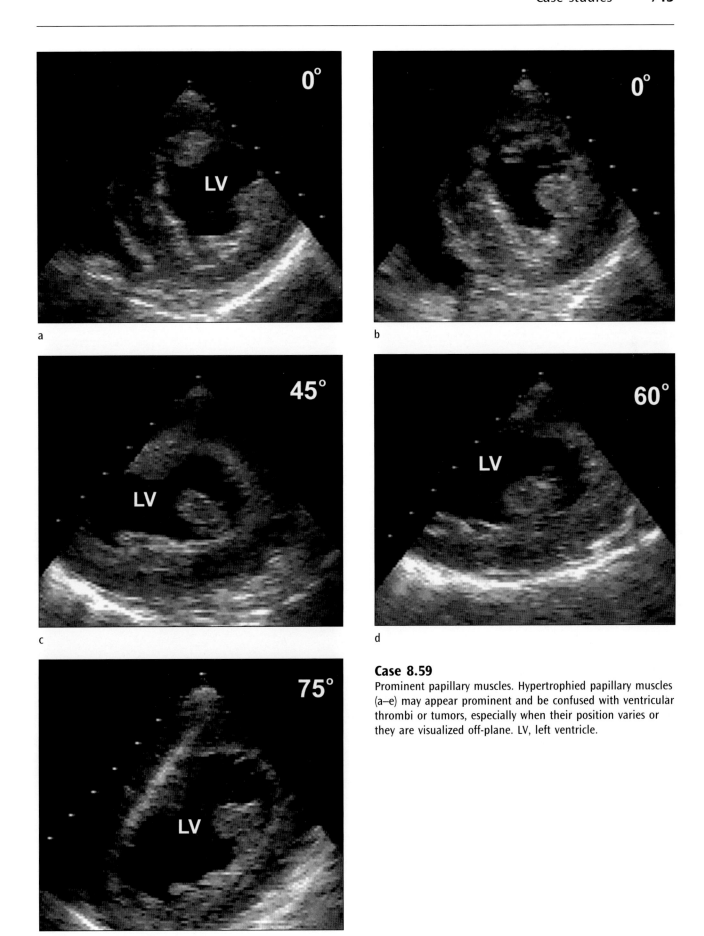

Case 8.59

Prominent papillary muscles. Hypertrophied papillary muscles (a–e) may appear prominent and be confused with ventricular thrombi or tumors, especially when their position varies or they are visualized off-plane. LV, left ventricle.

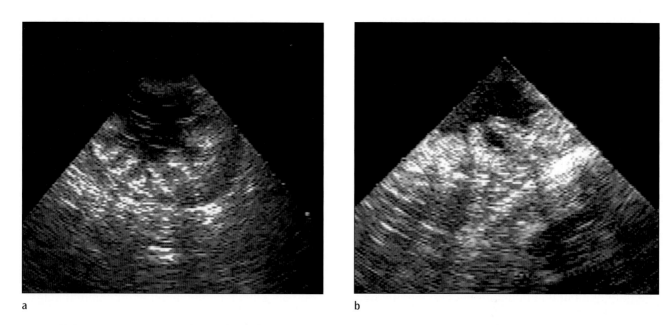

a   b

Case 8.60

Prominent gastric rugal folds. Hypertrophy of the gastric rugal folds (a, b) frequently appears in the proximal echocardiographic sector in between the transducer artifact and the posterior cardiac surface. The gastric rugal folds usually follow the contour of the stomach in a rather concave perimeter, delineating them from pericardial debris or mass.

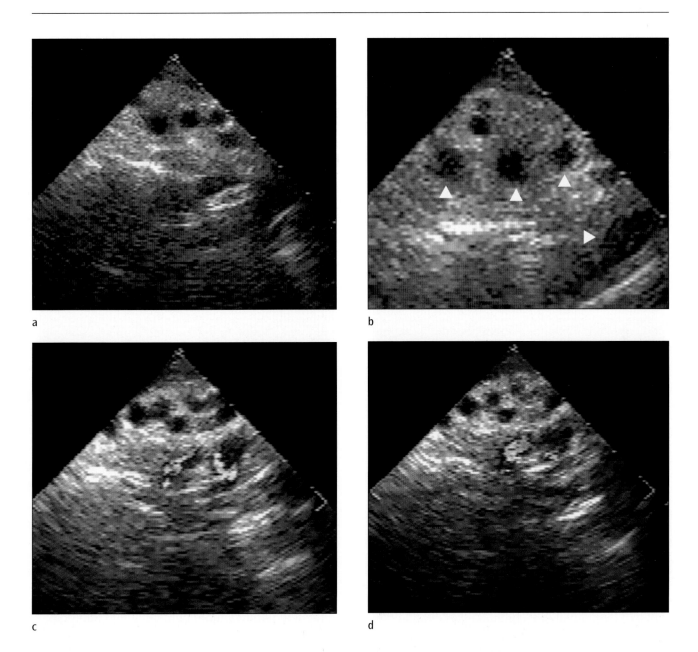

a

b

c

d

Case 8.61

Esophageal varicies. Occasionally in an unsuspected patient, esophageal varicies are demonstrated with TEE. Varicies (a–d) appears as small serpiginous vessels that are thrombosed with flow demonstrated with color flow Doppler. Esophageal varicies represent a contraindication to performing TEE, and when discovered require delicate maneuvering of the transducer and the decision to continue with the study should be weighed heavily.

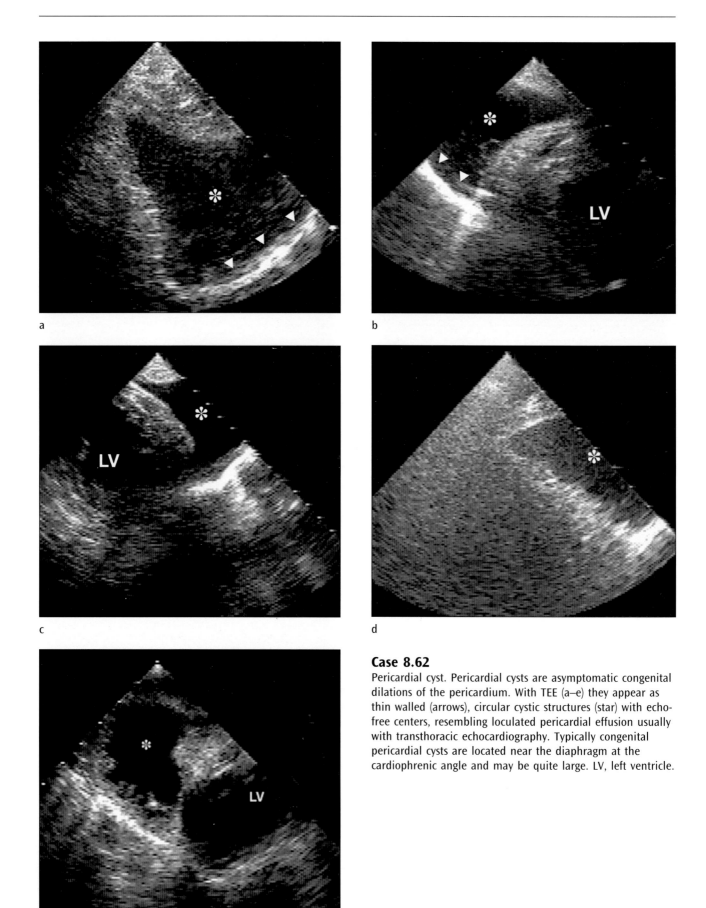

a

b

c

d

e

Case 8.62

Pericardial cyst. Pericardial cysts are asymptomatic congenital dilations of the pericardium. With TEE (a–e) they appear as thin walled (arrows), circular cystic structures (star) with echo-free centers, resembling loculated pericardial effusion usually with transthoracic echocardiography. Typically congenital pericardial cysts are located near the diaphragm at the cardiophrenic angle and may be quite large. LV, left ventricle.

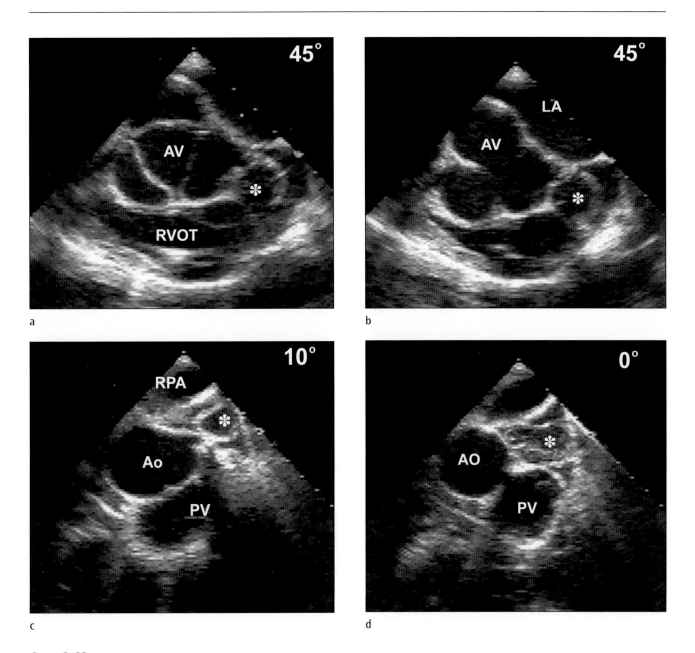

a

b

c

d

Case 8.63

Pericardial cyst. Small pericardial cysts (star) located in the region of the transverse sinus. Due to their echogenic feature the cysts may be difficult to visualize (a, b) which may be aided by multiplane TEE. The cystic walls are readily appreciated in the transverse sinus (c, d). AV, aortic valve; RVOT, right ventricular outflow tract; LA, left atrium; Ao, aorta; PV, pulmonary valve; RPA, right pulmonary artery.

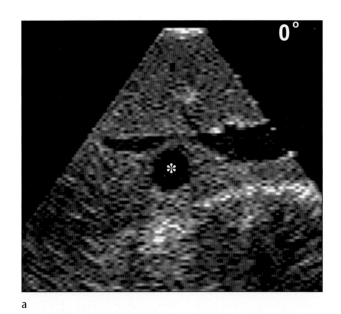

a

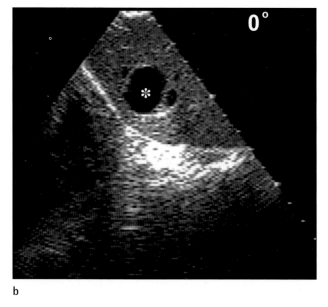

b

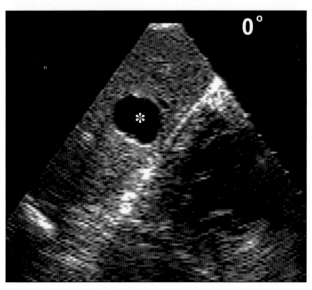

c

Case 8.64

Liver cyst. Small liver cysts (star) may be demonstrated with TEE, during routine visualization of the heart. They are occasionally visualized with congenital heart disease.

References

1. *Heart and Stroke Facts.* American Heart Association Statistical Supplement, Dallas Texas. (14) 1996.
2. Vaziri SM, Larson MG, Benjamin EJ, Levy D. Echocardiographic predictors of nonrheumatic atrial fibrillation: the Framingham Heart Study. *Circulation* 1994;89:724–30.
3. Brodsky MA, Allen BJ, Capparelli EJ, et al. Factors determining maintenance of sinus rhythm after chronic atrial fibrillation with left atrial dilatation. *Am J Cardiol* 1989;63:1065–8.
4. Morris JJ, Kong Y, North WC, McIntosh HD. Experience with cardioversion of atrial fibrillation and flutter. *Am J Cardiol* 1964;14:94–100.
5. Bjerkelund C, Orning OM. The efficacy of anticoagulant therapy in preventing embolism related to DC electrical conversion of atrial fibrillation. *Am J Cardiol* 1969;23:208–16.
6. Weinberg DM, Mancini GBJ. Anticoagulation for cardioversion of atrial fibrillation. *Am J Cardiol* 1989;63:745–6.
7. Arnold AZ, Mick MJ, Mazurek RP, Loop FD, Trohman RG. Role of prophylactic anticoagulation for direct cardioversion in patients with atrial fibrillation or atrial flutter. *J Am Coll Cardiol* 1992;19:851–5.
8. Roy D, Marchand E, Gagne P, Chabot M, Cartier R. Usefulness of anticoagulant therapy in the prevention of embolic complications of atrial fibrillation. *Am Heart J* 1986;112:1039–43.
9. Klein AL, Grimm RA, Black IW, et al, for the ACUTE Investigators. Cardioversion guided by transesophageal echocardiography: the ACUTE pilot study: a randomized, controlled trial. *Ann Intern Med* 1997;126:200–9.
10. Rokseth R, Storstein O. Quinidine therapy of chronic auricular fibrillation: the occurrence and mechanism of syncope. *Arch Intern Med* 1963;111:184–9.
11. Manning WJ, Silverman DI, Gordon SPF, Krumholz HM, Douglas PS. Cardioversion from atrial fibrillation without prolonged anticoagulation with the use of transesophageal echocardiography to exclude the presence of atrial thrombi. *N Engl J Med* 1993;328:750–5.
12. Shrestha NK, Moreno FL, Narciso FV, et al. Two-dimensional echocardiographic diagnosis of left atrial thrombus in rheumatic heart disease: a clinicopathologic study. *Circulation* 1983;67:341–7.
13. Schweizer P, Bardos P, Erbel R, et al. Detection of left atrial thrombi by echocardiography. *Br Heart J* 1981;45:148–56.
14. Masuda Y, Morooka M, Yoshida H, et al. Noninvasive diagnosis of thrombus in the heart and large vessels: usefulness of two-dimensional echocardiography and X-ray CT. *Jpn Circulation J* 1984;48:83–9.
15. Mugge A, Kuhn H, Daniel WG. The role of transesophageal echocardiography in the detection of left atrial thrombi. *Echocardiography* 1993;10:405–17.
16. Aschenberg W, Schluter M, Kremer P, et al. Transesophageal two-dimensional echocardiography for the detection of left atrial appendage thrombus. *J Am Coll Cardiol* 1986;7:163–6.
17. Fatkin D, Scalia G, Jacobs N, et al. Accuracy of biplane transesophageal echocardiography in detecting left atrial thrombus. *Am J Cardiol* 1996;77:321–3.
18. Mugge A, Daniel WG, Hausmann D, Godke J, Wagenbreth I, Lichtlen PR. Diagnosis of left atrial appendage thrombi by transesophageal echocardiography: clinical implications and follow-up. *Am J Card Imaging* 1990;4:173–9.
19. Hwang JJ, Chen JJ, Lin SC, et al. Diagnostic accuracy of transesophageal echocardiography for detecting left atrial thrombi in patients with rheumatic heart disease having undergone mitral valve operations. *Am J Cardiol* 1993;72:677–81.
20. Manning WJ, Weintraub RM, Waksmonsi CA, et al. Accuracy of transesophageal echocardiography for identifying left atrial thrombi: a prospective, intraoperative study. *Ann Intern Med* 1995;123:817–22.
21. Manning WJ, Leeman DE, Gotch PJ, Come PC. Pulsed Doppler evaluation of atrial mechanical function after electrical cardioversion of atrial fibrillation. *J Am Coll Cardiol* 1989;13:617–23.
22. Aronow WS, Ahn C, Kronzon I. Echocardiographic findings associated with atrial fibrillation in 1,699 patients ages > 60 years. *Am J Cardiol* 1995;76:1191–2.
23. Hoglund C, Rosenhamer G. Echocardiographic left atrial dimension as a predictor of maintaing sinus rhythm after conversion of atrial fibrillation. *Acta Med Scand* 1985;217:411–5.
24. Black IW, Fatkin D, Sagar KB, et al. Exlclusion of atrial thrombus by transesophageal echocardiography does not preclude embolism after cardioversion of atrial fibrillation: a multicenter study. *Circulation* 1994;89:2509–13.
25. Stoddard MF, Dawkins P, Prince CR, Longaker RA. Transesophageal echocardiography guidance of cardioversion in patients with atrial fibrillation. *Am Heart J* 1995;129:1204–15.
26. Olson JD, Goldenberg IF, Pedersen W, et al. Exclusion of atrial thrombus by transesophageal echocardiography. *J Am Soc Echocardiogr* 1992;5:52–6.
27. Silverman DI, Manning WJ. Role of echocardiography in patients undergoing elective cardioversion of atrial fibrillation. *Circulation* 1998;98:479–86.
28. Manning WJ, Silverman DI, Katz SE, et al. Impaired left atrial mechanical function after cardioversion: relationship to the duration of atrial fibrillation. *J Am Coll Cardiol* 1994;23:1535–40.
29. Corrado G, Tadeo G, Manzillo GF, Spata M, Tagllagambe LM, Santarone M. Atrial thrombus resolution due to anticoagulation: a transesophageal echocardiography study. Bologna, Italy: International Meeting on Atrial Fibrillation; 1997.
30. Collins LJ, Silverman DI, Douglas PS, Manning WJ. Cardioversion of non-rheumatic atrial fibrillation: reduced thromboembolic complications with 4 weeks of precardioversion anticoagulation are related to atrial thrombus resolution. *Circulation* 1995;92:160–3.
31. Mehta D, Ip JH, Mann N, et al. Incidence of atrial thrombi in patients with first presentation of atrial flutter undergoing electrical cardioversion: a prospective study. *Circulation* 1997;96(suppl I):I-453 (abstr.).
32. Weigner MJ, Caulfield TA, Canias PG, et al. Risk for clinical thromboembolism associated with conversion to sinus rhythm in patients with atrial fibrillation of less than 48 hours' duration. *Ann Intern Med* 1997;126:615–20.
33. Mitchell MA, Hughes GS, Ellenbogen KA, et al. Cardioversion-related stroke rates in atrial fibrillation and atrial flutter. *Circulation* 1997;96(suppl I):I-453 (abstr.).
34. Visser CA, Kan G, David GK, et al. Two-dimensional echocardiography in the diagnosis of left ventricular thrombus: a prospective study of 67 patients with anatomic validation. *Chest* 1983;83:228–32.
35. Stratton JR, Lighty GW, Pearlman AS, Ritchie JL. Detection of left ventricular thrombus by two-dimensional echocardiography: sensitivity, specificity and causes of uncertainty. *Circulation* 1982;66:156–66.
36. Parkinson J, Bedford DE. Cardiac infarction and coronary thrombosis. *Lancet* 1928;1:4–11.
37. Jordan RA, Miller RD, Edwards JE, Parker RL. Thromboembolism in acute and in healed myocardial infarction: intracardiac mural thrombosis. *Circulation* 1952;6:1–6.
38. Bean WB. Infarction of the heart: III. Clinical course and morphological findings. *Ann Intern Med* 1938;12:71–94.
39. Garvin CF. Mural thrombi in the heart. *Am Heart J* 1941;21:713–20.
40. Nixon JV. Left ventricular mural thrombus. *Arch Intern Med* 1983;143:1567–71.
41. Hellerstein HK, Martin JW. Incidence of thromboembolic lesions accompanying myocardial infarction. *Am Heart J* 1947;33:443–52.
42. Dubnow MH, Burchell HB, Titus JL. Postinfarction ventricular

aneurysm: clinicopathologic and electrocardiographic study of 80 cases. *Am Heart J* 1965;70:753–60.

43. Visser CA, Kan G, Meltzer RS, et al. Long-term follow-up of left ventricular thrombus after acute myocardial infarction: a two-dimensional echocardiographic study in 96 patients. *Chest* 1984;86:532–6.

44. Weinreich DJ, Burke JF, Pauletto FJ. Left ventricular mural thrombi complicating acute myocardial infarction. *Ann Intern Med* 1984;100:789–94.

45. Asinger RW, Mikell FL, Elsperger J, Hodges M. Incidence of left ventricular thrombosis after acute transmural myocardial infarction. *N Engl J Med* 1981;305:297–302.

46. Keating EC, Gross SA, Schlamowitz RA, et al. Mural thrombi in myocardial infarctions: prospective evaluation by two-dimensional echocardiography. *Am J Med* 1983;74:989–95.

47. Kinney EL. The significance of left ventricular thrombi in patients with coronary heart disease: a retrospective analysis of pooled data. *Am Heart J* 1985;109:191–4.

48. Haugland JM, Asinger RW, Mikell FL, et al. Embolic potential of left ventricular thrombi detected by two-dimensional echocardiography. *Circulation* 1984;70:588–98.

49. Visser CA, Kan G, Meltzer RS, et al. Embolic potential of left ventricular thrombus after myocardial infarction: a two-dimensional echocardiographic study of 119 patients. *J Am Coll Cardiol* 1985;5:1276–80.

50. Meltzer RS, Visser CA, Kan G, Roelandt J. Two-dimensional echocardiographic appearance of left ventricular thrombi with systemic emboli after myocardial infarction. *Am J Cardiol* 1984;53:1511–3.

51. Stratton JR, Resnick AD. Increased embolic risk in patients with left ventricular thrombi. *Circulation* 1987;75:1004–11.

52. Arvan S. Mural thrombi in coronary artery disease: recent advances in pathogenesis, diagnosis, and approaches to treatment. *Arch Intern Med* 1984;144:113–6.

53. Roberts WC, Seigel RJ, McManus BM. Idiopathic dilated cardiomyopathy: analysis of 152 necropsy patients. *Am J Cardiol* 1987;60:1340–55.

54. Fuster V, Gersh BJ, Giuliani ER, Tajik AJ, Bradenburg RO, Frye RL. The natural history of idiopathic dilated cardiomyopathy. *Am J Cardiol* 1981;47:525–31.

55. Al-Khadra AS, Salem DN, Rand WM, Udelson JE, Smith JJ, Konstam MA. Warfarin anticoagulation and survival: a cohort analysis from the studies of left ventricular dysfunction. *J Am Coll Cardiol* 1998;31:749–53.

56. Baker DW, Wright RF. Management of heart failure: IV anticoagulation for the patients with heart failure due to left ventricular systolic dysfunction. *JAMA* 1994;272:1614–8.

57. Koniaris LS, Goldhaber SZ. Anticoagulation in dilated cardiomyopathy. *J Am Cardiol* 1998;31:745–8.

58. Felner JM, Knopf WD. Echocardiographic recognition of intracadiac and extracardiac masses. *Echocardiography* 1985;2:3–55.

59. Roberts WE, Ferrans VJ. Pathologic anatomy of the cardiomyopathies: idiopathic dilated and hypertrophic types, infiltrative types and endomyocardial disease with and without eosinophilia. *Hum Pathol* 1975;6:287–342.

60. Felner JM, Churchwell AL, Murphy DA. Right atrial thromboemboli: clinical, echocardiographic, and pathophysiologic manifestations. *J Am Coll Cardiol* 1984;4:1041–5.

61. Come PC. Transient right atrial thrombus during acute myocardial infarction: diagnosis by echocardiography. *Am J Cardiol* 1983;51:1228–9.

62. Manno BV, Panidis IP, Kotler MN, et al. Two-dimensional echocardiographic detection of right atrial thrombi. *Am J Cardiol* 1983;51:615–6.

63. Stowers SA, Leiboff RH, Wasserman AG, et al. Right ventricular thrombus formation in association with acute myocardial infarc-

tion: diagnosis by 2–dimensional echocardiography. *Am J Cardiol* 1983;52:912–3.

64. Patel AK, Kroncke GM, Heltne CE, et al. Multiple calcified thrombi (rocks) in the right ventricle. *J Am Coll Cardiol* 1983;2:1224–7.

65. Riggs T, Paul MH, DeLeon S, Ilbawi M. Two-dimensional echocardiography in evaluation of right atrial masses: five cases in pediatric patients. *Am J Cardiol* 1981;48:961–6.

66. Kunze KP, Schluter M, Costard A, et al. Right atrial thrombus formation after transvenous catheter ablation of the atrioventricular node. *J Am Coll Cardiol* 1985;6:1428–30.

67. Schuster AH, Zugibe F Jr, Nanda NC, Murphy GW. Two-dimensional echocardiographic identification of pacing catheter-induced thrombosis. *PACE* 1982;5:124–8.

68. Wartmann WB, Hellerstein HK. The incidence of heart disease in 2000 consecutive autopsies. *Ann Intern Med* 1948;28:41–65.

69. Havig O. Deep vein thrombosis and pulmonary embolism. *Acta Chir Scand* 1977;478(suppl):1–120.

70. McAllister, HA, Fenoglio JJ. Tumors of the cardiovascular system. *Atlas of Tumor Pathology*. 2nd Series, Fascicle 15. Washington, D.C.: Armed Forces Institute of Pathology, 1978.

71. Burke A, Virmani R. Tumors of the heart and great vessels. *Atlas of Tumor Pathology*. 3rd Series, Fascicle 16. Washington, D.C.: Armed Forces Institute of Pathology, 1995.

72. Pricard RW, Tumours of the heart. *Arch Pathol* 1951;51:98–128.

73. Straus R, Merliss R. Primary tumors of the heart. *Arch Pathol* 1945;39:74–82.

74. Whorton CM. Primary malignant tumors of the heart. *Cancer* 1945;2:245–60.

75. Molina JE, Edwards JE, Ward HB. Primary cardiac tumors: experience at the University of Minnesota. *Thorac Cardiovasc Surg* 1990;38:183–91.

76. Hall JR, Cooley DA. Neoplastic disease of the heart. In: *The Heart*. (Hurst, W. ed). New York: McGraw-Hill, 1986.

77. Fyke FE, Seward JB, Edwards WD, et al. Primary cardiac tumors: experience with 30 consecutive patients since the introduction of two-dimensional echocardiography. *J Am Coll Cardiol* 1985;5:1465–73.

78. Salcedo EE, Adams KV, Lever HM, et al. Echocardiographic findings in 25 patients with left atrial myxoma. *J Am Coll Cardiol* 1983;I:1162–6.

79. Dashkoff N, Boersma REB, Nanda NC, et al. Bilateral atrial myxomas: echocardiographic considerations. *Am J Med* 1978;65:361–6.

80. Turlapati RV, Jacobs LE, Kotler MN. Right atrial myxoma casing total destruction of the tricuspid valve leaflets. *Am Heart J* 1990;120:1227–31.

81. Burakovsky VI, Zuckerman GI, Kossatch GA, et al. Surgical treatment of cardiac myxomas. *J Thorac Cardiovasc Surg* 1988;96:800–5.

82. Silverman NA. Primary cardiac tumors. *Ann Surg* 1980;191:127–38.

83. Fine G. Neoplasms of the pericardium and heart. In: Gould SE. (ed). *Pathology of the Heart and Blood Vessels*. Springfield, IL: Charles C Thomas, 1968:851.

84. Fyke FE, Tajik AJ, Edwards WD, Seward JB. Diagnosis of lipomatous hypertrophy of the atrial septum by two-dimensional echocardiography. *J Am Coll Cardiol* 1983;1:1352–7.

85. Pochis WT, Saeian K, Sagar KB. Usefulness of transesophageal echocardiography in diagnosing lipomatous hypertrophy of the atrial septum with comparison to transthoracic echocardiography. *Am J Cardiol* 1992;70:396–8.

86. LiMandri G, Homma S, DiTullio MR, et al. Detection of multiple papillary fibroelastomas of the tricuspid valve by transesophageal echocardiography. *J Am Soc Echocardiogr* 1994;7:315–7.

87. Lee KS, Topol EJ, Steward WJ. Atypical presentation of papillary fibroelastoma mimicking multiple vegetations in suspected subacute bacterial endocarditis. *Am Heart J* 1993;125:1443–5.

88. Richard J, Castello R, Dressler FA, et al. Diagnosis of papillary fibroelastoma of the mitral valve complicated by non Q-wave infaction with apical thrombus: transesophageal and transthoracic echocardiographic study. *Am Heart J* 1993;126:710–2.

89. Calderon M, Talledo O, Ott DA, et al. Left ventricular papillary fibroelastoma: an unusual cause of cerebral emboli. *Tex Heart Inst J* 1991;18:219–22.

90. Neerukonda SK, Jantz RD, Vijay NK, et al. Pulmonary embolization of papillary fibroelastoma arising from the tricuspid valve. *Tex Heart Inst J* 1991;18:132–5.

91. Hurle JM, Garcia-Martinez V, Sanchez-Quintana D. Morphologic characteristics and structure of surface excrescences (Lambl's Excrescences) in the normal aortic valve. *Am J Cardiol* 1986;58:1223–7.

92. Magarey FR. On the mode of formation of Lambl's excrescences and their relation to chronic thickening of the mitral valve. *J Pathol Bacteriol* 1949;61:203–8.

93. Roldan CA, Shively BK, Crawford MH. Valve excrescences: prevalence, evolution and risk for cardioembolism. *J Am Coll Cardiol* 1997;30:1308–14.

94. Armstrong WF. Valve excrescences: harmless and common or strokes-in-waiting?. *J Am Coll Cardiol* 1997;30:1315–6.

95. Cooley DA. Surgical treatment of cardiac neoplasms: 32-year experience. *Thorac Cardiovasc Surg* 1990;38:176–82.

96. Critchley M, Earl CJC. Tuberous sclerosis and allied conditions. *Brain* 1932;55:311.

97. Shaher RM, Mintzer J, Farina M, et al. Clinical presentation of rhabdomyoma of the heart in infancy and childhood. *Am J Cardiol* 1972;30:95.

98. Loffler H, Grille W. Classification of malignant cardiac tumors with respect to oncological treatment. *Thorac Cardiovasc Surg* 1990;38:173–5.

99. Ohtsuki Y, Kobayashi S, Hahashi T, Ohmori M. Angiosarcoma of the heart. Report of a case and review of the literature. *Acta Pathol Jpn* 1973;23:407.

100. Hollingsworth JH, Sturgill BC, Treatment of primary angiosarcomas of the heart. *Am Heart J* 1969;78:254.

101. DeLoach JF, Haynes JW. Secondary tumors of the heart and pericardium: review of the subject and report of 137 cases. *Arch Intern Med* 1953;91:224–49.

102. Goudie R. Secondary tumours of the heart and pericardium. *Br Heart J* 1955;17:183–8.

103. Abraham K, Reddy V, Gattuso P. Neoplasms metastatic to the heart: review of 3314 consecutive autopsies. *Am J Cardiovasc Path* 1990;3:195–8.

104. Glancy DL, Roberts WC. The heart in malignant melanoma: a study of 70 autopsy cases. *Am J Cardiol* 1968;21:555–71.

105. Applefeld MM, Pollock SH. Cardiac disease in patients who have malignancies. *Curr Probl Cardiol* 1980;4:1–37.

106. Heath D. Pathology of cardiac tumor. *Am J Cardiol* 1968;21:315–27.

107. Prichard RW. Tumors of the heart: review of the subject and report of one hundred and fifty cases. *Arch Pathol* 1951;51:98–128.

108. Lestuzzi C, Nicolosi GL, Mimo R, et al. Usefulness of transesophageal echocardiography in evaluation of paracardiac neoplastic masses. *Am J Cardiol* 1992;70:247–51.

109. Schiavone WA, Rice TW. Pericardial disease: current diagnosis and management methods. *Cleve Clin J Med* 1989;56:639–45.

110. Smalling RG, Alboronoz M, Tak T, et al. Role of transesophageal echocardiography in evaluating pericardial disease. *Circulation* 1992;86(suppl 4):I-726.

111. Chandraratna PAN, Aronow WS. Detection of pericardial metastases by cross-sectional echocardiography. *Circulation* 1981;63:197–9.

112. Kotler MN. Metastatic cardiac tumours: recognition of pericardial, myocardial, and endocardial involvement by two-dimensional echocardiography. In: Kapoor, AS (ed). *Cancer and the Heart.* New York: Springer, 1986:51–61.

113. Perry MC. Cardiac metastasis. In: Kapoor, AS (ed). *Cancer and the Heart.* New York: Springer, 1986:76–81.

9

Adult congenital heart disease

Congenital heart disease describes abnormalities of the heart and great vessels that are present from birth. With advancements in medical and surgical management of congenital heart defects, survival has been extended into adulthood. Presentation of congenital anomalies in adolescent and young adults differs from the typical presentation in the pediatric population.[1–3] Defects diagnosed in adulthood generally are less severe defects. These considerations have necessitated the division of congenital heart disease into pediatric and adult subspecialties.[4] This chapter describes the common lesions encountered in adults with transesophageal echocardiography.

In the pediatric population, transthoracic echocardiography is usually all that is required for definitive diagnosis.[5] The excellent image quality obtained with transthoracic echocardiographic imaging has virtually relegated cardiac catheterization to the role of therapeutics.[6–8] In older patients, especially with chest deformities or small stature, transthoracic imaging may be technically difficult,[9,10] and may not provide the image resolution or necessary views suitable to make the correct diagnosis of complex congenital anomalies.[11] Transesophageal echocardiography, with higher frequency transducers, provides the required resolution for displaying the detailed cardiac anatomy in congenital defects.[12–17] Transesophageal echocardiography is also useful in patients who have had palliative or corrective surgery for congenital heart lesions.[18] The role of transesophageal echocardiography for congenital heart disease is expanding in conjunction with interventional procedures performed in the cardiac catheterization laboratory for the correction of congenital lesions.

The major limitation of transesophageal echocardiography in the congenital heart disease population is the size of the probes.[10,16,19] Although smaller pediatric probes have been introduced and are currently available, they may not always be available in every laboratory. Currently, in the authors' experience, adult multiplane transesophageal echocardiography probes can usually be safely utilized in the average 15-year-old patient. The major consideration is whether the patient's oro-pharynx is large enough to accommodate the size and shape of the transducer in allowing the scope to pass beyond the soft palate. The shape and size of the transesophageal echocardiography probe from individual manufacturers may be of importance.

In some younger adults with congenital heart disease with mental retardation, consideration should be given as to whether the patient is capable of having the procedure performed with topical anesthesia and conscious intravenous sedation. In general these patients require added vigilance and support in preparation for the procedure. The experience of the operator and the sonographer are also extremely important, in order to avoid a prolonged examination and a traumatic experience for the young patient. Transthoracic echocardiographic examination should always be performed before the transesophageal echocardiographic examination in these patients, to obtain as much information as possible which may dramatically shorten the time required for the transesophageal examination. Even when the transthoracic echocardiography images are not diagnostic, the Doppler data obtained often enables calculation of the hemodynamics necessary for diagnosis.

As the heart grows and enlarges, defects may not appear the same as at a younger age. The echocardiographer must not only know all of the findings present in specific congenital heart lesions, but also be proficient in recognizing the various surgical corrections that may have been performed, which influence the appearance of original lesions. It is also extremely important to have knowledge of the associated congenital anomalies that occurs with each specific defect, allowing for a more complete examination.

Echocardiographic examination in congenital disease

To perform an echocardiographic examination in a patient with a suspected congenital heart defect, a detailed systematic and segmental approach is required, to obtain all the diagnostic information.[20] Most adult patients with complex congenital malformations will have been diagnosed in childhood and many will have had surgical correction, therefore it is important to obtain a detailed history prior to performing the transesophageal echocardiogram, in order to simplify and shorten the examination. Whether or not surgical modification of the cardiac anatomy has been performed, the echocardiogram should be approached in the same systematic manner as when first diagnosing the malformation. The study should demonstrate all four cardiac valves and all four cardiac chambers, when present. Specifically, it is important to establish atrial situs and morphology, venous inflow (systemic and pulmonary) connections, ventricular morphology and position, and ventriculo-arterial relationships. It is important to recognize that multiple defects may occur concurrently.

When performing a transesophageal echocardiogram it is essential to perform the study systematically, especially following surgical corrective procedures when anatomy may have been distorted. In the author's experience, most errors in diagnosis of adult congenital lesions result from incomplete or inadequate examinations performed in an unsystematic manner. The deep transgastric view, which is frequently overlooked, provides the best position for visualizing all four cardiac chambers and great vessels from a single window with minimal probe manipulation. The deep transgastric view is an optimal view to begin with, to establish a 'road map' of the circulation. The specific anatomic morphology of the cardiac chambers may not be ideally visualized due to the decreased resolution provided in this view, however each cardiac structure may be positively identified connected to either the pulmonary or systemic circuit. Starting with the deep transgastric probe position, the systemic inflow to the heart is identified. The direction of blood flow may be followed sequentially with the aid of color flow Doppler

or peripheral venous agitated saline contrast injections traversing each cardiac structure, defining the pulmonary circuit with corresponding atrium, ventricle and great artery.[21–25] Subsequently the position of the systemic atrium, ventricle and great vessel are deduced or directly visualized with echocardiographic contrast agents if difficulties arise in defining the pulmonary circuit. Abnormal communications between the cardiac chambers are usually easily demonstrated with the use of agitated saline or echo contrast agents. The size of each cardiac chamber may be assessed in relation to the other chambers. Mapping the pulmonary and systemic flow circuits, the position of each cardiac chamber is noted which allows morphological identification of each cardiac structure.

Determining atrial situs as defined by abdominal viscera (right-sided liver and left-sided stomach) is not always as facile with the transesophageal approach as it is with transthoracic echocardiography,[26,27] but is also probably best addressed in the deep transgastric views. Frequently the liver appears both on the left and the right with transesophageal echocardiography, so it is important to confirm visceral situs with transthoracic echocardiography or chest X-ray. With minor manipulations of the probe, the position of the descending aorta and inferior vena cava may be identified, with the inferior vena cava to the right of the spine with the descending aorta to the left of the spine. This anatomical relationship of the inferior vena cava and aorta defines situs solitus. When visualizing the liver from the deep transgastric position minor rotation of the probe to the right usually demonstrates the connection of the inferior vena cava to the right atrium, especially when a Eustachian valve remnant is identified. In the deep transgastric position minor rotation to the left identifies the connection of the superior vena cava. The left atrium is displayed to the left and posterior to the right atrium. It is important to determine echocardiographically that the chamber identified as the left atrium does not communicate with the inferior vena cava. Usually all four pulmonary veins can be demonstrated with transesophageal echocardiography and color flow Doppler, in short axis, in close proximity to and/or connecting to the left atrium as discussed in Chapter 6.

Atrial morphology is usually, easily determined with transesophageal echocardiography from the mid to upper esophagus between 0° and 120°. The right atrium is identified by the Eustachian valve originating from the inferior portion of the inferior vena cava and by the right atrial appendage with its short broad base originating near the orifice of the superior vena cava separated by a prominent atrial fold which identifies the crista terminalis. The left atrium is more globular with a long and narrow atrial appendage. Identification of the atrial appendage, enables atrial isomerism to be determined.[28] Rarely, the left appendage may be connected to the right atrium and the right appendage to the left atrium. Even rarer, both atria may possess appendages with identical right or left appendage morphologies.

Ventricular morphology can be defined by transesophageal echocardiography from multiple views. The right ventricle is identified by its trabeculated endocardial surface and triangular cavity shape and the more apical insertion of the tricuspid valve. Other characteristics of the right ventricle include chordal insertion into the ventricular septum, the infundibulum and the moderator band located near the apex of the ventricle. The left ventricle is identified by its smooth endocardial surface, circular configuration in the short-axis views, two papillary muscles and the ellipsoidal geometry in the long-axis views. The mitral valve insertion is more basal than the insertion of the tricuspid valve. The tricuspid valve is always part of the right ventricle and the mitral valve always identifies the left ventricle. In the four-chamber views, the basal–apical axis may be defined when the left ventricular apex is directed to the left as levocardia; and when the left ventricular apex is to the right as dextrocardia. The left ventricular apex directed towards the midline identifies mesocardia.

After defining ventricular morphology, the great ventriculo-arterial connections must be established. The identity of the great arteries is best performed at the basal heart levels from the mid and upper esophagus. In the normal heart the great arteries and corresponding semilunar valves do not lie in the same echocardiographic planes. Their anatomical position and identity may be established from the deep transgastric views, which demonstrates the normal spiral relationship of the great vessels. The pulmonary artery is identified by its primary bifurcation into the right and left pulmonary arteries. The aorta runs parallel to the sternum and appears longer than the pulmonary artery which courses obliquely before bifurcating. The aorta is identified by the origin of the brachiocephalic vessels. The semilunar valves correspond with their respective great arteries. The coronaries can be visualized in numerous planes with multiplane transesophageal echocardiography, with their origin best demonstrated in the basal short-axis views imaged from the upper esophagus.[29–31] In the normal heart, the pulmonary valve is the semilunar valve that is most leftward in position within the fibrous skeleton, with the aortic valve rightwards of the pulmonary valve.

Once identification of the morphology of each cardiac chamber has been achieved, atrioventricular and ventriculoarterial corrections can be determined. Atrioventricular concordance is defined when the right atrium is connected to the tricuspid valve and right ventricle and the left atrium is connected to the left ventricle and mitral valve. Ventriculoarterial concordance describes the connections between the right ventricle and pulmonary artery and the left ventricle and aorta. When the normal connections between cardiac structures do not occur at either the atrioventricular or ventriculoarterial positions they are described as discordant.

After determining the anatomical components of the pulmonary and systemic circulations, the individual lesions can be addressed in the optimal transesophageal views. For a detailed discussion of congenital valvular anomalies such as bicuspid aortic valve, subaortic stenosis, aneurysm of the sinus of Valsalva, congenital anomalies of the mitral valve, pulmonary valvular stenosis, the reader is referred to the respective chapters addressing these pathologies.

Atrial septal defect

Atrial septal defect comprises 5–10% of all congenital heart lesions, and is the most common defect in adults, after bicuspid aortic valve.[32–35] Spontaneous closure of atrial septal defects occurs in 40% of cases usually within the first year of life. Rarely, delayed closure of an atrial septal defect occurs by age 5, with most of the remaining defects decreasing in size, even if they do not close.[32] Atrial septal defects often remain asymptomatic until the fourth or fifth decade of life. Atrial septal defects are the most common congenital lesion identified by echocardiography in adults.[34] Atrial septal defect should be excluded by echocardiography in all patients over the age of 40, with mild-to-moderate pulmonary hypertension without an obvious etiology.

Atrial septal defect results from a defect in embryological development which provides free communication of blood between the left and right atrium as part of the normal fetal–placental circulation. Atrial septal defects are classified according to their anatomical location in the atrial septum with respect to the fossa ovalis. There are four types of atrial septal defects, ostium primum type, ostium secundum type, sinus venosus (superior and inferior types) and the rare unroofed coronary sinus atrial septal defect. All of these atrial septal defects may be encountered in the adult. In addition to true atrial septal defects, a patent foramen ovale may also be responsible for atrial shunting, and can be easily distinguished from true atrial septal defects with transthoracic as well as transesophageal echocardiography.

The physiological consequence of atrial septal defect shunting is the same irrespective of the location of the defect. The direction and magnitude of atrial shunting is determined by the size of the defect, the relative diastolic compliances of the right and left ventricles and the difference in vascular resistance between the pulmonary and systemic circulations. Patients with small atrial septal defects have normal hemodynamics and small left-to-right shunt flows ($Q_P:Q_S < 1.5$) and are usually free of symptoms. Larger atrial septal defects remain asymptomatic as long as the right ventricle remains compliant and there is no significant elevation in pulmonary vascular resistance. Persistent atrial septal shunt flow produces progressive right atrial, right ventricular and pulmonary artery dilatation and the increased pulmonary blood flow results in changes in pulmonary arteriolar walls resulting in increased pulmonary artery pressure. In the later stages, right ventricular compliance falls and right ventricular failure may ensue, resulting in the reversal of shunting in a right-to-left direction producing cyanosis. In addition to the physiological consequences that are produced by the atrial septal defect in the adult, the usual cardiac changes attributable to aging occur concurrently and account for the differences in presentation in individual patients, such as development of diastolic dysfunction, coronary artery disease and degenerative pathologies. Obstructive pulmonary vascular disease rarely occurs as a result of an atrial septal defect, even in the presence of large defects.

In contrast to children, atrial septal defects in adults may not be directly visualized with transthoracic echocardiography, depending on their location; however, they are usually suspected as a result of the consequences of the defect.[36–38] In the adult, transesophageal echocardiography readily identifies atrial septal defects if they are not visualized with the transthoracic examination, especially if the defect is of the sinus venosus or coronary sinus type. The major role of transesophageal echocardiography in the diagnosis of atrial septal defects is in defining the associated abnormalities including recognition of abnormal pulmonary venous drainage.[38]

Conventional and color flow Doppler may be utilized to demonstrate atrial shunt flow with transesophageal echocardiography similar to transthoracic echocardiography.[39–44] Atrial shunt flow begins in mid-systole, peaking in early diastole, before slowly decreasing to mid-diastole. The flow velocity increases again with atrial systole and ends in early systole often with minor flow reversal. Qualitative assessment of the magnitude of the atrial shunt is easily assessed with color flow Doppler and transesophageal echocardiography, by measuring the shunt jet diameter and the spatial area of the color flow jet.[41–44] Appropriate color Doppler gain settings are important to display the low velocity flows that characterize atrial septal defects and differentiate the shunt flow from the other flows to the right atrium. The width of the color Doppler shunt flow jet correlates with the size of the defect, with diameters greater than 15 mm corresponding to significant shunts with Q_P:Q_S flow ratios greater than 2:1.[43,44] In uncomplicated atrial septal defects, the pulmonary arterial systolic pressure can be calculated utilizing the modified Bernoulli equation and the systolic gradient of the right ventricular/right atrial gradient obtained with continuous wave Doppler of the tricuspid regurgitant jet.[45] The Q_P:Q_S ratio can be calculated by estimating the flow volume across the tricuspid inflow or pulmonary outflow (Q_P) and comparing these to the flow volume across the mitral inflow or aortic outflow tracts (Q_S).[42,46] The volume of flow is calculated as the product of the time velocity integral and the corresponding cross-sectional area of the inflow or outflow tract, respectively.

Ostium secundum atrial defects comprise the vast majority (70–80%) of atrial septal defects, resulting from deficient tissue in the septum in the central region of the atrial septum, the fossa ovalis.[1–3] Small secundum defects may be confused with a patent foramen ovale, especially by transthoracic echocardiograph. Ostium secundum atrial defects may occur as a single defect or multiple small defects in the septal tissue. Larger ostium secundum defects may extend directly posterior in the atrial septum to the posterior atrial wall, or may extend in a posterior–inferior direction to border the orifice of the inferior vena cava. Anomalous pulmonary venous return is associated with ostium secundum atrial defects in approximately 10% of cases. The most frequent anomaly is the right upper pulmonary vein draining into the superior vena cava or directly into the body of the right atrium.[1–3]

Ostium secundum atrial septal defects have also been associated with mitral valve prolapse in 10–20% of cases. In many cases, the mitral valve prolapse may be classified as pseudo-prolapse, since it frequently disappears following surgical correction of the atrial septal defect.[47]

Small ostium secundum atrial septal defects must be distinguished from a patent foramen ovale that occurs in the central portion of the secundum septum in approximately 25% of all adults.[48–50] Atrial septal aneurysms are frequently associated with a patent foramen ovale. The foramen ovale plays an important role during fetal development, allowing oxygenated placental blood flow to be directed from the inferior vena cava across the atrial septum in order to bypass the lungs, and proceeds to the fetal systemic circulation predominantly to the brachiocephalic vessels to facilitate growth of the head. The atrial septum is formed during embryological development from central union of the growing tissue from the left-sided septum primum and the right-sided septum secundum. The foramen ovale is formed from the union of the superior portion of the septum primum and the inferior portion of the septum secundum tissue, overlapping to produce a unidirectional tunnel, in a right to left direction, through the atrial septum. After birth, the foramen ovale tissue fuses, effectively forming a permanent seal in the atrial septum.

In cases where fusion is ineffective, a provocable communication is produced between the two atria. In certain physiological maneuvers (e.g. cough, Valsalva), when the right atrial pressure exceeds left atrial pressure, the tissue of the foramen ovale may separate to allow a right to left communication, and has been implicated in causation of cryptogenic stroke in young adults.[51–57] The propensity for separation of the foramen ovale may be enhanced, by discordant atrial enlargement, particularly of the left atrium, which produces inferior displacement (stretching) of the superior border of the primum septum. Patent foramen ovale defects can be easily differentiated from small atrial secundum defects with transesophageal echocardiography by the demonstration of persistent atrial shunt flow with color flow Doppler with true defects.[58] Although injection of agitated saline echocardiographic contrast is usually not necessary for the detection of true atrial septal defects, it may be utilized to detect a patent foramen ovale by demonstrating small bubbles crossing the atrial septum and entering the left atrium, as the patients performs a Valsalva maneuver, when color flow Doppler is inconclusive.

An atrial septal aneurysm is produced by redundancy of septal tissue and is demonstrated by excessive motion of the primum septal tissue. Echocardiographically, an atrial septal aneurysm is defined by excessive motion of the atrial septal tissue, producing protrusion of the septum towards the right or left atrium of at least 10 mm during the cardiac cycle.[59] Atrial septum aneurysms are frequently associated with a patent foramen ovale.[60] Transesophageal echocardiography is extremely helpful in delineating atrial septal defects from patent foramen ovale and from atrial septal aneurysm by directly visualizing the defect present in the atrial septum and the typical atrial septal shunt flow pattern with Doppler echocardiography.

Ostium primum atrial septal defects occur in 20–25% of cases and lie inferior to the fossa ovalis towards the crux of the heart.[1–3] Ostium primum atrial septal defects usually present as part of an atrioventricular canal defect, so that they are usually diagnosed in childhood.[5] Isolated primum atrial septal defects therefore rarely present in adulthood. The most common feature of ostium primum atrial septal defects is the demonstration of both atrioventricular valves lying in the same anatomical plane within the fibrous skeleton, which is usually readily detectable by transthoracic echocardiography.[61] Defects in the primum atrial septum commonly extend into atrioventricular valvular tissue, which produce clefts in the leaflet tissue. Atrioventricular clefts may not be visualized by transthoracic echocardiography, but are suggested by the association of significant central atrioventricular regurgitation. Although mitral valve clefts are more common, clefts in either valve may produce significant valvular regurgitation in addition to the shunt flow. Direct visualization of atrioventricular valvular clefts is readily accomplished with transesophageal echocardiography.

Sinus venosus atrial septal defects are produced by the non-union of the atrial septal components during embryological development, resulting in the overriding of the superior or inferior vena cava to the free interatrial septal margin.[62] Sinus venosus atrial septal defects are frequently associated with anomalous pulmonary venous return as a result of the location of the defect. Although transthoracic echocardiography is good for diagnosing secundum and primum atrial septal defects, the sensitivity and specificity for detecting sinus venosus defects is considerably less in adults. Numerous reports have demonstrated the superiority of transesophageal echocardiography in diagnosing sinus venous defects and its associated abnormalities.[63–66]

The most common type of sinus venosus defect is the superior type with the defect located in the superior limbus of the atrial septum, inferior to the superior vena cava and the right pulmonary artery. The sinus venous defects usually involve the right upper and mid-pulmonary veins and rarely the right lower pulmonary vein, emptying into the superior vena cava and/or directly into the body of the right atrium. Defects also occur in the superior septal aspect of the atrial septum, which may not be associated with anomalous pulmonary venous return.

Transesophageal echocardiography best demonstrates the superior type sinus venosus defect in the longitudinal (bicaval) view of the right atrium at 90° from the mid to upper esophagus. The typical defect demonstrates the lack of septal tissue lying adjacent to the orifice of the superior vena cava, inferior to the right pulmonary artery. The hallmark of the superior type is the lack of superior atrial septal tissue adjacent to the wall of the pulmonary artery, which differentiates it from a superiorly placed secundum atrial septal defect. The lack of the superior fatty limbus attachment of the septum produces an echocardiographic appearance of the orifice of the superior vena cava overriding or above the left and right atrium.

The anomalous drainage of the right upper pulmonary vein to the superior vena cava, can usually be seen entering the superior vena cava inferiorly, proximal to its ostium. The addition of color flow Doppler, demonstrates flow from the pulmonary vein emptying into the superior vena cava, confirming the diagnosis of anomalous drainage. Anomalous drainage of the upper or the middle pulmonary veins to the superior vena cava may also be demonstrated in short axis views of the superior vena cava at 0°. With minor advancement or withdrawal of the transesophageal probe at the level of the origin of the superior vena cava to the right atrium, the anomalous pulmonary vein may be seen entering the superior vena cava distorting its normal circular shape. The normal azygous vein should not be misinterpreted as anomalous pulmonary drainage. Anomalous pulmonary veins usually enter the superior vena cava inferior to the azygous vein in short-axis image orientation. Although it is important to identify anomalous drainage of right-sided pulmonary veins preoperatively, it is as important to identify anomalous drainage of the left-sided pulmonary veins, since the drainage of the left pulmonary veins are not easily appreciated by the cardiac surgeon, from the standard surgical approach.

The inferior type of sinus venous defect is less frequent[67] and is demonstrated in the bicaval longitudinal view at 90°–120° with the image directed toward the inferior vena cava. The defect appears in the cephalad portion of the atrial septum adjacent to the inferior vena cava. In this view care must be taken to distinguish the sinus venous defect from the normal origin of the coronary sinus. Fine manipulation of the probe enables the coronary sinus to be demonstrated in a different plane than the sinus venous defect. Rotation of the transducer to 0°, demonstrates the defect in close approximation to the inferior vena cava overriding the atrial septum and distinct from the coronary sinus orifice.

The coronary sinus atrial septal defect is the rarest type of atrial septal defect occurring with a prevalence of 1–2%, and is frequently associated with a left-sided superior venae cava[1-3,36] and an enlarged coronary sinus.[68-71] The diagnosis of a coronary sinus atrial septal defect should be entertained in patients in whom an atrial septal defect is suspected and a secundum, primum, or sinus venous defect is not visualized with echocardiography. In coronary sinus atrial septal defects or an unroofed coronary sinus, free communication between the right and left atrium is produced by a small, slit-like sinoseptal defect between the roof of the coronary sinus and the posterior left atrial wall. Coronary sinus defects are frequently associated with tricuspid atresia and detected after Fontan procedures as a new right to left atrial shunt. Detection of the defect of a coronary sinus atrial septal defect and the left superior vena cava usually requires the use of transesophageal echocardiography in the adult, since the resolution of transthoracic imaging is usually not adequate for the posterior position of the coronary sinus and left superior vena cava.[72,73] Echocardiographically the small defect in the coronary sinus is usually, easily appreciated with the edges of the defect freely vibrating, in views demonstrating the posterior left atrial wall. With color flow Doppler shunt flow may be demonstrated in both a right to left or left to right direction depending on the respective atrial pressures. A persistent left superior vena cava and a coronary sinus atrial septal defect may be diagnosed by intravenous injection of agitated saline contrast in the left arm. Echocardiographic contrast is visualized in the left superior vena cava draining into the dilated coronary sinus with bubbles appearing simultaneously in the left atrium from the defect.

Transesophageal echocardiography is extremely useful during the repair of atrial septal defects whether performed surgically or by device closure in the cardiac catheterization laboratory. Preoperatively, transesophageal echocardiography defines cardiac anatomy, semiquantitates hemodynamics for estimating shunt size and pulmonary artery pressure. Additionally, intraoperative transesophageal echocardiography may demonstrate abnormalities that were not anticipated preoperatively, including anomalous pulmonary venous drainage, multiple septal defects and the unroofed coronary sinus

defect. Postoperatively, transesophageal echocardiography determines successful closure and also demonstrates residual shunting. Surgical repair of an atrial septal defect may be performed either by direct suture closure or placement of a surgical patch, dictated by the size and the shape of the defect. Shunt flow is not expected, after successful surgical closure of uncomplicated atrial septal defect. Occasionally small suture leaks may be demonstrated initially with patch repairs, which disappear in the early postoperative period. In patients with the surgical correction of anomalous pulmonary venous return, color flow Doppler determines the adequacy of the redirection of blood flow. Following successful surgical correction of a sinus venosus atrial defect, transesophageal echocardiography should demonstrate an intact, atrial septal patch, an unobstructed opening for the ostium of the appropriate vena cava, and a baffle directing flow to the left atrium from the anomalous pulmonary venous return.

The resolution of right heart dilatation and pulmonary hypertension is usually related to the preoperative size of the defect and the age at which it was repaired. In contrast to the surgical closure of atrial septal defects in children, right heart dimensions do not usually normalize postoperatively, but should decrease substantially in the majority of adult patients.[74,75] Despite the persistence of these structural changes, life expectancy is prolonged in adult patients, through the normalization of left heart dynamics and by improved left ventricular ejection fraction.[76] There is improvement in New York Heart Association functional class in patients even with severe preoperative right heart failure. The risk of cardiac systemic embolization does not appear to be affected by surgical atrial septal defect (ASD) closure, in patients who exhibit atrial tachyarrhythmias.

Transesophageal echocardiography is extremely useful in the catheterization laboratory during the interventional closure of an atrial septal defect with an occluder device.[77-79] Transesophageal echocardiography allows, location of the defect, and assessment of the suitability of closure with an occluder device as well as guiding proper deployment of the device. The appropriate size of the occluder device may be determined by the direct measurement of the defect size. During deployment of the occluder device, transesophageal imaging aids in determining the ideal position for the occluder in relation to the septal borders of the defect, and elimination of the shunt after device deployment. The use of transesophageal echocardiography during transcatheter closure of septal defects is described in Chapter 10.

Ventricular septal defect

Ventricular septal defects are the most common congenital defect in infants and children.[1-3] The majority of ventricular septal defects close spontaneously in child-hood within the first year of life, with 90% of ventricular septal defects closing by age 10.[80–84] However, individual cases of late spontaneous closure have been reported in adulthood.[85–88] The majority of ventricular septal defects that do not undergo spontaneous closure, usually produce symptoms and should be diagnosed in childhood.

Ventricular septal defects that are discovered in adult-hood are generally small and restrictive. Larger moder-ately restrictive or non-restrictive ventricular septal defects with significant left-to-right shunting are rarely detected in adulthood.[89,90] In contrast to atrial septal defects, ventricular septal defects are only occasionally discovered in the adult as an isolated defect, but usually co-exist with other congenital anomalies such as pulmonic stenosis or following palliative or corrective procedures of complex congenital defects.

The ventricular septum is derived from the union of several embryological structures, which produce specific segments of the septum. The terminology for labeling the ventricular septal segments originate from the anatomical divisions of the septum, viewed from the right ventricu-lar septal surface as listed in Table 9.1.[91] The anatomical configuration of the right ventricle produces a true anatomical inflow tract and outflow tract. This configura-tion produces a curvilinear shape to the ventricular septum, which often leads to difficulty in identifying the precise location of the individual segments of the septum, with two-dimensional echocardiograph imaging. Multi-plane transesophageal echocardiography is helpful in providing multiple views of the ventricular septum in adults, to identify each segment of the ventricular septum.

The right ventricular septum is divided into two major components, the membranous septum and the muscular septum. The membranous septum is thin and small (approximately 5 mm in diameter) and attached to the base of the heart below the right and non-coronary cusps of the aortic valve, in between the mitral and tricuspid valves. The membranous septum can be divided into two segments by a plane defined by the insertion point of the tricuspid septal leaflet. The pars atrioventricularis membranous septum lies above and the pars interventric-ularis membranous lies below the septal insertion of the tricuspid valve.

The muscular septum is divided into two components, the inlet component and the outlet component. The right ventricular septal band defines the separation of each component, with each component originating from the inferior border of the membranous septum.

The inlet component is made up of the atrioventricu-lar and inlet septal segments. The atrioventricular septal segment is smooth walled and lies below the atrioventric-ular valve plane. The inlet septal segment comprises the lower third of the ventricular septum and extends to the apex and is limited by the tricuspid valve chordal inser-tion on the septal wall. The inlet septal segment consists of lightly trabeculated muscular tissue that becomes thicker towards the apex.

The outlet component of the muscular ventricular septum includes the trabecular septal segment and the infundibular or outlet septal segment. The trabecular septal segment is the largest segment of the ventricular septum and is demarcated by heavy trabeculation and the right ventricular septal band in the inferior border. The infundibular septal segment is smooth walled and forms the superior portion of the outflow tract below the semilunar valves. The infundibular septum may be further divided into two segments by the crista supraventricularis. The area immediately below the pulmonary valve and above the crista is labeled the supracristal portion and the area below the crista is the infracristal portion.

Most ventricular septal defects occur as the result of the non-union of the septal components during embryologi-cal development. These ventricular septal defects are denoted by their location in the septum and named by the components that border them, i.e. perimembranous-inlet or perimembranous-outlet septal defects. Ventricular septal defects may also occur as the result of deficient tissue within a segment of the septum, as represented by muscular septal defects. Ventricular septal defects are rarely isolated to the membranous septum and usually extend to segments of the muscular septum. Perimem-branous defects are the most common type of ventricular septal defects and occur in approximately 70% of cases.[92] Trabecular muscular septal defects are usually multiple and vary in size, shape and location. Defects in the inlet and outlet ventricular septum are much less frequent, accounting for approximately 5% of defects.[92]

Inlet ventricular septal defects are frequently large, usually associated with atrioventricular canal type defects and only rarely present as an isolated defect. Isolated inlet

---

Table 9.1 Subdivisions of the ventricular septum

Membranous ventricular septum
Pars atrioventricularis
Pars interventricularis

Muscular ventricular septum
Inlet component
   Atrioventricular septum
   Inlet septum
Outlet component
   Trabecular (muscular) septum
   Infundibular (outlet) septum
      Supracristal septum
      Infracristal septum

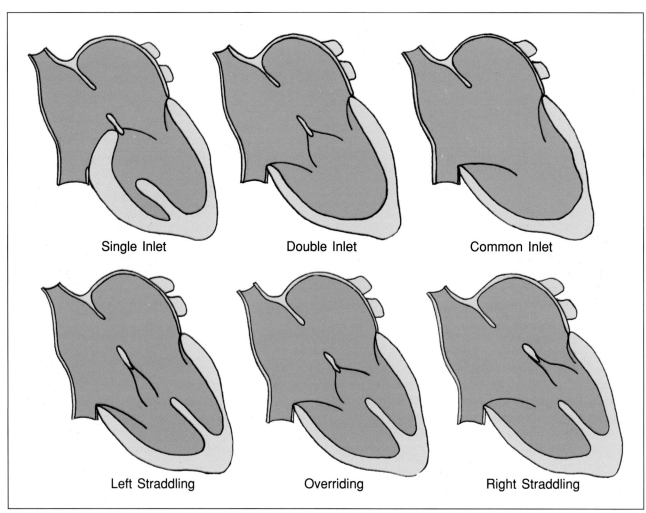

Single Inlet Double Inlet Common Inlet

Left Straddling Overriding Right Straddling

Figure 9.1
Inlet septal defects frequently alter the normal anatomical relationship of the atrioventricular valves to the ventricular septum. Malalignment of either atrioventricular valve may result from the defect and override the ventricular septum, committing the annulus to both ventricles. A double-inlet ventricle is denoted when more than 50% of the atrioventricular valve annulus overrides the contralateral ventricle. In addition to overriding of the annulus, the malalignment may be responsible for producing abnormal chordae tendinae insertion. Straddling of the atrioventricular valve results when chordae from the overriding valve cross over the defect and insert into the opposite ventricle. Both atrioventricular valves may be committed to a single ventricle producing the double inlet configuration or a single valve is committed to a single ventricle as a common inlet or single inlet when one valve is atretic.

defects may be recognized by observing the normal apical displacement of the tricuspid valve, in distinction to atrioventricular canal defects in which the atrioventricular valves lie in the same plane. Inlet septal defects frequently alter the normal anatomical relationship of the atrioventricular valves to the ventricular septum as depicted in Figure 9.1. Malalignment of either atrioventricular valve may result from the defect and override the ventricular septum, committing the annulus to both ventricles. A double-inlet ventricle is denoted when more than 50% of the atrioventricular valve annulus overrides the contralateral ventricle. In addition to overriding of the annulus, the malalignment may be responsible for

producing abnormal chordae tendineae insertion. Straddling of the atrioventricular valve results when chordae from the overriding valve cross over the defect and insert into the opposite ventricle.[91,93]

Outlet ventricular septal defects are usually small defects, and are closely associated with the semilunar valves. Defects may occur in either the supracrista or infracrista septal segments. When supracristal ventricular septal defects involve both semilunar valves, it is referred to as a doubly committed subarterial defect. The outflow defects including infundibular or supracristal types are often associated with complex syndromes that result in malalignment of the outflow tracts and ventriculo-arterial

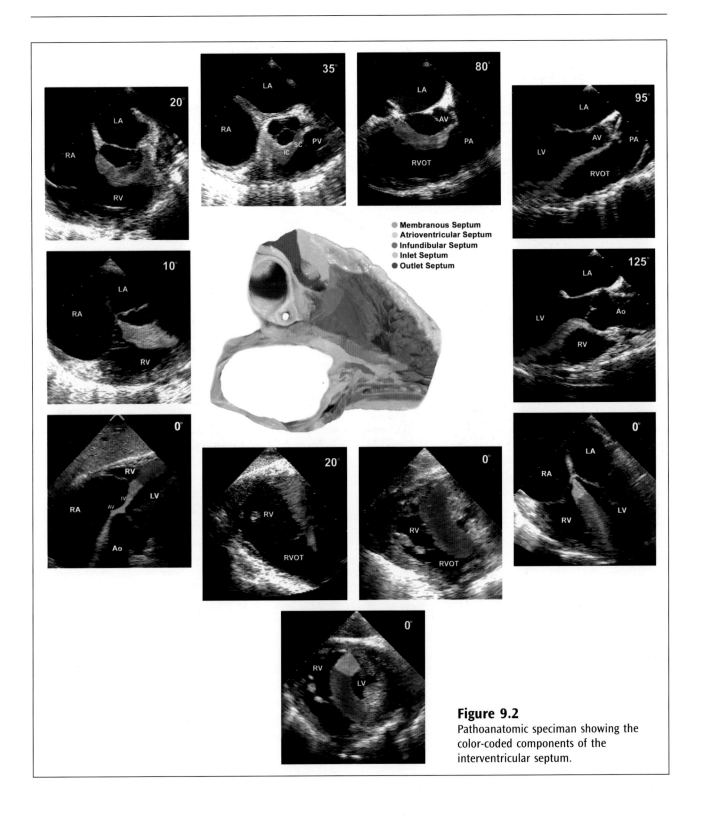

● Membranous Septum
● Atrioventricular Septum
● Infundibular Septum
● Inlet Septum
● Outlet Septum

Figure 9.2
Pathoanatomic speciman showing the
color-coded components of the
interventricular septum.

connections. Malalignment is defined with respect to the semilunar valves and the trabecular septum. Malalignment to the left of the trabecular septum is noted in defects such as tetralogy of Fallot, double outlet ventricles, truncus arteriosus and occasionally transposition of the great arteries.

The precise location of the ventricular septal defect may be identified in several different views with multiplane transesophageal echocardiography as illustrated in Figure 9.2. Perimembranous and infundibular septal defects are usually best identified in short-axis and long-axis views at the base of the heart in a plane below the level of the aortic annulus. The membranous septum is visualized in close proximity to the septal leaflet of the tricuspid valve below the aortic valve level in short-axis images obtained between 15° and 45°. Rotation of the transducer to approximately 125° and fine manipulation of the probe enables visualization of the thin membranous septum which may be visualized as the superior portion of the muscular septum in direct continuity with the right coronary cusp of the aortic valve. In deep transgastric views at 0°–15°, the membranous septum is visualized in detail, demonstrating the levels above and below the tricuspid septal insertion plane.

Infundibular defects may be visualized in views similar to perimembranous defects. In short-axis views at the base of the heart the infundibular septum surrounds the inferior border of the aortic valve annulus. The segments of the infundibular septum are demonstrated with the supracristal septum lying closest to the pulmonary valve, and the infracristal septum in between the supracristal and membranous septum closer to the midline of the aorta. Rotating the transducer from 80° to 100° produces long-axis views of the right ventricular outflow tract and the pulmonary valve, and demonstrates the infundibular septum as the superior portion of the ventricular septum in direct continuity with the inferior portion of the pulmonary valve annulus. In deep transgastric, gastric views and views from the lower esophagus, several different long-axis images of the right ventricular outflow tract may be obtained from 0° to 30° and from 125° to 135° demonstrating the infundibular septum and its relationship to the aortic and pulmonary valves. These views allow assessment of the degree of involvement of the aortic and pulmonary valves, malalignment and overriding of the semilunar valves with the infundibular septum. The degree of aortic insufficiency resulting from the lack of support of the aortic annulus below the right sinus of Valsalva by the defect can also be determined. Narrowing or obstruction of the right and left ventricular outflow tracts resulting from malalignment may also be recognized, in the long-axis views that demonstrate both outflow tracts.

Atrioventricular and inlet septal defects are optimally demonstrated in obliquely cut short-axis views obtained from the mid to upper esophagus at 0°–30°. The inlet septum is demonstrated close to the tricuspid septal leaflet insertion point as the superior portion of the ventricular septum. These views are ideal for demonstrating ventricular septal aneurysms and the degree of involvement of the septal leaflet of the tricuspid value. In the mid to lower esophageal views obtained at 0°, a four-chamber view is obtained showing the inlet septum lying between both atrioventricular views, and is the best view for demonstrating the normal anatomical relationships of the crux of the heart. The apical displacement of the tricuspid valve, septal leaflet insertion into the ventricular crest, and

the anterior mitral leaflet associated with the lower border of the left atrium are appreciated using the zoom feature. These are ideal views for assessing atrioventricular alignment and determining overriding and straddling of the atrioventricular valves. In short-axis gastric views at 0°–15° both the inlet and trabecular ventricular septum are imaged in short-axis projections from multiple planes in breadloaf fashion.

The trabecular septum is the largest septal segment, and is visualized in most views of the ventricular septum, as the inferior portion of the ventricular septum. As described previously, defects of the trabecular septum are usually multiple small defects towards the apex. Defects in the trabecular septum may be difficult to visualize because of their small size and because they may close and be totally obscured during ventricular contraction. Trabecular septal defects may also be difficult to detect since the defect in the septum usually takes an oblique path through the septum with the entrance to the defect occurring at a different level than the exit of the defect. Trabecular ventricular defects can be demonstrated by color flow Doppler as aliased flow entering the right ventricle from the left ventricle.[94,95]

In addition to identifying the location of the ventricular septal defect, the magnitude of the shunt and pulmonary artery pressure can be quantitated by echocardiography.[96,97] Once shunt flow is detected with color flow Doppler, pulsed or continuous wave Doppler can be guided to measure the maximum velocity of the shunt jet. The shunt gradient between the left and right ventricles may be calculated using the modified Bernoulli method, incorporating the maximum jet velocity determined by pulsed or continuous wave Doppler ($4v^2$).[98–103] The right ventricular systolic pressure can be calculated from the shunt gradient determination and the measurement of the systolic arm blood pressure (SBP_{arm}) provided that there is no left ventricular outflow tract obstruction present ($RVSP = SBP_{arm} - 4v^2_{TR\ JET}$).[36] The right ventricular systolic pressure may also be estimated in patients with tricuspid regurgitation, by measurement of the right ventricular/right atrial gradient from the maximal velocity of the tricuspid regurgitation jet ($RVSP = 4(v_{RV/RA})^2 + RA_{pres}$).[36] In cases without significant right ventricular outflow obstruction the right ventricular systolic pressure equals the pulmonary arterial systolic pressure.

The magnitude of the shunt may also be estimated from the determination and comparison of the right and left ventricular stroke volumes as the $Q_P:Q_S$ ratio.[104–109] The Q_P can be determined from the pulmonary outflow tract and the Q_S measurement from the aortic outflow tract. The stroke volume measurement can be made from the time velocity integral and the corresponding annular cross-sectional area. With ventricular septal defects the shunt ratio calculation can be simplified by substituting the time velocity integral with the maximal systolic jet velocity in the outflow tract. Small ventricular septal defects are usually denoted by ratios of less than 1.5:1, and larger defects are associated with ratios of greater than 1.5:1.0. The accuracy of shunt ratios determined with transthoracic echocardiography are limited by the ability to measure accurately the pulmonary annulus, which may be difficult in adults with transesophageal echocardiography. Ventricular septal defect shunt flow may also be estimated with color flow Doppler, utilizing the proximal flow convergence method[110,111] together with the continuous-wave Doppler time velocity integral of the ventricular septal defect during systole.[106,108,109]

Conventional Doppler of the ventricular septal defect shunt jet usually demonstrates holosystolic flow; with the exception of trabecular muscular defects that frequently obliterate during mid-to-late systole. Low velocity continuous shunt flow is also recorded during diastole in larger shunts, suggesting higher left ventricular end-diastolic pressures than right ventricular end-diastolic pressures which imply low pulmonary artery pressures and pulmonary vascular resistance.[45,94,98,106,107] This finding may disappear, however, in the presence of tricuspid or pulmonary insufficiency. In moderate-to-large defects, flow reversal may be recorded denoting a small degree of right to left shunting in late systole.

The magnitude of the shunt is determined by the size of the defect and the level of the pulmonary vascular resistance, and is not related to the location of the defect. Since the flow of blood is directed by the path of least resistance, the magnitude of the ventricular septal defect shunting is determined by the size of the defect and by the pulmonary vascular resistance. Two types of ventricular septal defects may be identified with echocardiography by direct measurement of the size of the defect, or more importantly, measurement of the ventricular gradient across the defect. There are restrictive and non-restrictive defects.[91,112–114]

In small and intermediate size ventricular septal defects, resistance to shunt flow is provided directly by the size of the defect, and results in high velocity shunt gradient, normal cardiac chamber dimensions, near normal right ventricular systolic pressure and normal pulmonary vascular resistance. When the defect is larger, but still restrictive, there may be elevated right ventricular systolic pressures, mild enlargement of the main pulmonary artery and left atrium, mild-to-moderate enlargement of the left ventricular chamber, and normal right ventricular chamber dimensions. The location of the septal defect may produce left ventricular dilatation, when aortic insufficiency is associated most notably with infundibular defects.

Larger ventricular septal defects provide less resistance to flow and the pulmonary vascular resistance determines the magnitude of the shunt. The lower the pulmonary vascular resistance, the greater the magnitude of shunt flow. The second group includes non-restrictive ventricular septal defects with nearly equal right and left ventricular systolic pressures and no systolic shunt gradient. In addition to dilation of the main pulmonary artery and the left sided cardiac chambers, the right ventricle also becomes enlarged due to the increasing pulmonary artery pressures reflecting increased pulmonary vascular resistance. Shunting of blood flow through the defect may be difficult to detect with color flow Doppler, and when detected exhibits low velocity. Pulmonary vascular obstructive disease develops early with large ventricular septal defects, however, right-to-left shunts do not develop until later stages of adolescence and early adulthood with the onset of Eisenmenger's reaction. Most notably, left-to-right shunting is not detectable, but right-to-left shunting may be present. Enlargement of the right ventricle and main pulmonary artery occurs in response to elevation of pulmonary systolic pressures and pulmonary systemic resistance. Additionally, left atrial and ventricular dilatation decreases in isolated ventricular septal defects, due to the decrease in shunt flow. Left ventricular enlargement remains when significant aortic insufficiency is present.

Transesophageal echocardiography is extremely important in the pre and postoperative evaluation and follow-up of the surgical repair of ventricular septal defect in both pediatric and adult patients. During the preoperative transesophageal examination it is important to asess the position of the ventricular septal defect and also identify the presence of multiple defects that may not have been visible on transthoracic echocardiography. Identifying the precise position of the defect aids the surgeon in choosing his or her surgical approach. Perimembranous ventricular septal defects are now routinely closed through a right atrial approach. Muscular ventricular defects are closed usually through the right atrium. However, a right ventricular approach may be necessary and for the rare apical muscular defect a left ventricular approach may be required. Infundibular defects may be closed through a transverse incision of the right ventricular infundibulum or through the pulmonary valve depending on its size or occasionally through the aorta. In addition, the presence of significant aortic regurgitation suggesting aortic valve prolapse or atrioventricular valve regurgitation associated with leaflet clefts in atrioventricular canal defects should be excluded with transesophageal echocardiography.

In contrast to closure of atrial septal defects, ventricular septal defects frequently leak in the early post-operative period. Residual shunting has been attributed to many factors including the anatomy of the defect as well as the expertise of the surgeon performing the closure. Ventricular septal defects are generally harder to close in comparison to atrial septal defects due to limitations in surgical exposure and most notable the irregular shape of the defect associated with the nonplanar surface of the ventricular septum. Further confounding patch closure of ventricular septal defect is the dynamic nature of the ventricular septum during the cardiac cycle. The position of the defect and the comparison of the margins of the defect whether they are primarily muscular or membranous contribute to patch deformity during contraction and relaxation, which promotes residual shunting through the patch edges or suture lines (i.e. a smaller muscular margin may pull away from the membranous portion with contraction). Furthermore, during systole the ventricular septal patch may balloon slightly towards the right ventricle as seen with the increased resolution of transesophageal echocardiography, which becomes less prominent after healing has occurred.

When residual shunting is detected postoperatively, they frequently appear as multiple high velocity turbulent jets denoting leaking through the restrictive patch usually along the suture lines. Owing to the high velocity and spatial display of the flow along with the reflective artifact produced by the patch initially the tendency is to over interpret the shunt as being worse than that preoperatively. As experience is obtained in the postoperative assessment of ventricular septal defect repairs this tendency decreases. It is important to remember the more restrictive the patch or septal defect the higher the velocity obtained if the pulmonary pressures are normal. An unsuccessful repair is usually determined by observing suture dehiscence, suture break or a flail patch. New or worsening of the degree of especially aortic or tricuspid insufficiency may suggest aberrant suture placement in securing the patch and should be relayed to the surgeon. Simply establishing the presence or absence of an overload pattern to the left heart and the determination of the pulmonary pressure assesses the magnitude of the shunt. If the left heart chambers remain small following defect closure and weaning from bypass and the pulmonary pressures remain normal the residual shunt may be determined to be acceptable especially when considering the difficulty in placing the patch. Discretion should be exercised in determining an unsuccessful repair and requires that the transesophageal echocardiographic findings be carefully discussed with the surgeon. Additionally, it should be remembered that shunt determinations are difficult to perform in the operating suite following surgery and are frequently inaccurate and therefore often only add to confusion in the decision making process.

Multiple defects may occasionally be missed preoperatively and become apparent only after closure of the primary septal defect. New septal defects observed postoperatively may not have exhibited significant shunt flow preoperatively especially if they were smaller than the original defect and may not necessarily have been detected by the surgeon during the primary repair. With closure of the first defect and change in hemodynamics, shunting through the new defect occurs that was always present but not identified as contributing a significant role.

Tetralogy of Fallot

Tetralogy of Fallot is the most common cause of cyanotic congenital heart disease encountered in the adult other than Eisenmenger's syndrome.[115] Tetralogy of Fallot is produced by the anterior and rightward deviation of the infundibular ventricular septum.[116-118] The infundibular ventricular septal defect produced is large and results in malalignment and dextroposition of an enlarged aorta. The aorta overrides both ventricles consequently narrowing the right ventricular outflow tract. Obstruction of the right ventricular outflow tract may occur in the subvalvular, valvular, supravalvular levels or in the pulmonary artery branches. Tetralogy of Fallot is similar so may be confused with pulmonary atresia with a ventricular septal defect or truncus arteriosus in children.

Tetralogy of Fallot is frequently associated with several other anomalies,[119-124] such as a right-sided aortic arch (25%), atrial septal defect (10%), multiple muscular ventricular septal defects, coronary artery anomalies (10%), patent ductus arteriosus, absent left pulmonary artery, and absent pulmonary valve.

Tetralogy of Fallot usually produces a significant right-to-left shunt; therefore most patients present in childhood with symptoms and have a palliative or complete correction at an early age. Although cases of unrepaired tetralogy of Fallot may be seen in adults, the majority have had some type of repair performed. Adult survival is largely determined by the degree of right ventricular outflow obstruction which protects the lungs from pulmonary vascular disease. The so called 'pink Fallots' usually have a doubly committed subarterial ventricular septal defect. In patients with congenital absence of the pulmonary valve and tetralogy of Fallot, there is usually a sufficient degree of infundibular stenosis to protect the lungs, and delay presentation until adulthood.[125,126]

Echocardiography readily demonstrates the morphological and physiological features of tetralogy of Fallot.[127-131] Transthoracic and/or transesophageal echocardiography usually confirm the clinical diagnosis of tetralogy of Fallot and its associated anomalies and are used routinely to follow patients after surgical repair. The infundibular ventricular septal defect with overriding of a large aorta is readily demonstrated by both techniques. The greater the degree of anterior and rightward deviation of the malaligned outflow septum, the more severe the right ventricular outflow tract obstruction and the greater the propensity for aortic insufficiency. In tetralogy of Fallot associated with pulmonary atresia, aortic insufficiency is usually significant. The anatomy of the right ventricular outflow tract in adults is best visualized with transesophageal echocardiography from the mid-esophagus in long axis views between 75° and 90° or from the deep transgastric views at 0°–15°. Color flow Doppler imaging visualizes the right-to-left shunting through the ventricular septal defect in most views. The severity of obstruction to the right ventricular outflow tract may be assessed with conventional Doppler, and the right ventricular systolic pressure calculated using the peak velocity of the tricuspid regurgitation jet. In adult patients, transesophageal echocardiography provides better visualization of the presence or absence of aortopulmonary collateral vessels, the pulmonary artery and its proximal branches, and the path of the proximal coronary arteries. Frequently aortopulmonary collaterals may be demonstrated in views of the descending aorta with color flow Doppler. Although transesophageal echocardiography provides good information, cardiac catheterization or magnetic resonance angiography are still required for a complete evaluation of the coronary arteries, distal branches of the pulmonary arteries and definition of the aortopulmonary collateral vessels.

Adults who have undergone either a palliative or complete surgical repair require serial echocardiographic evaluations, and constitute a large percentage of adult congenital cases in our laboratory. Currently, complete surgical reparative procedures are performed in pediatric patients; however, older adults may have only had palliative procedures performed because of prohibitive morphology in early childhood.[132–141]

Some of the more common, palliative surgical procedures for tetralogy of Fallot include the Blalock–Taussig shunt, Waterston shunt and the Potts anastomosis. Echocardiographic assessment of these procedures includes noting the asymmetry of the pulmonary arteries, detecting distortion at the site of the anastomosis of the shunt, measuring the velocity of flow through the shunt. Function is assessed of both the right and left ventricles, especially for the development of restrictive diastolic filling pattern. The tricuspid valve is evaluated for structural abnormalities and tricuspid insufficiency.

Transesophageal echocardiography is extremely valuable for the postoperative assessment of total correction of tetralogy of Fallot, both in pediatric and adult patients.[137–141] Complete surgical correction includes closure of the ventricular septal defect and relief of the right ventricular outflow obstruction. Postoperatively the right ventricular outflow tract should be assessed for residual recurrent obstruction. Pulmonary regurgitation may develop as a consequence of the repair with or without patch placement and enlargement of the infundibulum. Patients with severe pulmonary regurgitation usually do well, however, it may contribute to right ventricular failure in the long term. In patients with distal pulmonary artery stenosis and severe pulmonary regurgitation severe volume overload of the right ventricle may develop. Earlier corrective techniques of the right ventricular outflow tract often resulted in aneurysmal formation of the wall at the incision site, which may occasionally enlarge or even rupture. Residual ventricular septal patch leaks may occur and increase in severity overtime. Left ventricular dysfunction may occur as a result of poor myocardial preservation at the time of surgery or as a result of volume overload, especially in patients that have had a palliative shunt. Aortic insufficiency may develop postoperatively which is usually mild.

Patent ductus arteriosus

Patent ductus arteriosus (PDA) is a frequent congenital cardiovascular abnormality that occurs in approximately 10% of all congenital cases.[1–3,142,143] It may occur as an isolated lesion or is frequently associated with more complex malformations.[142–150] In the fetus, the ductus arteriosus provides the obligatory connection between the descending thoracic aorta and the left pulmonary artery, permitting right-sided blood flow to bypass the unexpanded lungs and enter the systemic circulation via the aorta, to be returned to and oxygenated in the placenta. The ductus arteriosus usually closes spontaneously by the third day after birth. The ductus arteriosus may remain persistently patent producing a left-to-right shunt, with continuous flow from the aorta to the pulmonary artery. Large patent ductus arteriosus is usually diagnosed in infancy, however, small or moderate patent ductus arteriosus may not be detected until adulthood. Symptoms in early adulthood such as fatigue, dyspnea, palpitations or frank left ventricular failure may ensue. In addition to the hemodynamic effects of the shunt flow, patients are at an increased risk for the development of infective endocarditis, endarteritis, aneurysmal dilatation and calcification of the ductus that may precipitously rupture.[149,150] Due to the risk of complications especially endarteritis, closure of small patent ductus arteriosus when discovered, is often advocated since the risk of surgical correction or percutaneous interventional closure is minimal.

Diagnosis of a persistently PDA by transthoracic echocardiography may be extremely difficult in adolescents and adults due to the relative posterior position of the ductus and the descending aorta which is usually obscured by the lungs and ribs. Transesophageal echocardiography has a high sensitivity and specificity for the diagnosis of PDA and is superior to transthoracic echocardiography in the adult, especially in patients with pulmonary hypertension.[151–159]

Patent ductus arteriosus is visualized in both the horizontal and longitudinal planes, from the upper esophagus windows with transesophageal echocardiography.

The bifurcation of the pulmonary artery is visualized with the transducer at 0°, and the probe rotated counterclockwise towards the descending aorta. The ductus is visualized between the descending aorta and the left pulmonary artery with a length of approximately 8 mm (5.5–13 mm) and diameter of 1.5–13 mm at the aortic origin. To aid in recognition of the ductus anatomy, color flow Doppler may be utilized to substantiate flow in the duct. Once visualized the full dimensional aspect of the ductus may be observed with rotation of the transducer through 90°. Aneurysmal dilatation or calcification should be noted, and is easily assessed by scanning from the horizontal to longitudinal plane.[149,150] Thrombus or vegetations may be detected near the ductus in the left pulmonary artery.

Color flow Doppler permits the direct visualization of the turbulent aliased flow from the descending aorta through the duct into the pulmonary artery which is diagnostic for PDA. Flow convergence is detected at the origin of the ductus arteriosus on the aortic side. A mosaic flow in the pulmonary artery without demonstration of its origin from the aorta is not definitive for PDA. Pulsed-wave or continuous wave Doppler of the ductus flow demonstrates high velocity flow. In cases with Eisenmenger's syndrome complicating PDA bi-directional flow is detected with flow from the pulmonary artery to the aorta during systole and flow from the aorta to the pulmonary artery in diastole.

Flow convergence is usually detected toward the ductus from the descending aorta in early diastole, and the finding is helpful in determining patency as well as the size of the PDA. Shiota and colleagues, have demonstrated that small ductus < 4 mm exhibited a flow convergence radius of ≤ 3 mm, and moderate-to-large ductus had a flow convergence radius of > 3 mm, confirmed during surgical repair.[160] Peak shunt flow rates and shunt flow volumes may also be estimated with the flow convergence method and correlate with those determined at cardiac catheterization. Identification of the flow convergence for a patent ductus is also useful for following the results of surgical or interventional closure of the ductus arteriosus.[160–163]

Coarctation of the aorta

Coarctation of the aorta is a common congenital lesion, which accounts for approximately 5% of all congenital heart disease cases and predominates in males.[1–3,164,165] Coarctation of the aorta exhibits numerous anatomical variations with a wide range of clinical presentations. The symptoms of coarctation of the aorta appear either early in infancy or not until the third or fourth decade.[164–166]

Coarctation of the aorta is frequently associated with other congenital malformations.[167,168] A bicuspid aortic valve is the most commonly associated malformation occurring in 40–80% of post-ductal coarctation. Hypoplasia of the aorta and abnormalities of the aortic arch are usually associated with preductal coarctation. Ventricular septal defect with posterior deviation of the outflow septum, subaortic stenosis, and mitral valve anomalies are also associated with coarctation.

Coarctation of the aorta may occur at any level in the thoracic aorta, but most commonly occurs distal to the origin of the left subclavian artery in the vicinity of the insertion of the ligamentum arteriosum known as the cardiac isthmus. When the coarctation occurs proximal to the ductus arteriosum level it is termed a preductal or infantile type coarctation. If the coarctation occurs distal to the ductus arteriosum it is termed a postductal or adult type coarctation. The infantile or adult type terminology can be misleading, however, since either presentation of coarctation defect may be visualized in adulthood. The defect in aortic coarctation either produces a discrete and localized indentation to the aortic lumen or a diffuse narrowing, which may involve the whole isthmus and even extend into the aortic arch.

Echocardiographically, coarctation of the aorta appears as a discrete narrowing of the aortic lumen contour, with a posterior echodense shelf protruding into the aortic lumen.[168–174] In short-axis transesophageal views at 0°, slow advancement or withdrawal of the probe enables the location of the narrowing, proximal or distal to the left subclavian artery to be detemined. In wide plane, longitudinal views at 90° (increasing the depth to 10–12 cm), isthmus hypoplasia in the area of coarctation produces an hourglass deformity. The area of the coarctation possesses increased echogenicity with a 'fuzzy' appearance to the aortic lumen due to the hyperplasia of the aortic wall, in contast to the normal aortic segments. The aortic segments proximal to the coarctation segment are usually dilated, with dilatation extending into the brachiocephalic vessels. Poststenotic dilatation is noted in a short segment of the aorta distal to the coarctation. Noticeable aortic pulsations are detected in the proximal aortic segments, with no detectable pulsation in the poststenotic segment. Conventional Doppler is usually not helpful with transesophageal echocardiography, since reliable parallel flow interrogation planes are not obtainable of the aortic arch or descending aorta. Turbulent flow is detected in the whole area of the coarctation with color flow Doppler.[169,171,172] The diameter of the color flow jet in the coarctation site helps determine the size and extent of the area of coarctation. In addition, the zone of flow convergence may be visualized proximal to the coarctation which identifies the site and severity of the constriction.[171]

In infants and younger patients transthoracic echocardiography provides direct visualization of the site of coarctation from the suprasternal window, in the majority of patients. In older patients, when adequate visualization of the aorta is not possible from the suprasternal approach, transesophageal echocardiography is usually necessary.[166,169] Although transesophageal may allow direct visualization of aortic coarctation, it requires a meticulous and often prolonged examination, in order to evaluate the aorta in its entirety. In addition, hemodynamic information may be very difficult or impossible to obtain with transesophageal echocardiography, and necessitate MRI (magnetic resonance imaging) or contrast aortography for complete evaluation of aortic coarctation. MRI gated spin-echo and cine techniques provide excellent images for detailing anatomy, severity of obstruction (stenosis diameter), identifying pre and poststenotic dilatations, collateral arteries, and determining the site of leakage in late postoperative pseudoaneurysm in adult patients.[172,175,176] The major role of transesophageal echocardiography is in the evaluation of left ventricular systolic function, the complications of coarctation (aneurysm, dissection and rupture) and the associated congenital cardiac anomalies.

Transesophageal echocardiography is helpful as an adjunct to interventional reparative procedures such as balloon angioplasty or stent placement for aortic coarctation.[177,178] Transesophageal echocardiography is also invaluable in assessing the short- and long-term results and complications that may occur following surgical or interventional repair of aortic coarctation.[172–174]

Transposition of the great arteries

Transposition of the great arteries describes discordant ventriculoarterial connection with the aorta arising from the morphological right ventricle and the pulmonary artery arising from the morphological left ventricle.[1–3] The pulmonary artery is parallel to the aorta in a posterior position, producing a 'double barrel' appearance with echocardiography.[179–181] Transposition occurs commonly with situs inversus or situs solitus. The most common form is D-transposition, in which there is normal atrial arrangement (atrioventricular concordance), with discordant ventriculoarterial connection with the aorta lying anterior and to the right of the pulmonary artery. Systemic venous return drains into the right atrium, the right ventricle and immediately re-enters the systemic circulation through the aorta. Pulmonary venous return enters the left atrium, the left ventricle and returns via the pulmonary artery. This arrangement allows two independent blood flow circuits and without an associated abnormal connection such as an atrial or ventricular septal defect, the systemic blood flow never reaches the lungs, resulting in severe cyanosis at birth. This congenital abnormality is incompatible with life if a shunt (atrial or ventricular septal defect or patent ductus arteriosus) is not present. D-transposition is commonly associated with a perimembranous ventricular septal defect, pulmonary stenosis, pulmonary atresia or subvalvular pulmonary stenosis. Uncorrected D-transposition with a large ventricular septal defect with either pulmonary vascular disease or pulmonary stenosis may be encountered in adults.

The parallel orientation of the great vessels is readily demonstrated in long-axis views by echocardiography, with the aorta and pulmonary artery lying side-by-side, lacking the normal spiral relationship. The aorta is distinguished by the brachiocephalic vessels and the pulmonary artery by the bifurcation into the right and left pulmonary arteries. In short-axis views, a direct antero-posterior relationship is demonstrated, with a centrally located pulmonary artery and valve visualized simultaneously with the aortic valve and aorta. The aorta is usually larger than the pulmonary artery. In addition, the short-axis views demonstrate the direct continuity of the aorta with the right ventricular outflow tract. When subpulmonary stenosis is present, diffuse hypertrophy of the infundibulum may resemble the appearance of idiopathic hypertrophic subaortic stenosis. Four-chamber views demonstrate the pulmonary artery bifurcation and the relationship of the pulmonary artery to the septum. Subpulmonary stenosis is frequently associated with a ventricular septal defect, which is usually visualized in the same views.

Most adult patients with D-transposition will have had surgical correction and present for echocardiographic evaluation of the sequelae of the correction. The two most common surgical procedures for correction of D-transposition, which are usually performed after a palliative atrial septostomy, include the atrial switch procedures and the arterial switch procedure.[182] In transposition associated with ventricular septal defect and severe pulmonary stenosis an external valve conduit between the right ventricle and the pulmonary artery may be created as in the Rastelli or Damus–Kaye–Stanus procedure.[183]

The atrial switch includes the Mustard or Senning procedures. In the atrial switch procedure, a baffle is created in the atrium through the atrial septum to redirect venous returns to their appropriate circulations, i.e. the systemic venous flow is directed to the left ventricle and the pulmonary artery with the pulmonary venous return directed to the right ventricle and to the aorta.[182–188] After removing the atrial septum, an oblong patch is sewn over the orifice of both the superior vena cava and the inferior vena cava, usually incorporating the coronary sinus and extends to the orifice of the mitral valve. Pulmonary venous blood flows over and around the baffle towards the tricuspid valve. Echocardiographically, the baffle creates a pulmonary venous atrium and a systemic venous atrium best visualized in the four-chamber views. In adult patients, transesophageal echocardiography is usually necessary to evaluate the atrial switch procedure. The pulmonary venous baffle is demonstrated originating from the pulmonary veins crossing obliquely towards the right ventricle. The systemic venous atrium is demonstrated originating from the right atrium and criss-crossing the pulmonary venous atrium towards the mitral valve. The pulmonary venous atrium is usually larger when visualized from the mid-esophagus and deep transgastric four-chamber views. The direction of blood flow is determined either with color flow Doppler or agitated saline echocardiographic contrast. Complications of atrial switch procedures include ventricular dysfunction (especially right ventricular dysfunction), baffle obstruction, tricuspid and/or aortic regurgitation.[187,188]

Atrial switch procedures have been largely replaced by the arterial switch procedure.[189] The Jatene procedure restores the normal structural and functional relationships between the ventricles and arterial connections. The aorta and the pulmonary arteries are divided in their proximal portions and rotated and re-anastomosed to their appropriate positions. The coronary arteries are removed from the pulmonary artery and attached to the aorta. Complications include supravalvular narrowing at the anastomotic sites, narrowing or kinking of the re-implanted coronary arteries, and distortion of the left and right pulmonary arteries as a result of rotating the pulmonary artery for anastomosis. Obstruction at the anastomotic sites can be defined echocardiographically, and most commonly occurs at the pulmonary anastomosis. The aorta is frequently dilated, which results in aortic insufficiency. The development of regional wall motion abnormalities of the left ventricle suggests obstruction at the site of re-implantation of the coronary arteries.

In congenitally corrected or L-transposition, there is discordant ventriculoarterial connection with ventricular inversion and atrioventricular discordance.[190] Systemic venous returns drain into the right atrium, left ventricle and pulmonary artery. Pulmonary venous return enters the left atrium, right ventricle and aorta. The anomaly essentially 'corrects' itself due to the ventricular inversion with the morphological right ventricle lying to the left of the morphological left ventricle. Coexisting cardiac anomalies frequently associated with L-transposition include tricuspid valve structural abnormalities producing an Ebstein-like deformity, perimembranous ventricular septal defect, left ventricular outflow tract obstruction and subvalvular pulmonic stenosis.[191–193] The development of right ventricular dysfunction is the rule in adulthood; due to the systemic load imposed on a morphological right ventricle and its inability to meet those demands over a protracted period of time, i.e. the right ventricle 'wears out', with increasing systemic atrio-ventricular valve regurgitation.

Echocardiographically the pulmonary artery arises posteriorly from the left ventricle, producing a lower position of the pulmonary valve as compared to the aortic valve. The aorta arises anteriorly and from the right ventricle. The aorta and the pulmonary artery appear to lie side by side, similar to D-transposition. The diagnosis of L-transposition includes the identification of ventricular inversion with echocardiography. The left-sided systemic ventricle is a morphological right ventricle denoted by the apical position of the tricuspid valve in relationship to the internal cardiac crux, and the moderator band. The right-sided pulmonary ventricle exhibits the fish-mouth shape of the mitral valve and the left ventricular papillary muscle configuration.

Ebstein's anomaly of the tricuspid valve

Ebstein's anomaly results from a malformation of the tricuspid valve, which produces significant tricuspid regurgitation resulting in a variable degree of right ventricular dysfunction.[194–199] Embryologically, the tricuspid valve leaflets and subvalvular apparatus are derived from delamination of the inner layers of the inlet region of the right ventricle, which is interrupted with Ebstein's anomaly. The presentation of Ebstein's anomaly depends on the severity of the tricuspid valve malformation and the degree of right ventricular dysfunction. Ebstein's anomaly in less severe forms may present asymptomatically in the adult and is discovered incidentally by echocardiography often during the evaluation of supraventricular arrhythmia.

In Ebstein's anomaly, the tricuspid valve is displaced downwards, the annular attachment of the septal and posterior leaflets are within the body of the right ventricle. The apical displacement of the leaflets usually exceeds 20 mm or 8 mm/m^2 in the adult. Tricuspid leaflet displacement results in atrialization of the proximal portion of the right ventricle and reduction in size of the functional right ventricle. In the most florid cases of Ebstein's anomaly, the right heart is effectively divided into three chambers, the true right atrium, the atrialized right ventricle and the functional right ventricle, with an effective tricuspid orifice that is displaced downward into the right ventricular cavity. The atrialized right ventricle is anatomically the right ventricle but functions as the right atrium, which predisposes the thin walled atrialized portion to dilate and may result in an aneurysm between the tricuspid annulus and the displaced posterior leaflet. Although the annular attachment of the anterior leaflet may be normal, the leaflet is malformed as the result of thickening and redundancy. The anterior leaflet may be dysplastic and frequently adherent to the right ventricular free wall which may result in right ventricular inflow or outflow tract obstruction. Tricuspid regurgitation accompanies the structurally abnormal valve and is frequently severe. Variations in the degree of the tricuspid valve malformation dictates the natural history of Ebstein's anomaly. Ebstein's anomaly is associated with either an atrial septal defect or patent foramen ovale in over 80% of cases. In patients with elevated right atrial pressure, right-to-left shunting may occur.

Echocardiography accurately identifies Ebstein's anomaly in the majority of cases, and is currently the method of choice for establishing the diagnosis.[200–205] Transthoracic echocardiography is usually sufficient for most patients provided that image quality is adequate. For the less severe forms of the anomaly careful scanning is important, to establish the diagnosis. The most important diagnostic echocardiographic findings for Ebstein's anomaly is the apical displacement of the septal tricuspid valve leaflet ≥ 8 mm/m^2 along with a redundant and elongated anterior tricuspid leaflet. Ammash and colleagues, found that these two findings most consistently identified patients with Ebstein's anomaly.[202] Echocardiography with the addition of color flow Doppler identifies the degree of tricuspid regurgitation and demonstrates inflow or outflow stenosis when present. The position of the flow convergence associated with the tricuspid regurgitant jet is helpful for demonstrating the level of apical displacement of the effective tricuspid orifice within the right ventricle, especially when there is difficulty in determining the level of insertion of the septal leaflet. Dilated tricuspid annulus and paradoxical ventricular septal motion are usually present producing alteration in left ventricular geometry and function. Histological studies have demonstrated increased fibrosis in the left ventricular wall and ventricular septum distinguishing the abnormal wall motion from pressure or volume overload.

Carpentier has proposed a functional classification for the severity of Ebstein's anomaly, to assist in defining the surgical correction technique.[206,207] Type A lesions occur in approximately 5% of cases and exhibit mild displacement of the septal leaflet, with a small atrialized chamber. Type B lesions (35%) exhibit massive displacement of the septal leaflet, normal motion of the anterosuperior leaflet and a large atrialized chamber. In type C lesions (51%), the mural leaflet is absent, the anterosuperior leaflet is severely restricted by muscular trabeculations and short chordae tendineae, the anterolateral papillary muscle is incorporated in the right ventricular wall, the atrialized chamber is markedly enlarged with dyskinetic wall motion, hypokinesis of the functional right ventricle and stenosis of the tricuspid valve. In type D lesions (8%), the most severe type, the tricuspid leaflet tissue is extremely dysplastic; the ventricular walls are thin and exhibit severe contraction abnormality. Type D lesions probably require valve replacement while type B and C lesions can be adequately repaired with valvuloplasty.

Numerous reports have described the beneficial effects of valve preservation techniques in the treatment of Ebstein's anomaly.[206–211] The Carpentier technique of tricuspid valvuloplasty for Ebstein's anomaly includes the mobilization of the restrictive anterosuperior leaflet and the longitudinal plication of the inlet component of the right ventricle with or without the placement of a tricuspid annuloplasty ring. In addition a partial Glenn anastomosis (cavo-bipulmonary anastomosis) is performed in the most severe cases with right ventricular failure. Echocardiography postvalvuloplasty demonstrates elimination or reduction of tricuspid regurgitation to mild severity. There is marked improvement in the ratio of the atrialized chamber to functional right ventricle associated with improvement in right ventricular function.

Partial anomalous pulmonary venous return

Partial anomalous pulmonary venous return is described when one or more pulmonary veins, but not all are connected to the right atrium, the superior vena cava or rarely the inferior vena cava.[1–3] Partial anomalous pulmonary venous return may occur as an isolated defect with an intact atrial septum, but is uncommonly discovered in adults.[212–214] Partial anomalous pulmonary venous return is more frequently associated with sinus venosus than secundum atrial septal defects and persistent left superior vena cava is common.

Numerous reports have described the benefit of transesophageal echocardiography for detection of partial anomalous pulmonary venous return; however, a high index of suspicion is usually necessary in order not to miss the defect.[215–217] With transesophageal echocardiography, all four pulmonary veins with their origin to the left atrium may be consistently visualized as described in Chapter 6. The right upper and middle lobe pulmonary veins are most commonly involved and reports have described anomalous connections to all of the systemic veins. The shunt produced by anomalous pulmonary venous return may not be hemodynamically significant, and is dictated by the difference between the right atrial and left atrial pressures. Generally in isolated pulmonary venous return, when only one pulmonary vein is involved, the shunt is small as evidenced by normal dimensions of the right atrium and ventricle; two anomalous veins may be associated with mild right atrial and ventricular enlargement.[217]

Pulmonary vein stenosis

Pulmonary vein stenosis may be occasionally seen with transesophageal echocardiography, usually as an incidental finding.[218-224] Pulmonary vein stenosis may be congenital or acquired as a result of extracardiac external compression from an enlarged descending aorta or pulmonary mass or following atrial fibrillation ablations. Congenital pulmonary vein stenosis may be isolated in one vein or in all four pulmonary veins. Pulmonary venous flow is usually laminar in quality despite increased flow or flow reversal. With pulmonary venous stenosis, high velocity flow is detected with transesophageal echocardiography, conventional and color flow Doppler techniques.

Persistent left superior vena cava

Persistent left superior vena cava is a common anomaly frequently visualized in adults by both transthoracic and transesophageal echocardiography. A persistent left superior vena cava may be present in 3–10% of cases with congenital heart disease.[1-3] In approximately 90% of cases the left superior vena cava drains directly into the coronary sinus. Left superior vena cava may also connect directly to the left atrium, specifically to the roof of the left atrium interposed between the upper and lower pulmonary veins at the level of the left atrial appendage.[225-227] In the remainder of cases, the left superior vena cava connects to the left pulmonary veins along the lateral border of the left atrium. A persistent left superior vena cava is commonly associated with secundum atrial septal defects, tetralogy of Fallot and tricuspid atresia.

Echocardiographically, a persistent left superior vena cava is suspected when the coronary sinus is dilated, and the cause is not related to an increase in the right atrial pressure or increased coronary flow states. The enlarged coronary sinus lies in the atrioventricular groove anterior to the posterior pericardial space. The persistent left superior vena cava is demonstrated in short axis near the left atrial appendage coursing anterior to the main pulmonary artery toward the atrioventricular groove. In cases where the persistent left superior vena cava enters the left atrium directly, the vessel appears interposed between the left atrial appendage and the left upper pulmonary vein, in the region of the 'Q-tip'. Doppler interrogation of the persistent left superior vena cava demonstrates low flow velocities, with a typical venous pattern. Agitated saline echocardiographic injection from the left arm, defines the persistent superior vena cava and demonstrates its connection to either the coronary sinus, left atrium or pulmonary vein.

Cor triatriatum

Cor triatriatum is a rare congenital cardiac defect that may present in adulthood.[1-3] When significant obstruction is present, the lesion is diagnosed in infancy or early childhood. The diagnosis of cor triatriatum is frequently an incidental finding discovered with transesophageal echocardiography when evaluating patients for unexplained pulmonary hypertension or congestive heart failure. In adults, the membrane that separates the left atrium into anterior and posterior chambers is usually non-obstructive in comparison to that seen in symptomatic pediatric patients.[228-240] The membrane is visualized stretching from the junction of the left atrial appendage and the left superior pulmonary vein orifice to the area of the fossa ovalis of the atrial septum, and is usually the same thickness as the atrial wall, and is seen undulating (trampoline-like) with the opening and closing of the mitral valve. The atrium is divided into a superior pulmonary venous chamber that drains all four pulmonary veins, and an inferior chamber includes the foramen ovale and the atrial appendage. The membrane is usually fenestrated in the adult with one large orifice close to the atrial septum.

The site of obstruction is identified with color flow Doppler as a high velocity jet, with an area of flow convergence on the superior surface of the membrane. Continuous wave Doppler may be used to calculate the gradient using the modified Bernoulli formula.

Very occasionally, small masses may be visualized with transesophageal echocardiography in close proximity to the membrane, which may represent thrombus and/or vegetation.[241,242]

Cor triatriatum must be distinguished from a supravalvular mitral ring or membrane. A mitral supravalvular ring is usually identified by transesophageal echocardiography as a thin membrane with a central orifice, close to the mitral annulus (usually within 1 cm). Supravalvular mitral stenosis is usually associated with other mitral valve abnormalities and other left-sided obstructive lesions.

Cor triatriatum dexter may rarely occur in the right atrium.[243-248] Abnormal persistence of the sinus venosus valve, results in a two-chambered right atrium. The resultant membrane extends from the inferior vena cava to the superior vena cava and separates the right atrial appendage and the tricuspid valve to the lower right atrial chamber. Blood flow empties from the vena cava through perforations in the membrane, producing a similar physiological situation as tricuspid atresia, however, with a well formed tricuspid valve and right ventricle. Cor triatriatum dexter is frequently associated with a secundum atrial septal defect. In the adult patient the membrane is demonstrated by flow disturbance with color flow Doppler. Careful echocardiographic examination delineates cor triatriatum dexter from a prominent Chiari's network or prominent atrial wall fold that does not produce significant flow disturbance as described in Chapter 6.

Anomalous coronary artery

Coronary artery anomalies are rare, but when present are responsible for producing myocardial ischemia, and are a common cause of sudden cardiac death in young adults.[249,250] Variations include patients in whom the anomalous coronary artery courses between the aorta and pulmonary artery or there is distortion of the ostia of the anomalous vessel.

Echocardiography may be helpful in evaluating anomalous coronary arteries.[251–271] The anomalous origin of the coronary arteries may be detected with either transthoracic or transesophageal echocardiography. Frequently, the origin of the right coronary artery and the left main coronary artery including its bifurcation into the left anterior descending and circumflex artery are visualized in their proximal segments. Varied success has been reported for the consistent visualization of the coronary arteries with both transthoracic and transesophageal echocardiography. The sensitivity of transesophageal echocardiography for the evaluation of the left main coronary artery is between 77 and 100%, with a sensitivity for the right coronary artery of 26%. Therefore, cardiac catheterization is usually required to confirm the diagnosis for anomalous coronary arteries.[253] When the coronary arteries are well visualized, the diagnosis of anomalous coronary arteries can be made with certainty, with transesophageal echocardiography. Recognition of coronary artery anomalies with echocardiography requires knowledge of the multiple variations and their respective frequencies (Figure 9.3).

An important coronary anomaly that usually presents in neonates is the origin of the left coronary artery from the pulmonary artery. The anomalous left main coronary artery connects above the left or posterior cusp and rarely from the right cusp of the main pulmonary artery. The left main coronary artery is usually of normal length before it divides into the left anterior descending and circumflex artery. The right coronary artery arises normally from the aorta and gives off numerous collaterals to the left coronary artery resulting in retrograde blood flow from the left coronary artery to the pulmonary artery. Most patients die in the first year of life if the diagnosis is not made, although few may live to the fifth or sixth decade and sustain sudden death. Echocardiographically, the continuity of the left main coronary artery with the aorta is not demonstrated even though the left main coronary artery appears in its proper location. The right coronary artery usually dilates over time, providing a clue towards the presence of the anomaly. The anomalous left coronary artery also produces global dilatation of the left ventricle with decreased cardiac function, resembling a dilated cardiomyopathy.

Anomalous origin of the right coronary artery may also be visualized with transesophageal echocardiography, especially when it originates directly from the left coronary artery. Whether the anomalous coronary artery passes between the aorta and pulmonary trunk, is important but this is not reliably demonstrated echocardiographically.

Other common variations include: anomalous origin of the left main coronary artery from the right coronary cusp or directly from the right coronary artery; left anterior descending or left circumflex originating from the right cusp or directly from the right coronary artery; origin of the right coronary artery from the left cusp or directly from the left coronary artery; origin of the right coronary artery from the proximal portion of the ascending aorta (high origin); single coronary artery; or all three coronary vessels with separate ostia from either the right or left coronary cusp. Some variations are more susceptible to distorted ostia, or tunneling in between the aorta and pulmonary artery.

Coronary arterial fistulae

A congenital coronary arteriovenous fistula is a direct, connection between a coronary artery and another cardiac structure. Communications usually enter the right heart chambers (90%) but have been described to all four cardiac chambers, the coronary sinus, cardiac veins, proximal superior vena cava, proximal pulmonary artery and pulmonary veins near their connection to the heart. Coronary arteriovenous fistulae involve the right coronary artery or its branches in 55% of cases, the left coronary artery in 35% of cases and both coronaries are involved in 5%.[272–274] The fistulous connection may be attached in a side-to-side fashion or extend from the end of a normal anatomical coronary artery.[275] The coronary artery dilates and elongates frequently in a serpiginous fashion as a result of the shunt flow produced through the fistula. The dilatation is uniform throughout and often produces a huge coronary artery. At the point of fistulous connection, the coronary artery dilates out of proportion to the rest of the artery in an aneurysmal fashion. Despite progressive dilatation of the coronary artery with advancing age, the arteries do not appear prone to rupture.[276] Frequently the fistulous opening is multiple and produces a confluence of multiple tracts to the receiving chamber. The coronary artery distal to the fistulous connection usually is normal size or frequently smaller than expected. The true incidence of coronary arteriovenous fistula is not known since the majority are probably small and inconsequential findings on coronary arteriography, which resembles a small blush in the vicinity of the receiving chamber, with no significant coronary artery dilatation.

In 25% of cases, the coronary arteriovenous fistula enters the right atrium, 40% enter the right ventricle, 15–20% enter the main pulmonary artery, 7% to the coronary sinus and 1% to the superior vena cava.[272,273,277] Fistulae entering the right heart produce a left-to-right

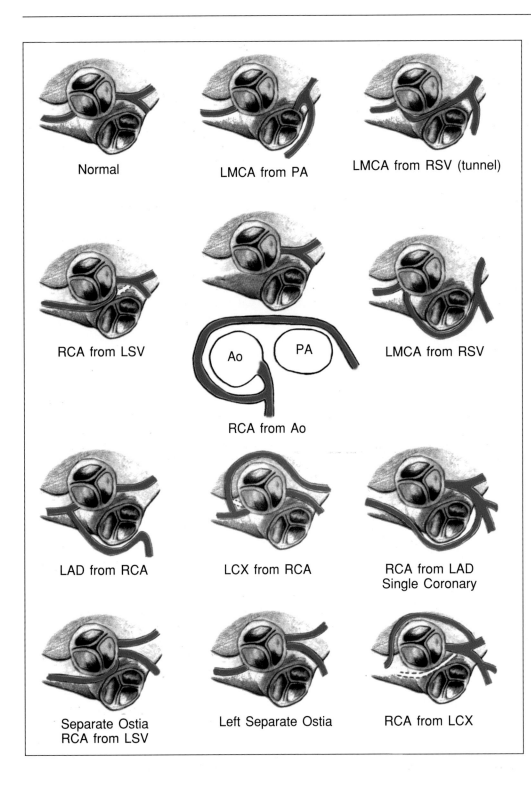

Normal

LMCA from PA

LMCA from RSV (tunnel)

RCA from LSV

Ao   PA

RCA from Ao

LMCA from RSV

LAD from RCA

LCX from RCA

RCA from LAD
Single Coronary

Separate Ostia
RCA from LSV

Left Separate Ostia

RCA from LCX

Figure 9.3
Artist's rendition of some of the more common coronary anomalies as might be visualized from the upper esophageal short-axis view at 45° at the base of the heart with multiplane transesophageal echocardiography. When the coronary arteries are adequately visualized with transesophageal echocardiography an accurate diagnosis of anomalous origin may be made precisely. Varied success has been reported for the consistent visualization of the coronary arteries with both transthoracic and transesophageal echocardiography.

shunt pattern which seldom results in a $Q_p:Q_s$ ratio larger than 1.8. The remaining fistula produce a communication to the left atrium, and rarely to the left ventricle or proximal pulmonary veins, which produces an increase in overload to the left ventricle.

Coronary arteriovenous fistulas are usually well demonstrated with multiplane transesophageal echocardiogra-

phy.[278-280] Occasionally older patients evaluated for a cause of congestive heart failure, are shown to have congenital arteriovenous fistula, with a continuous murmur and systolic thrill when the fistula is anterior and emptying into the right atrium or right ventricle. Coronary artery dilatation with or without aneurysm formation is easily seen. When the receiving chamber is the right or left atrium or coronary sinus these structures are generally dilated. When the left ventricle is the receiving chamber, it is dilated with volume overload pattern similar to aortic regurgitation. Five percent of cases are associated with bacterial endocarditis. Transesophageal echocardiography is especially helpful in identifying the receiving chamber as well as determining a successful operative repair. Due to the low operative risk of surgical repair, the risk of bacterial endocarditis and the probability that the fistulae will increase in size eventually precipitating congestive failure, surgery is indicated when the Q_p:Q_s is greater than 1.3 when entering a right-sided chamber or when a significant left ventricular overload pattern is present.

Congenital surgeries

Transesophageal echocardiography is invaluable in adult patients for analysis of the results of surgical correction of congenital heart disease.[280] It is mandatory that a thorough history be obtained including the surgical technique utilized prior to performing the transesophageal examination, in order to assess the results of surgical correction.

Surgical procedures for congenital heart disease have greatly modified the natural history of most congenital defects. The success of surgery is determined not only by increased survival into adulthood but also by improvement in quality of life. Surgical procedures may be classified as palliative or corrective depending on whether the morphological anomaly is cured or only modified, which is important when assessing the results of surgical procedures with echocardiography. Knowledge of the type of surgical repair and the ramifications for each repair are important in order to obtain all the information necessary during the echocardiographic examination and are illustrated in Appendix 1. The following discussion of the congenital surgeries is a brief review and for a more comprehensive discussion the reader is directed to both surgical and echocardiographic texts dealing with congenital heart disease.

Pulmonary artery banding

Pulmonary artery banding is a palliative procedure, initially utilized in the 1950s and 1960s for infants with large ventricular septal defects as a measure to delay corrective surgery until the child grew older.[281–286] Drawbacks to pulmonary artery banding included a high hospital mortality of 16%, difficulty in adjusting the tightness of the band, and the need for a second surgery for adjusting the band. De-banding is not technically easy and is frequently more challenging than primary repair. The banding procedure may result in infundibular and valvular pulmonary stenosis, subaortic stenosis and migration

of the band to the pulmonary artery bifurcation. Restenosis of the pulmonary artery sometimes follows the de-banding operation.

Pulmonary artery banding may still be indicated with severe heart failure from Swiss cheese septum. A 3–4 mm wide silastic tape impregnated with Dacron is used. Distal pulmonary artery pressure should be less than 50% of systemic pressure with the band in place. The pulmonary artery band is usually left in place for 6 months, if left longer then reconstruction of the pulmonary artery is frequently necessary. Echocardiographically, the band appears as a bright white linear echo across the mid-portion of the main pulmonary artery. If the band moves forward, the pulmonary valve is often distorted and if the band slips backward the distal pulmonary artery is distorted. Tight bands often produce pulmonary valve prolapse, and poststenotic dilatation. It is often difficult to tell if the band has been removed echocardiographically, since a residual area of stenosis and echogenicity is still seen following removal of the band secondary to the scar tissue that remains. The pulmonary systolic pressure may be estimated with subtraction of the velocity across the band from the systolic arm blood pressure. In cases without left ventricular outflow tract obstruction, the right ventricular systolic pressure equals the systemic systolic blood pressure. Doppler detects a high velocity, mosaic jet distal to the band.

Atrial septostomy

The Blalock–Hanlon atrial septectomy operation may occasionally be performed in seriously ill neonates or infants with complex types of congenital heart disease, including complex types of transposition of the great vessels through a right lateral thoracotomy. Atrial septostomy may also be performed within the catheterization laboratory with a Rashkind procedure utilizing a balloon tipped catheter or by the Park procedure with blade atrial septostomy.

Echocardiographic assessment is basically the same as for any atrial septal defect. The diameter of the atrial opening should be measured and the direction and volume of the bi-directional shunting should be evaluated with pulsed and color flow Doppler. Left and right ventricular function should be assessed. The right and left atrium should be assessed for thrombus.

Systemic artery to pulmonary artery shunt

Systemic arterial to pulmonary artery shunts are usually performed to correct or control malformations producing decreased pulmonary blood flow such as tetralogy of

Fallot. These shunts are created surgically and interposed between the aorta and the pulmonary artery branches. Examples include the Waterson shunt, Potts shunt, central shunt and the Blalock–Taussig shunt.[287–291]

The Waterson shunt is created between the ascending aorta and the right pulmonary artery. The Potts shunt is created between the descending, thoracic aorta and the left pulmonary artery. The central shunt connects the ascending aorta with the main pulmonary artery. The Blalock–Taussig shunt connects the right subclavian artery to the right pulmonary artery. Occasionally a Blalock–Taussig shunt is created between the left subclavian artery and the left pulmonary artery, but is prone to shunt kinking.

Shunts are best visualized in the deep transgastric and upper esophageal views, using non-standard views. In all types of shunts, kinking of the shunt and the pulmonary artery should be identified. This may resemble constriction or distortion usually at the connection to the pulmonary artery. Color flow Doppler demonstrates high velocity mosaic flow in the shunt, which continues for a short distance into the pulmonary artery. Continuous wave Doppler may be obtained in the deep transgastric or high esophageal windows, and may be utilized to measure the velocity of the shunt flow to determine size of the shunt, the peak pressure gradient from the aorta to the pulmonary artery and the pulmonary artery pressure.

Right ventricular to pulmonary artery conduits

Today, shunts are usually created from cryopreserved aortic and pulmonary homograft incorporating a valve, which have largely replaced porcine heterografts and woven Dacron tube grafts.

Echocardiographically, all types of shunts appear highly echogenic in comparison to the normal cardiac structures, and the incorporated valves are usually difficult to visualize. Discrete areas of calcification within the shunt are frequently visualized, and do not always indicate obstruction of the conduit.

Over time, a neointimal layer of tissue lines the shunt, and may involve the valve and increases the velocity of flow detected in the shunt, as the internal caliber of the shunt decreases. With homograft shunts, stenosis is usually at the proximal and distal anastomotic sites.

Glenn shunt

The classic Glenn shunt was originally utilized for tricuspid atresia, created surgically by dividing and connecting the end of the superior vena cava to the side of the right pulmonary artery after division from the main pulmonary artery.[292–297] The modified 'bi-directional' Glenn shunt is produced by connecting the superior vena cava to the right pulmonary artery without dividing the pulmonary artery. The bi-directional Glenn shunt is thought to improve systemic oxygen saturation without significantly adding to the volume overload to the subaortic ventricle.

Transesophageal echocardiography demonstrates the right atrium with the stump of the divided superior vena cava in the biatrial view obtained from the mid-to-upper esophagus at 90°–115°. Rotation of the probe to the right, enables visualization of the direction and course of the superior vena cava and the anastomotic site of the superior vena cava to the right pulmonary artery. The size of the anastomosis and degree of obstruction of the anastomotic site should be assessed. The development of right lower lobe small pulmonary arteriovenous fistulae may occur as a complication of the classic Glenn shunt procedure. These fistulae are readily detected by echocardiography with the administration of agitated saline and the rapid appearance of bubbles in the left atrium from the right lower pulmonary vein. Contrast appearing in the right atrium may denote a collateral connection between the azygous vein and the inferior vena cava.

Atrial switch repairs

Atrial switch repairs were frequently performed for transposition of the great vessels, to direct venous return flow to the appropriate circulation. Initially the Senning technique was introduced, and a technically easier modification of the baffle procedure was accomplished with the Mustard technique. In the Senning technique, a septal flap is constructed to direct the blood flow from the pulmonary veins to the right atrium. The Mustard technique utilizes a baffle created from pericardial tissue with excision of the true atrial septum. With refinement of the arterial switch procedure, the atrial switch repairs are performed less frequently.

Echocardiographically, both the pulmonary venous flow and the superior and inferior vena cava are identified and followed through the heart to assess postoperative caval obstruction or pulmonary venous obstruction.[298–301] Surgically produced obstruction is most commonly noted as narrowing at the superior vena caval–right atrial junction and at the pulmonary venous inflow area. The baffle is interrogated for obstruction or leak, with the notation of residual atrial shunting, which is the rule. Obstruction of the atrial baffle is demonstrated with color flow or conventional Doppler as turbulent, biphasic or continuous flow within the pulmonary or systemic venous atrium. The presence and severity of tricuspid regurgitation should be assessed which is usually trivial or mild, tricuspid regurgitation is rarely severe. It is important to assess right ventricular function although progression of right ventricular failure is uncommon.

Arterial switch repairs

The Jatene or arterial switch procedure with re-implantation of the coronary arteries to the ascending aorta is currently the operation of choice in patients for transposition of the great arteries.[302–305] The procedure is most successful when there is no coexistent left ventricular outflow tract obstruction. The aorta and pulmonary artery are transected and a 'button' attachment of the coronary arteries is performed attaching them to the aorta. Following the removal of the coronary arteries, the pulmonary artery is patched. This procedure produces a great artery orientation with pulmonary artery anteriorly and the aorta posteriorly. Echocardiographically, the pulmonary artery and branches should be assessed for normal flow velocity, to rule out obstruction. Obstruction most commonly occurs with the pulmonary anastomosis, and kinking may result in distortion of the left or right pulmonary arteries due to the anastomosis. The re-implanted coronary arteries should be assessed for unobstructed flow, regional wall motion abnormality or worsening left ventricular function suggesting abnormal coronary flow. The presence and severity of aortic valvular regurgitation should be noted, along with right and left ventricular dilatation and dysfunction.

Fontan

In tricuspid atresia and malformations producing a single ventricle or univentricular heart, systemic caval blood flow is directed to the pulmonary artery through a total cavopulmonary connection, so that the single ventricle serves as a systemic pump only. Essentially the main pulmonary artery segment to the right pulmonary artery is removed and ligated. The right superior vena cava is subdivided and both ends are sewn in an interposed fashion to the right pulmonary artery. An intra-atrial baffle is created from inferior vena cava to the right pulmonary artery.

Echocardiographically,[306–314] this repair produces biphasic pulmonary artery flow, and the right pulmonary artery dimension increases. The superior and inferior

vena cava should be interrogated with pulsed and color flow Doppler, to detect baffle stenosis and baffle leaks. The atrial septum should be assessed for septal shunt. In certain patients an adjustable atrial septal shunt is created and adjusted in the early postoperative period under the direction of echocardiography and color flow Doppler or agitated saline contrast. The proximal pulmonary artery is assessed for obstruction from distortion or thrombosis, which is visualized in both short-axis and long-axis views with transesophageal echocardiography. The thickness and function of the single ventricle should be noted.

Rastelli procedure

The Rastelli procedure is performed in patients with truncus arteriosus or transposition with a ventricular septal defect and pulmonary stenosis. A ventricular–pulmonary artery conduit with an external valve is placed between the right ventricle and the main pulmonary artery. The external conduit is composed of a woven double velour Dacron tubular graft with a homograft valve. Right ventricular blood flow is routed through a surgically created intraventricular conduit or tunnel extending through the ventricular septal defect and directed to the aorta.

Echocardiographically, the external valve conduit is assessed for obstruction and the incorporated valve for regurgitation with color and conventional Doppler. The pressure gradient may be determined with the usual Doppler technique. The external valve conduit and the intraventricular conduit are assessed for thrombus formation and pseudoaneurysm formation. Due to the composition of the external conduit, both horizontal and longitudinal views obtained with transesophageal echocardiography are frequently required for a complete analysis. The functioning atrioventricular valve is assessed for the development and/or the severity of regurgitation.

Damus–Kaye–Stansel

The Damus–Kaye–Stansel procedure[183] is performed in single ventricle with subaortic obstruction or transposition of the great vessel with a ventricular septal defect and pulmonary valve stenosis. A window is created between aorta and pulmonary artery, by anastomosis of the proximal pulmonary artery to the side of the aorta. The proximal aorta is over sewn above the aortic valve and a patch is applied to the ventricular septal defect when present. An external valved conduit is placed between the right ventricle and the distal main pulmonary artery. Echocardiographically the severity of pulmonary insufficiency is assessed, along with the integrity of the septal defect patch, and the flow is assessed for obstruction of the external conduit anastomotic site.

Case 9.1

Secundum atrial septal defect. (a) Moderate size atrial septal defect as demonstrated from the bicaval view at 95°. (b, c) Corresponding color flow Doppler frame demonstrating left-to-right shunt flow (arrow) directed into the right atrium. (d) Two-dimensional image from a modified bicaval view advancing the probe with mild retroflexion demonstrating the tricuspid valve orifice and mild prolapse (arrow) with the corresponding color flow Doppler image (e) demonstrating tricuspid regurgitation (open arrow). This view is particularly useful for convention Doppler interrogation of the tricuspid regurgitant jet and estimation of the pulmonary artery systolic pressure since the jet is presented in a parallel orientation in the imaging sector as well as differentiating a tricuspid regurgitant jet from atrial shunt flow. (f) Pulsed Doppler image of the left-to-right shunt flow jet demonstrating flow during systole and diastole. RA, right atrium; LA, left atrium; RV, right ventricle; SVC, superior vena cava.

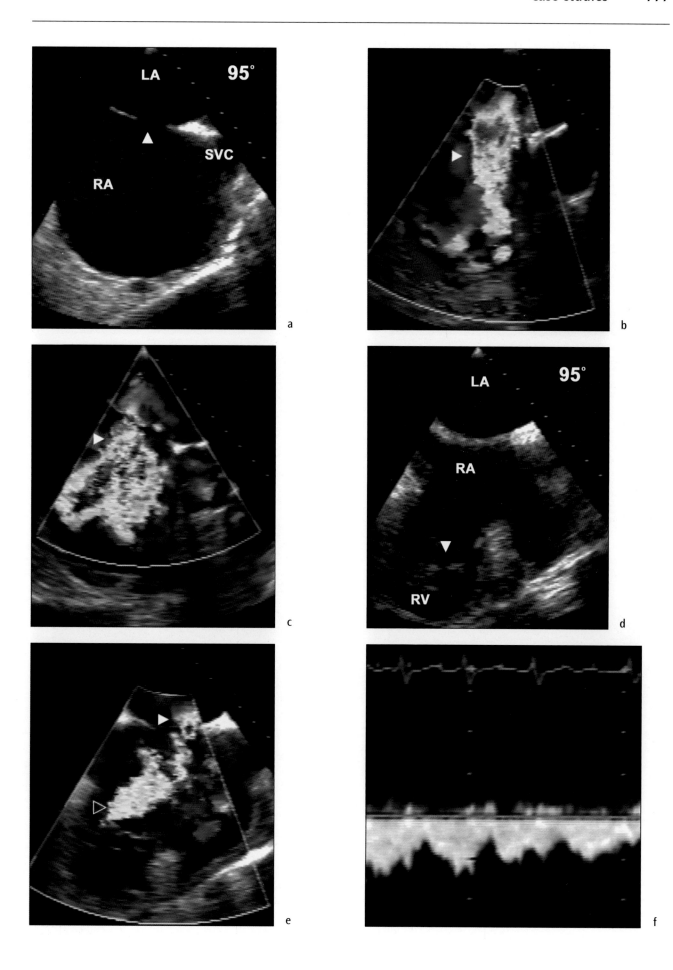

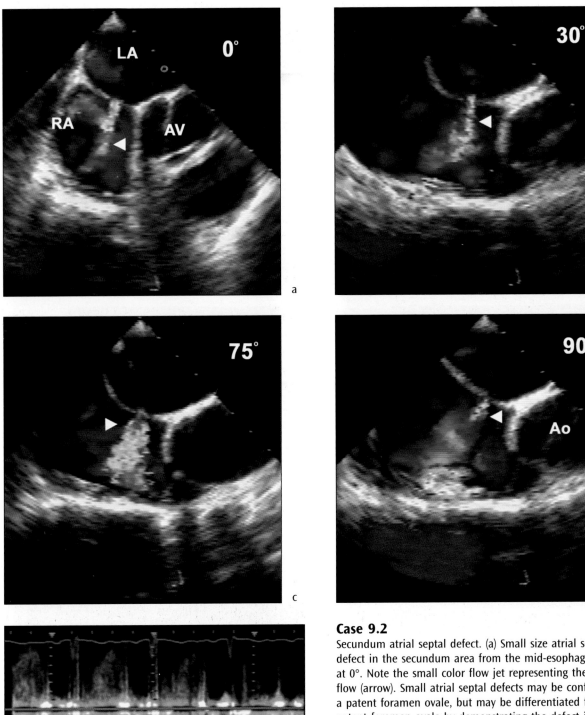

Case 9.2

Secundum atrial septal defect. (a) Small size atrial septal defect in the secundum area from the mid-esophageal window at 0°. Note the small color flow jet representing the shunt flow (arrow). Small atrial septal defects may be confused with a patent foramen ovale, but may be differentiated from a patent foramen ovale by demonstrating the defect in the atrial septum. (b) Color flow Doppler obtained at 30°, (c) 75°, and (d) 90° demonstrating the shunt jet with multiplane echocardiography. In addition to demonstrating the shunt flow, the size of the septal defect may be appreciated from multiple views, note the defect varies in shape when visualized from different angles. (e) Pulsed Doppler of the atrial shunt flow, atrial shunt flow begins in mid-systole (arrow), peaking in early diastole, before slowly decreasing to mid-diastole. The flow velocity increases again with atrial systole and ends in early systole frequently with minor flow reversal. RA, right atrium; LA, left atrium; AV, aortic valve; Ao, aorta.

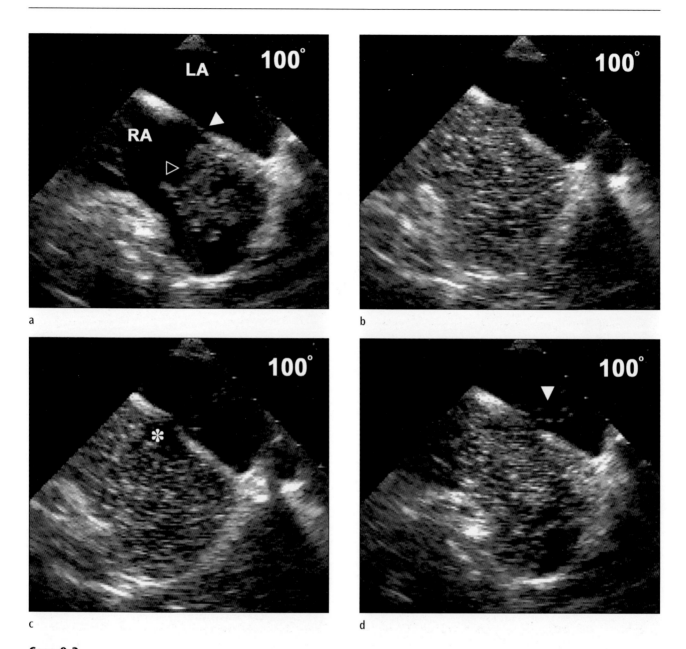

Case 9.3

Secundum atrial septal defect. In addition to color flow Doppler an atrial shunt may be demonstrated with a saline contrast injection. (a–d) A moderate size secundum atrial defect is demonstrated during the cardiac cycle in a modified bicaval view at 100°. Contrast is seen initially entering the right atrium from the superior vena cava (a), and totally fills the right atrium (b). (c) Once the right atrium is filled with contrast a negative contrast image is produced by the left-to-right shunt flow (star) in close proximity to the anatomical defect in the atrial septum. (d) With reversal of the shunt flow a small right-to-left shunt is depicted as contrast entering the left atrium (arrow). LA, left atrium; RA, right atrium.

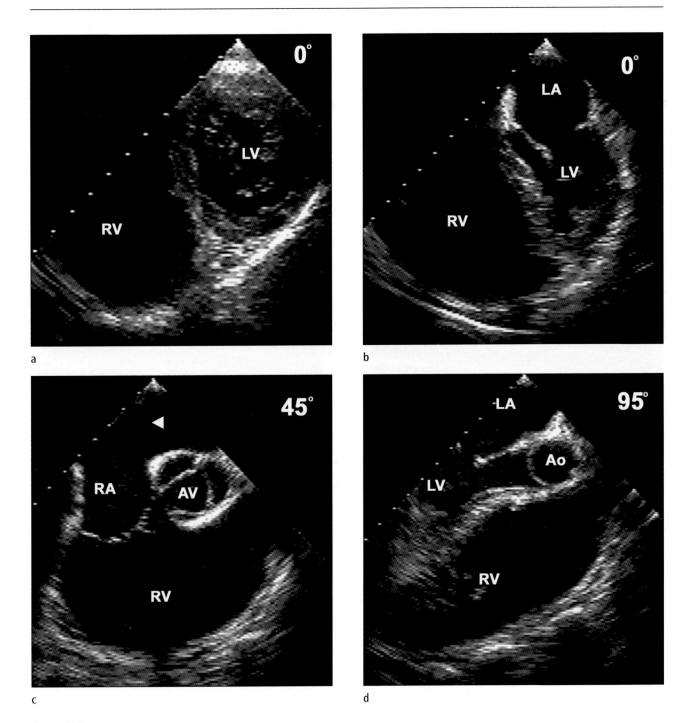

Case 9.4

Secundum atrial septal defect. Large secundum atrial septal defect. Right ventricular enlargement develops as sequelae of significant shunting and is demonstrated in multiple views. (a) Transgastric short-axis view at 0° of the ventricular chambers, (b) Lower esophageal four-chamber view at 0°, (c) mid-esophageal view at 45° with visualization of the atrial septal defect (arrow), and (d) mid-esophageal view at 90°. The defect which comprises the majority of the atrial septum is appreciated in multiple views with and without color flow Doppler.

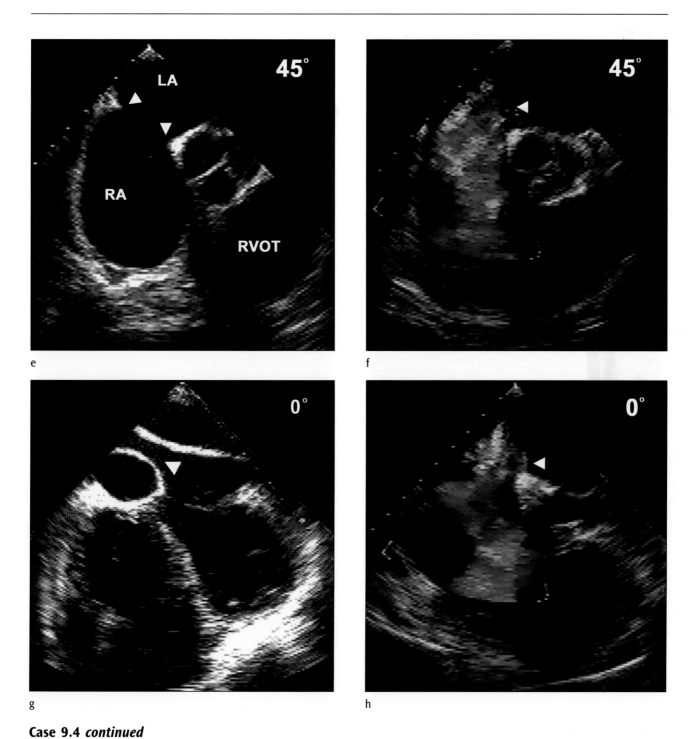

e

f

g

h

Case 9.4 *continued*
(e, f) Upper esophageal window at 45°. (g, h) Lower esophageal window four-chamber view at 0°. RA, right atrium; LA, left atrium; LV, left ventricle; RV, right ventricle; Ao, aorta; AV, aortic valve; RVOT, right ventricular outflow tract.

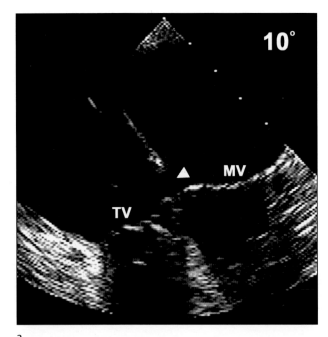

a

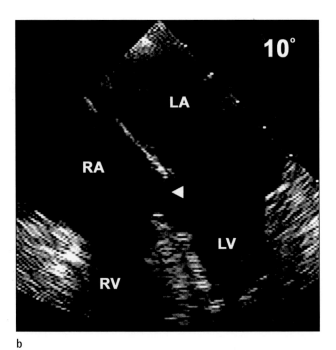

b

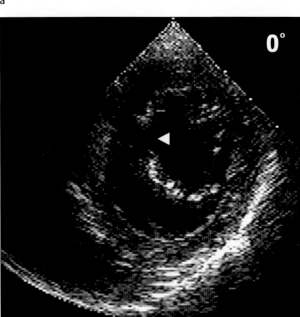

c

Case 9.5

Ostium primum atrial septal defect. (a) Four-chamber view at 10° demonstrating an ostium primum atrial defect as a lack of continuity of the atrial septum with the superior portion of the cardiac crux. The usual offset of the tricuspid and mitral valve is missing both the tricuspid and mitral valve annulus lie in the same plane due to the defect in systole.

(b) Diastolic frame in the same view. Cleft defects of the atrioventricular valves are frequently associated with ostium primum defects, are frequently associated with significant regurgitation and are readily demonstrated with multiplane transesophageal echocardiography (TEE). (c) In the short-axis transgastric view at 0° a cleft (arrow) is demonstrated in the anterior mitral leaflet.

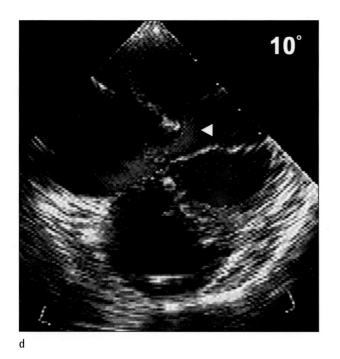

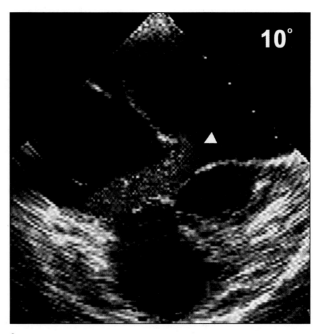

d

e

Case 9.5 *continued*

(d, e) Color Doppler frames from the four-chamber view
demonstrating atrial shunt flow in a left-to-right direction.
TV, tricuspid valve; MV, mitral valve. LA, left atrium; RA, right
atrium; LV, left ventricle; RV, right ventricle.

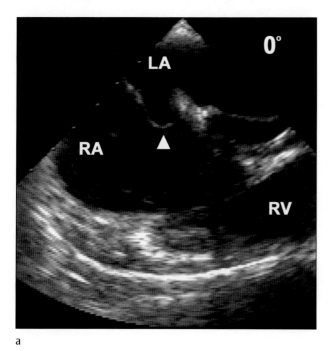

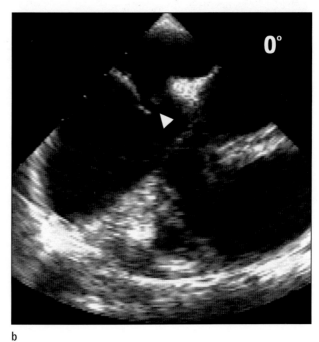

a

b

Case 9.6

Atrial septal aneurysm and a moderate secundum defect. Multiplane TEE frequently demonstrates floppy margins to the septal
defect denoting associated atrial septal aneurysm. (a, b) Mid-esophageal four-chamber view at 0° demonstrating floppy redundant
atrial septal tissue surrounding the margins of the defect (arrow) during the cardiac cycle.

continued

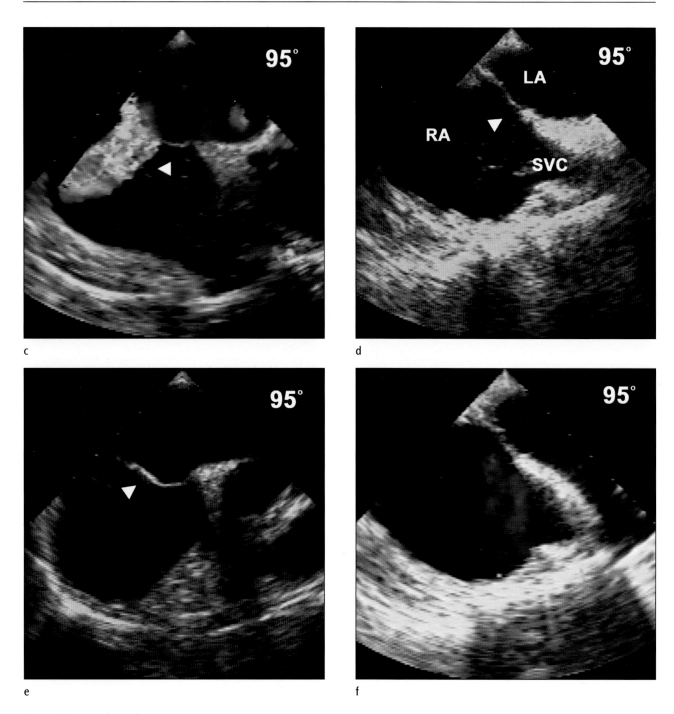

Case 9.6 *continued*

(c) Color flow Doppler of left-to-right atrial shunt flow through the defect. (d–f) Postoperative TEE imaging demonstrating an atrial surgical patch denoted as a thicker, echogenic structure in the region of the atrial septum. (f) Color flow Doppler demonstrating an intact atrial septal surgical patch. RA, right atrium; LA, left atrium; RV, right ventricle; SVC, superior vena cava.

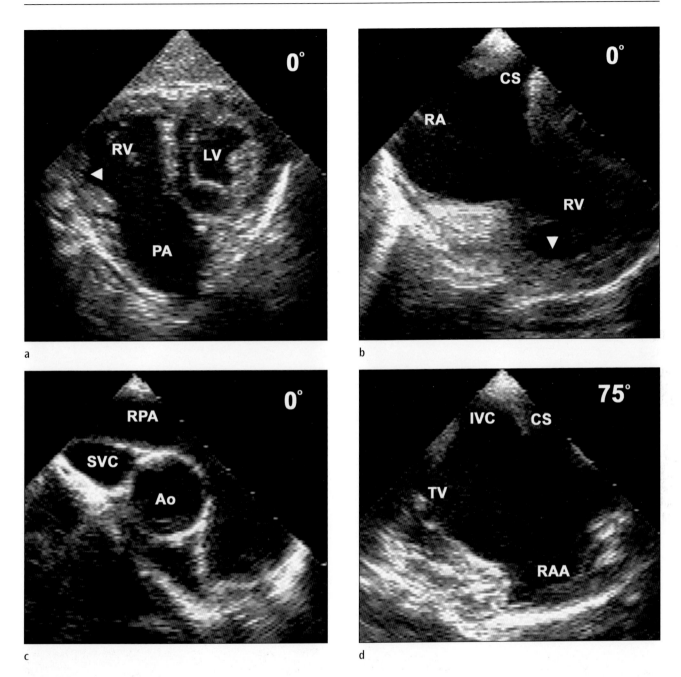

a

b

c

d

Case 9.7

Superior-type, sinus-Venosus atrial septal defect. The hallmark of the diagnosis of the superior type is the lack of superior septal tissue adjacent to the wall of the pulmonary artery, which differentiates it from a superiorly placed secundum atrial septal defect. The lack of the superior fatty limbus attachment of the septum produces an echocardiographic appearance of the orifice of the superior vena cava overriding or centered above both the left and right atrium. (a) Transgastric short-axis view at 0°, (b) four-chamber view at 0°, (c) upper esophageal window short-axis view at the base of the heart at 0° and (d) at 75° demonstrates enlargement of the right ventricle and main pulmonary artery with right ventricular hypertrophy (arrow).

continued

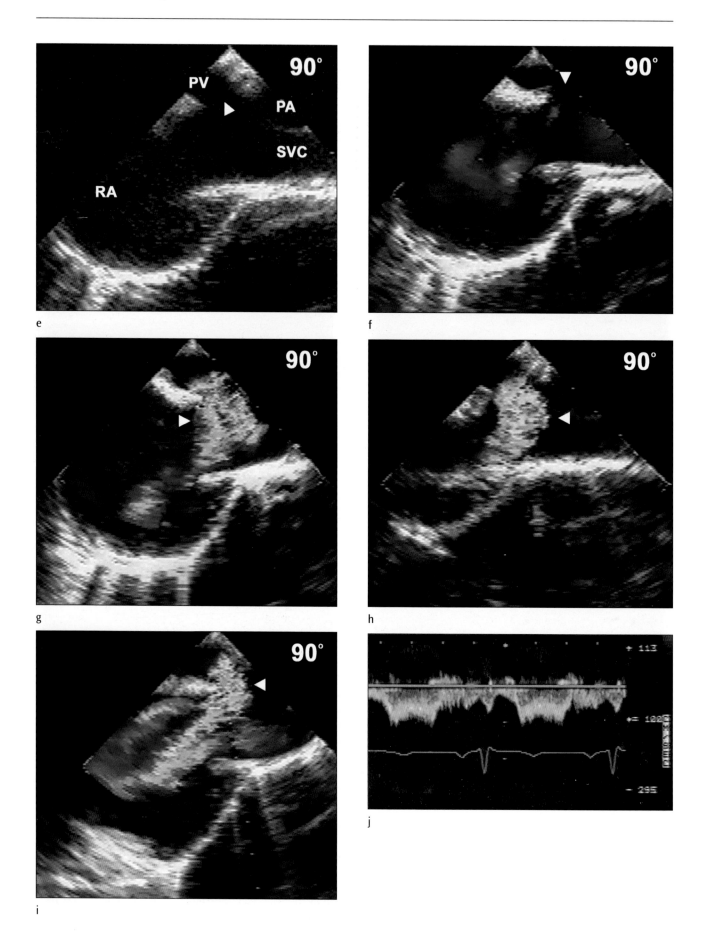

Case 9.7 *continued*

(e) Upper esophageal bicaval view at 90° demonstrates a defect near the origin of the superior vena cava and the right upper pulmonary vein. (f–i) Color flow Doppler demonstrating a left-to-right shunt through the sinus of Venosus defect during the cardiac cycle with multiplane TEE. (j) Pulsed Doppler flow interrogation of the sinus venosus shunt. RV, right ventricle; LV, left ventricle; PA, pulmonary artery; Ao, aorta; CS, coronary sinus; RPA, right pulmonary artery; SVC, superior vena cava; IVC, inferior vena cava; TV, tricuspid valve; RA, right atrium; PV, pulmonary vein; RAA, right atrial appendage.

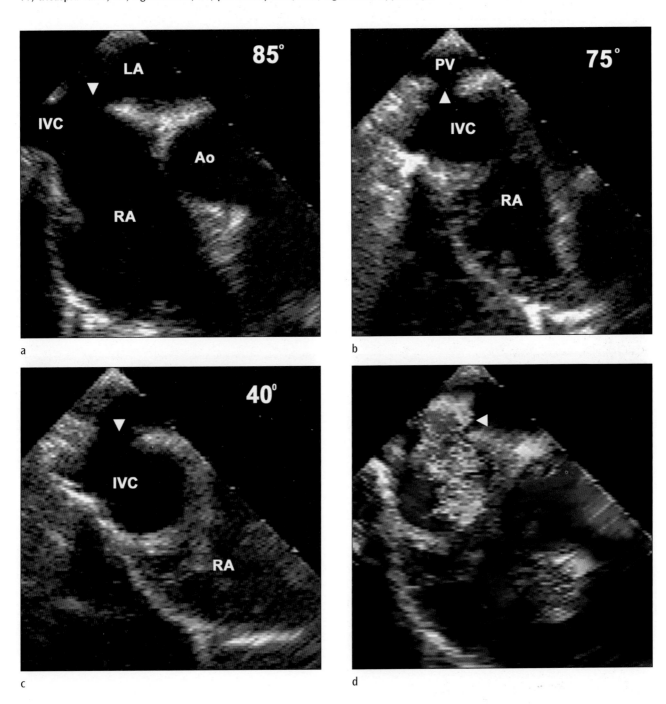

Case 9.8

Inferior-type, sinus of Venosus atrial septal defect. (a) Mid-esophageal window of a modified four-chamber view at 85° and (b) and (c) at 75° obtained with rotation of the probe clockwise to visualize the orifice of the inferior vena cava demonstrates a defect (arrow) in the inferior portion of the venosus area in close proximity to the inferior vena cava. (d) Color flow Doppler demonstration of the atrial shunt flow in a left-to-right direction of an inferior-type sinus of Venosus atrial septal defect. RA, right atrium; IVC, inferior vena cava; PV, pulmonary vein; LA, left atrium; Ao, aorta.

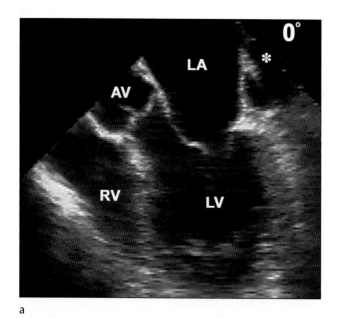

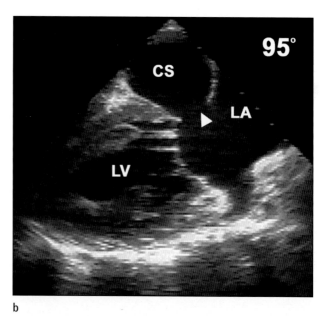

a   b

Case 9.9

Coronary sinus atrial septal defect. (a) Lower esophageal window five-chamber view at 0° demonstrating an echolucent structure (star) near the left atrial appendage representing a left superior vena cava. The increased flow to the coronary sinus from left superior vena cava produces dilatation of the sinus making it prominent, aiding in its detection during imaging. Echocardiographically, the small defect in the coronary sinus is usually, easily appreciated with the edges of the defect freely vibrating, in views demonstrating the posterior left atrial wall. (b) Lower esophageal window two-chamber view at 95° demonstrating an enlarged coronary sinus with a defect (arrow) which emptied into the left atrium. AV, aortic valve; RV, right ventricle; LV, left ventricle; LA, left atrium; CS, coronary sinus.

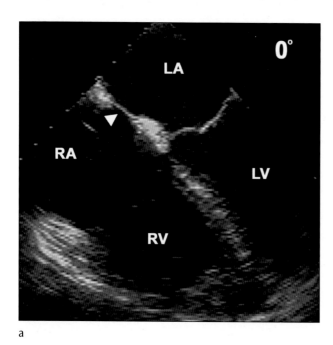

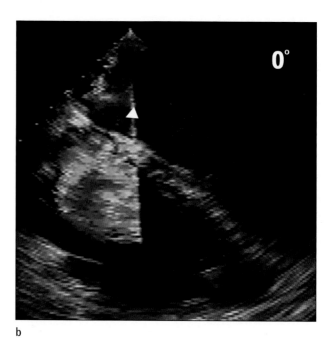

a   b

Case 9.10

Postoperative secundum surgical repair. Atrial septal defects are surgically closed by direct closure or by placement of a patch. The resolution of right heart dilatation and pulmonary hypertension is usually related to the preoperative size of the defect and the age at which it was repaired. In contrast to surgical closure of atrial septal defects in children, right heart dimensions do not usually normalize postoperatively, but should substantially decrease in the majority of adult patients. (a) Four-chamber view at 0° demonstrating an atrial septal surgical patch denoted as the bright echogenic area of thickening of the atrial septum (arrow). (b) Corresponding color Doppler image demonstrating surgical patch integrity.

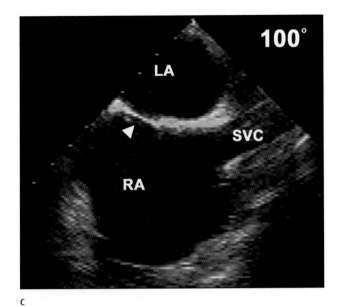

c

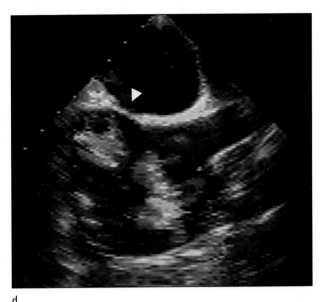

d

Case 9.10 *continued*

(c) Bicaval view at 100° demonstrating atrial septal surgical patch (arrow). LA, left atrium; RA, right atrium; LV, left ventricle; RV, right ventricle; SVC, superior vena cava.

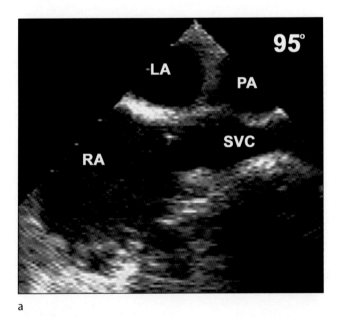

a

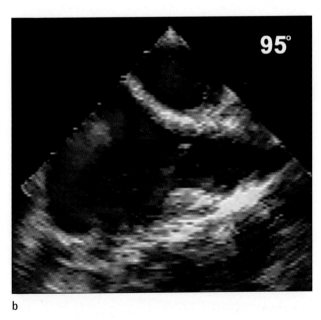

b

Case 9.11

Postoperative sinus Venosus atrial septal defect surgical repair. Interrogation of the repair of a sinus venosus atrial septal defect requires meticulous inspection of the repair site due to the numerous surrounding structures that may be falsely labeled as a defect. Multiplane TEE provides the necessary views in order to determine thoroughly the success of the repair and the absence of anomalous venous return. (a) Standard bicaval view and modified views (b–f) demonstrating a successful surgical repair of a sinus venosus defect. RA, right atrium; LA, left atrium; SVC, superior vena cava; PA, pulmonary artery; PV, pulmonary vein; arrow, surgical repair.

continued

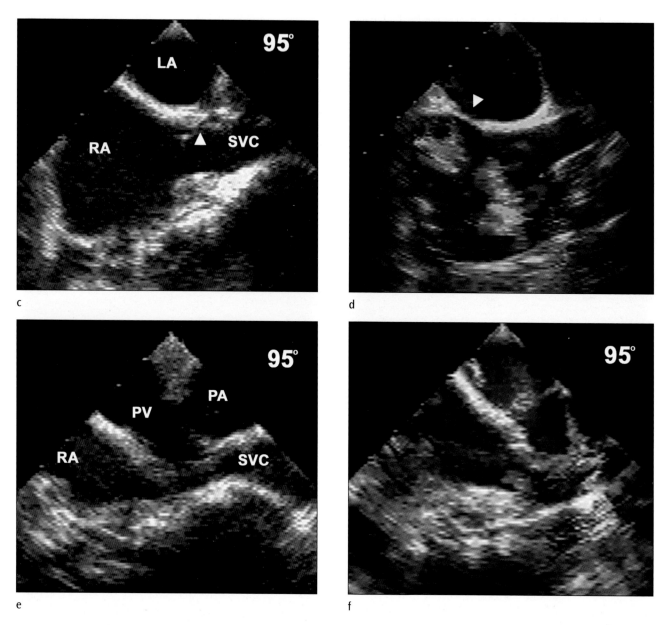

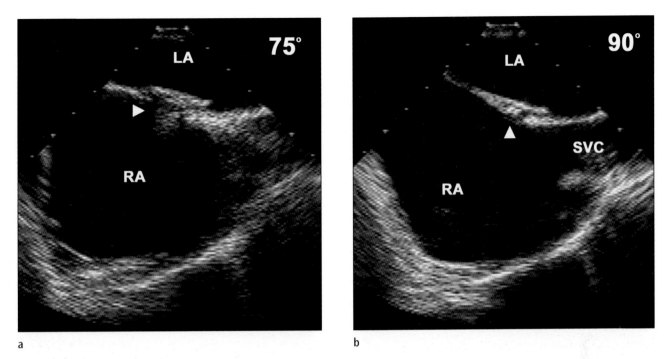

a   b

Case 9.12
Atrial septal defect closure device. (a) Bi-atrial view at 75° and (b) bicaval view at 90° demonstrating proper position and appearance of an atrial septal closure device of a secundum atrial septal defect. LA, left atrium; RA, right atrium; SVC, superior vena cava.

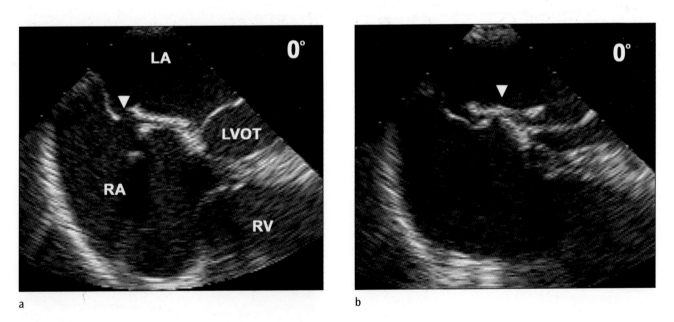

a   b

Case 9.13
Atrial septal defect closure device. (a, b) Mid-esophageal window in a modified four-chamber view demonstrating malalignment of an atrial septal closure device (arrow) with the atrial septal defect due to strut fracture.

continued

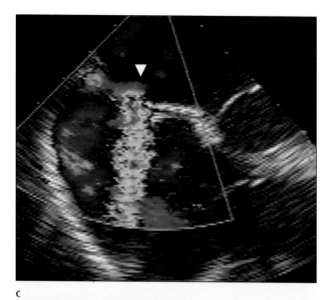

c

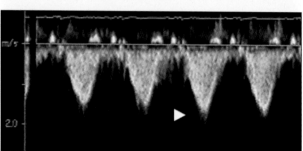

d

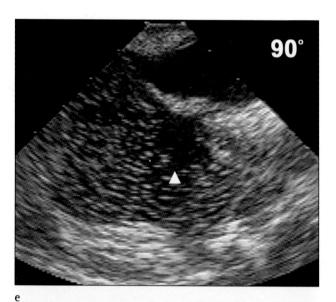

e

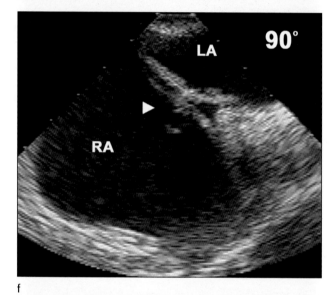

f

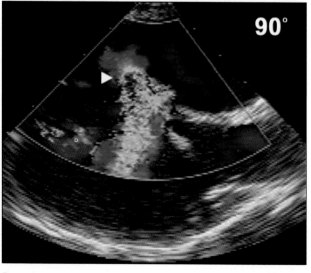

g

Case 9.13 *continued*

(c) Color flow Doppler demonstration and (d) pulsed Doppler interrogation of atrial shunt flow (arrow) in a left-to-right orientation through the malpositioned atrial septal closure device. (e) Bicaval view with saline echocardiographic contrast, with negative contrast in the vicinity of the closure device. (f, g) Bicaval view at 90° demonstrating the malposition of the closure device and color flow Doppler demonstration of residual atrial shunt flow. LA, left atrium; RA, right atrium; RV, right ventricle; LVOT, left ventricular outflow tract.

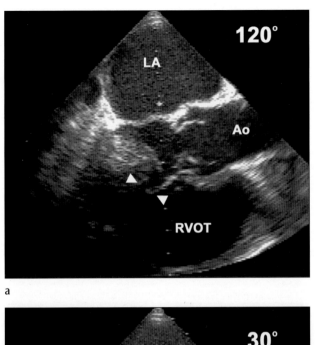

a

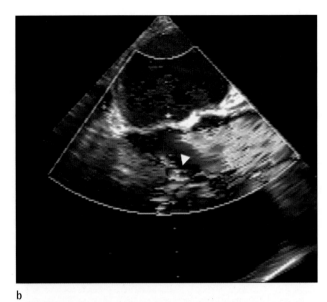

b

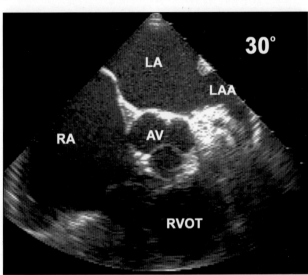

c

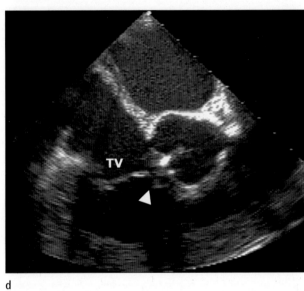

d

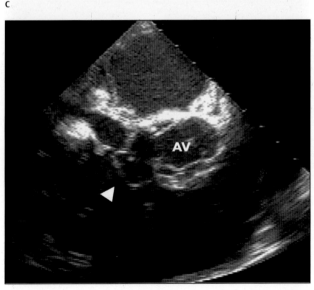

e

Case 9.14

Perimembranous ventricular septal defect. (a, b) Defects in the vicinity of the membranous septum are usually easily seen in the longitudinal view at 120° with imaging and color flow Doppler, once the defect is documented then the other views obtained with multiplane TEE are helpful for determining the exact position of the ventricular septal defect. (c) Short-axis view of the base of the heart at 30° illustrating the aortic valve. This view helps place the defect in the membranous, infracristal or supracristal region of the septum. (d, e) With minor rotation of the probe the tricuspid valve septal leaflet is well visualized, and exhibits redundant tissue (arrow) outlining the defect which is referred to as a septal aneurysm.

continued

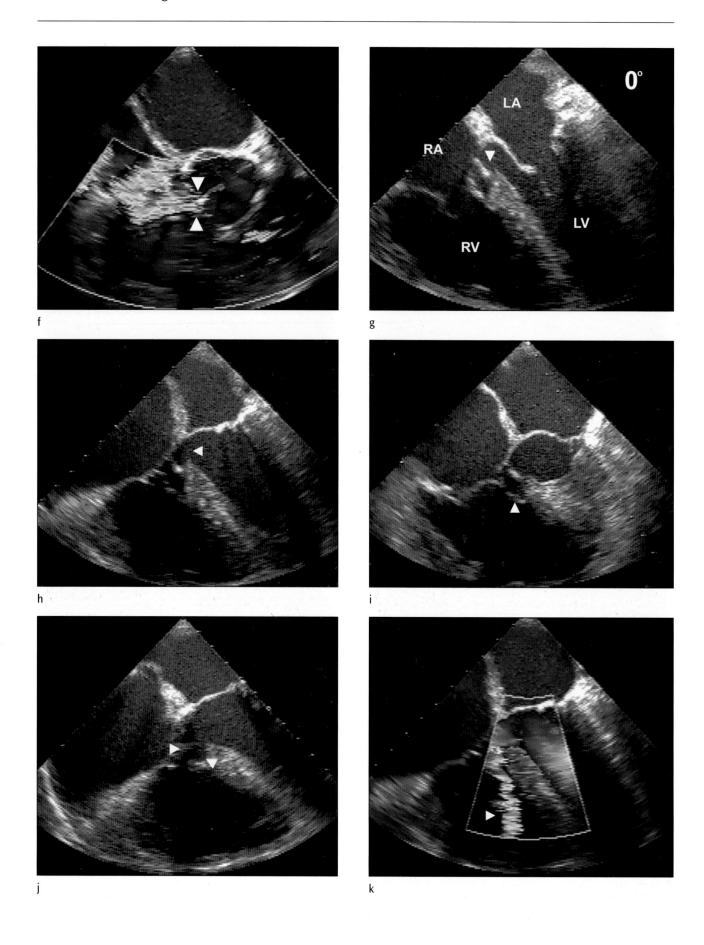

f

g

h

i

j

k

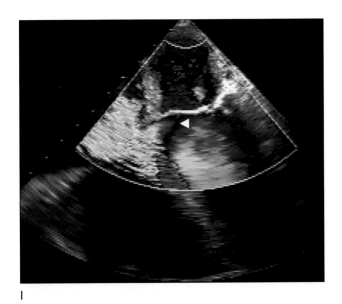

l

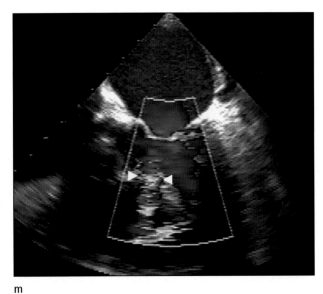

m

Case 9.14 continued

(f) Color flow Doppler is utilized to demonstrate shunt flow through the defect. (g, h) Four-chamber view at 0° demonstrates septal dropout in the vicinity of the ventricular septum in the region of the cardiac crux. In many cases documentation of the defect is not always easy in this view due to the thinness of the ventricular septum in this area. (i–m) Minor rotation of the TEE probe to the right with mild advancement orients the ventricular septum at the internal cardiac crux in a near perpendicular presentation delineating the defect (arrow) with imaging and demonstrating shunt flow (arrow) with color flow Doppler. In addition shunt flow may be delineated from tricuspid regurgitation (k) which may result from an associated cleft in the tricuspid leaflets, involvement of the tricuspid septal leaflet with aneurysm formation or in shunts that lie above the plane of the septal tricuspid annulus plane (pars atrioventricularis type). LA, left atrium; RA, right atrium; Ao, aorta; AV, aortic valve; RVOT, right ventricular outflow tract; LAA, left atrial appendage; TV, tricuspid valve; LV, left ventricle; RV, right ventricle.

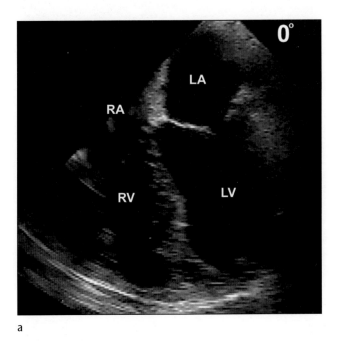

a

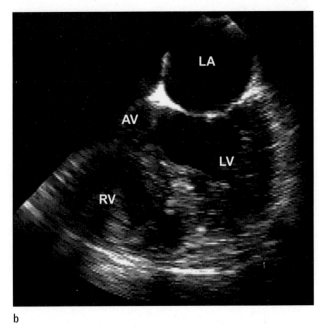

b

Case 9.15

Moderate perimembranous ventricular septal defect. (a) Four-chamber view of the heart from the low esophageal window demonstrating an intact appearing ventricular septum with imaging. (b) Orienting the probe to a five-chamber view with the aortic valve again demonstrates an intact septum.

continued

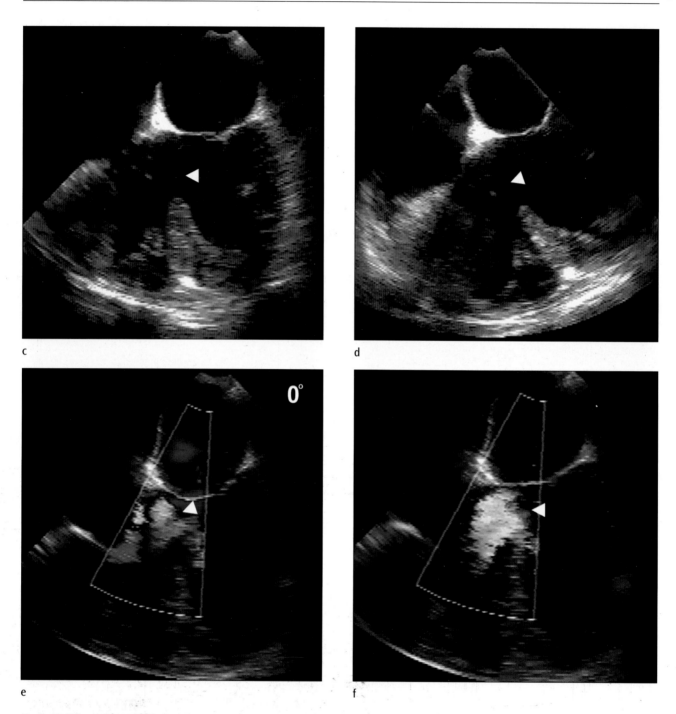

c

d

0°

e

f

Case 9.15 *continued*

(c, d) Midway between the four-chamber and five-chamber view demonstrate a moderate size defect (arrow) with mild rotation of the probe to the right. (e–g) Color flow Doppler demonstrates shunt flow (arrow) through the area of the defect through the cardiac cycle.

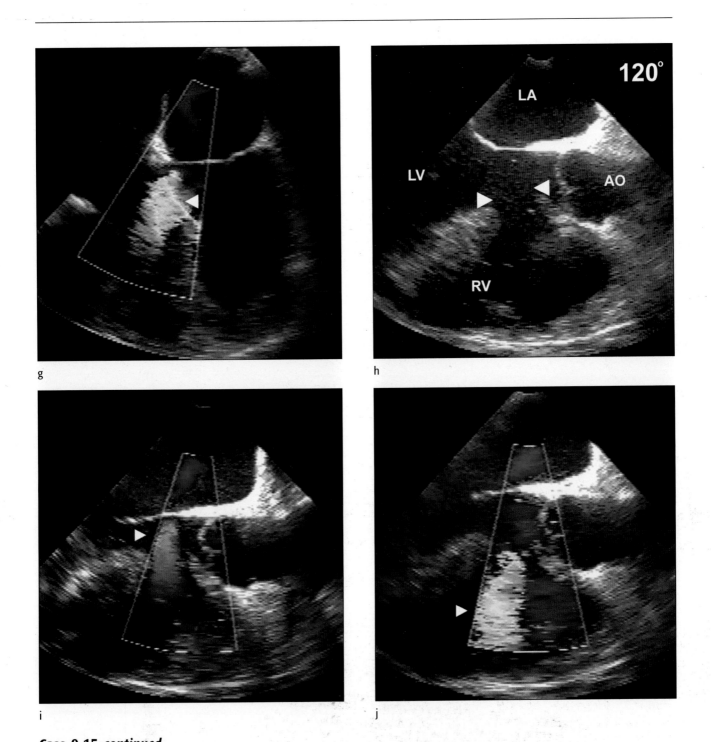

g

h

i

j

Case 9.15 *continued*

(h) Longitudinal view at 120° demonstrates both the superior and inferior borders (arrows) in the ventricular septum. (i, j) Color flow Doppler demonstrates shunt flow in the longitudinal views during the cardiac cycle which presents the shunt flow jet in a parallel orientation in this view for interrogation with conventional Doppler. Although not usually necessary for demonstrating shunt flow due to the multiple imaging planes and excellent resolution, saline echocardiographic contrast may be utilized.

continued

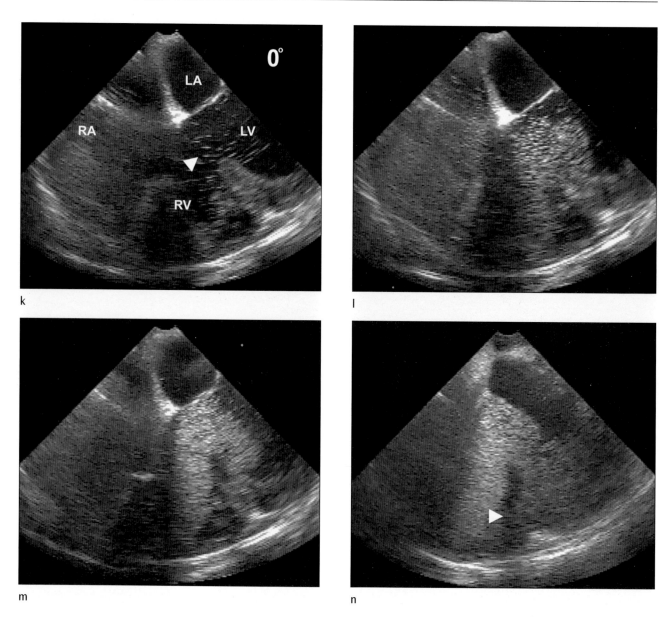

Case 9.15 *continued*

(k–n) Saline contrast injection in the modified four-chamber view at 0°. Bubbles are demonstrated crossing the defect following opacification of the right heart chambers demonstrating flow in a right-to-left direction. (n) Negative contrast (arrow) is demonstrated with opacification demonstrating the predominant left-to-right shunt. RA, right atrium; LA, left atrium; RV, right ventricle; LV, left ventricle; AV, aortic valve; Ao, aorta.

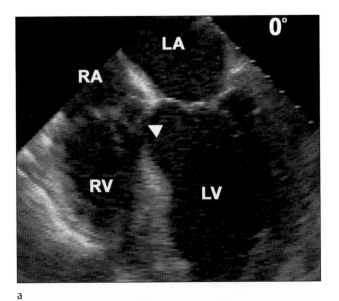

a

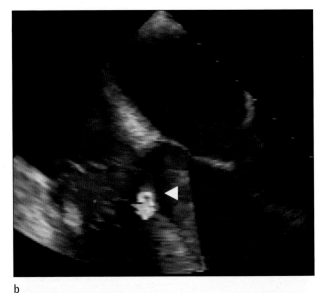

b

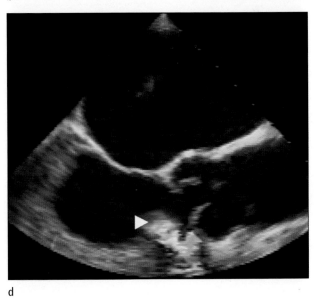

c

d

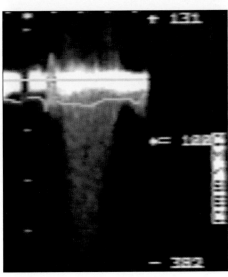

e

Case 9.16

Small perimembranous ventricular septal defect with tricuspid valve cleft. (a) Four-chamber view at 0° demonstrates a small defect (arrow) in the ventricular septum. (b) Color flow Doppler demonstrates a small left-to-right shunt jet through the defect. (c, d) Small defect noted inferior to the aortic valve in a longitudinal projection at 95° with imaging and color flow Doppler. Note the flow convergence of the shunt jet on the left ventricular septal surface. (e) Continuous wave Doppler demonstrates a systolic jet (3.82 m/second).

continued

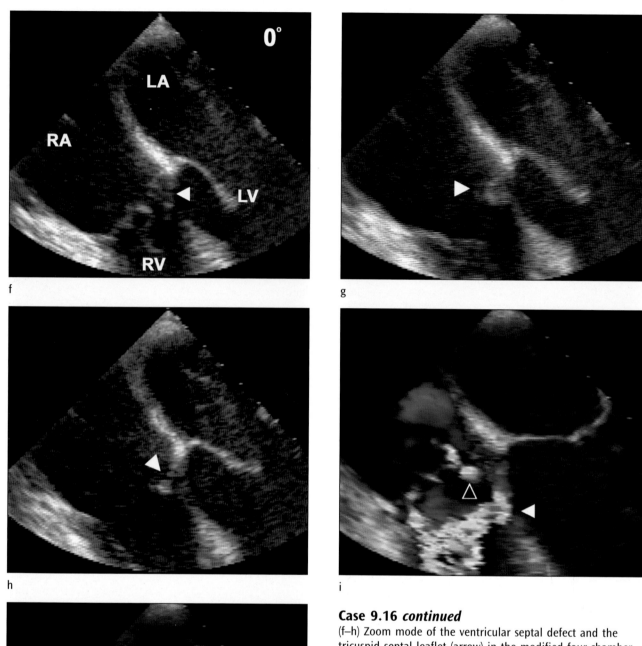

Case 9.16 *continued*

(f–h) Zoom mode of the ventricular septal defect and the tricuspid septal leaflet (arrow) in the modified four-chamber view at 0°. (h–j) A cleft (arrow) is demonstrated within the tricuspid septal leaflet with a tricuspid regurgitant jet through the cleft (arrow) with color flow Doppler. LA, left atrium; LV, left ventricle; RA, right atrium; RV, right ventricle; LVOT, left ventricular outflow tract; Ao, aorta.

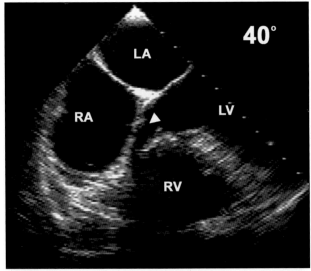

a

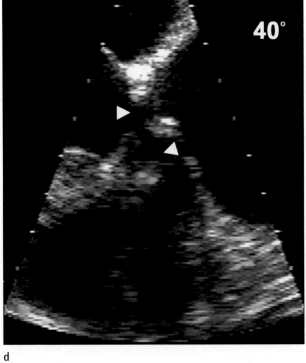

b

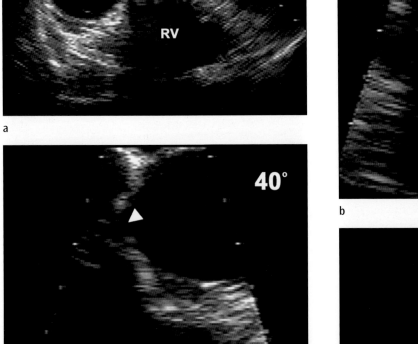

c

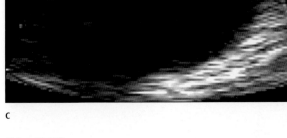

d

Case 9.17
Small perimembranous ventricular septal defect. (a) Small perimembranous ventricular septal defect visualized from the modified four-chamber view. The defect exhibits jagged edges (arrow) in zoom mode (b–c). (d) With further mild rotation of the probe a pars atrioventricularis defect is noted.

continued

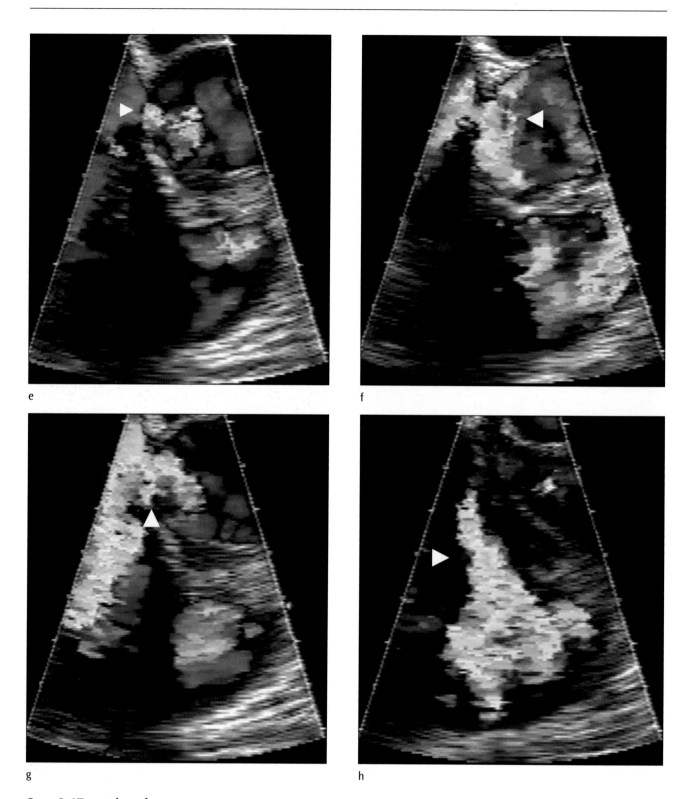

e

f

g

h

Case 9.17 *continued*

(e–g) Color flow Doppler demonstrates shunt flow (arrow) from the left ventricle to the right atrium. Care must be taken to identify shunt flow of this type and not to mistake the shunt flow with a pars atrioventricularis defect with tricuspid regurgitation. (h) Shunt flow (arrow) is also demonstrated from the left ventricle to the right ventricle with color flow Doppler. LA, left atrium; RA, right atrium; RV, right ventricle; LV, left ventricle.

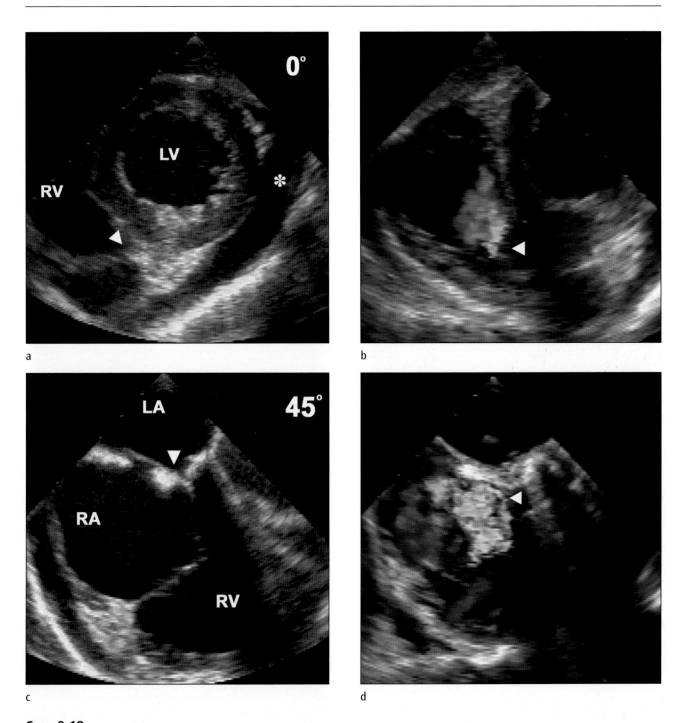

Case 9.18

Small ventricular septal defect. A small residual ventricular septal defect is detected following repair of a perimembranous ventricular septal defect and an atrial septal defect. (a) Short-axis gastric view demonstrating a surgical ventricular septal patch (arrow). Note a small pericardial effusion (star) is also demonstrated. (b) Color flow Doppler demonstrates a small left to right shunt (arrow). (c) Modified four-chamber view at 45° demonstrating the atrial septal surgical patch and defect in the ventricular septum. (d) Color flow Doppler demonstrating associated tricuspid regurgitation.

continued

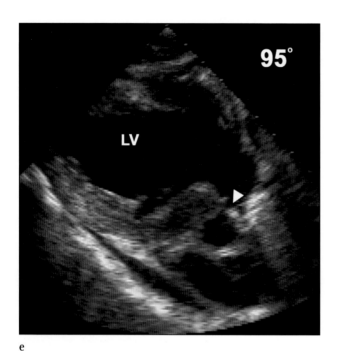

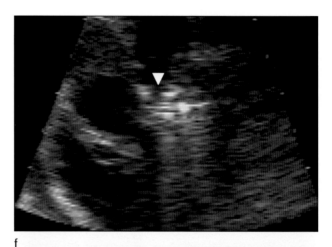

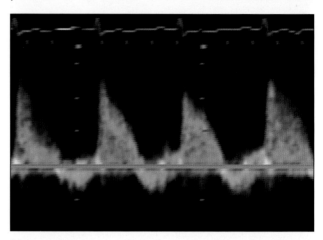

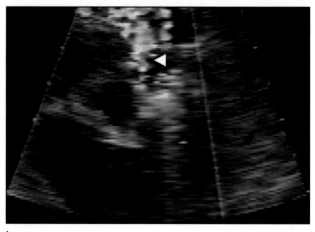

Case 9.18 *continued*

(e) Imaging from the gastric window at 95° demonstrates the ventricular septal surgical patch in more detail. (f) Zoom mode demonstrating the residual defect which was repaired from the right side. (g, h) Continuous wave and color flow Doppler of the residual ventricular shunt (arrow). LA, left atrium; RA, right atrium; RV, right ventricle; LV, left ventricle.

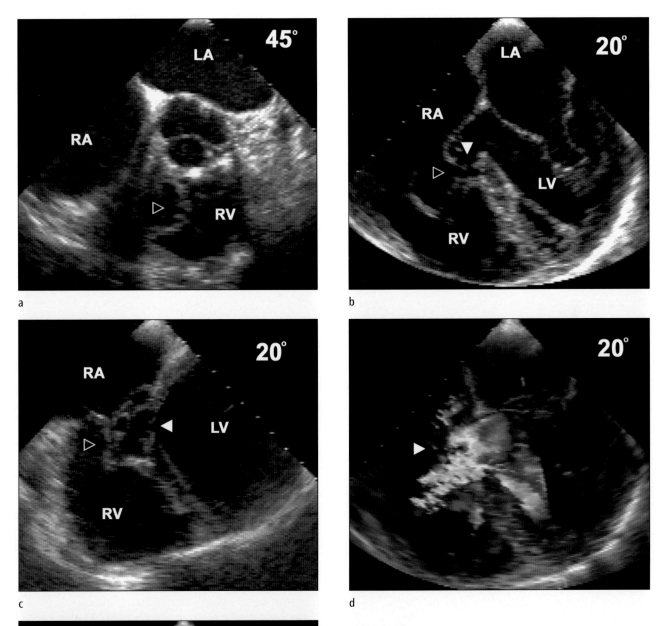

Case 9.19

Ventricular septal aneurysm. (a) Short-axis view of the base of the heart at the aortic valve level at 45°. Redundant tissue (arrow) from closure of a membranous ventricular septal defect. (b, c) Modified four-chamber view demonstrating the typical appearance of a ventricular septal aneurysm (closed arrow). Tricuspid valvular tissue involved in the aneurysm (open arrow). (d, e) Color flow Doppler demonstrating mild tricuspid regurgitation and small residual shunting (arrow).

continued

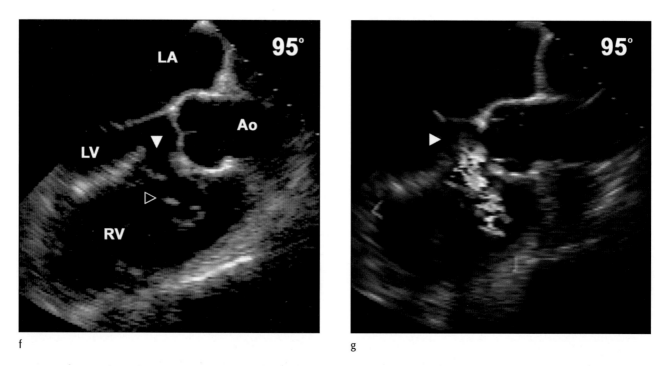

f

g

Case 9.19 *continued*

(f, g) Longitudinal view at 95° demonstrating the area of a perimembranous ventricular septal defect with redundant tissue (open arrow) with imaging and a small residual shunt (closed arrow) with color flow Doppler, note most of the shunt is contained by the aneurysm. LA, left atrium; RA, right atrium; RV, right ventricle; LV, left ventricle; Ao, aorta.

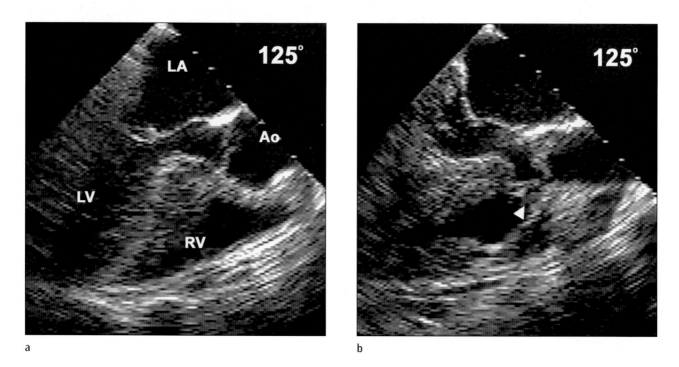

a

b

Case 9.20

Infracristal perimembranous ventricular septal defect. (a, b) Longitudinal view demonstrating a small ventricular septal defect. In diastole (a) the defect is not easily seen, however, it is readily apparent in systole (b).

continued

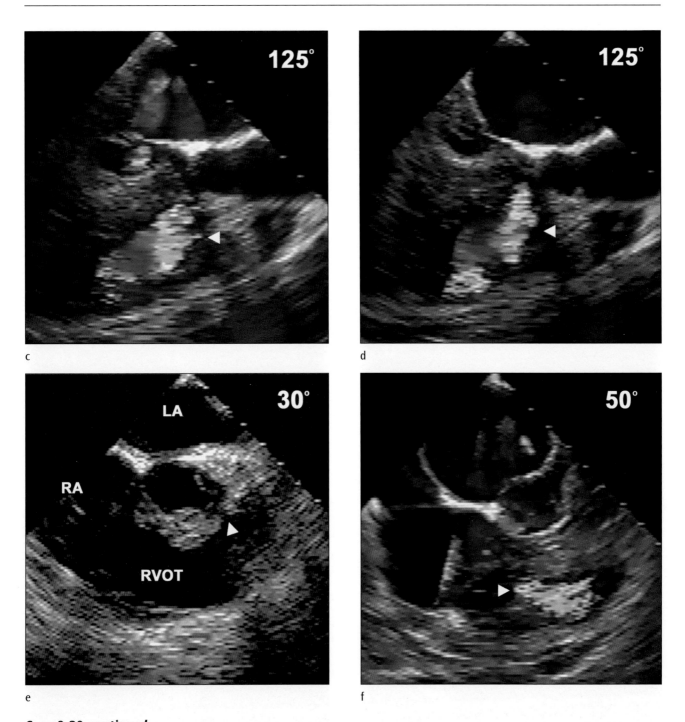

Case 9.20 *continued*

(c, d) A left-to-right shunt (arrow) is demonstrated with color flow Doppler documenting a ventricular septal defect in that area. (e) Short-axis view at the base of the heart demonstrating the membranous ventricular septum and a defect in the infracristal region (arrow). (f) Color flow Doppler demonstration of a left-to-right shunt from the infracristal ventricular septal defect. LA, left atrium; LV, left ventricle; Ao, aorta; RV, right ventricle; RA, right atrium; RVOT, right ventricular outflow tract.

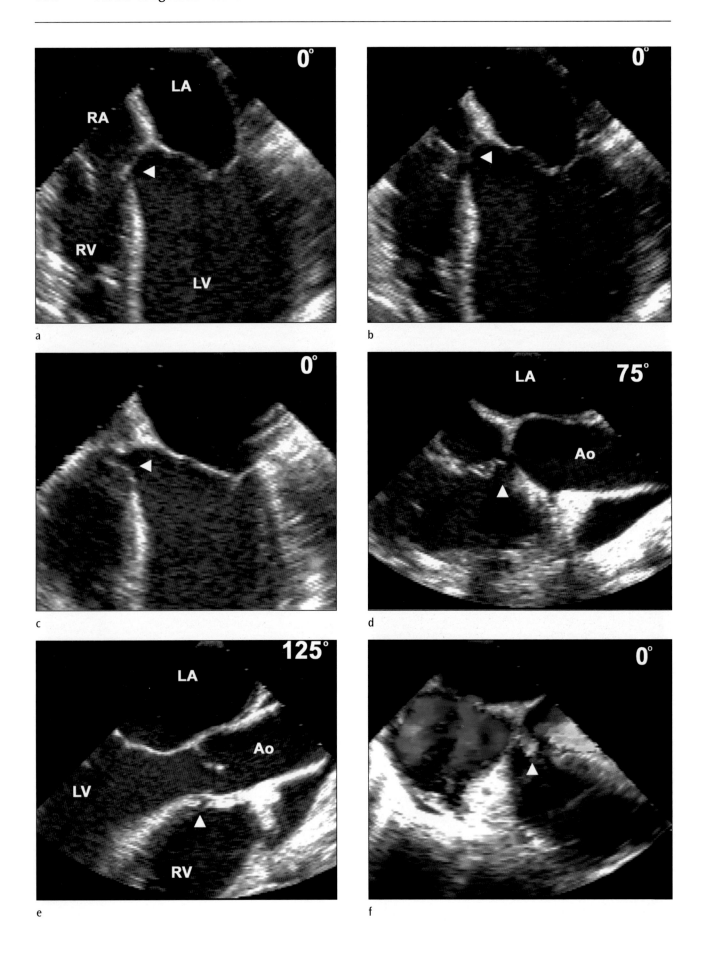

Case 9.21

Small ventricular septal aneurysm. (a–c) Four-chamber view demonstrating a small perimembranous defect that closed with a ventricular septal aneurysm comprised of the tricuspid septal leaflet as seen during the cardiac cycle. (d, e) Longitudinal view from 75° to 125° demonstrating a small ventricular aneurysm. F. Color flow Doppler demonstrating shunt flow (arrow) restrained by the septal aneurysm. LA, left atrium; RA, right atrium; RV, right ventricle; LV, left ventricle; Ao, aorta.

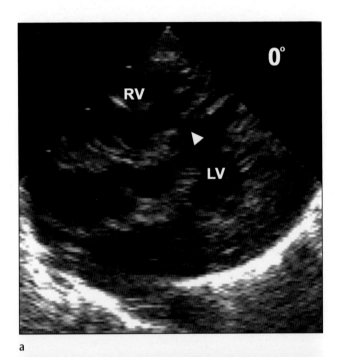

a

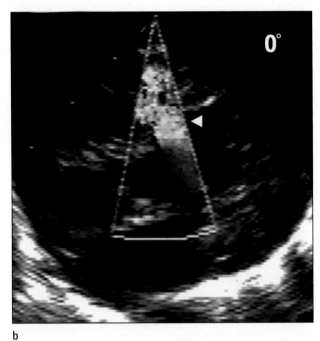

b

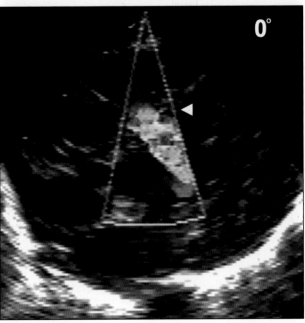

c

Case 9.22

Muscular ventricular septal defect. (a) Deep transgastric view demonstrating a moderate defect in the muscular ventricular septum in a modified five-chamber view. (b, c) Color flow Doppler demonstrating a left-to-right shunt through the muscular defect throughout the cardiac cycle. Ao, aorta; LA, left atrium; LV, left ventricle; RV, right ventricle.

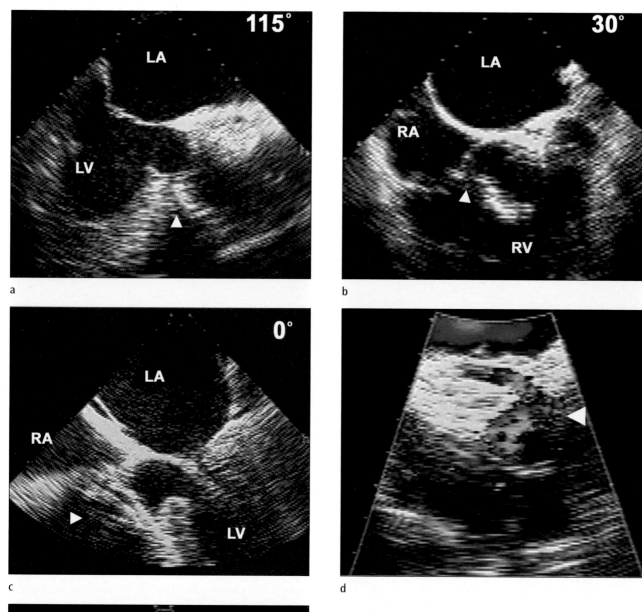

Case 9.23

Surgical patch. Postoperative study following surgical repair with patch of a perimembranous ventricular septal defect. Mild distortion of the superior portion of the ventricular septum with a surgical patch (arrow) demonstrated as a highly refractile area from 115° to 0° with multiplane TEE. (d, e) Color flow Doppler demonstrating integrity of the ventricular septal patch repair (arrow). LA, left atrium; LV, left ventricle; RA, right atrium; RV, right ventricle.

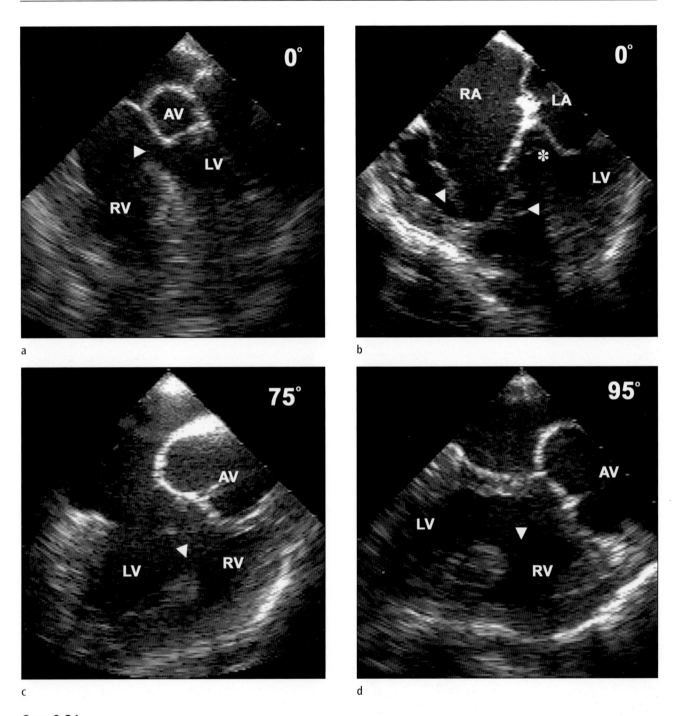

Case 9.24

Tetralogy of Fallot. (a–d) The infundibular ventricular septal defect (arrow) with overriding of a large aorta is readily demonstrated by multiplane TEE. The greater the degree of anterior and rightward deviation of the misaligned outflow septum, the more severe the right ventricular outflow tract obstruction and the greater the propensity for detecting aortic insufficiency.

continued

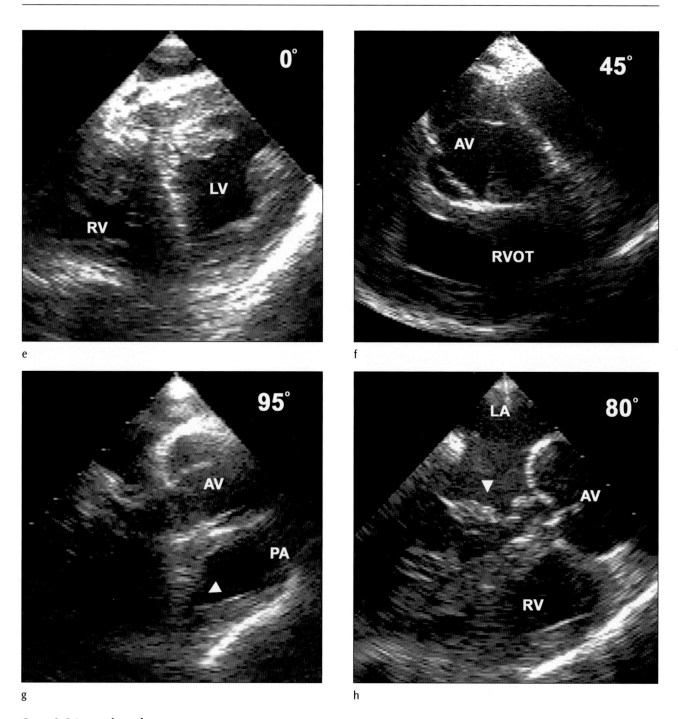

Case 9.24 *continued*

(e) Short-axis gastric view at 0° demonstrating significant right ventricular hypertrophy with septal flattening. (f) Short-axis view at the base of the heart at the aortic valve level displaying enlarged aortic root with displacement of the aortic annulus and valve. In tetralogy of Fallot associated with pulmonary atresia, the most severe malformation, aortic insufficiency is usually significant.

(g–j) Anatomy of the right ventricular outflow tract in adults is best visualized with transesophageal echocardiography in the mid-esophageal long-axis views between 75° and 90° or the deep transgastric views from 0° to 15°. Color flow Doppler imaging visualizes the right-to-left shunting through the ventricular septal defect in most views. The severity of the obstruction of the right ventricular outflow tract may be assessed with conventional Doppler, and the right ventricular systolic pressure may be calculated utilizing the tricuspid regurgitation jet method described previously. AV, aortic valve; LV, left ventricle; RV, right ventricle; PA, pulmonary artery; RA, right atrium; LA, left atrium; RVOT, right ventricular outflow tract.

continued

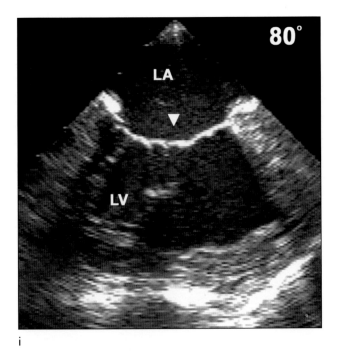

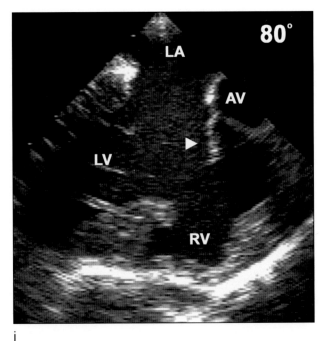

i

j

Case 9.24 *continued*

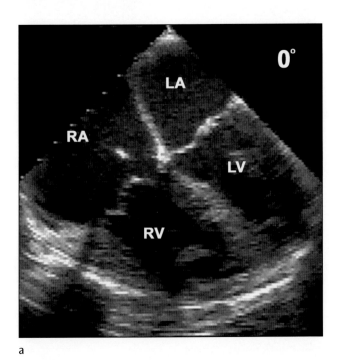

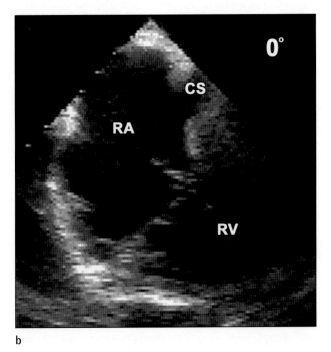

a

b

Case 9.25

Tetralogy of Fallot postsurgical repair. Transesophageal echocardiography is extremely valuable for the postoperative assessment of total correction of tetralogy of Fallot in adult patients. Complete surgical correction includes closure of the ventricular septal defect and relief of the right ventricular outflow obstruction. Postoperatively the right ventricular outflow tract should be assessed for residual or recurrent obstruction. Pulmonary regurgitation may develop as a consequence of the repair with or without patch placement of the infundibulum. Patients with severe pulmonary regurgitation usually do well, however, it may contribute to right ventricular failure in the long term. In patients with distal pulmonary artery stenosis and severe pulmonary regurgitation severe volume overload of the right ventricle may result. (a–c) Four-chamber and modified four-chamber view evaluating the repair and tricuspid regurgitation (arrow) postoperatively.

continued

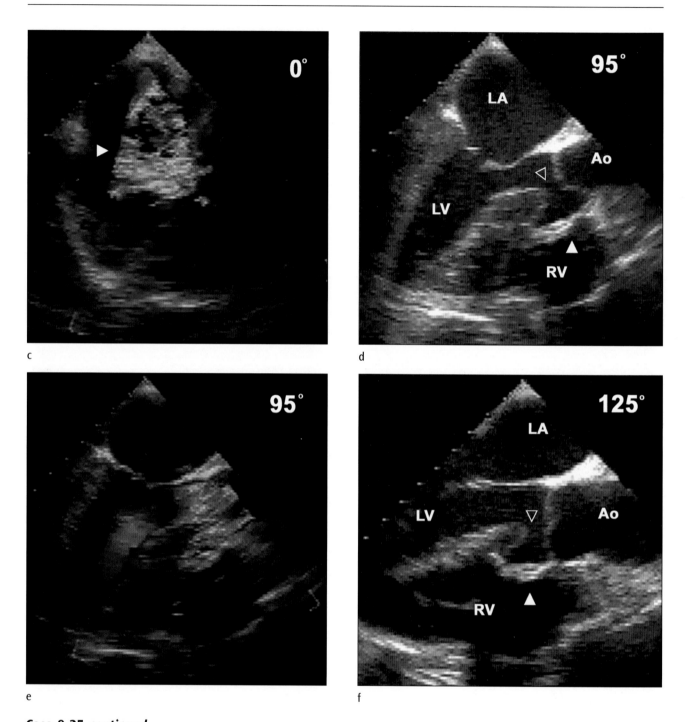

Case 9.25 *continued*
(d–j) Multiple views obtained with TEE demonstrating the ventricular septal surgical patch (arrow).

continued

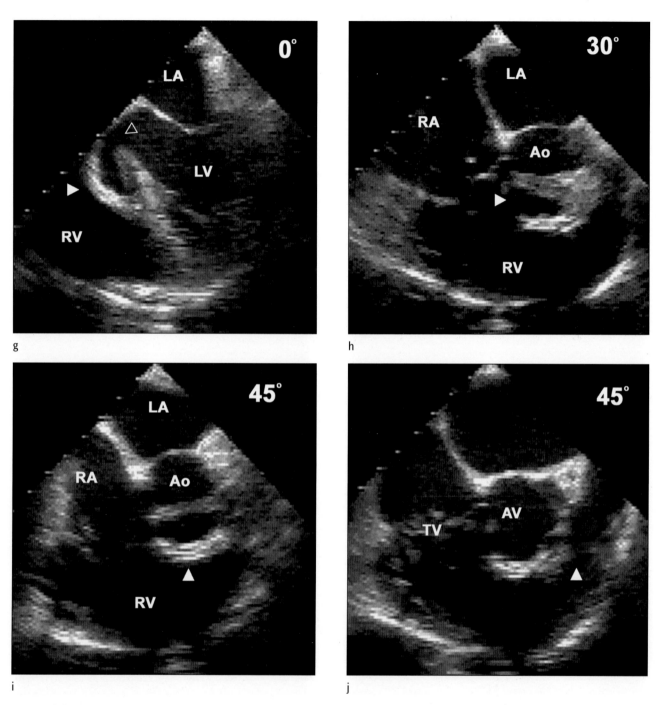

g

h

i

j

Case 9.25 *continued*

continued

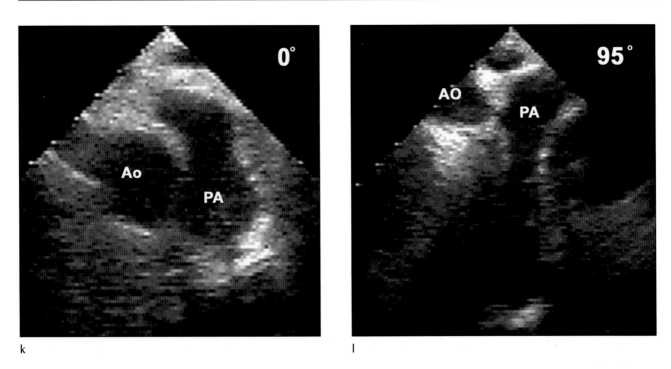

k   l

Case 9.25 *continued*

(k, l) Frontal and longitudinal views of the right ventricular outflow tract. Note residual narrowing suggested by the waist in the main pulmonary artery superior to the pulmonary valve. RA, right atrium; LA, left atrium; RV, right ventricle; LV, left ventricle; CS, coronary sinus; Ao, aorta; TV, tricuspid valve; AV, aortic valve; PA, pulmonary artery.

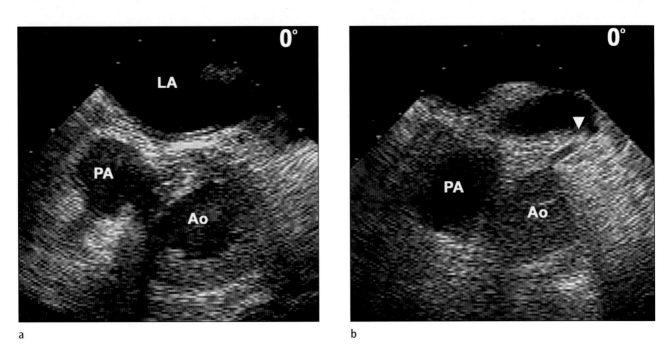

a   b

Case 9.26

Transposition of great arteries. With echocardiography the parallel orientation of the great vessels is readily demonstrated in long axis views, imaging the aorta and pulmonary artery simultaneously, lying side by side, with the lack of the usual spiral relationship of normal anatomy. The aorta is distinguished by the brachiocephalic vessels and the pulmonary artery by the branching of the right and left pulmonary arteries. (a, b) In short-axis views, a direct anterior–posterior relationship is demonstrated with a central located pulmonary valve or artery simultaneously visualized with the aortic valve or aorta. The aorta usually exhibits a larger diameter in comparison to the pulmonary artery. In addition, the short axis views demonstrate the direct continuity of the aorta with the right ventricular outflow tract. Ao, aorta; PA, pulmonary artery; LA, left atrium.

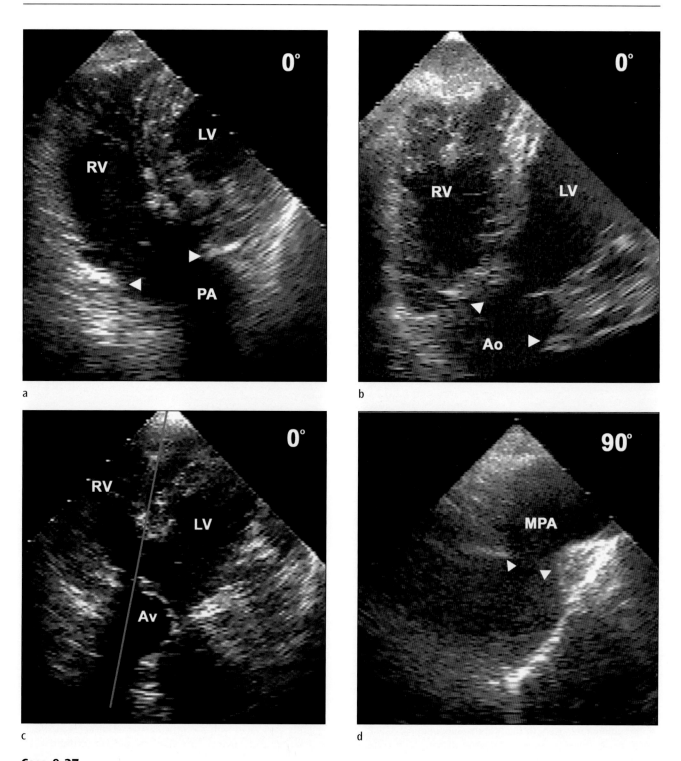

Case 9.27

Transposition of great arteries. The Jatene procedure restores the normal structural and functional relationships between the ventricles and arterial connections. The aorta and the pulmonary arteries are divided in their proximal portions and rotated and re-anastomosed to their appropriate positions. The coronary arteries are removed from the pulmonary artery and attached to the aorta. Complications include supravalvular narrowing at the anastomotic sites and narrowing or kinking of the re-implanted coronary arteries, and distortion to the left and pulmonary arteries as a result of rotating the pulmonary artery for anastomosis. Obstruction occurring at the anastomotic sites is readily defined by echocardiography, and most commonly occurs at the pulmonary anastomosis. (a–d) Evaluation of the great vessel anastomotic sites from the deep transgastric views.

continued

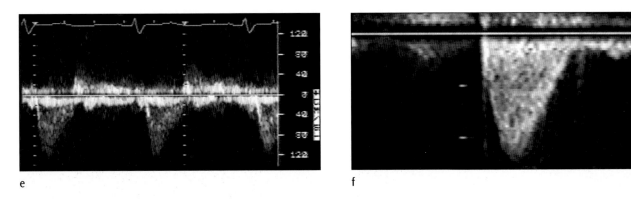

e   f

Case 9.27 *continued*

Conventional Doppler interrogation is also readily accessible from this view for both the aortic (e) and pulmonary artery (f) anastomosis sites. Mild obstruction at the pulmonary anastomosis site. RV, right ventricle; LV, left ventricle; PA, pulmonary artery; Ao, aorta; AV, aortic valve.

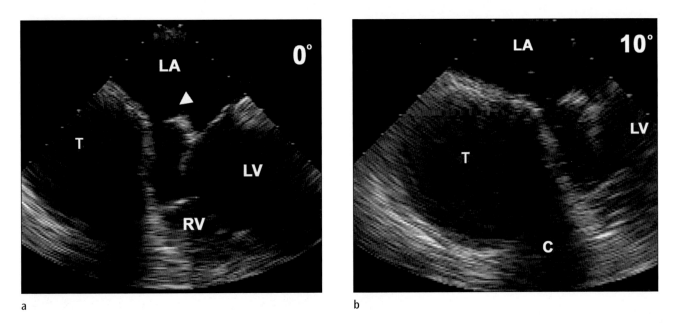

a   b

Case 9.28

Transposition of the great arteries with an infundibular ventricular septal defect and subpulmonary stenosis postsurgical correction. When subpulmonary stenosis is present, diffuse hypertrophy of the infundibulum resembles the appearance of idiopathic hypertrophic subaortic stenosis. Four-chamber views demonstrate the pulmonary artery bifurcation and the relationship of the pulmonary artery to the septum. Subpulmonary stenosis is frequently associated with a ventricular septal defect, which is visualized in the same views. Most adult patients with D-transposition will have had surgical correction and present for the echocardiographic evaluation of residua and sequelae of the correction.

continued

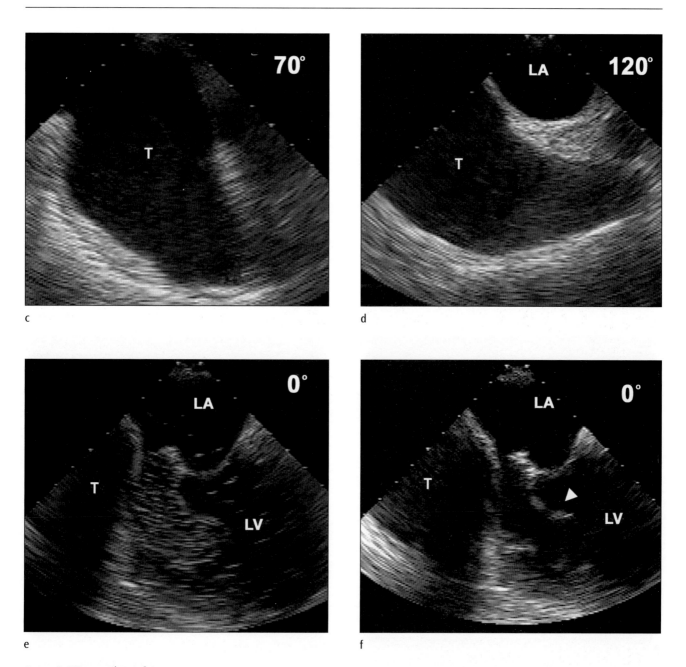

c

d

e

f

Case 9.28 *continued*
The two most common surgical procedures seen for correction of D-transposition, which are usually performed after a palliative atrial septostomy, include the atrial switch procedures and the arterial switch procedure. In transposition associated with ventricular septal defect and severe pulmonary stenosis an external valve conduit may be placed between the right ventricle and the pulmonary artery as in either the Rastelli or Damus–Kaye–Stamus procedures. (a) Four-chamber view demonstrating a small remnant right ventricle with an infundibular ventricular septal defect. (b–f) Tunnel created in the right atrium as viewed in multiple planes.

continued

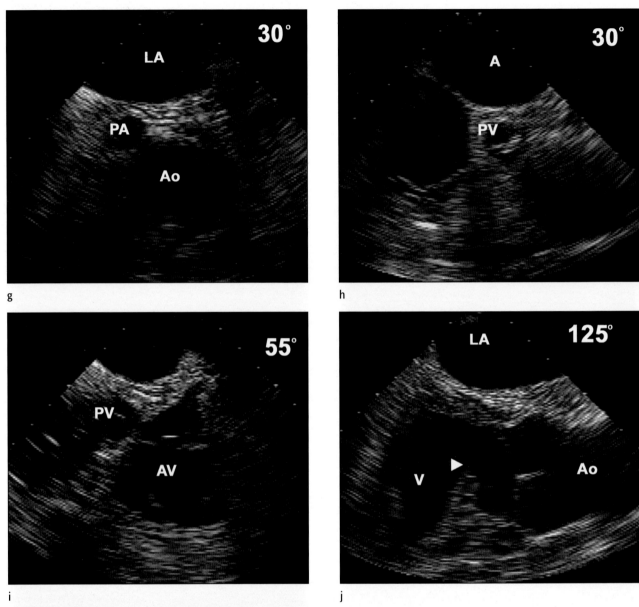

Case 9.28 *continued*
(g–i) Short-axis view at the base of the heart demonstrating a small pulmonary artery and aorta in the typical transposition orientation. (j, k) Longitudinal views of the ventricular septal defect and the enlarged aorta. (l–q) A valved conduit was created between the tunnel and the right pulmonary artery and is visualized in multiple planes. LA, left atrium; LV, left ventricle; RV, right ventricle; T, tunnel; C, conduit; V, ventricle; Ao, aorta; PA, pulmonary artery; PV, pulmonary vein.

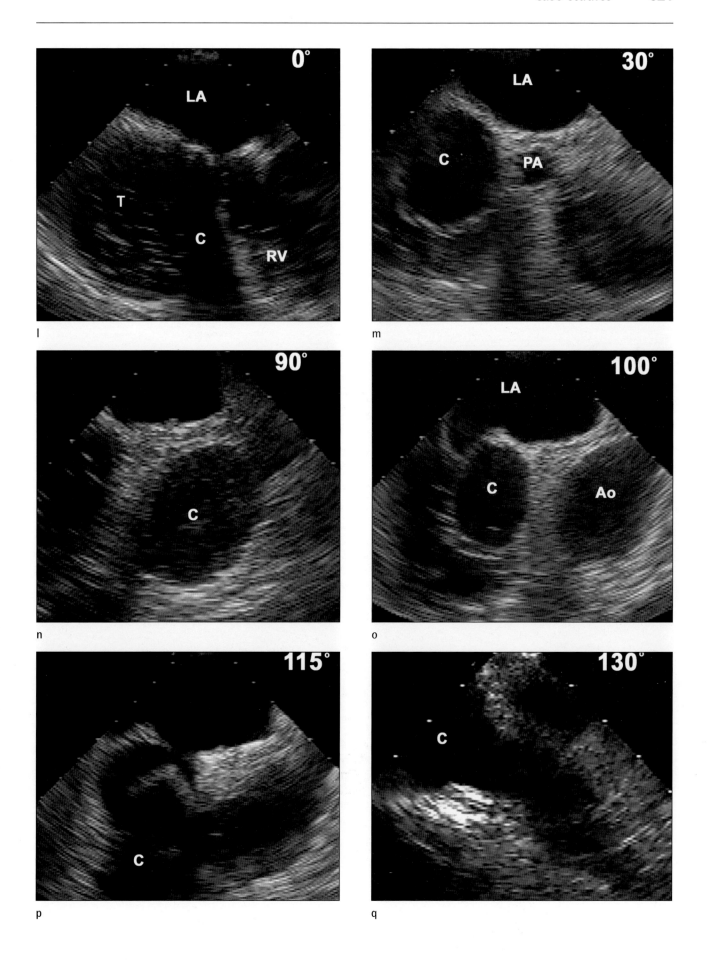

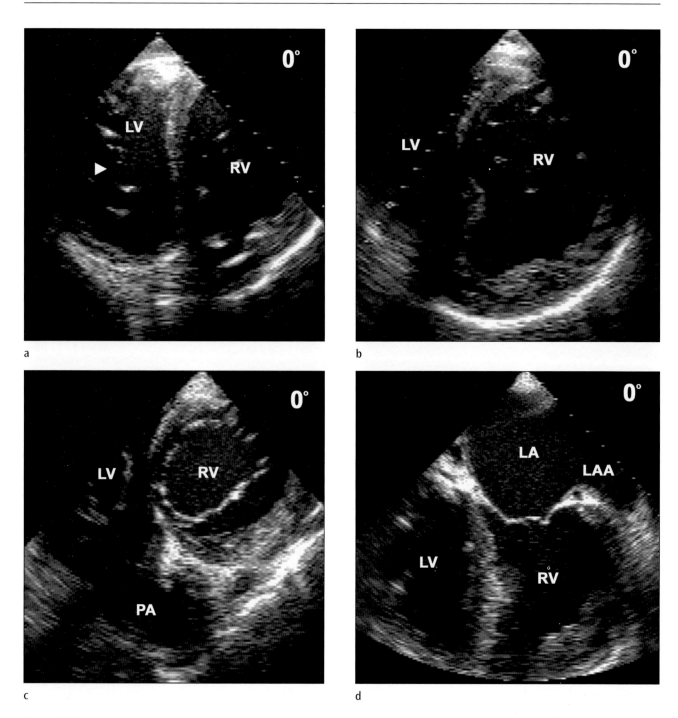

Case 9.29

Congenitally corrected transposition of great arteries. The pulmonary artery arises posteriorly from the left ventricle. The aorta arises anteriorly and from the right ventricle. The aorta and the pulmonary artery appear to lie side by side, in a similar fashion as in D-transposition. The diagnosis of L-transposition includes the identification of ventricular inversion with echocardiography. The left-sided systemic ventricle exhibits the morphology of the right ventricle and is denoted by the apical position of the tricuspid valve in relationship to the internal cardiac crux, and the moderator band. (a–c) Short-axis views demonstrating ventricular inversion with the pulmonary artery arising from the left ventricle. The right-sided pulmonary ventricle exhibits the fish-mouth shape of the mitral valve and the left ventricular papillary muscle configuration. (d) Ventricular inversion in the four-chamber view.

continued

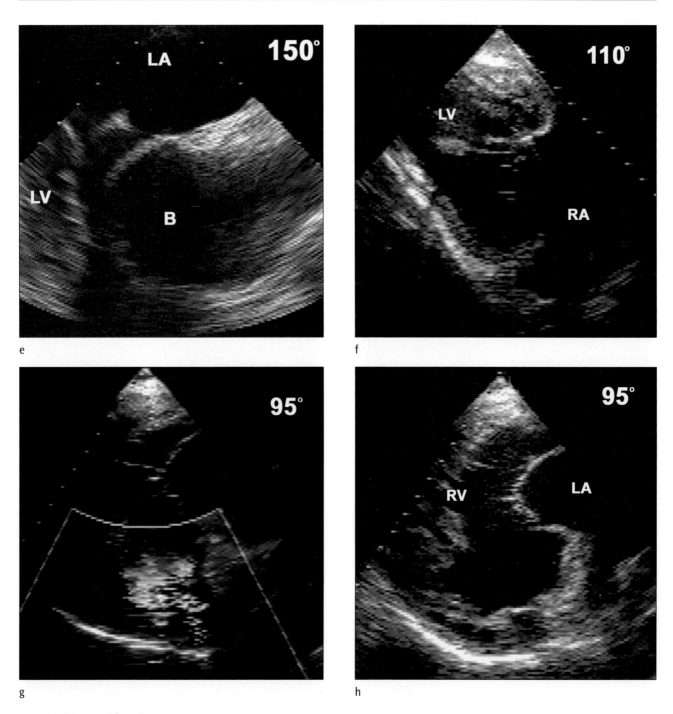

Case 9.29 *continued*

(e–g) Longitudinal views of the right and left heart. (h–p) Short-axis views of the base of the heart from 30° to 160° illustrating the position of the aorta and the pulmonary artery from a lower position of the pulmonary valve to a side-by-side orientation of the great vessels in the longitudinal views with imaging and color flow Doppler. RV, right ventricle; LV, left ventricle; PA, pulmonary artery. LA, left atrium; LAA, left atrial appendage; RA, right atrium; RAA, right atrial appendage; PV, pulmonary vein; Ao, aorta; SVC, superior vena cava.

continued

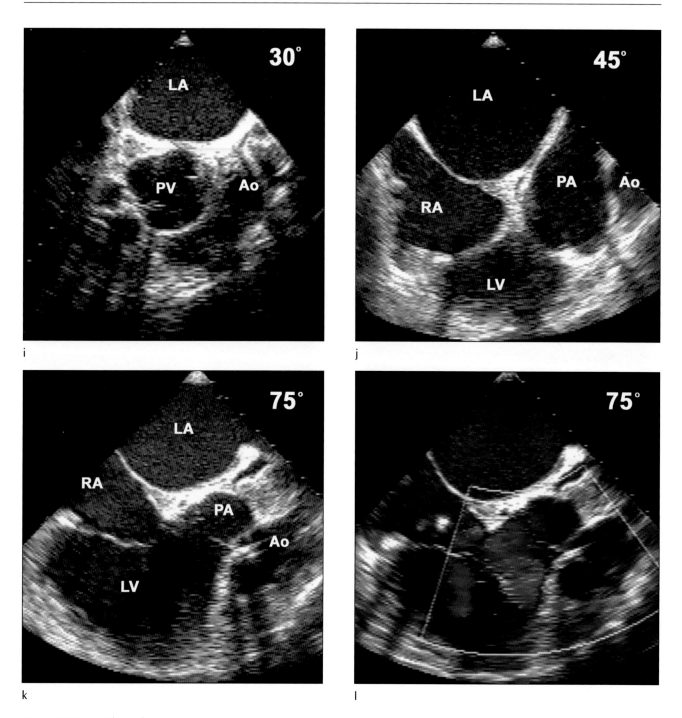

Case 9.29 *continued*

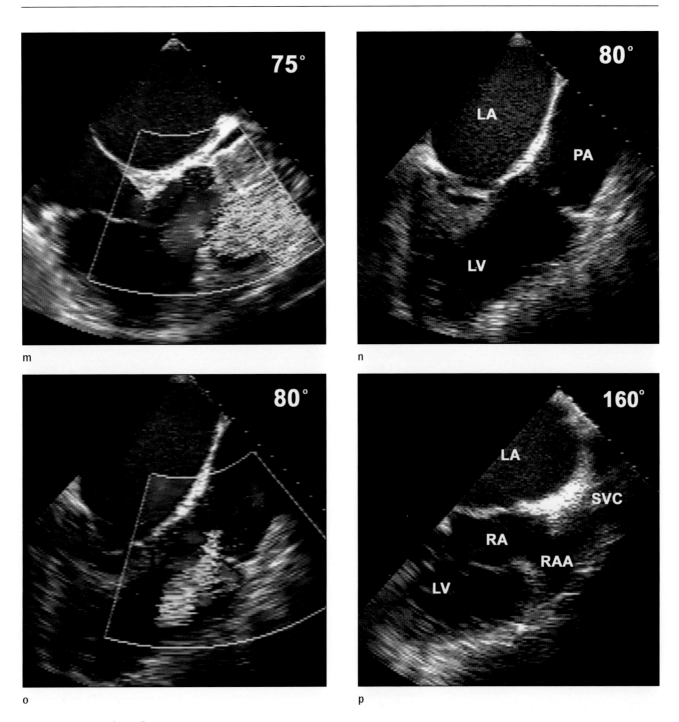

Case 9.29 *continued*

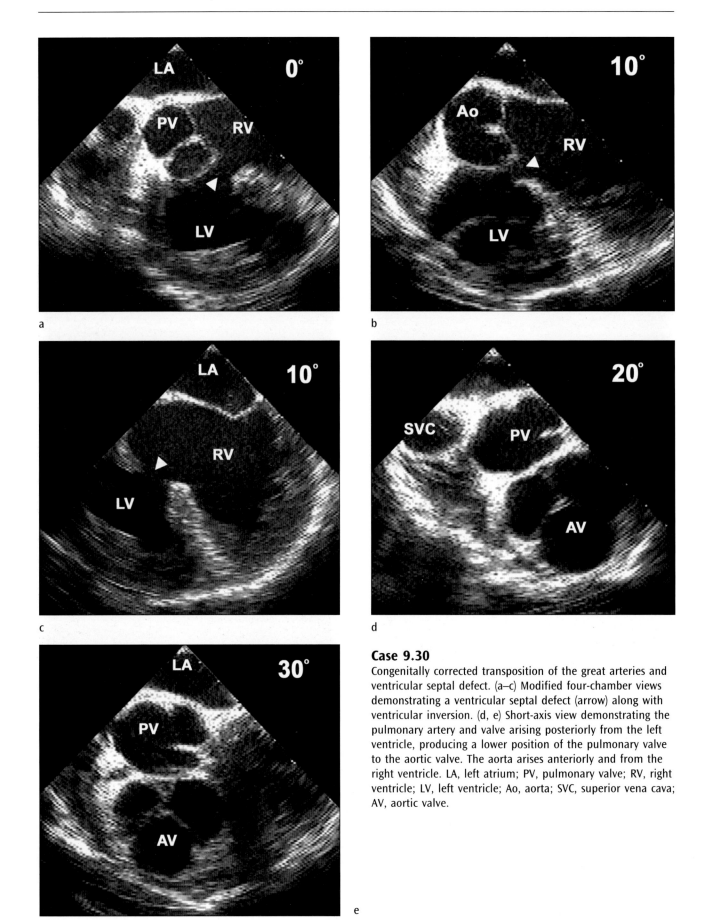

Case 9.30
Congenitally corrected transposition of the great arteries and ventricular septal defect. (a–c) Modified four-chamber views demonstrating a ventricular septal defect (arrow) along with ventricular inversion. (d, e) Short-axis view demonstrating the pulmonary artery and valve arising posteriorly from the left ventricle, producing a lower position of the pulmonary valve to the aortic valve. The aorta arises anteriorly and from the right ventricle. LA, left atrium; PV, pulmonary valve; RV, right ventricle; LV, left ventricle; Ao, aorta; SVC, superior vena cava; AV, aortic valve.

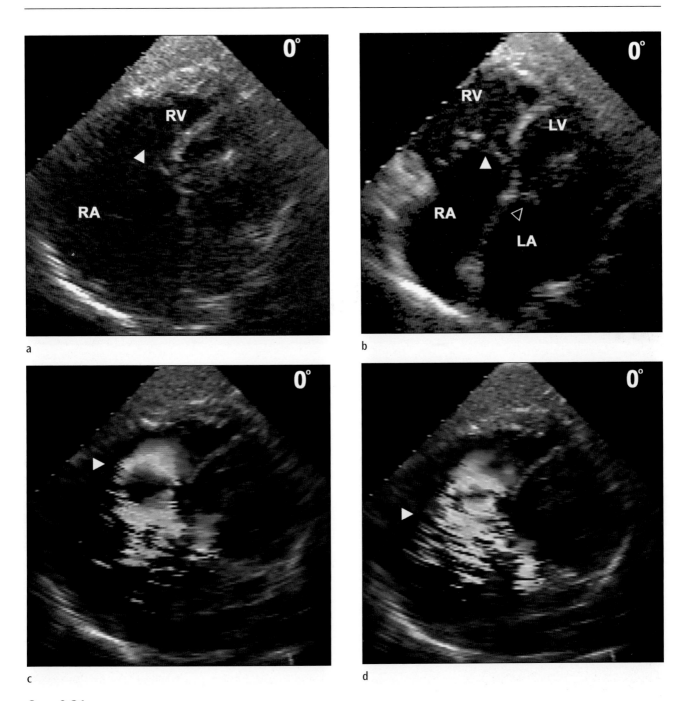

a

b

c

d

Case 9.31

Ebstein's anomaly. In Ebstein's anomaly, the tricuspid valve exhibits the downward displacement of the annular attachment of the septal and posterior leaflets within the body of the right ventricle. (a, b) Deep transgastric view in Ebstein's anomaly readily demonstrates apical displacement of the tricuspid valve (closed arrow) in comparison to the mitral annular plane (open arrow). The apical displacement of the leaflets usually exceeds 20 mm or 8 mm/m^2 in the adult. (c, d) The addition of color flow Doppler aids in determining the true plane of the tricuspid orifice (arrow) by visualizing flow convergence as a result of forward flow or regurgitant flow. Tricuspid leaflet displacement results in atrialization of the proximal portion of the right ventricle, which results in a reduction in the functional size of the right ventricle. As a consequence, the right heart is effectively divided into three chambers, the true right atrium, the atrialized right ventricle and the functional right ventricle, with an effective tricuspid orifice that is displaced downward into the right ventricular cavity. The atrialized right ventricle is anatomically the right ventricle but functions as the right atrium, which predisposes the thin walled atrialized portion to dilate and may result in an aneurysm between the tricuspid annulus and the displaced posterior leaflet. Although the annular attachment of the anterior leaflet is normal, the leaflet is malformed as the result of thickening and redundancy. The anterior leaflet may be dysplastic and frequently adheres to the right ventricular free wall. This may result in right ventricular inflow or outflow tract obstruction. Tricuspid regurgitation accompanies the structurally abnormal valve and frequently is severe.   *continued*

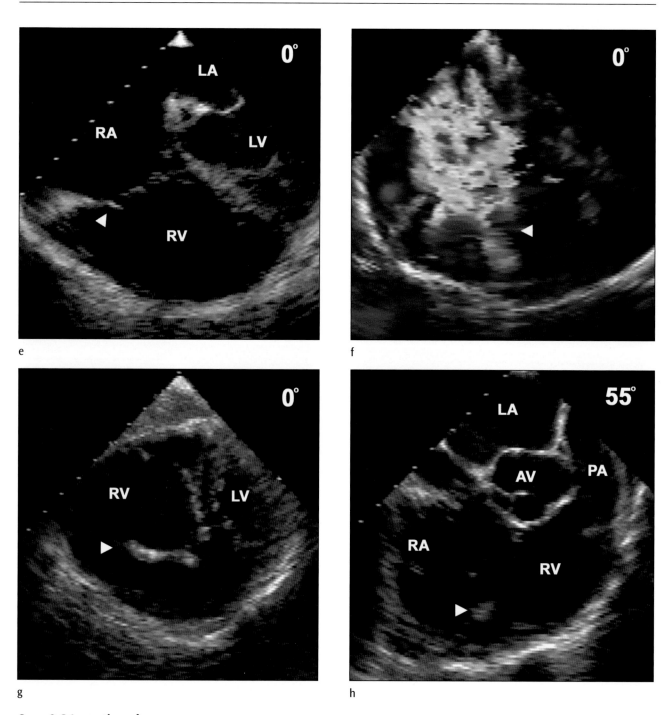

e

f

g

h

Case 9.31 *continued*

(e, f) Modified four-chamber view demonstrating the tricuspid apparatus with imaging and severe tricuspid regurgitation with color flow Doppler. (g–l) Multiple views focusing on the right atrial enlargement due to the atrialization of the right ventricle and the effective decrease right ventricular size. RA, right atrium; RV, right ventricle; LA, left atrium; LV, left ventricle; AV, aortic valve; PA, pulmonary artery.

continued

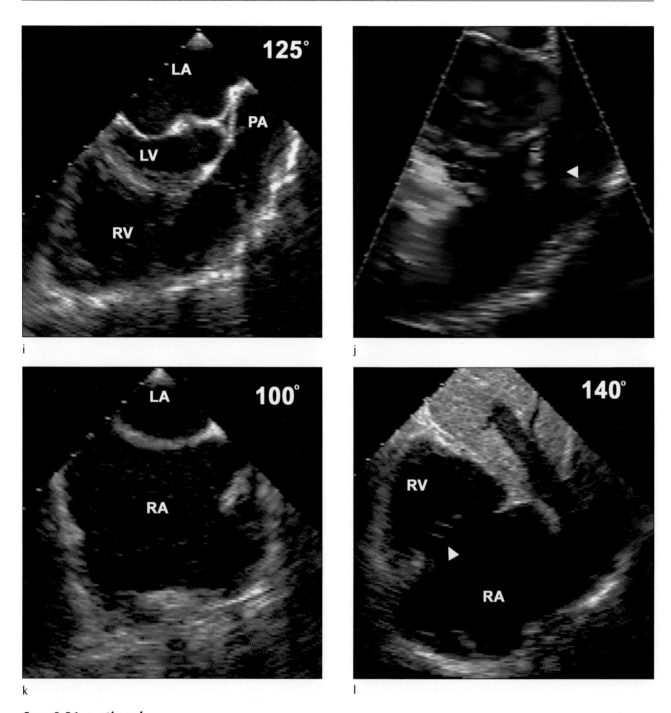

i

j

k

l

Case 9.31 *continued*

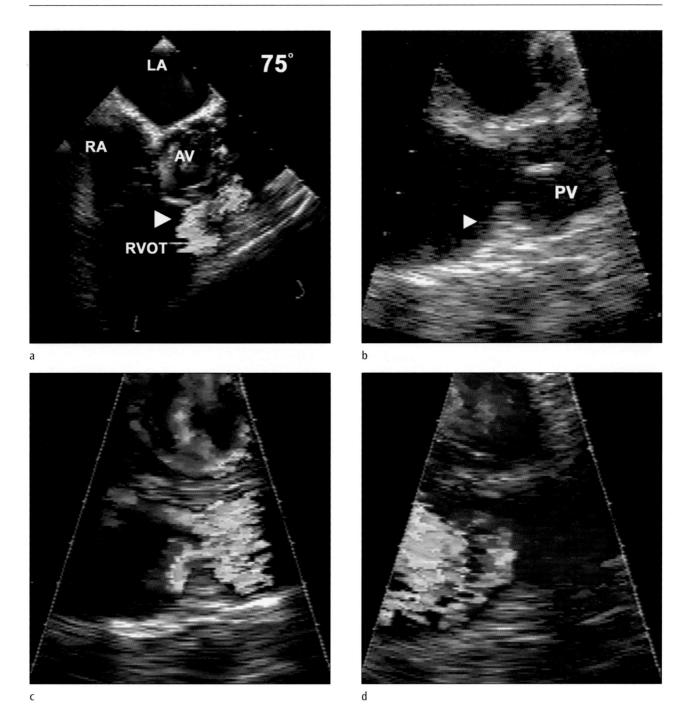

Case 9.32

Infundibular stenosis. (a) Discrete infundibular stenosis visualized from a short-axis view from the mid-esophageal window at 75°. Color flow Doppler documents the obstruction which may not be obvious from imaging alone. Flow convergence (arrow) is demonstrated near an area of discrete enlargement proximal to the pulmonary valve. (b–d) Zoom mode demonstrating the discrete narrowing (arrow) of the infundibulum and area of obstruction of outflow with color flow Doppler during the cardiac cycle. LA, left atrium; RA, right atrium; AV, aortic valve; RVOT, right ventricular outflow tract; PV, pulmonary vein.

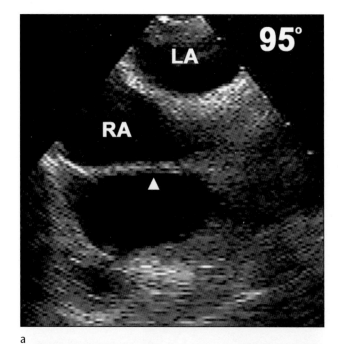

a

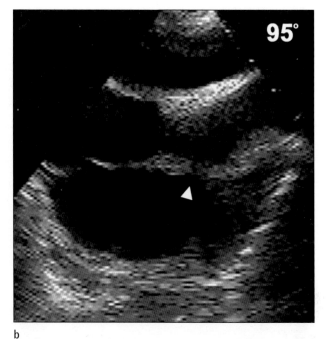

b

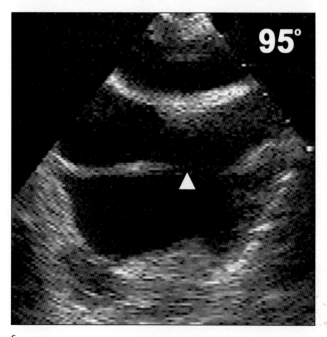

c

Case 9.33

Cor triatriatum dexter. Cor triatriatum dexter is rarer than cor triatriatum on the left side. (a–c) Abnormal persistence of the sinus venosus valve, results in a two-chambered right atrium as demonstrated in a bicaval view. The resultant membrane extends from the inferior vena cava to the superior vena cava and relegates the right atrial appendage and the tricuspid valve to the lower right atrial chamber. Blood flow empties from the vena cava through perforations in the membrane, producing a similar physiological situation as tricuspid atresia, however, with a well-formed tricuspid valve and right ventricle.

continued

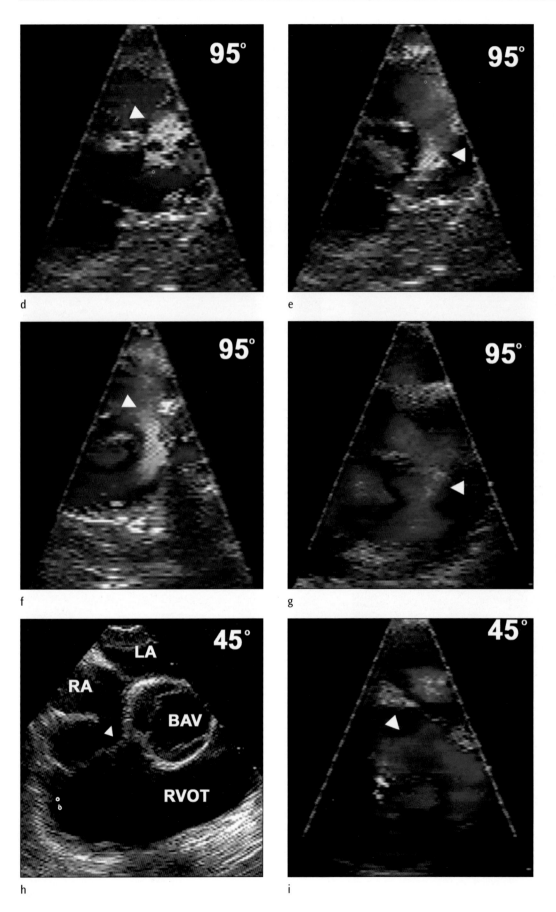

(d–g) Color flow Doppler documenting obstruction to flow through fenestrations in the membrane. In the adult patient the membrane is highly perforate, and is demonstrated to have flow disturbance and obstructing qualities with color flow Doppler. (h, i) Short-axis view at 45° demonstrates a bicuspid valve at the aortic valve level and evidence of the membrane in the right atrium. The membrane should be visualized in two opposite planes in order to confirm the presence of cor triatriatum dexter and to rule out the presence of just a prominent atrial wall ridge. LA, left atrium; RA, right atrium. RVOT, right ventricular outflow tract.

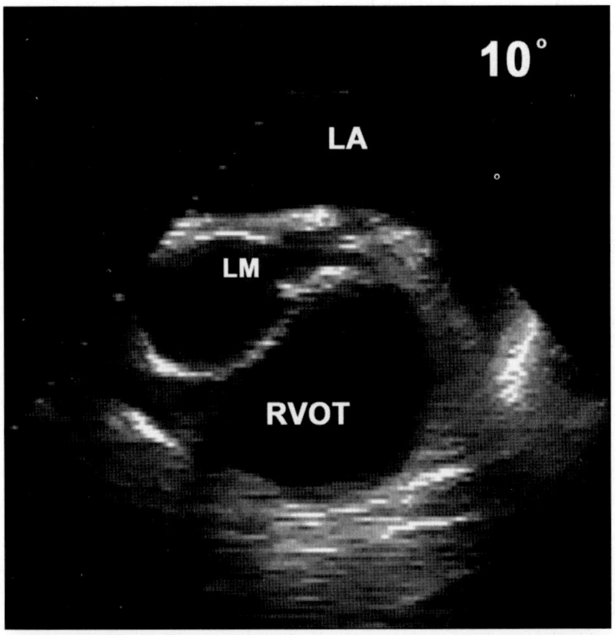

a

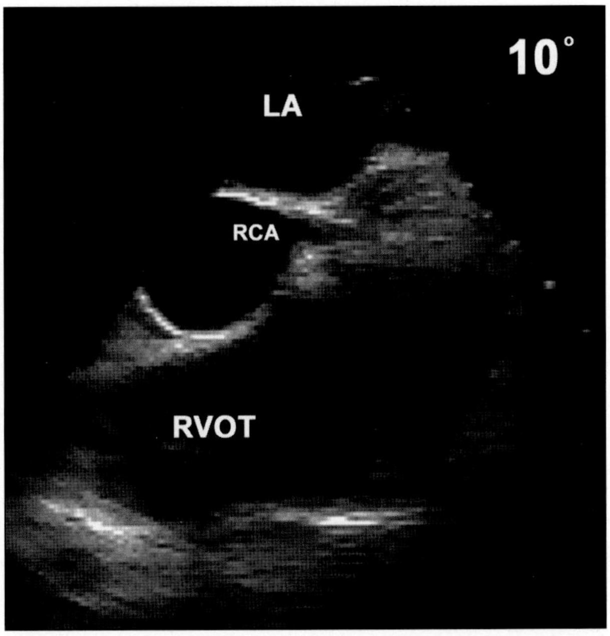

b

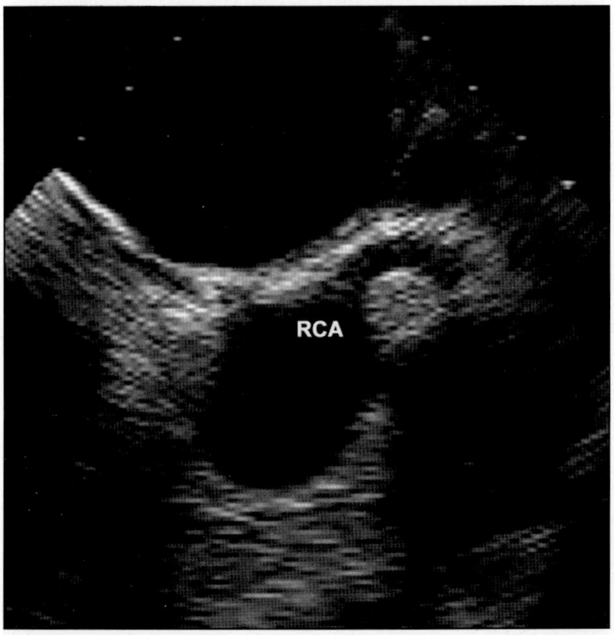

c

Case 9.34

Coronary artery anomalies. The sensitivity of transesophageal echocardiography for the evaluation of the left main coronary artery is between 77 and 100%, with a sensitivity for the right coronary artery of 26%, therefore, cardiac catheterization is usually required to confirm the diagnosis of anomalous coronary arteries. When the coronary arteries are well-visualized the diagnosis of anomalous coronary arteries can be made with certainty, especially with TEE in adults and younger patients. The accurate recognition of coronary artery anomalies with echocardiography requires the knowledge of the variations that may be expected and the frequency that they occur. (a) Short left main with mild dilatation branching to left anterior descending and left circumflex arteries. (b) Same patient the right coronary artery originates from the left coronary cusp. (c) High take off and origin of the right coronary artery from the level of the sinotubular junction. The direction of the coronary artery appears to be between the aorta and pulmonary artery.

continued

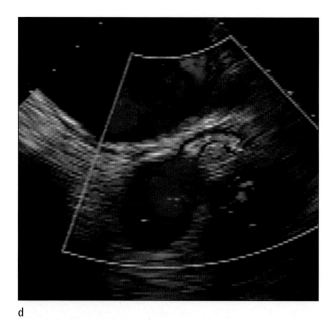
d

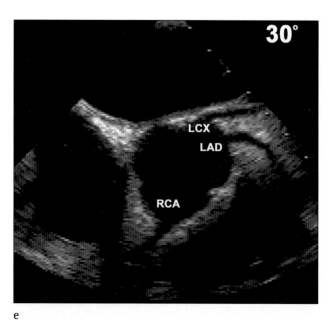
e

Case 9.34 *continued*

(d) Color flow Doppler demonstrating flow in the right coronary artery which helps determine the direction of the coronary even though the artery falls out of plane and is not adequately visualized. (e) Separate ostia of the left anterior descending artery and the left circumflex arteries. Note the origin of the right coronary artery is visualized in the same plane as the left coronary artery. Usually minor manipulation of the probe is required to see the right and left coronary artery and they are not usually visualized simultaneously. LA, left atrium; LM, left main coronary artery; RVOT, right ventricular outflow tract; RCA, right coronary artery; LCX, left circumflex artery; LAD, left anterior descending artery.

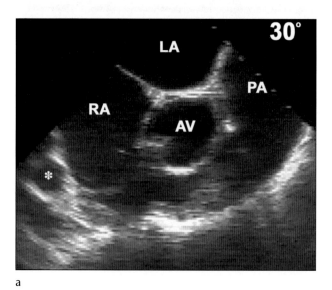
a

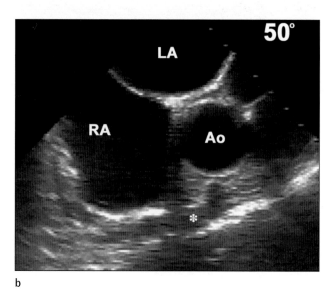
b

Case 9.35

Coronary artery fistula. A congenital coronary arteriovenous fistula is a direct, anomalous connection between a coronary artery and another cardiac structure. Communications usually enter the right heart chambers (90%) but have been described to all four cardiac chambers, the coronary sinus, cardiac veins, proximal superior vena cava, proximal pulmonary artery and pulmonary veins near their connection to the heart. The coronary dilates and elongates frequently in a serpiginous fashion as a result of the shunt flow produced through the fistula. The dilatation is uniform throughout and often produces a huge coronary artery. At the point of fistulous connection, the coronary artery dilates out of proportion to the rest of the artery in an aneurysmal fashion. Frequently the fistulous opening is multiple and produces a confluence of multiple tracts to the receiving chamber. The coronary artery distal to the fistulous connection usually is normal size or frequently smaller than expected. (a) Short-axis view of the base of the heart at 30° demonstrating a dilated right coronary artery (star). (b) Longitudinal plane of a dilated right coronary artery (star).

continued

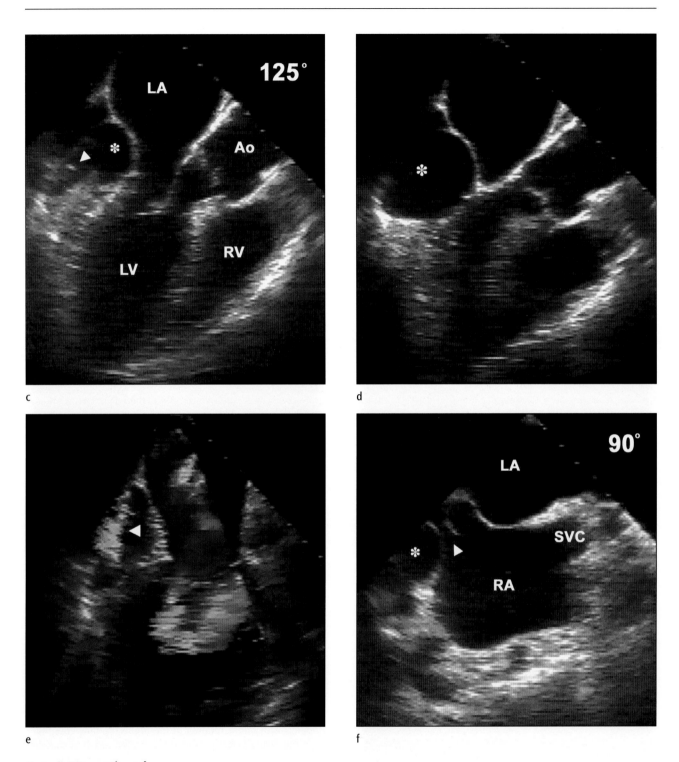

Case 9.35 *continued*

(c) Dilated coronary sinus demonstrating aneurysmal formation (start) as the fistula enters the coronary sinus (arrow) at 125°.
(d) Minor rotation of the probe demonstrates the full breadth of the aneurysmal dilatation (star). (e) Color flow Doppler
demonstrating blood flow in the aneurysm. (f) Modified bicaval view at 90° demonstrating aneurysmal dilation (star).

continued

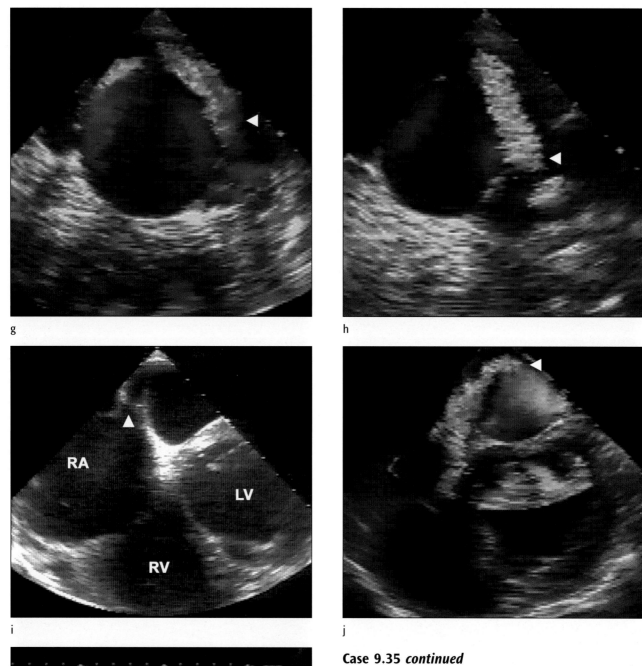

g

h

i

j

k

Case 9.35 *continued*

(g) Zoom mode of a four-chamber view demonstrating the enlarged coronary sinus and aneurysm with color flow Doppler, with minor rotation of the probe the flow entering from the fistula is demonstrated (h). (i) Modified four-chamber view demonstrating the origin of the coronary sinus and (j) flow from the coronary sinus emptying into the right atrium with color Doppler. (k) Conventional Doppler of the coronary sinus flow into the right atrium representing the shunt flow. PA, pulmonary artery; LA, left atrium; RA, right atrium; LV, left ventricle; RV, right ventricle; AV, aortic valve; Ao, aorta; SVC, superior vena cava.

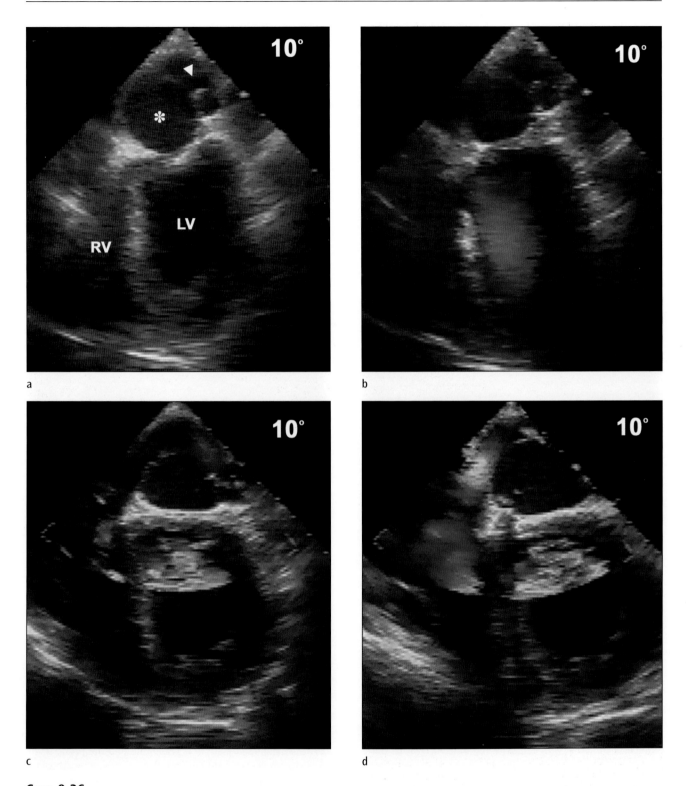

a

b

c

d

Case 9.36

Postoperative coronary artery fistula repair. TEE is extremely useful for demonstrating a successful result following surgical ligation of the coronary artery. Success is demonstrated by the lack of flow from the area of the fistula entering the aneurysmal pouch. (a–d) Two-dimensional imaging and color flow Doppler from a modified four-chamber view demonstrating the continued presence of the aneurysmal pouch (star) and the approximate area of the fistulous ligation (arrow) with normal color flow Doppler and the lack of fistulous flow as visualized preoperatively. LV, left ventricle; RV, right ventricle.

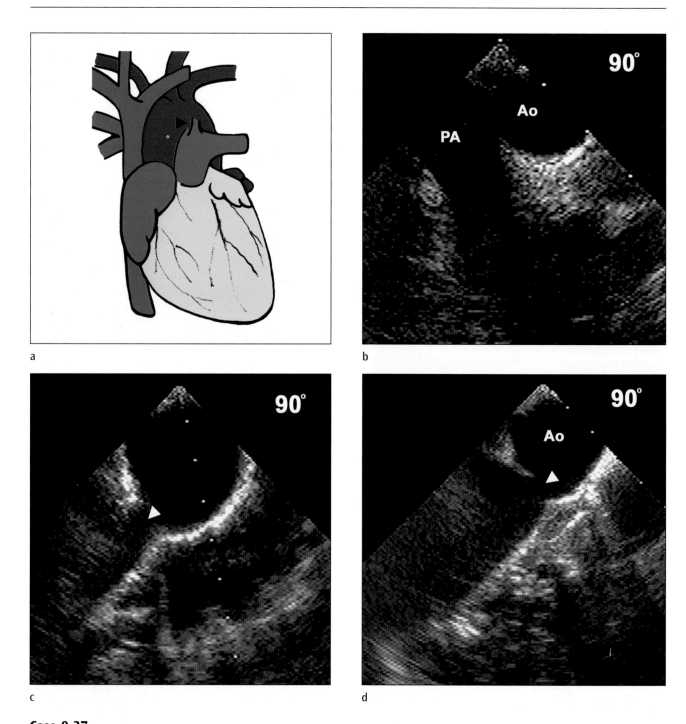

a

b

c

d

Case 9.37

Patent ductus arteriosus. Patent ductus arteriosus is visualized in both the horizontal and longitudinal planes, from the upper esophageal windows with TEE. With the transducer at 0° the bifurcation of the pulmonary artery is visualized, and the probe is rotated in a counterclockwise direction towards the descending aorta. The ductus is visualized between the descending aorta and the left pulmonary artery with a length of approximately 8 mm (5.5–13 mm) and diameter of 1.5–13 mm at the aortic origin. To aid in recognition of the ductus anatomy, color flow Doppler may be utilized to substantiate flow in the ductal structure. Once visualized the full dimensional aspect of the ductus may be observed with rotation of the transducer through 90°. (a) Artists rendition of ductus arteriosus anatomy. (b–d) Serial multiplane transesophageal echocardiography imaging with color flow Doppler demonstrating a patent ductus arteriosus (arrow).

continued

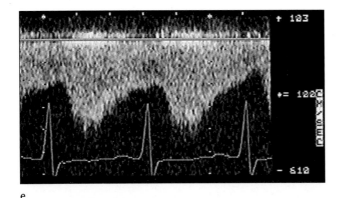

e

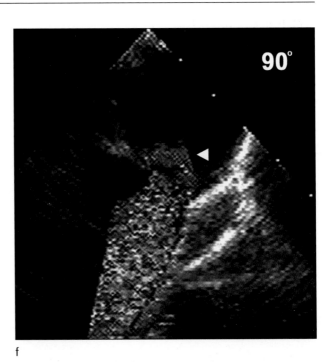

f

Case 9.37 *continued*

(e) Pulsed Doppler of shunt flow through the ductus. (f) Color flow Doppler frequently helps determine the presence of ductal flow between the aorta and pulmonary artery by demonstrating flow convergence on the aortic side and a mosaic, highly turbulent flow jet towards the pulmonary artery. Ao, aorta; PA, pulmonary artery.

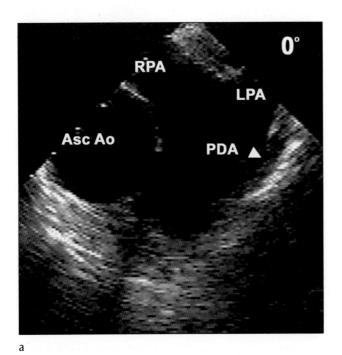

a

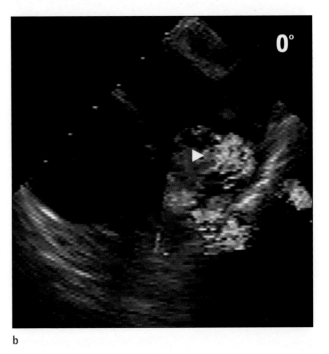

b

Case 9.38

Patent ductus arteriosus. (a) Short-axis view from the upper esophagus demonstrating the pulmonary tree and origin of the patent ductus (arrow). (b–e) Color flow Doppler demonstrating ductal flow into the pulmonary artery.

continued

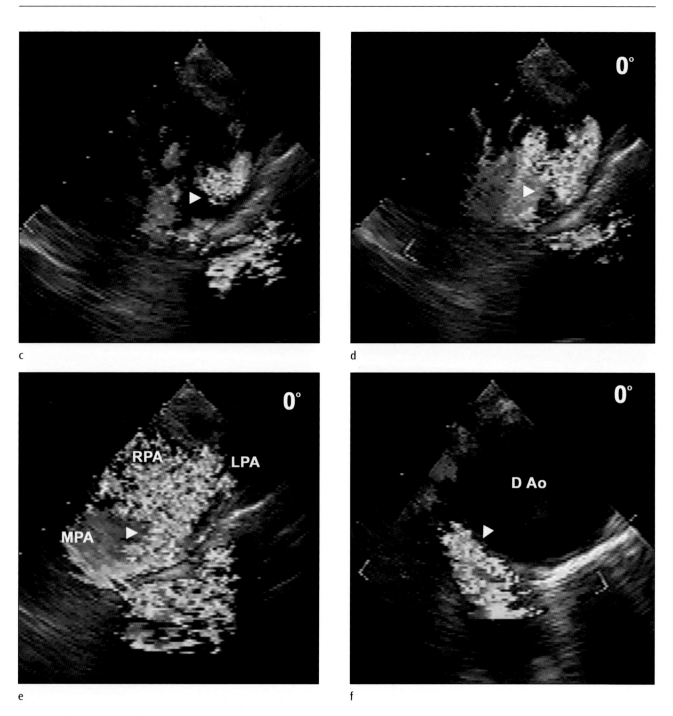

Case 9.38 *continued*

(f–h) Rotating the probe to the back demonstrates the origin of the ductus from the aorta. Asc Ao, ascending aorta; PDA, patent ductus arteriosus; LPA, left pulmonary artery; RPA, right pulmonary artery; MPA, main pulmonary artery; D Ao, descending aorta.

continued

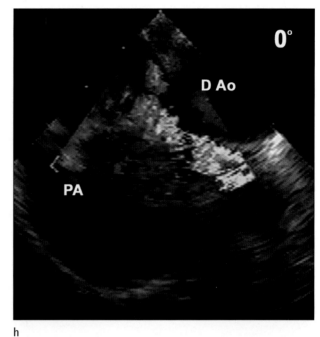

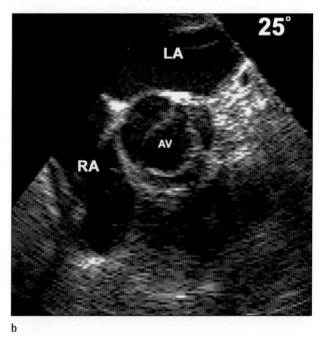

g

h

Case 9.38 continued

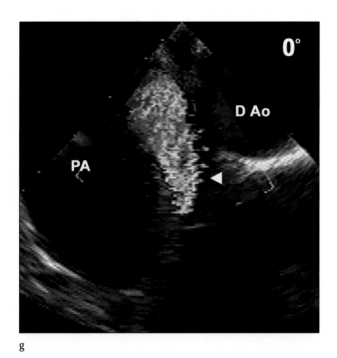

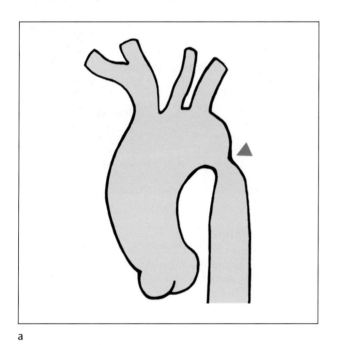

a

b

Case 9.39

Discrete coarctation of the aorta. (a) Artists rendition of a discrete coarctation at the area of the cardiac isthmus. Echocardiographically, coarctation of the aorta appears as a definite narrowing of the aortic lumen contour, with a posterior echodense shelf protruding into the aortic lumen. In short-axis transesophageal views at 0°, slow advancement or withdrawal of the probe define the narrowing as proximal or distal to the left subclavian artery. In wide plane, longitudinal views at 90° (increasing the depth to 10–12 cm), if isthmus hypoplasia is present the area of coarctation produces an hourglass deformity. The area of the coarctation possesses increased echogenicity with a fuzzy appearance to the aortic lumen due to the hyperplasia of aortic wall distinct to the normal aortic segments. The aortic segments proximal to the coarctation segment are usually dilated, with dilatation extending into the brachiocephalic vessels. Poststenotic dilatation is noted in a short segment of the aorta distal to the coarctation. Noticeable aortic pulsations are detected in the proximal aortic segments, with no detectable pulsation in the poststenotic segment. (b) Short-axis image demonstrating a bicuspid valve.   *continued*

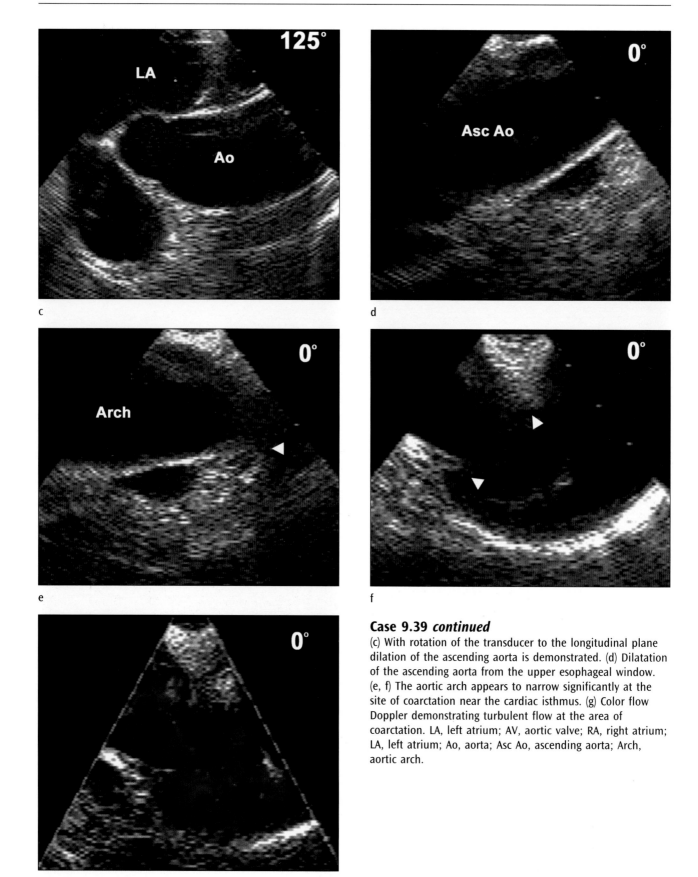

Case 9.39 *continued*

(c) With rotation of the transducer to the longitudinal plane dilation of the ascending aorta is demonstrated. (d) Dilatation of the ascending aorta from the upper esophageal window. (e, f) The aortic arch appears to narrow significantly at the site of coarctation near the cardiac isthmus. (g) Color flow Doppler demonstrating turbulent flow at the area of coarctation. LA, left atrium; AV, aortic valve; RA, right atrium; LA, left atrium; Ao, aorta; Asc Ao, ascending aorta; Arch, aortic arch.

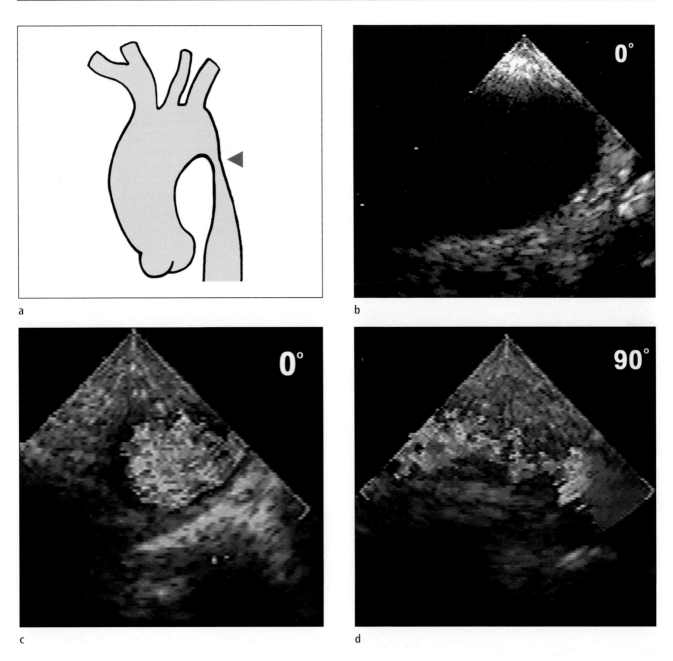

a

b

c

d

Case 9.40

Diffuse coarctation of the aorta. The defect in aortic coarctation either produces a discrete and localized indentation to the aortic lumen or a diffuse narrowing, which may involve the whole isthmus and/or extend into the aortic arch. (a) Artists rendition of a diffuse coarctation. (b) The aortic arch visualized from the upper esophageal window. (c, d) Color flow Doppler demonstrates disturbed flow through a long narrow portion of the aortic coarctation.

continued

e

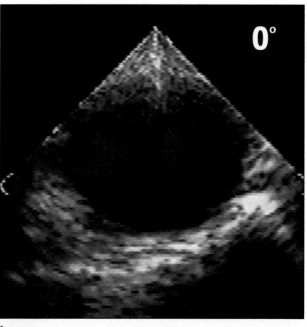

f

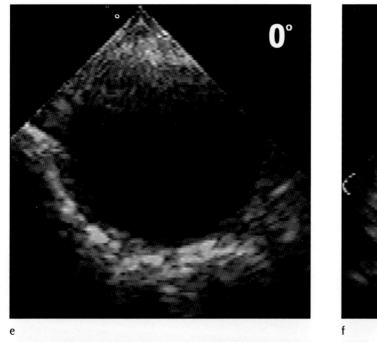

90°

g

Case 9.40 *continued*
(e) Short-axis descending aorta distal to the coarctation demonstrating normal diameter and (f) normal color flow Doppler. (g) Longitudinal view of the descending aorta distal to the coarctation demonstrating normal color flow Doppler in the aorta.

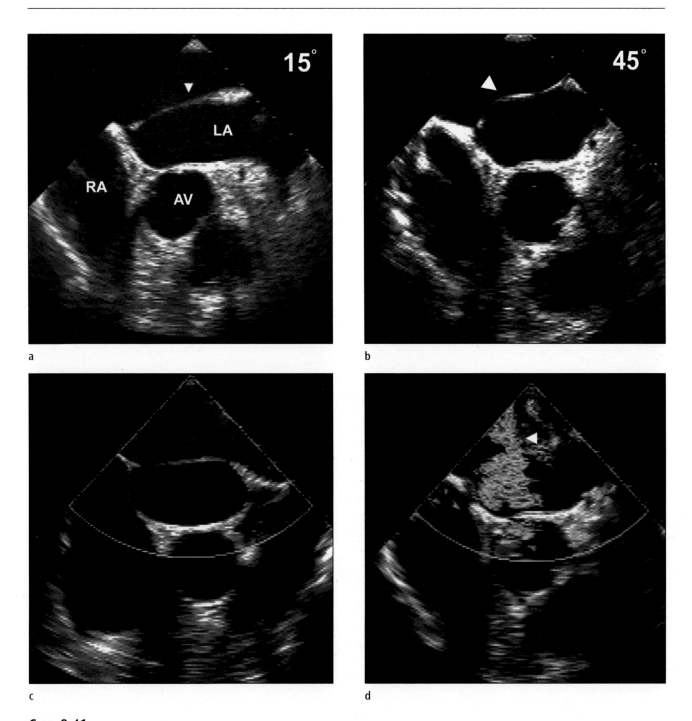

a
b
c
d

Case 9.41

Cor Triatriatum. In adults the membrane that separates the left atrium into anterior and posterior chambers is usually nonobstructive in comparison to that seen in symptomatic pediatric patients. (a–f) The membrane is visualized stretching from the junction of the left atrial appendage and the left superior pulmonary vein orifice to the area of the fossa ovalis of the atrial septum, and is usually the same thickness as that of the atrial wall, and is seen undulating (trampoline-like) with the opening and closing of the mitral valve with the cardiac cycle.

continued

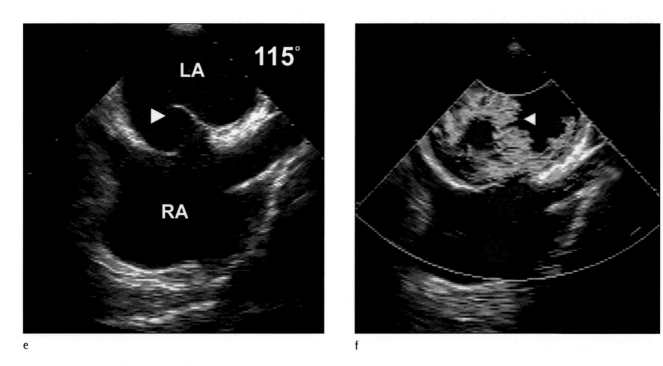

e   f

Case 9.41 *continued*

The atrium is divided into a superior pulmonary venous chamber that drains all four pulmonary veins, and an inferior chamber includes the foramen ovale and the atrial appendage. The membrane is usually fenestrated in the adult with one large orifice usually in close proximity to the atrial septum. (c,d,f) The site of obstruction is identified with color flow Doppler as a high velocity jet, with an area of flow convergence on the superior surface of the membrane. Continuous wave Doppler may be used to calculate the gradient utilizing the modified Bernoulli formula.

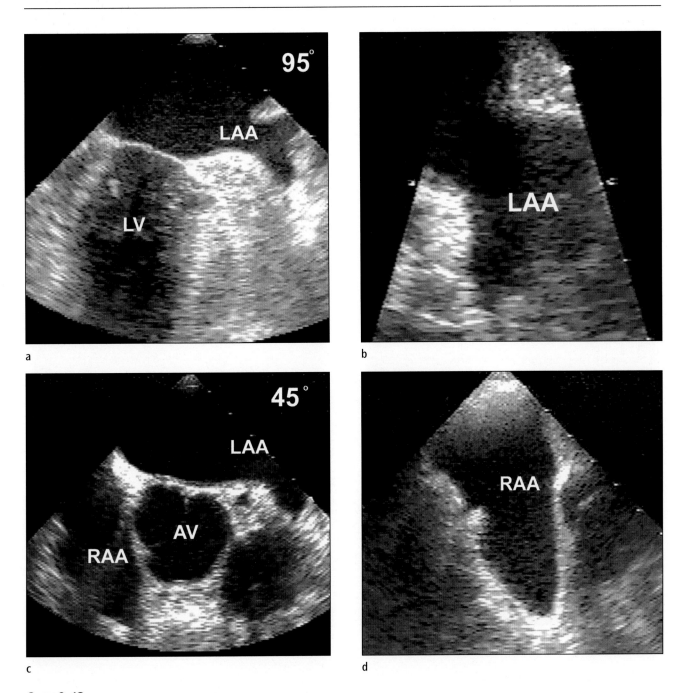

a   b

c   d

Case 9.42

Double left atrial appendage. Atrial morphology is usually, easily determined with transesophageal echocardiography in the mid- to upper esophageal views from 0 to 120 degrees, however the importance of atrial morphology has a lesser role in adult congenital heart disease. The right atrium is identified by noting the Eustachian valve remnant originating from the inferior portion of the inferior vena cava and the right atrial appendage with its short, broad configuration originating near the superior vena cava with a prominent atrial fold or projection identifying the crista terminalis. The left atrium (a–c) in distinction from the right atrium is usually more globular with a long and narrow appendage. With identification of the atrial appendage, isomerism or the proper relationship of the corresponding appendage with the respective atrium may be determined. Rarely the left appendage may be connected to the right atrium and the right appendage to the left atrium. Even rarer, both atria may possess appendages with identical right or left appendage morphologies. (a–d) Transesophageal echocardiographic views of the right and left atrial appendage. This patient presented for evaluation of a right atrial mass noted on a transthoracic echocardiographic examination. The left atrial appendage is visualized in the normal two-chamber view with and without zoom mode. The morphology of the left atrial appendage is bilobed. (c) The right atrial appendage in the short-axis basal view is long and wraps around the heart in an atypical direction. (d) In zoom mode the right atrial appendage exhibits a single lobe left atrial appendage with a narrow and long morphology. RAA, right atrial appendage; LAA, left atrial appendage. LA, left atrium; LV, left ventricle.

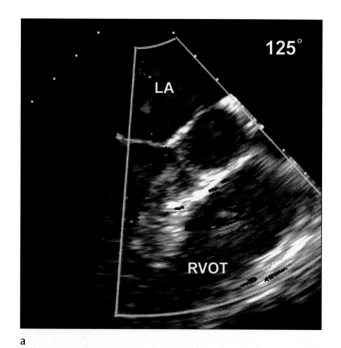

a

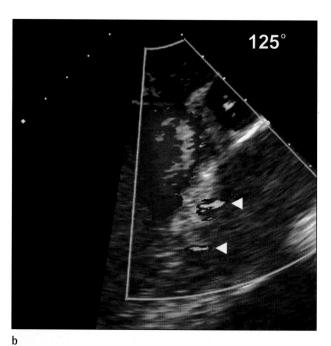

b

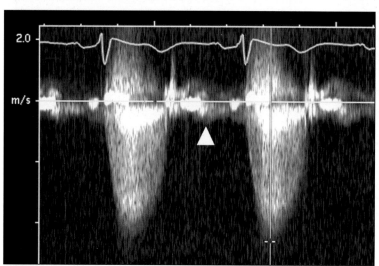

c

Case 9.43

Muscular ventricular septal defect. (a,b) Multiple small muscular ventricular septal defects in the region of the outflow trabecular septum. Frequently the defects are small, multiple (arrows) and only truly identified with the aid of color-flow Doppler. (c) Continuous-wave Doppler demonstrates high velocity flow emanating from the shunt with a maximum velocity over 4m/sec. Since ventricular septal defect flow takes the path of lease resistance, diastolic flow recorded (arrow) through the defect is often a reassuring sign that the compliance of the right ventricle is lower than the left ventricle suggesting a lower pulmonary vascular resistance. LA, left atrium; RVOT, right ventricular outflow tract.

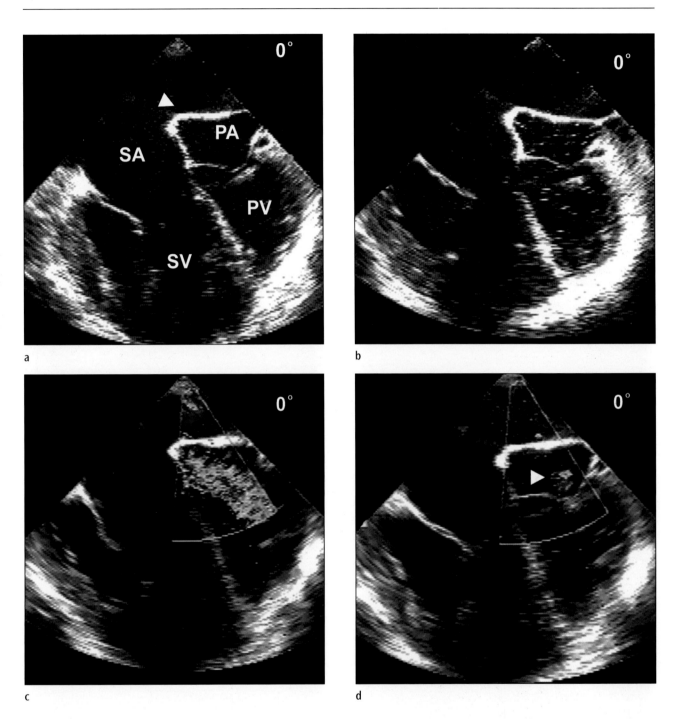

a

b

c

d

Case 9.44

The Mustard technique utilizes a baffle created from pericardial tissue with excision of the true atrial septum. With refinement of the arterial switch procedure, the atrial switch repairs are seen less frequently. (a–m) A normal example in multiple transesophageal views illustrating a Mustard repair created with a baffle (arrows) in the atrial cavities to redirect pulmonary and systemic venous flow to the appropriate ventricle. (b) Saline echocardiographic contrast injected through a peripheral venous site identifies the systemic venous drainage and the functional right ventricle. Echocardiographically, both the pulmonary venous return flow and the superior and inferior vena cava is identified and followed through the heart to assess post-operative caval obstruction or pulmonary venous obstruction.

continued

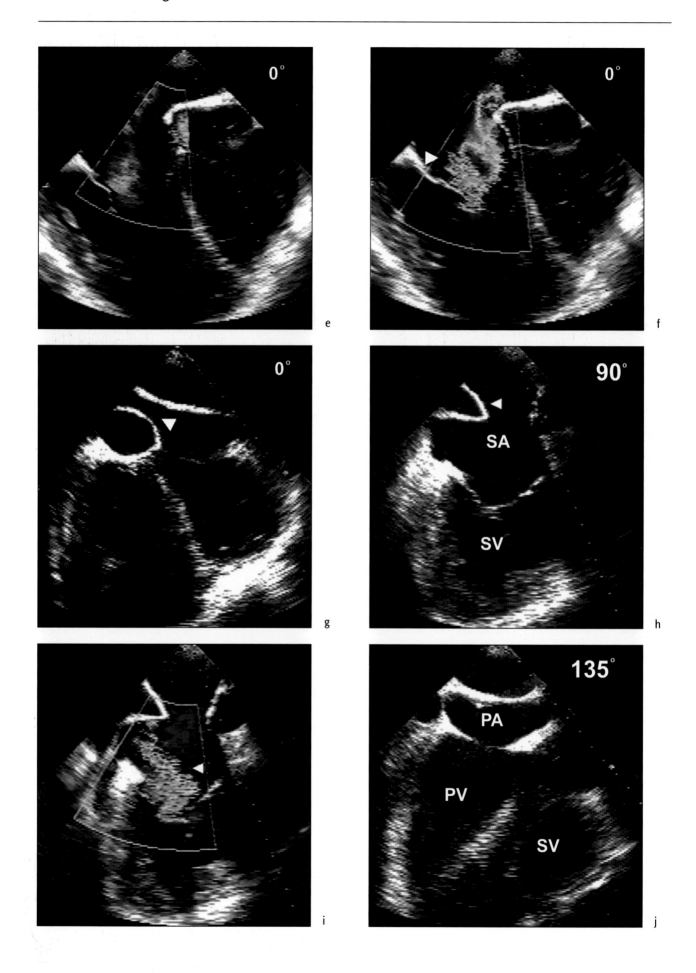

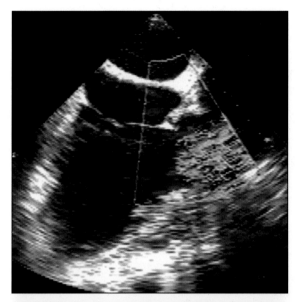

k

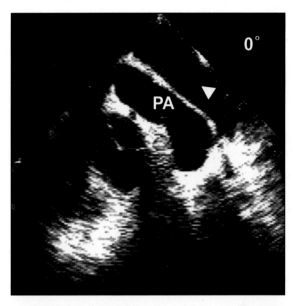

l

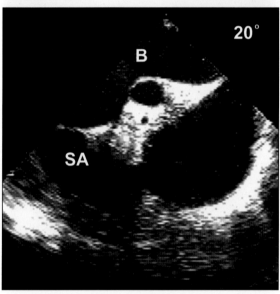

m

Case 9.44 *continued*

Surgically produced obstruction is most commonly noted as narrowing at the superior vena caval – right atrial junction and at the pulmonary venous inflow area. The baffle is interrogated for obstruction or leak, with the notation of residual atrial shunting, which is the rule. Obstruction of the atrial baffle is demonstrated with color flow or conventional Doppler as turbulent, biphasic or continuous flow within the pulmonary or systemic venous atrium. (f) The presence and severity of tricuspid regurgitation (arrow) is noted, trivial or mild tricuspid regurgitation, rarely mod to severe regurgitation is seen. It is important to assess right ventricular function although progression of right ventricular failure is uncommon. SA, systemic atrium; SV, systemic ventricle (morphologic right ventricle); PA, pulmonary atrium; PV, pulmonic ventricle (morphologic left ventricle); B, baffle.

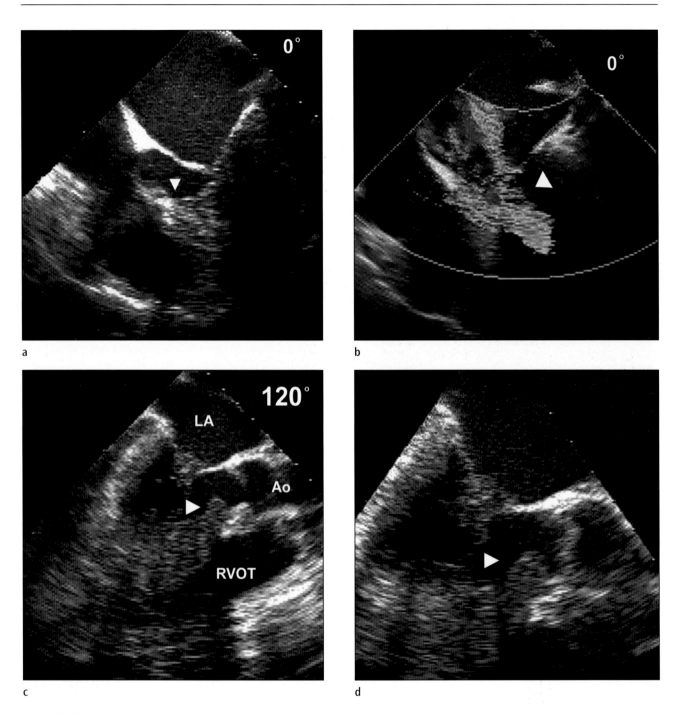

Case 9.45

Subaortic stenosis pre and post-op. In discrete subaortic stenosis, obstruction to flow occurs inferior to or below the aortic valve. Sub aortic stenosis may be caused by a subvalvular membrane, by a fibromuscular ridge opposite the level of the mitral annulus, a combination of a membrane and fibrous ridge and a subvalvular fibromuscular collar or tunnel. Subvalvular membranes usually occur just below the aortic valve as a thin fibrous membrane within a normal outflow tract. Subvalvular fibrous rings or ridges occur approximately 1–2 cm beneath the aortic valve and may extend into the left ventricular outflow for another 1 to 2 cm. The obstructing tissue is comprised of white fibroelastic tissue and may form a discrete band, or accumulation of tissue bands, or a diffuse ridge, which may extend across the outflow tract onto the base of the anterior mitral leaflet. The area of outflow tract narrowing may extend for several centimeters affecting all borders of the outflow tract. (a–d) Discrete diffuse ridge (arrow) type sub aortic stenosis identified in multiple view with transesophageal echocardiography from 0 to 120 degrees with obstruction noted by color Doppler.

continued

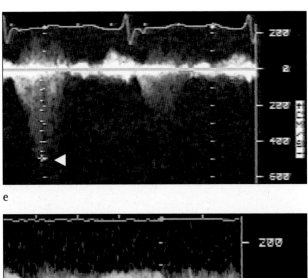

e

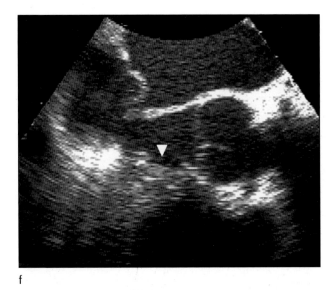

f

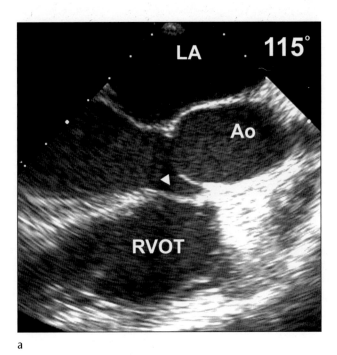

g

Case 9.45 *continued*

(e) Continuous-wave Doppler demonstrates the typical appearance of left ventricular outflow tract obstruction with a maximum velocity of 5m/sec. This patient was misdiagnosed as a hypertrophic cardiomyopathy with obstruction by transthoracic echocardiography. (f) Following post-operative removal of the obstructing tissue an obvious deformity (arrow) in the proximal ventricular septum is noted. (g) Continuous-wave Doppler demonstrates a markedly reduced flow from the left ventricular outflow tract following surgery. LA, left atrium; RVOT, right ventricular outflow tract.

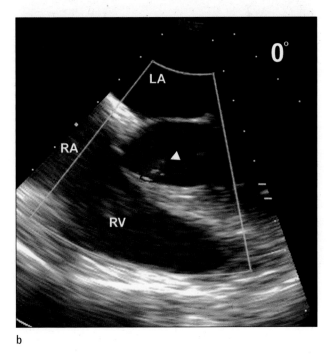

a

b

Case 9.46

Healed subpulmonic VSD with mild infundibular stenosis and a bicuspid aortic valve. (a, b) Thinning in the area of the ventricular outflow septal segment (arrow) in the area of a ventricular septal defect followed with serial echocardiographic studies.

continued

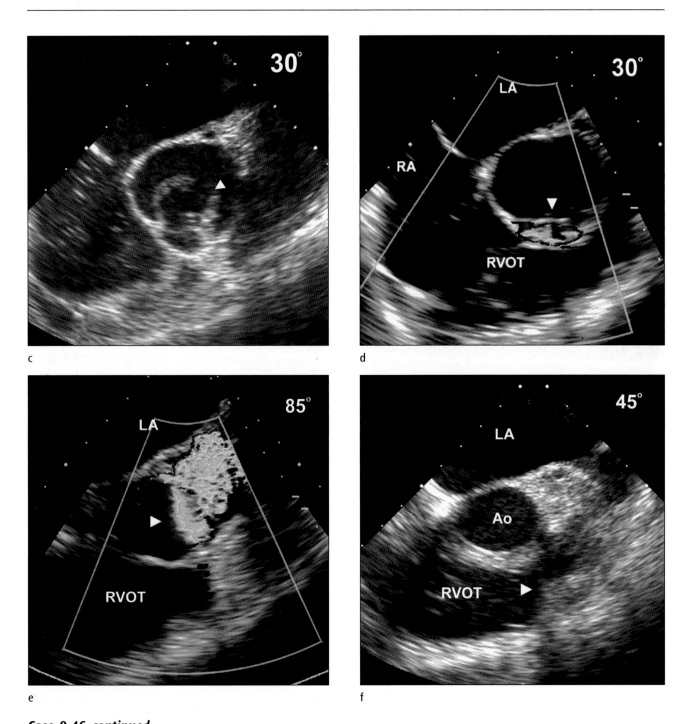

Case 9.46 *continued*

(c–e) A bicuspid aortic valve as well as aortic coarcation is frequently associated with these types of defects. (e) Color flow Doppler is consistent with aortic stenosis produced by the bicuspid valve. (f) There was also mild associated infundibular stenosis as denoted by a muscular protuberance (arrow) in the right ventricular outflow tract. A thorough examination is mandatory in patients with congenital heart disease as not to miss multiple associated defects. LA, left atrium; RVOT, right ventricular outflow tract; Ao, aorta; RA, right atrium; RV, right ventricle.

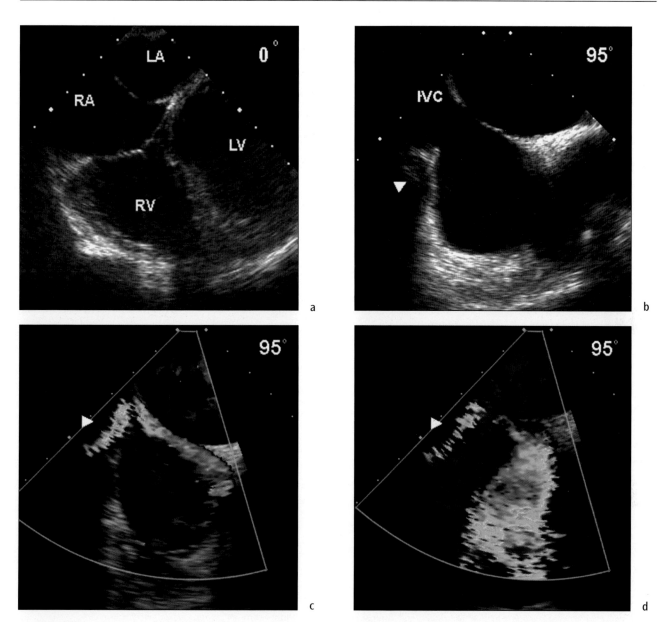

Case 9.47

Isolated partial anomalous pulmonary venous return with an intact atrial septum. Partial anomalous pulmonary venous return is described when one or more pulmonary veins, but not all are adherently connected to the right atrium or rarely the inferior vena cava. Partial anomalous pulmonary venous return may occur as an isolated defect with an intact atrial septum, but is uncommonly discovered in adults. Numerous reports have described the benefit of transesophageal echocardiography for detection of partial anomalous pulmonary venous return; however a high index of suspicion is usually necessary in order not to miss the defect. With transesophageal echocardiography, all four pulmonary veins with their origin to the left atrium may consistently be visualized. The right pulmonary veins are most commonly involved and reports have described anomalous connections to all of the systemic veins. The shunt produced by anomalous pulmonary venous return may not be significant, and is dictated to a large degree by the pressure difference between the right atrial and left atrial pressures. Generally in isolated pulmonary venous return, when only one pulmonary vein is involved the shunt is small as substantiated by normal dimensions of the right atrium and ventricle, with two anomalous veins producing mild overload to the right heart and mild right atrial and ventricular enlargement. (a) Four-chamber view at 0 degrees from the lower esophageal window in a patient who exhibited the characteristics of an atrial septal defect clinically and by transthoracic echocardiography however shunt flow or an atrial septal defect was not seen echocardiographically. (b–d) Modified bicaval view of the atria centered on the inferior vena cava demonstrating an abnormal area suggesting a vessel (arrow) anomalous pulmonary vein near the orifice of the IVC and significant flow (arrow) entering from the vessel emptying into the right atrium. Note the atrial septum appears intact. Also during the study the right lower pulmonary vein could not be identified with transesophageal echocardiography. RA, right atrium; LA, left atrium; RV, right ventricle; LV, left ventricle; IVC; inferior vena cava.

References

1. Mitchell SC, Korones SB, Berendes HW. Congenital heart disease in 56,109 births: incidence and natural history. *Circulation* 1971;41:323–32.

2. Hoffman JIE, Christianson R. Congenital heart disease in a cohort of 19,502 births with long-term follow up. *Am J Cardiol* 1978;42:641–7.

3. Fyler DC. Report of the New England Regional Infant Cardiac Program. *Pediatrics* 1980;65(suppl. 2):375.

4. Webb GD, Williams RG. 32nd Bethesda Conference: care of the adult with congenital heart disease. *J Am Coll Cardiol* 2001;37:1166.

5. Child JS. Echo-Doppler and color-flow imaging in congenital heart disease. *Cardiol Clin* 1990;8:289–313.

6. Shub C, Tajik AJ, Seward JB, et al. Surgical repair of uncomplicated atrial septal defect without 'routine' preoperative cardiac catheterization. *J Am Coll Cardiol* 1985;6:49–54.

7. Tumbarello R, Sanna A, Cardu G, et al. Usefulness of transesophageal echocardiography in the pediatric catheterization laboratory. *Am J Cardiol* 1993;71:1321–5.

8. Stumper O, Witsenburg M, Sutherland GR, et al. Transesophageal echocardiographic monitoring of interventional cardiac catheterization in children. *J Am Coll Cardiol* 1991;18:1506–14.

9. Stumper O, Kaulitz R, Elzenga NJ, et al. The value of transesophageal echocardiography in children with congenital heart disease. *J Am Soc Echocardiogr* 1991;4:164–76.

10. Fyfe DA, Ritter SB, Snider AR, et al. Guidelines for transesophageal echocardiography in children. *J Am Soc Echocardiogr* 1992;5:640–4.

11. Hoppe UC, Dederichs B, Deutsch HJ, et al. Congenital heart disease in adults and adolescents: comparative value of transthoracic and transesophageal echocardiography and MR imaging. *Radiology* 1996;199:669–77.

12. Sreeram N, Sutherland GR, Geuskens R, et al. The role of transesophageal echocardiography in adolescents and adults with congenital heart defects. *Eur Heart J* 1991;12:231–40.

13. Fyfe DA. Multiplane transesophageal echocardiography for congenital heart disease: leveling the playing field. *Echocardiography* 1996;13:651–2.

14. Fyfe DA, Kline CH. Transesophageal echocardiography for congenital heart disease. *Echocardiography* 1991;8:573–84.

15. Marelli AJ, Child JS, Perloff JK. Transesophageal echocardiography in congenital heart disease in the adult. *Cardiol Clin* 1993;11:505–20.

16. Seward JB, Khandheria BK, Oh JK, et al. Critical appraisal of transesophageal echocardiography: limitations, pitfalls, and complications. *J Am Soc Echocardiogr* 1992;5:288–305.

17. Stümper O, Elzenga NJ, Hess J, Sutherland GR. Transesophageal echocardiography in children with congenital heart disease: an initial experience. *J Am Coll Cardiol* 1990;16:433–41.

18. Stevenson JG, Sorenson GK, Gartman DM, et al. Transesophageal echocardiography during repair of congenital cardiac defects: identification of residual problems necessitating reoperation. *J Am Soc Echocardiogr* 1993;6:356.

19. Sloth E, Hasenkam JM, Sorensen KE, et al. Pediatric multiplane transesophageal echocardiography in congenital heart disease: new possibilities with a miniaturized probe. *J Am Soc Echocardiogr* 1996;9:626–8.

20. Hagler DJ. Echocardiographic segmental approach to complex congenital heart disease in the neonate. *Echocardiography* 1991;8:467.

21. Stümper O, Vargas-Barron J, Rijlaarsdam M, et al. Assessment of anomalous systemic and pulmonary venous connections by transesophageal echocardiography in infants and children. *Br Heart J* 1991;66:411–18.

22. Seliem MA. Echocardiographic and color flow Doppler assessment of systemic and pulmonary venous connection and drainage in the neonate with congenital heart disease. *Echocardiography* 1991;8:477–85.

23. Andrade JL, Leal SMG, Campos Filho O, et al. Contrast echocardiography during cardiac catheterization in patients with congenital heart diseases. *Cathet Cardiovasc Diagn* 1993;29:117–21.

24. Hajduczok ZD, Winniford MD, Kerber RE. Sensitivity of contrast ultrasound in the detection of atrial septal defect with predominant left to right shunting. *J Am Soc Echocardiogr* 1992;5:475–80.

25. Waggoner AD, Davila-Roman VG, Hopkins WE, et al. Comparison of color flow imaging and peripheral venous saline contrast during transesophageal echocardiography to evaluate right-to-left shunt at the atrial level. *Echocardiography* 1993;10:59–66.

26. Silverman NH, De Araujo LML. An echocardiographic method for the diagnosis of cardiac situs and malpositions. *Echocardiography* 1987;4:35.

27. Stümper OFW, Sreeram N, Elzenga NJ, et al. Diagnosis of atrial situs by transesophageal echocardiography. *J Am Coll Cardiol* 1990;16:442–6.

28. Stümper O, Rijlaarsdam M, Vargas-Barron J, et al. The assessment of juxtaposed atrial appendages by transesophageal echocardiography. *Int Cardiol* 1990;29:365–71.

29. Fernandes R, Alam M, Smith S, Khaga R. The role of transesophageal echocardiography in identifying anomalous coronary arteries. *Circulation* 1993;88:2532–40.

30. Girannoccaro PJ, Sochowski RA, Morton BC, Chan KL. Complementary role of transesophageal echocardiography to coronary angiography in the assessment of coronary artery anomalies. *Br Heart J* 1993;70:70–4.

31. Gaither NS, Rogan KM, Stajduhar K, et al. Anomalous origin and course of coronary arteries in adults: identification and improved imaging utilizing transesophageal echocardiography. *Am Heart J* 1991;122:69–75.

32. Craig RJ, Selzer A. Natural history and prognosis of atrial septal defect. *Circulation* 1968;37:805–15.

33. Shub C, Tajik AJ, Seward JB. Clinically 'silent' atrial septal defect: diagnosis by two-dimensional and Doppler echocardiography. *Am Heart J* 1985;110:665–7.

34. Gault JH, Morrow AAF, Gay WA, Ross J. Atrial septal defect in patients over the age of forty years: clinical and hemodynamic studies and the effects of operation. *Circulation* 1968;37:261.

35. St. John Sutton MG, Tajik AJ, McGoon DC. Atrial septal defect in patients ages 60 years or older: operative results and long-term postoperative follow-up. *Circulation* 1981;64:402–9.

36. Shub C, Dimopoulos IN, Seward JB, et al. Sensitivity of two-dimensional echocardiography in the direct visualization of atrial septal defect utilizing the subcostal approach: experience with 154 patients. *J Am Coll Cardiol* 1983;2:127–35.

37. Hausmann D, Daniel WG, Mügge A, et al. Value of transesophageal color Doppler echocardiography for detection of different types of atrial septal defect in adults. *J Am Soc Echocardiogr* 1992;5:481–8.

38. Child JS. Multiplane transesophageal echocardiography of the atria and related structures. In: Roelandt JR, Pandian N. (eds). *Multiplane Transesophageal Echocardiography*. New York: Churchill-Livingston, 1996.

39. Khandheria BK, Shub C, Tajik AJ, et al. Utility of color flow imaging for visualizing shunt flow in atrial septal defect. *Int J Cardiol* 1989;23:91–8.

40. Morimoto K, Matsuzaki M, Tohma Y, et al. Diagnosis and quantitative evaluation of secundum-type atrial septal defect by transesophageal Doppler echocardiography. *Am J Cardiol* 1990;66:85–91.

41. Faletra F, Scarpini S, Moreo A, et al. Color Doppler echocardiographic assessment of atrial septal defect size: correlation with surgical measurements. *J Am Soc Echocardiogr* 1991;4:429–34.

42. Dittmann H, Jacksch R, Voelker W, et al. Accuracy of Doppler echocardiography in quantitation of left to right shunts in adult patients with atrial septal defects. *J Am Coll Cardiol* 1988;11:338–42.

43. Mehta RH, Helmcke F, Nanda NC, et al. Transesophageal Doppler color flow mapping assessment of atrial septal defect. *J Am Coll Cardiol* 1990;16:1010–16.

44. Pollick C, Sullivan H, Cujec B, Wilansky S. Doppler color flow imaging assessment of shunt size in atrial septal defect. *Circulation* 1988;78:522–8.

45. Currie PJ, Seward JB, Chan KL, et al. Continuous wave Doppler determination of right ventricular pressure: a simultaneous. Doppler-catheterization study in 127 patients. *J Am Coll Cardiol* 1985;6:750–6.

46. Kitabatake A, Inoue, M, Asao M, et al. Noninvasive evaluation of the ratio of pulmonary to systemic flow in atrial septal defect by duplex Doppler echocardiography. *Circulation* 1984;69:73–9.

47. Schreiber TL, Feigenbaum H, Weyman AE. Effect of atrial septal defect repair on left ventricular geometry and degree of mitral valve prolapse. *Circulation* 1980;61:888–96.

48. Patten BM. The closure of the foramen ovale. *Am J Anat* 1931;48:19.

49. Hagen PT, Scholz DG, Edwards WD. Incidence and size of patent foramen ovale during the first 10 decades of life: an autopsy study of 965 normal hearts. *Mayo Clin Proc* 1984;59:17–20.

50. Sweeny LJ, Rosenquist GC. The normal anatomy of the atrial septum in the human heart. *Am Heart J* 1979;98:194-9.

51. Mügge A, Daniel WG, Klopper JW, Lichtlen PR. Visualization of patent foramen ovale by transesophageal color-coded Doppler echocardiography. *Am J Cardiol* 1988;62:837–8.

52. Hausmann D, Mügge A, Becht I, Daniel WG. Diagnosis of patent foramen ovale by transesophageal echocardiography and association with cerebral and peripheral embolic events. *Am J Cardiol* 1992;70:668–72.

53. Meissner I, Whisnant JF, Khandheria BK, et al. Prevalence of potential risk factors for stroke assessed by transesophageal echocardiography and carotid ultrasonography: the SPARC study. Stroke Prevention: assessment of risk in a community. *Mayo Clin Proc* 1999;74:862–9.

54. Sacco RL, Ellenberg JH, Mohr JP, et al. Infarcts of undetermined cause: the NINCDS Stroke Data Bank. *Ann Neurol* 1989;25:382–90.

55. Steiner MM, Di Tullio MR, Rundek T, et al. Patent foramen ovale size and embolic brain imaging findings among patients with ischemic stroke. *Stroke* 1998;29:944–8.

56. Webster MW, Chancellor AM, Smith HJ, et al. Patent foramen ovale in young stroke patients. *Lancet* 1988;ii:11–12.

57. Lechat P, Mas JL, Lascault G, et al. Prevalence of patent foramen ovale in patients with stroke. *N Engl J Med* 1988;318:1148–52.

58. De Belder MA, Tourikis L, Leech G, Camm AJ. Risk of patent foramen ovale for thromboembolic events in all age groups. *Am J Cardiol* 1992;69:1316–20.

59. Mügge A, Daniel WG, Angermann C, et al. Atrial septal aneurysm: atrial septal aneurysm in adult patients: a multicenter study using transthoracic and transesophageal echocardiography. *Circulation* 1995;91:2785–92.

60. Cabanes L, Mas JL, Cohen A, et al. Atrial septal aneurysm and patent foramen ovale as risk factors for cryptogenic stroke in patients less than 55 years of age. A study using transesophageal echocardiography. *Stroke* 1993;24:1865–73.

61. Dhar PK, Fyfe DA, Sharma S. Multiplane transesophageal echocardiographic evaluation of defects of the atrioventricular septum: the crux of the matter. *Echocardiography* 1996;13:663–76.

62. Ettedgui JA, Siewers RD, Anderson RH, et al. Diagnostic echocardiographic features of the sinus venosus defect. *Br Heart J* 1990;64:329–31.

63. Kronzon I, Tunick PA, Freedberg RS, et al. Transesophageal echocardiography is superior to transthoracic echocardiography in the diagnosis of sinus venosus atrial septal defect. *J Am Coll Cardiol* 1991;17:537–42.

64. Maxted W, Finch A, Nanda NC, et al. Multiplane transesophageal echocardiographic detection of sinus venous atrial septal defect. *Echocardiography* 1995;12:139–43.

65. Pascoe RD, Oh JK, Warnes CA, et al. Diagnosis of sinus venosus atrial septal defect with transesophageal echocardiography. *Circulation* 1996;94:1049–55.

66. Pascoe RD, Oh JK, Warnes CA, et al. Heart disease in the young: diagnosis of sinus venosus atrial septal defect with transesophageal echocardiography. *Circulation* 1996;94:1049–55.

67. Becker AE, Anderson RH (eds). *Cardiac Pathology: An Integrated Text and Colour Atlas.* New York: Raven Press, 1983.

68. Yeager SB, Chin AJ, Sanders SP. Subxyphoid two-dimensional echocardiographic diagnosis of coronary sinus defects. *Am J Cardiol* 1984;54:686–7.

69. Hamada Y, Ebihara H, Tanimoto Y, et al. Unroofed coronary sinus demonstrated by two-dimensional echocardiography. *Am Heart J* 1984;108:1558–60.

70. Schmidt KG, Silverman NH. Cross-sectional and contrast echocardiography in the diagnosis of interatrial communications through the coronary sinus. *Int J Cardiol* 1987;16:193–9.

71. Sunaga Y, Hayashi K, Okubo N, et al. Transesophageal echocardiographic diagnosis of coronary sinus type atrial septal defect. *Am Heart J* 1992;124:1657–9.

72. Lei MH, Chang CI, Lo CY. Coronary sinus septal defect mimicking left atrial membrane. *Am Heart J* 1994;127:1621–4.

73. Child JS. Echocardiographic evaluation of the adult with postoperative congenital heart disease. In: Otto C. (ed). *The Practice of Clinical Echocardiography.* Philadelphia, PA: WB Saunders Co, 1997.

74. Mejjboom F, Hess J, Szatmari A, et al. Long-term follow-up (9–20 years) after surgical closure of atrial septal defect at a young age. *Am J Cardiol* 1993;72:1431–4.

75. Meyer RA, Korfhagen JC, Covitz W, Kaplan S. Long-term follow-up study after closure of secundum atrial septal defect in children: an echocardiographic study. *Am J Cardiol* 1982;50:143–8.

76. Attie F, Rosas M, Granados N, et al. Surgical treatment for secundum atrial septal defects in patients >40 years old. *J Am Coll Cardiol* 2001;38:2035–42.

77. Minich LL, Snider AR. Echocardiographic guidance during placement of the buttoned double-disc device for atrial septal defect closure. *Echocardiography* 1993;10:567–72.

78. Hellenbrand WE, Fahey JT, McGowen FX, et al. Transesophageal echocardiographic guidance of transcatheter closure of atrial septal defect. *Am J Cardiol* 1990;66:207–13.

79. Lloyd TR, Vermilion RP, Zamora R, et al. Influence of echocardiographic guidance on positioning of the buttoned occluder for transcatheter closure of atrial septal defects. *Echocardiography* 1996;13:117–21.

80. Moe DG, Guntherorth WG. Spontaneous closure of uncomplicated ventricular septal defect.*Am J Cardiol* 1987;60:674–8.

81. Bloomfield DK. The natural history of ventricular septal defect in patients surviving infancy. *Circulation* 1964;29:914.

82. Hoffman JIE, Rudolph AM. The natural history of ventricular septal defects in infancy. *Am J Cardiol* 1965;16:634–53.

83. Wise JR, Wilson WS. The natural history of the so-called aneurysm of the membranous ventricular septum in childhood. *Circulation* 1979;75:90.

84. Glancy DL, Roberts WC. Complete spontaneous closure of ventricular septal defect. *Am J Med* 1967;43:846–53.

85. Schott GD. Documentation of spontaneous functional closure of a ventricular septal defect during adult life. *Br Heart J* 1973;35:1214–16.

86. Campbell M. Natural history of ventricular septal defect. *Br Heart J* 1971;33:246.

87. Keith JD, Rose V, Collins G, Kidd BSL. Ventricular septal defect: incidence, morbidity, and mortality in various age groups. *Br Heart J* 1979;33:246–57.

88. Hu DCK, Giuliani ER, Downing TP, et al. Spontaneous closure of congenital ventricular septal defect in an adult. *Clin Cardiol* 1986;9:587–8.

89. Otterstad JE, Nitter-Hauge S, Myhre E. Isolated ventricular septal defects in adults: clinical and haemodynamic findings. *Br Heart J* 1983;50:343–8.

90. Weidman WH, Blount SG, DuShane JW, et al. Clinical course in adults with ventricular septal defect. *Circulation* 1977;56:I-78.

91. Hagler DJ, Edwards WD, Seward JB, Tajik AJ. Standardized nomenclature of the ventricular septum and ventricular septal defects, with applications for two-dimensional echocardiography. *Mayo Clin Proc* 1985;60:741–52.

92. Graham TP Jr, Gutgesell HP. Ventricular septal defects. In: Emmanouilides GC, Riemenschneider TA, Allen HD, Gutgesell HP (eds). *Moss and Adams Heart Disease in Infants, Children and Adolescents*. Baltimore, MD: Williams & Wilkens, 1995:724.

93. Milo S, Yen S, Macartney FJ, et al. Straddling and overriding atrioventricular valves: morphology and classification. *Am J Cardiol* 1979;14:1122–34.

94. Spevak PJ, Mandell VS, Colan SD, et al. Reliability of Doppler color flow mapping in the identification and localization of multiple ventricular septal defects. *Echocardiography* 1993;10:573–81.

95. Reeder GS, Seward JB, Hagler DJ, Tajik AJ. Color flow imaging in congenital heart disease. *Echocardiography* 1986;3:533.

96. Ritter SB. Recent advances in color-Doppler assessment of congenital heart disease. *Echocardiography* 1988;5:457.

97. Reeder GS, Currie PJ, Hagler DJ, et al. Use of Doppler techniques (continuous-wave, pulsed-wave, and color flow imaging) in the noninvasive hemodynamic assessment of congenital heart disease. *Mayo Clin Proc* 1986;61:725–44.

98. Murphy DJ Jr, Ludomirsky A, Huhta JC. Continuous wave Doppler in children with ventricular septal defect: noninvasive estimation of interventricular pressure gradient. *Am J Cardiol* 1986;57:428–32.

99. Hatle L, Angelsen B. *Doppler Ultrasound in Cardiology*. Edn 2. Philadelphia, PA: Lea & Febiger, 1985.

100. Hatle L, Rokseth R. Noninvasive diagnosis and assessment of ventricular septal defect by Doppler ultrasound. *Acta Med Scand* 1981;645:47–56.

101. Rahko PS. Doppler echocardiographic evaluation in ventricular septal defects in adults. *Echocardiography* 1993;10:517–31.

102. Andrade JL. The role of Doppler echocardiography in the diagnosis, follow-up, and management of ventricular septal defects. *Echocardiography* 1991;8:501–16.

103. Chan KL, Currie PJ, Seward JB, et al. Comparison of three Doppler ultrasound methods in the prediction of pulmonary artery pressure. *J Am Coll Cardiol* 1987;9:549–54.

104. Kurokawa S, Takahashi M, Katoh Y, et al. Noninvasive evaluation of the ratio of pulmonary to systemic flow in ventricular septal defect by means of Doppler two-dimensional echocardiography. *Am Heart J* 1988;116:1033–44.

105. Stevenson JG. The use of Doppler echocardiography for detection and estimation of severity of patent ductus arteriosus, ventricular septal defect, and atrial septal defect. *Echocardiography* 1987;4:321.

106. Kronzon I, Cziner DG, Rosenzweig BP, Tunick PA. Diastolic left-to right shunting in uncomplicated ventricular septal defect. *Echocardiography* 1995;12:457.

107. Pieroni DR, Nishimura RA, Bierman FZ, et al. Second natural history study of congenital heart defects: ventricular septal defect: echocardiography. *Circulation* 1993;87(Suppl 2):I-80–8.

108. Sabry AF, Reller MD, Silberbach M, et al. Comparison of four Doppler echocardiographic methods for calculating pulmonary-to-systemic shunt flow ratios in patients with ventricular septal defect. *Am J Cardiol* 1995;75:611–14.

109. Teien D, Karp K, Wendel H, et al. Quantification of left-to-right shunts by echo Doppler cardiography in patients with ventricular septal defects. *Acta Paediatr Scand* 1991;80:335–60.

110. Moises VA. A new method for noninvasive estimation of ventricular septal defect shunt flow by color Doppler flow mapping: imaging of the laminar flow convergence on the left septal surface. *J Am Coll Cardiol* 1991;18:824–32.

111. Levine RA. Doppler color mapping of the proximal flow convergence region: a new quantitative physiologic tool. *J Am Coll Cardiol* 1991;18:833–6.

112. Valdes-Cruz LM, Cayre RO. Ventricular septal defects. In: Valdes-Cruz LM, Cayre RO (eds). *Echocardiographic Diagnosis of Congenital Heart Disease: An Embryologic and Anatomic Approach*. Philadelphia, PA: Lippincott-Raven, 1999; 199.

113. Kidd L, Driscoll DJ, Gersony WM, et al. Second natural history study of congenital heart defects: results of treatment of patients with ventricular septal defects. *Circulation* 1993;87:(suppl 2):I-38–51.

114. Neumayer U, Stone S, Somerville J. Small ventricular septal defects in adults. *Eur Heart J* 1998;19:1573–82.

115. Fallot A. Contribution a l'anatomie pathologique de la maladie bleue (cyanose cardiaque). *Marseille Med* 1888;25:77.

116. Rao BN, Anderson RC, Edwards JE. Anatomic variations in the tetralogy of Fallot. *Am Heart J* 1971;81:361–71.

117. Soto B, Pacifico AD, Ceballos R, et al. Tetralogy of Fallot: an angiographic–pathologic correlative study. *Circulation* 1981;64:558–66.

118. Becker AE, Connor M, Anderson RH. Tetralogy of Fallot: a morphometric and geometric study. *Am J Cardiol* 1975;35:402–12.

119. Rowe RD, Vlad P, Keith JD. Experiences with 180 cases of tetralogy of Fallot in infants and children. *Can Med Assoc J* 1955;73:23.

120. Dabizzi RP, Teodori G, Barletta GA, et al. Associated coronary and cardiac anomalies in the tetralogy of Fallot: an angiographic study. *Eur Heart J* 1990;11:692–704.

121. Marino B, Di Giulio MC, Grazioli S, et al. Associated cardiac anomalies in isolated and syndromic patients with tetralogy of Fallot. *Am J Cardiol* 1996;77:505–8.

122. Donofrio MT, Jacobs ML, Rychik J. Tetralogy of Fallot with absent pulmonary valve: echocardiographic morphometric features of the right-sided structures and their relationship to presentation and outcome. *J Am Soc Echocardiogr* 1997;10:556–61.

123. Rowland DG, Caserta T, Foy P, et al. Congenital absence of the pulmonary valve with tetralogy of Fallot with associated aortic stenosis and patent ductus arteriosus: a prenatal diagnosis. *Am Heart J* 1996;132:1075–7.

124. Vargas-Barron J, Espinola-Zavaleta N, Rijlaarsdam M, et al. Tetralogy of Fallot with absent pulmonary valve and total anomalous pulmonary venous connection. *J Am Soc Echocardiogr* 1999;12:160–3.

125. Capelli H, Somerville J. Atypical Fallot's tetralogy with doubly committed subarterial ventricular septal defect. *Am J Cardiol* 1983;51:282–5.

126. Di Segni E, Einzig S, Bass JL, Edwards JE. Congenital absence of pulmonary valve associated with tetralogy of Fallot: diagnosis by 2–dimensional echocardiography. *Am J Cardiol* 1983;51:1798–800.

127. Child JS. Echocardiographic assessment of adults with tetralogy of Fallot. *Echocardiography* 1993;10:629–40.

128. Geibel A. Echocardiographic evaluation in unoperated congenital heart disease in adults. *Herz* 1999;24:276–92.

129. Gatzoulis MA, Soukias N, Ho SY, et al. Echocardiographic and morphological correlations in tetralogy of Fallot. *Eur Heart J* 1999;20:221–31.

130. Xu J, Shiota T, Ge S, et al. Intraoperative transesophageal echocardiography using high-resolution biplane 7.5 MHz probes with continuous-wave Doppler capability in infants and children with tetralogy of Fallot. *Am J Cardiol* 1996;77:539–42.

131. Miller-Hance WC, Silverman NH. Transesophageal echocardiography (TEE) in congenital heart disease with focus on the adult. *Cardiol Clin* 2000;18:861–92.

132. Presbitero P, Prever SB, Contrafatto I, Morea M. Results of total correction of tetralogy of Fallot performed in adults. Updated in 1996. *Ann Thorac Surg* 1996;61:1870–3.

133. Karube M, Utsunomiya H, Iida T, et al. Total repair of tetralogy of Fallot in an adult: report of a case without prior treatment at 59 years of age. *Jpn J Thorac Surg* 1996;49:395–9.

134. Stellin G, Milanesi O, Rubino M, et al. Repair of tetralogy of Fallot in the first six months of life: transatrial versus transventricular approach. *Ann Thorac Surg* 1995;60(suppl 6):S588–91.

135. Norgard G, Gatzoulis MA, Josen M, et al. Does restrictive right ventricular physiology in the early postoperative period predict subsequent right ventricular restriction after repair of tetralogy of Fallot? *Heart* 1998;79:481–4.

136. Kurosawa H, Morita K, Yamagishi M, et al. Conotruncal repair for tetralogy of Fallot: midterm results. *J Thorac Cardiovasc Surg* 1998;115:351–60.

137. Rosenfeld HM, Gentles TL, Wernovsky G, et al. Utility of intraoperative transesophageal echocardiography in the assessment of residual cardiac defects. *Pediatr Cardiol* 1998;19:346–51.

138. Yang SG, Novello R, Nicolson S, et al. Evaluation of ventricular septal defect repair using intraoperative transesophageal echocardiography: frequency and significance of residual defects in infants and children. *Echocardiography* 2000;17:681–4.

139. Roberson DA, Muhiudeen IA, Cahalan MK, et al. Intraoperative transesophageal echocardiography of ventricular septal defect. *Echocardiography* 1991;8:687–97.

140. Kaushal SK, Radhakrishanan S, Dagar KS, et al. Significant intraoperative right ventricular outflow gradients after repair for tetralogy of Fallot: to revise or not to revise? *Ann Thorac Surg* 1999;68:1705–12.

141. Joyce JJ, Hwang EY, Wiles HB, et al. Reliability of intraoperative transesophageal echocardiography during Tetralogy of Fallot repair. *Echocardiography* 2000;17:319–27.

142. Campbell M. Natural history of persistent ductus arteriosus. *Br Heart J* 1968;30:4–13.

143. Campbell M. Patent ductus arteriosus: some notes on prognosis and on pulmonary hypertension. *Br Heart J* 1955;17:511.

144. Kelly DT. Patent ductus arteriosus in adults. *Cardiovasc Clin* 1979;10:321–6.

145. Fisher RG, Moodie DS, Sterba R, Gill CC. Patent ductus arteriosus in adults — long-term follow-up: nonsurgical versus surgical treatment. *J Am Coll Cardiol* 1986;8:280–4.

146. Espino-Vela J, Cardenas N, Cruz R. Patent ductus arteriosus: with special reference to patients with pulmonary hypertension. *Circulation* 1968;38(suppl I):I-45–60.

147. Musewe NN, Smallhorn JF. Benson LN, et al. Validation of Doppler-derived pulmonary arterial pressure in patient with ductus arteriosus under different hemodynamic states. *Circulation* 1987;76:1081–91.

148. Coggin CJ, Parker KR, Keith JD. Natural history of isolated patent ductus arteriosus and the effect of surgical correction: twenty years' experience at the Hospital for Sick Children, Toronto. *Can Med Assoc J* 1970;102:718–20.

149. Ohtsuka S, Kakihana M, Ishikawa T, et al. Aneurysm of patent ductus arteriosus in an adult case: findings of cardiac catheterization, angiography, and pathology. *Clin Cardiol* 1987;10:537–40.

150. Lund JT, Jensen MB, Hjelms E. Aneurysm of the ductus arteriosus: a review of the literature and the surgical implications. *Eur J Cardiothorac Surg* 1991;5:566–70.

151. Shyu KG, Lai LP, Lin SC, et al. Diagnostic accuracy of transesophageal echocardiography for detecting patent ductus arteriosus in adolescents and adults. *Chest* 1995;108:1201–5.

152. Mügge A, Daniel WG, Lichtlen PR. Imaging of patent ductus arteriosus by transesophageal color-coded Doppler echocardiography. *J Clin Ultrasound* 1991;19:128–9.

153. Takenaka K, Sakamota T, Shiota T, et al. Diagnosis of patent ductus arteriosus in adults by biplane transesophageal color Doppler flow mapping. *Am J Cardiol* 1991;68:691–3.

154. John S, Muralidharan S, Jairaj PS, et al. The adult ductus: review of surgical experience with 131 patients. *J Thorac Cardiovasc Surg* 1981;82:314–19.

155. Sahn DJ, Allen HD. Real-time cross-sectional echocardiographic imaging and measurement of the patent ductus arteriosus in infants and children. *Circulation* 1978;58:343–54.

156. Andrade A, Vargas-Barron J, Rijlaarsdam M, et al. Utility of transesophageal echocardiography in the examination of adult patients with patent ductus arteriosus. *Am Heart J* 1995;130:543–6.

157. Szulc M, Ritter SB. Patent ductus arteriosus in an infant with atrioventricular septal defect and pulmonary hypertension: diagnosis by transesophageal color flow echocardiography. *J Am Soc Echocardiogr* 1991;4:194–8.

158. Krauss D, Weinert L, Lang RM. The role of multiplane transesophageal echocardiography in diagnosing PDA in an adult. *Echocardiography* 1996;13:95–8.

159. Ryan K, Sanyal RS, Pinheiro L, Nanda NC. Assessment of aortic coarctation and collateral circulation by biplane transesophageal echocardiography. 1992;9:277–85.

160. Shiota T, Omoto R, Cobanoglu A, et al. Usefulness of transesophageal imaging of flow convergence region in the operating room for evaluating isolated patent ductus arteriosus. *Am J Cardiol* 1997;80:1108–12.

161. Ho, AC, Tan PP, Yang MW, et al. The use of multiplane transesophageal echocardiography to evaluate residual patent ductus arteriosus during video-assisted thoracoscopy in adults. *Surg Endosc* 1999;13:975–9.

162. Wang KY, Hsieh KS, Yang MW, et al. The use of transesophageal echocardiography to evaluate the effectiveness of patent ductus arteriosus ligation. *Echocardiography* 1993;10:53–7.

163. Lavoie J, Javorski JJ, Donahue K, et al. Detection of residual flow by transesophageal echocardiography during video-assisted thoracoscopic patent ductus arteriosus interruption. *Anes Analg* 1995;80:1071–5.

164. Keith JD, Rowe RD, Vlad P. *Heart Disease in Infancy and Childhood*. New York: Macmillan, 1978.

165. Friedman WF. Congenital heart disease in infancy and childhood. In: Braunwald E, ed. *Heart Disease: A Textbook of Cardiovascular Medicine*, 5th edn. Philadelphia, PA: WB Saunders, 1997:877–962.

166. Cyran SE. Coarctation of the aorta in the adolescent and adult: echocardiographic evaluation prior to and following surgical repair. *Echocardiography* 1993;10:553–63.

167. Shone JD, Sellers RD, Anderson RD, et al. The development complex of 'parachute mitral valve' supravalvular ring of left atrium and coarctation of aorta. *Am J Cardiol* 1963;11:714.

168. Stern HC, Locher D, Wallnofer K, et al. Noninvasive assessment of coarctation of the aorta: comparative measurements by two-dimensional echocardiography, magnetic resonance and angiography. *Pediatr Cardiol* 1991;12:1–5.

169. Stern H, Erbel R, Schreiner G. Coarctation of the aorta: quantitative analysis by transesophageal echocardiography. *Echocardiography* 1987;4:387.

170. Vicente T, Pinar E, Garcia A, et al. The usefulness of transesophageal echocardiography in the diagnosis of atypical aortic coarctation. *Rev Esp Cardiol* 1997;50:802–5.

171. Duffy CI, Plehn JF. Transesophageal echocardiographic assessment of aortic coarctation using color, flow-directed Doppler sampling. *Chest* 1994;105:286–8.

172. Crepaz R, Knoll P, Paulmichl R, Pitscheider W. The utility of various Doppler parameters at rest and during exercise for the diagnosis of residual stenosis after operation for aortic coarctation. A Doppler–nuclear magnetic resonance comparison. *G Ital Cardiol* 1998;28:369–76.

173. Teien D, Wendel H, Holm S, Hallberg ML. Estimation of Doppler gradients at rest and during exercise in patients with recoarctation of the aorta. *Br Heart J* 1991;65:155–7.

174. Cyran SE, Grzeszczak M, Kaufman K, et al. Aortic 'recoarctation' at rest versus at exercise in children as evaluated by stress Doppler echocardiography after a 'good' operative result. *Am J Cardiol* 1993;71:963–70.

175. Marelli AJ, Julsrud R, Breen JF, Felmlee JP, et al. Coarctation of the aorta: collateral flow assessment with phase-contrast MR angiography. *Am J Roentgenol* 1997;189:1735.

176. Riquelme C, Laissy JP, Menegazzo, et al. MR imaging of coarctation of the aorta and its postoperative complications in adults: assessment with spin-echo and cine-MR imaging. *Magn Reson Imaging* 1999;17:37–46.

177. Cheung YF, Leung MP, Lee J, Yung TC. An evolving role of transesophageal echocardiography for the monitoring of interventional catheterization in children. *Clin Cardiol* 1999;22:804–10.

178. Lee CP, Lin TS, Chan P. Successful percutaneous transluminal angioplasty in native recoarctation of aorta in young adult: a case report. *Chin Med J* 1995;55:258–62.

179. Henry WL, Maron BJ, Griffith JM, et al. Differential diagnosis of anomalies of the great arteries by real-time two-dimensional echocardiography. *Circulation* 1975;51:283.

180. Daskalopoulus DA, Edwards WD, Driscoll DJ, et al. Correlation of two-dimensional echocardiographic and autopsy findings in complete transposition of the great arteries. *Am J Cardiol* 1982;2:1151–7.

181. Roberson DA, Silvermann NH. Malaligned outlet septum with subpulmonary ventricular septal defect and abnormal ventriculoarterial connection: a morphologic spectrum defined by echocardiography. *J Am Coll Cardiol* 1990;16:459–68.

182. Kirklin JW, Colvin EV, McConnell ME, Bargeron LM Jr. Complete transposition of the great arteries: treatement in the current era. *Pediatr Clin North Am* 1990;37:171–7.

183. Child JS. Echocardiographic evaluation of adult postoperative congenital heart disease: complex cyanotic congenital heart disease amenable to biventricular repair. *Echocardiography* 1995;12:509.

184. Aziz KU, Paul MH, Bharati S, et al. Two dimensional echocardiographic evaluation of Mustard operation for d-transposition of the great arteries. *Am J Cardiol* 1981;47:654–64.

185. Schmidt KG, Coez JL, Silverman NH. Assessment of right ventricular performance by pulsed Doppler echocardiography in patients after intraatrial repair of aortopulmonary transposition in infancy and childhood. *J Am Coll Cardiol* 1989;13:1578–85.

186. Smallhorn JF, Gow JL, Freedom RM, et al. Pulsed Doppler echocardiographic assessment of the pulmonary venous pathway after Mustard or Senning procedure for transposition of the great arteries. *Circulation* 1986;73:765–74.

187. Hurwitz RA, Caldwell RL, Dirod DA, Brown J. Right ventricular systolic function in adolescents and young adults after Mustard operation for d-transposition of the great arteries. *Am J Cardiol* 1996;77:294.

188. Mee RB. Severe right ventricular failure after Mustard or Senning operation. Two stage repair: pulmonary artery banding and switch. *J Thorac Cardiovasc Surg* 1986;92:385–90.

189. Losay J, Planche C, Gerardin B, et al. Midterm surgical results of arterial switch operation for transposition of the great arteries with intact septu. *Circulation* 1990;82(suppl IV):146–50.

190. Hopkins WE, Waggoner AD, Davila-Roman V, Perez JE. Two-dimensional Doppler color flow imaging in adults with L-transposition of the great arteries. *Echocardiography* 1993;10:611–17.

191. Caso P, Ascione LK, Lange A, et al. Diagnostic value of transesophageal echocardiography in the assessment of congenitally corrected transposition of the great arteries in adult patients. *Am Heart J* 1998;135:43–50.

192. Celermajer DS, Cullen S, Deanfield JE, Sullivan ID. Congenitally corrected transposition and Ebstein's anomaly of the systemic atrioventricular valve: association with aortic arch obstruction. *J Am Coll Cardiol* 1991;18:1056–8.

193. Silverman NH, Gerlis LM, Horowitz ES, et al. Pathologic elucidation of the echocardiographic features of Ebstein's malformation of the morphologically tricuspid valve in discordant atrioventricular connections. *Am J Cardiol* 1995;76:1277–83.

194. Anderson KR, Zurberbuhler JR, Anderson RH, et al. Morphologic spectrum of Ebstein's anomaly of the heart: a review. *Mayo Clin Proc* 1979;54:174–80.

195. Frescura C, Angelini A, Daliento L, Thiene G. Morphologic aspects of Ebstein's anomaly in adults. *Thorac Cardiovasc Surg* 2000;48:203–8.

196. Attie F, Rosas M, Rijlaarsdam M, et al. The adult with Ebstein anomaly. Outcome in 72 unoperated patients. *Medicine* 2000;79:27–36.

197. Celermajer DS, Bull C, Till JA, et al. Ebstein's anomaly: presentation and outcome from fetus to adult. *J Am Coll Cardiol* 1994;23:170–6.

198. Giuliani ER, Fuster V, Brandenburg RO, Mair DD. Ebstein's anomaly: the clinical features and natural history of Ebstein's anomaly of the tricuspid valve. *Mayo Clin Proc* 1979;54:163–73.

199. Mair DD. Ebstein's anomaly: natural history and management. *J Am Coll Cardiol* 1992;19:1047–8.

200. Oberhoffer R, Cook AC, Lang D, et al. Correlation between echocardiographic and morphological investigations of lesions of the tricuspid valve diagnosed during fetal life. *Br Heart J* 1992;68:580–5.

201. Shiina A, Seward JB, Edwards WD, et al. Two-dimensional echocardiographic spectrum of Ebstein's anomaly: detailed anatomic assessment. *J Am Coll Cardiol* 1984;3:356–70.

202. Ammash NM, Warnes CA, Connolly HM, et al. Mimics of Ebstein's anomaly. *Am Heart J* 1997;134:508–13.

203. Gussenhoven EJ, Stewart PA, Becker AE, et al. 'Offsetting' of the septal tricuspid leaflet in normal hearts and in hearts with Ebstein's anomaly: anatomic and echocardiographic correlation. *Am J Cardiol* 1984;54:172–6.

204. Oechslin E, Buchholz S, Jenni R. Ebstein's anomaly in adults: Doppler-echocardiographic evaluation. *Thorac Cardiovasc Surg* 2000;48:209–13.

205. Maxted W, Nanda NC, Kim KS, et al. Transesophageal echocardiographic identification and validation of individual tricuspid valve leaflets. *Echocardiography* 1994;11:585–96.

206. Chauvaud S. Ebstein's malformation. surgical treatment and results. *Thorac Cardiovasc Surg* 2000;48:220–3.

207. Senni M, Chauvaud S, Crupi G, et al. Early and intermediate term results of Carpentier's repair for Ebstein's anomaly. *G Ital Cardiol* 1996;26:1415–20.

208. Augustin N, Schmidt-Habelmann P, Wottke M, et al. Results after surgical repair of Ebstein's anomaly. *Ann Thorac Surg* 1997;63:1650–6.

209. Vargas FJ, Mengo G, Granja MA, et al. Tricuspid annuloplasty and ventricular plication for Ebstein's malformation. *Ann Thorac Surg* 1998;65:1755–7.

210. Kiziltan HT, Theodoro DA, Warnes CA, et al. Late results of bioprosthetic tricuspid valve replacement in Ebstein's anomaly. *Ann Thorac Surg* 1998;66:1539–45.

211. Kupilik N, Simon P, Moidl R, et al. Valve-preserving treatment of Ebstein's anomaly: perioperative and follow-up results. *Thorac Cardiovasc Surg* 1999;47:229–34.

212. Alpert JS, Dexter L, Vieweg WVR, et al. Anomalous pulmonary venous return with intact atrial septum. *Circulation* 1977;56:870–5.

213. Dupuis C, Charaf LAC, Breviere G, et al. The adult form of scimitar syndrome. *Am J Cardiol* 1992;70:502–7.

214. McGaughey MD, Trail TA, Brinker JA. Partial left anomalous pulmonary venous return: a diagnostic dilemma. *Cathet Cardiovasc Diagn* 1986;12:110–15.

215. Mehta RH, Jain SP, Nanda NC, et al. Isolated partial anomalous pulmonary venous connection: echocardiographic diagnosis and a new color Doppler method to assess shunt volume. *Am Heart J* 1991;122:870–3.

216. Miller DS, Schwartz SL, Geggel RL, et al. Detection of partial anomalous right pulmonary venous return with an intact atrial septum by transesophageal echocardiography. *J Am Soc Echocardiogr* 1995;8:924–7.

217. Snider AR, Serwer GA. Abnormal vascular connection and structures. In: Snider AR, Serwer GA (eds). *Echocardiography in Pediatric Heart Disease.* Chicago, IL: Chicago Year Book Medical Publishers, Inc. 1990, p.287.

218. Obeid AI, Carlson RJ, Evaluation of pulmonary vein stenosis by transesophageal echocardiography. *J Am Soc Echocardiogr* 1995;8:888–96.

219. Samdarshi TE, Morrow R, Helmcke FR, et al. Assessment of pulmonary vein stenosis by transesophageal echocardiography. *Am Heart J* 1991;122:1495–8.

220. Sadr IM, Tan PE, Kieran MW, et al. Mechanism of pulmonary vein stenosis in infants with normally connected veins. *Am J Cardiol* 2000;86:577–9, A10.

221. Breinholt JP, Hawkins JA, Minich LA, et al. Pulmonary stenosis with normal connection: associated cardiac abnormalities and variable outcome. *Ann Thorac Surg* 1999;68:164–8.

222. Bini RM, Cleveland DC, Ceballos R, et al. Congential pulmonary vein stenosis. *Am J Cardiol* 1984;54:369–75.

223. Ha JW, Chung N, Yoon J, et al. Pulsed wave and color Doppler echocardiography and cardiac catheterization findings in bilateral pulmonary vein stenosis. *J Am Soc Echocardiogr* 1998;11:393–6.

224. Webber SA, de Souza E, Patterson MW. Pulsed and color Doppler findings in congenital pulmonary vein stenosis. *Pediatr Cardiol* 1992;13:112–15.

225. Bourdillon PD, Foale RA, Sommerville J. Persistent left superior vena cava with coronary sinus and left atrial connection. *Eur J Cardiol* 1979;11:227–34.

226. Nanda NC, Pinheiro L, Sanyal R, et al. Transesophageal echocardiographic examination of left-sided superior vena cava and azygous and hemiazygous veins. *Echocardiography* 1991;8:731–40.

227. Podolsky LA, Jacobs LE, Schwartz M, et al. Transesophageal echocardiography in the diagnosis of the persistent left superior vena cava. *J Am Soc Echocardiogr* 1992;5:159–62.

228. Buchholz S, Jenni R. Doppler echocardiographic findings in 2 identical variants of a rare cardiac anomaly, 'subtotal' cor triatriatum: a critical review of the literature. *J Am Soc Echocardiogr* 2001;14:846–9.

229. Tantibhedhyangkul W, Godoy I, Karp R, Lang RM. Cor triatriatum in a 70-year-old woman: role of transesophageal echocardiography and dynamic three-dimensional echocardiography in diagnostic assessment. *J Am Soc Echocardiogr* 1998;11:837–40.

230. Hogue CW Jr, Barzilai B, Forstot R, et al. Intraoperative echocardiographic diagnosis of previously unrecognized cor triatriatum. *Ann Thorac Surg* 1992;54:562–3.

231. Fagan LF Jr, Penick DR, Williams GA, et al. Two-dimensional, spectral Doppler, and color flow imaging in adults with acquired and congenital cor triatriatum. *J Am Soc Echocardiogr* 1991;4:177–84.

232. Jeong JW, Tei C, Chang KS, et al. A case of cor triatriatum in an eighty-year-old man: transesophageal echocardiographic observation of multiple defects. *J Am Soc Echocardiogr* 1997;10:185–8.

233. Takeuchi Y, Kurogane K, Nishimura Y, et al. Asymptomatic cor triatrium in an elderly patient—observation by biplanar transesophageal Doppler echocardiography. *Jpn Circ J* 1997;61:189–91.

234. Sadiq M, Sreeram N, Silove ED. Congenitally divided left atrium: diagnostic pitfalls in cross-sectional echocardiography. *Int J Cardiol* 1995;48:99–101.

235. Shuler CO, Fyfe DA, Sade R, Crawford FA. Transesophageal echocardiographic evaluation of cor triatriatum in children. *Am Heart J* 1995;129:507–10.

236. Bartel T, Muller S, Geibel A. Preoperative assessment of cor triatriatum in an adult by dynamic three dimensional echocardiography was more informative than transoesophageal echocardiography or magnetic resonance imaging. *Br Heart J* 1994;72:498–9.

237. Kacenelenbogen R, Decoodt P. Biplane transesophageal echocardiographic diagnosis of cor triatriatum. *Chest* 1994;105:601–2.

238. Hoffmann R, Lambertz H, Flachskampf FA, Hanrath P. Transoesophageal echocardiography in the diagnosis of cor triatriatum; incremental value of colour Doppler. *Eur Heart J* 1992;13:418–20.

239. Vuocolo LM, Stoddard MF, Longaker RA. Transesophageal two-dimensional and Doppler echocardiographic diagnosis of cor triatriatum in the adult. *Am Heart J* 1992;124:791–3.

240. Hogue CW, Barzilai B, Forstot R, et al. Intraoperative echocardiographic diagnosis of previously unrecognized cor triatriatum. *Ann Thorac Surg* 1992;54:562–3.

241. Darbar D, Bridges AB, Roberts R, Pringle TH. Cor triatriatum: unusual cause of transient ischaemic attacks in a 67-year-old man. *Br J Clin Prac* 1995;49:166–7.

242. Huang TY, Sung PH. Transesophageal echocardiographic detection of cardiac embolic source in cor triatriatum complicated by aortic saddle emboli. *Clin Cardiol* 1997;20:294–6.

243. Lanzarini L, Lucca E, Fontana A, Foresti S. Cor triatriatum dextrum resulting from the persistence of embryonic remnants of the right valve of the sinus venosus: prevalence and echocardiographic aspects in a large consecutive non-selected patient population. *Ital Heart J* 2001;2(Suppl 11):1209–16.

244. Dobbertin A, Warnes CA, Seward JB. Cor triatriatum dexter in an adult diagnosed by transesophageal echocardiography: a case report. *J Am Soc Echocardiogr* 1995;8:952–7.

245. Fiorilli R, Argento G, Tomasco B, Serino W. Cor triatriatum dexter diagnosed by transesophageal echocardiography. *J Clin Ultrasound* 1995;23:502–4.

246. Lanzarini L, Raineri C, Bertoletti A. Broad Chiari's network simulating a right cor triatriatum in a transthoracic echocardiogram correctly diagnosed with transesophageal echocardiography. *Ital Heart J* 2000;1(suppl 9):1208–9.

247. Corno AF, Bron C, von Segesser LK. Divided right atrium. Diagnosis by echocardiography, and considerations on the functional role of the Eustachian valve. *Cardiol Young* 1999;9:427–9.

248. Roldan FJ, Vargas-Barron J, Espinola-Zavaleta N, et al. Cor triatriatum dexter: transesophageal echocardiographic diagnosis and 3-dimensional reconstruction. *J Am Soc Echocardiogr* 2001;14:634–6.

249. Click RL, Holmes DR, Vlielstra RE, et al. Anomalous coronary arteries: location, degree of atherosclerosis, and effect on survival – A report from the Coronary Artery Surgery Study. *J Am Coll Cardiol* 1989;13:531–7.

250. Maron BJ, Epstein SE, Roberts WC. Causes of sudden death in competitive athletes. *J Am Coll Cardiol* 1986;7:204–14.

251. Ishikawa T, Brandt PW. Anomalous origin of the left main coronary artery from the right anterior aortic sinus: angiographic definition of anomalous course. *Am J Cardiol* 1985;55:770–6.

252. Plehn JF, Ruggie N, Liebson PR, Messer JV. Visualization of an anomalous left main coronary artery with two-dimensional echocardiography. *Am Heart J* 1988;115:468–70.

253. Yamagishi M, Miyatke K, Beppu S, et al. Assessment of coronary blood flow by transesophageal two-dimensional pulsed Doppler echocardiography. *Am J Cardiol* 1988;62:641–4.

254. Gaither NS, Rogan KM, Stayduchar K, et al. Anomalous origin and course of coronary arteries in adults: identification and improved imaging utilizing transesophageal echocardiography. *Am Heart J* 1991;122:69–75.

255. Levin DC, Fellows KE, Abrams HL. Hemodynamically significant primary anomalies of the coronary arteries. Angiographic aspects. *Circulation* 1978;58:25–34.

256. Tolley PM, Bolsin SN. Intraoperative transesophageal echocardiogram of the coronary ostia. *J Cardiothorac Vasc Anes* 2001; 15:793–4.

257. Hildreth B, Junkel P, Allada V, et al. An uncommon echocardiographic marker for anomalous origin of the left coronary artery from the pulmonary artery: visualization of intercoronary collaterals within the ventricular septum. *Pediatr Cardiol* 2001;22:406–8.

258. Frommelt PC, Berger S, Pelech AN, et al. Prospective identification of anomalous origin of left coronary artery from the right sinus of valsalva using transthoracic echocardiography: importance of color Doppler flow mapping. *Pediatr Cardiol* 2001;22:327–32.

259. Lauer B, Thiele H, Schuler G. A 'new' coronary anomaly: origin of the right coronary artery below the aortic valve. *Heart* 2001;85:486.

260. Youn HJ, Foster E. Transesophageal echocardiography (TEE) in the evaluation of the coronary arteries. *Cardiol Clin* 2000;18:833–48.

261. Jureidini SB, Singh GK, Marino CJ, Fiore AC. Aberrant origin of the left coronary artery from the right aortic sinus: surgical intervention based on echocardiographic diagnosis. *J Am Soc Echocardiogr* 2000;13:1117–20.

262. Nanda NC, Bhambore MM, Jindal A, et al. Transesophageal three-dimensional echocardiographic assessment of anomalous coronary arteries. *Echocardiography* 2000;17:53–60.

263. Stefanelli CB, Stevenson JG, Jones TK, et al. A case for routine screening of coronary artery origins during echocardiography: fortuitous discovery of a life-threatening coronary anomaly. *J Am Soc Echocardiogr* 1999;12:769–72.

264. Frommelt PC, Friedberg DZ, Frommelt MA, Williamson JG. Anomalous origin of the right coronary artery from the left sinus of valsalva: transthoracic echocardiographic diagnosis. *J Am Soc Echocardiogr* 1999;12:221–4.

265. Goswami KC, Das GS, Shrivastava S. Cross-sectional and Doppler echocardiographic diagnosis of anomalous origin of the left coronary artery from the pulmonary artery and right coronary artery from posterior aortic sinus. *Int J Cardiol* 1998;66:81–3.

266. Zeppilli P, dello Russo A, Santini C, et al. In vivo detection of coronary artery anomalies in asymptomatic athletes by echocardiographic screening. *Chest* 1998;114:89–93.

267. Hsu SY, Lin FC, Chang HJ, et al. Multiplane transesophageal echocardiography in diagnosis of anomalous origin of the left coronary artery from the pulmonary artery: a case report. *J Am Soc Echocardiogr* 1998;11:668–72.

268. Kasprzak JD, Kratochwil D, Peruga JZ, et al. Coronary anomalies diagnosed with transesophageal echocardiography: complementary clinical value in adults. *Int J Card Imag* 1998;14:89–95.

269. Vicente T, Lopez J, Valdes M. Usefulness of transoesophageal echocardiography in showing the route of anomalous coronary arteries. *Heart* 1996;76:183–4.

270. O'Rourke DJ, Flanagan M, Berman N, et al. Stenosis at the origin of an anomalous left main coronary artery arising from the pulmonary artery in a symptom-free adolescent girl: transesophageal echocardiographic findings. *J Am Soc Echocardiogr* 1996;9:724–6.

271. Aliabadi D, Icenogle M, Samaan S, et al. Transesophageal echocardiographically guided angiography of an anomalous coronary artery. *Am Heart J* 1995;129:193–5.

272. Lowe JE, Oldham HN, Sabiston DC. Surgical management of congenital coronary artery fistulas. *Ann Surg* 1981;194:373–80.

273. Baim DS, Kline H, Silverman JF. Bilateral coronary artery–pulmonary artery fistulas. Report of five cases and review of the literature. *Circulation* 1982;65:810–15.

274. Urrutia-S CO, Falaschi G, Ott DA, Cooley DA. Surgical management of 56 patients with congenital coronary artery fistulas. *Ann Thorac Surg* 1983;35:300–7.

275. Lim CH, Tan NC, Tan L, Seah CS, Tan D. Congenital aneurysm of the right coronary artery. *Am J Cardiol* 1977;39:598.

276. Liberthson RR, Sagar K, Berkoben JP, et al. Congenital coronary arteriovenous fistula. Report of 13 patients, review of the literature and delineation of management. *Circulation* 1979;59:849–54.

277. Horiuchi T, Abe T, Tanake S, Koyamada K. Congenital coronary arteriovenous fistulas. *Ann Thorac Surg* 1971;11:102–12.

278. Lin FC, Chang HJ, Chern MS, et al. Multiplane transesophageal echocardiography in the diagnosis of congenital coronary artery fistula. *Am Heart J* 1995;130:1236–44.

279. Samdarshi TE, Mahan EF III, Nanda NC, Sanyal R. Transesophageal echocardiographic assessment of congenital coronary artery to coronary sinus fistulas in adults. *Am J Cardiol* 1991;68:263–6.

280. Santini R, Bonato R, Pittarello D, et al. Intraoperative transesophageal echocardiography during surgery for congenital heart disease. *Cardiovasc Imag* 1992;4:127–32.

281. Menahem S, Venables AW. Pulmonary artery banding in isolated or complicated ventricular septal defects: results and effects on growth. *Br Heart J* 1972;34:87–94.

282. Oldham HN Jr, Kakos GS, Jarmakani MM, Sabiston DC Jr. Pulmonary artery banding in infants with complex congenital heart defects. *Ann Thorac Surg* 1971;13:342–50.

283. Patel RG, Ihenacho HNC, Abrams LD, et al. Pulmonary artery banding and subsequent repair in ventricular septal defect. *Br Heart J* 1973;35:651–6.

284. Kirklin JW, Appelbaum A, Bargeron LM Jr. Primary repair versus banding for ventricular septal defects in infants. In: BSI Kidd, RD Rowe (eds). *The Child with Congenital Heart Disease after Surgery*. Mount Kisco, NY: Futura, 1976:3.

285. Subramanian S, Wagner HR. Pulmonary artery banding and debanding in patients with ventricular septal defects. In: BG Barratt-Boyes, JM Neutze, EA Harris (eds). *Heart Disease in Infancy: Diagnosis and Surgical Treatment*. London: Churchill Livingstone, 1973:141.

286. Freed MD, Rosenthal A, Plauth WH Jr, Nadas AS. Development of subaortic stenosis after pulmonary artery banding. *Circulation* 1973;47/48(suppl 3):7–10.

287. Yoshimura N, Yamaguchi M, Ohashi H, et al. Classic Blalock–Taussig shunt in neonates. *J Cardiovasc Surg* 1999;40:107–10.

288. Jan SL, Hwang B, Fu YC, Chi CS. Pseudoaneurysm formation after infected modified Blalock–Taussig shunt: echocardiographic findings. *Echocardiography* 2000;17:187–91.

289. Corno AF, Hurni M, Payot M, von Segesser LK. Modified Blalock–Taussig shunt with compensatory properties. *Ann Thorac Surg* 1999;67:269–70.

290. Al Jubair KA, Al Fagih MR, Al Jarallah AS, et al. Results of 546 Blalock-Taussig shunts performed in 478 patients. *Cardiol Young* 1998;8:486–90.

291. Godart F, Qureshi SA, Simha A, et al. Effects of modified and classic Blalock–Taussig shunts on the pulmonary arterial tree. *Ann Thorac Surg* 1998;66:512–17.

292. Murthy KS, Coelho R, Naik SK, et al. Novel techniques of bidirectional Glenn shunt without cardiopulmonary bypass. *Ann Thorac Surg* 1999;67:1771–4.

293. Mavroudis C, Backer CL, Kohr LM, et al. Bidirectional Glenn shunt in association with congenital heart repairs: the 1(1/2) ventricular repair. *Ann Thorac Surg* 1999;68:976–81.

294. Konstantinov IE, Alexi-Meskishvili VV. Cavo-pulmonary shunt: from the first experiments to clinical practice. *Ann Thorac Surg* 1999;68:1100–6.

295. Chang RK, Alejos JC, Atkinson D, et al. Bubble contrast echocardiography in detecting pulmonary arteriovenous shunting in children with univentricular heart after cavopulmonary anastomosis. *J Am Coll Cardiol* 1999;33:2052–8.

296. Reeder GS, Currie PJ, Fyfe DA, et al. Extracardiac conduit obstruction: intial experience in the use of Doppler echocardiography for noninvasive estimation of pressure gradient. *J Am Coll Cardiol* 1984;4:1006–11.

297. McElhinney DB, Reddy VM, Hanley FL, Moore P. Systemic venous collateral channels causing desaturation after bidirectional cavopulmonary anastomosis: evaluation and management. *J Am Coll Cardiol* 1997;30:817–24.

298. Kaulitz R, Stümper OFW, Geuskens R, et al. Comparative values of the precordial and transesophageal approaches in the echocardiographic evaluation of atrial baffle function after an atrial correction procedure. *J Am Coll Cardiol* 1990;16:686–94.

299. Myridakis DJ, Ehlers KH, Engle MA. Late followup after venous switch operation (Mustard procedure) for simple and complex transposition of the great arteries. *Am J Cardiol* 1994;74:1030–6.

300. Aziz KU, Paul MH, Bharati S, et al. Two-dimensional echocardiographic evaluation of Mustard operation for d-transposition of the great arteries. *Am J Cardiol* 1981;47:654–64.

301. Chin AJ, Sanders SP, Williams RG, et al. Two-dimensional echocardiographic assessment of caval and pulmonary venous pathways after the Senning operation. *Am J Cardiol* 1983;52:118–26.

302. Blakenberg F, Rhee J, Hardy C, et al. MRI vs echocardiography in the evaluation of the Jatene procedure. *J Comput Assist Tomogr* 1994;18:749–54.

303. Martin MM, Snider AR, Bove EL, et al. Two-dimensional and Doppler echocardiographic evaluation after arterial switch operation for transposition of the great arteries. *Am J Cardiol* 1995;76:153.

304. Webb GD, McLaughlin PR, Gow RM, et al. Transposition complexes. *Cardiol Clin* 1993;11:651–64.

305. Jatene FB, Bosisio IB, Jatene MB, et al. Late results (50 to 182 months) of the Jatene operation. *Eur J Cardio Thorac Surg* 1992;6:575–7.

306. Castaneda AR. From Glenn to Fontan: a continuing evolution. *Circulation* 1992;86(Suppl 5):180–4.

307. Sluysmans T, Sanders SP, Van-der-Velde M, et al. Natural history and patterns of recovery of contractile function in single left ventricle after Fontan operation. *Circulation* 1992;86:1753–61.

308. Fyfe DA, Kline CH, Sade RM, Gilette PC. Transesophageal echocardiography detects thrombus formation not identified by transthoracic echocardiography after the Fontan operation. *J Am Coll Cardiol* 1991;18:1733–7.

309. Bridges ND, Mayer JE Jr, Lock JE, et al. Effect of baffle fenestration on outcome of the modified Fontan operation. *Circulation* 1992;86:1762–9.

310. Hijazi ZM, Fahey JT, Kleinman CS, et al. Hemodynamic evaluation before and after closure of fenestrated Fontan: an acute study of changes in oxygen delivery. *Circulation* 1992;86:196–202.

311. Stümper O, Sutherland GR, Geuskens R, et al. Transesophageal echocardiography in evaluation and management after a Fontan procedure. *J Am Coll Cardiol* 1991;17:1152–60.

312. Gundry SR, Razzouk AJ, del Rio MJ, Shirali G, Bailey LL. The optimal Fontan connection: a growing extracardiac lateral tunnel with pedicled pericardium. *J Thorac Cardiovasc Surg* 1997;114:552–8 (discussion 558).

313. McElhinney DB, Reddy VM, Silverman NH, Hanley FL. Modified Damus–Kaye–Stansel procedure for single ventricle, subaortic stenosis, and arch obstruction in neonates and infants: midterm results and techniques for avoiding circulatory arrest. *J Thorac Cardiovasc Surg* 1997;114:718–25 (discussion 725–6).

314. Kirklin JW, Barratt-Boyes BG. *Cardiac Surgery.* New York: Wiley 1986.

Appendix A

Artist's rendition of the most common, modern surgical procedures for congenital heart disease that would be expected to be encountered and present for evaluation with transesophageal echocardiography. Cardiac surgical procedures have greatly modified the natural history of various congenital cardiac lesions allowing with patients living to adulthood. Knowledge of the type of surgery performed along, with the various modifications of each procedure is extremely important before evaluating the post-operative congenital patient in order to perform a thorough and complete transesophageal echocardiographic examination.

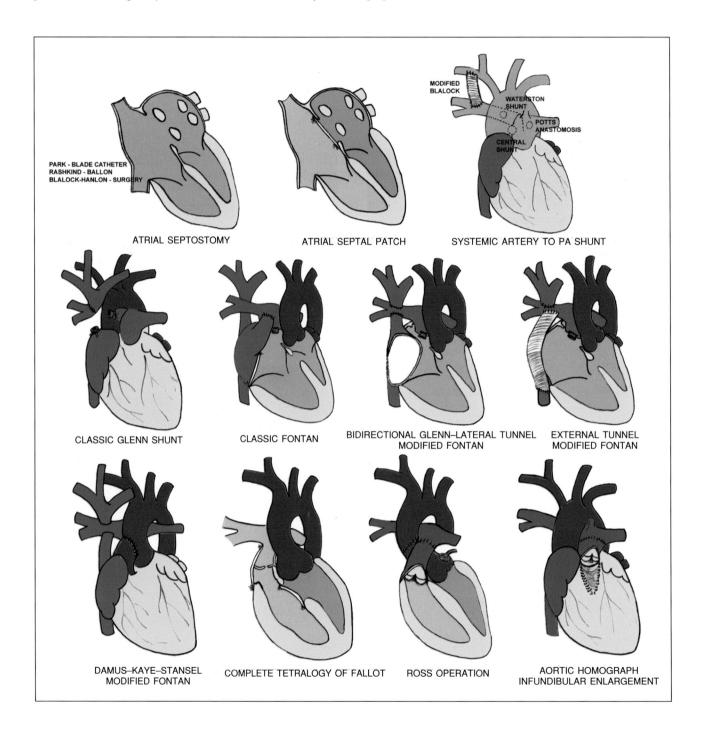

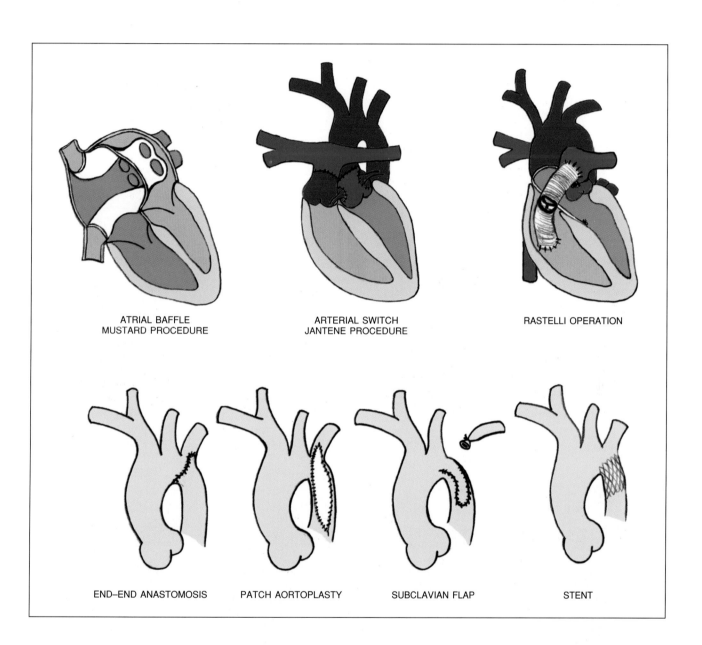

ATRIAL BAFFLE
MUSTARD PROCEDURE

ARTERIAL SWITCH
JANTENE PROCEDURE

RASTELLI OPERATION

END–END ANASTOMOSIS

PATCH AORTOPLASTY

SUBCLAVIAN FLAP

STENT

10

Transesophageal echocardiography and specific interventions

Since its widespread availability in the late 1980s transesophageal echocardiography has been used more than other imaging tools because of its ease of performance and the minimal number of complications associated with the technique. Transesophageal echocardiography has become established in the evaluation of cardiac source of embolus, diagnosis of endocarditis especially prosthetic valve endocarditis, as a screening tool for thrombus before cardioversion, the evaluation of valvular anatomy and function, defining cardiac tumors and masses, the rapid evaluation of the critical ill patient and trauma patient, the demonstration of aortic pathology and the evaluation of congenital heart disease. In addition to providing a routine cardiac examination for the diagnosis and management of cardiovascular disease, multiplane transesophageal echocardiography has been utilized to monitor cardiac function during cardiac interventions and cardiac surgery. Transesophageal echocardiography already has an established role in certain types of cardiac surgery such as valvular repair, prosthetic valve surgery, and repair of complex congenital heart disease in children and adults.[1–10] In many institutions it has been estimated that transesophageal echocardiography may be utilized in between 50 and 75% of all cardiac surgical cases, especially since cardiac anesthesiologists and critical care specialists perform intraoperative transesophageal echocardiography. Transesophageal echocardiography is invaluable in recognizing the complications and sequelae of cardiac surgical procedures and is replacing fluoroscopy during certain cardiac interventions in the cardiac catheterization laboratories such as balloon valvuloplasty and septal defect closure devices reducing radiation to the patient and eliminating the need for radiographic contrast. This chapter addresses the role of transesophageal echocardiograph during specific interventions that are utilized in our laboratories.

Numerous studies have addressed the safety of transesophageal echocardiography in adult and pediatric patients during long monitoring periods such as may be required during specific interventions discussed in this chapter.[11–19] Hulyalkar and colleagues, in 281 patients with continuous transesophageal echocardiography, have demonstrated a low risk of gastrointestinal injury associated with prolonged monitoring periods during cardiac surgery.[16] Greene and colleagues performed endoscopy after intraoperative transesophageal echocardiography was used for monitoring congenital heart surgery and demonstrated only mild mucosal injury and no long-term complications.[17] Minor injury of the esophagus was noted predominately in patients weighing less than 9 kg. Owall and colleagues, found no difference in the prevalence of pharyngitis following cardiac surgery, and no delay in endotracheal extubation in the perioperative period.[18] Andropoulos and colleagues have demonstrated that ventilatory compromise is infrequent in small infants undergoing transesophageal echocardiography, and thus transesophageal monitoring during cardiac surgery is feasible and safe in children.[19]

Routine coronary artery bypass surgery

Transesophageal echocardiography may have a role during routine coronary artery bypass surgeries[20–35] for the early detection of complications that may be addressed in the operating room. It has been suggested that performing transesophageal echocardiography during routine coronary artery bypass surgery is associated with decrease of morbidity and mortality, shortened operative time and duration of hospitalization.[20-35]

Transesophageal echocardiographic examination during cardiac surgery includes a complete examination in the preoperative and postoperative period with monitoring during the intraoperative period until weaning from cardiopulmonary bypass.

Preoperative examination is performed immediately after induction of anesthesia prior to sternotomy. This includes assessment of left and right ventricular function and hemodynamics, regional wall motion abnormalities, valvular structure and function, the presence of shunts particularly patent foramen ovale and recognition of intracardiac thrombus. The entire aorta is assessed for calcification, plaque and thrombus.[36-38]

Interoperative transesophageal echocardiography detects new findings in approximately 8–25% of cases and in a proportion of these, the planned surgical procedure has been altered.[39-43] New findings include new or worsening myocardial ischemia, aortic atheroma, valvular abnormalities, intracardiac shunts and thrombi.

New and unsuspected findings by interoperative transesophageal echocardiography may be classified as information that results in a primary interventional modification or secondary modification. Primary interventional modification is defined when transesophageal echocardiography provided new information, which results in an unplanned additional surgical procedure; modification of a planned procedure or cancellation of surgery. A secondary modification is defined as new information that does not alter the surgical procedural approach but assists in the intraoperative management of the anesthesia and or hemodynamics.

Mendelsohn and colleagues prospectively studied 233 patients undergoing routine coronary artery bypass grafting surgery, with no previously known valvular disease.[39] Transesophageal echocardiography provided important new information in 51 patients. In these patients, 42 (19%) had primary modifications and 9 (4%) had secondary modifications following transesophageal echocardiography.

Sousa and colleagues studied 130 cardiac surgical procedures which included 39 routine coronary bypass surgeries. Unsuspected preoperative findings on transesophageal echocardiography were detected in 8.5%, which altered the surgical plan in 5.4% of cases.[40] Asakura and colleagues studied 500 consecutive cardiac surgeries and discovered unsuspected findings in 21% of preoperative studies.[41] Sheikh and colleagues found that 2% of patients presenting for routine coronary bypass surgery had unexpected or a higher degree of mitral regurgitation

than was expected from preoperative workup and required concomitant mitral valvular surgery.[42] Over a 5-year period at the Mayo Clinic, new information supplied by the transesophageal echocardiogram in all cardiac surgical cases occurred in 15%, with change in surgical plan in 14%.[43]

The risk of perioperative stroke may be decreased in cardiac surgery through the transesophageal echocardiographic documentation of intimal thickening of the aortic arch. Mizuno and colleagues demonstrated that patients with intimal thickening greater than 5 mm, had a significantly greater incidence of perioperative stroke (p=0.007).[44] Davila-Roman utilized intraoperative transesophageal echocardiography and epiaortic ultrasound to assess atherosclerosis of the thoracic aorta undergoing cardiac surgery and found that both techniques were superior to palpation of the aorta by the cardiac surgeon. Imaging of the aorta helped determine optimal aortic cannulation and cross-clamping sites.[45] Trehan and colleagues, studied 792 patients undergoing coronary artery bypass grafting and identified 114 patients with atheroma involving the ascending aorta and aortic arch.[46] Modification of cardiac surgery in these patients included change in cannulation or cross-clamp site, use of hypothermic circulatory arrest with aortic arch atherectomy, and bypass grafting without cardiopulmonary arrest (beating heart surgery). The overall stroke rate in this group was 0.76% with only six patients suffering stroke following surgery.

Transesophageal echocardiography is continuously monitored until the heart is arrested, and again monitored following the release of the aortic cross-clamp until the sternal wires are placed and the chest closed. During the intraoperative assessment, changes in cardiac function and hemodynamics are noted including the development of new regional wall motion abnormalities that may occur before the institution of cardiopulmonary bypass. Echocardiography is also useful for directing line placement, i.e. coronary sinus catheter placement and the initial assessment of cardiopulmonary bypass flows.[47]

The postoperative examination determines the volume status and the presence of intracardiac air before weaning from cardiopulmonary bypass.[48] After discontinuation of the cardiopulmonary bypass. systolic and diastolic ventricular function is evaluated and compared to preoperative values, new or worsening regional wall motion abnormalities or valvular regurgitation are identified, following removal of the aortic cannula.[49-54]

Although rare, numerous studies have reported the detection of aortic dissection by transesophageal echocardiography that occurs following the removal of the aortic cross-clamp and aortic cannula.[55-58] The successful management of aortic dissection postcoronary artery bypass requires prompt recognition with a high index of suspicion especially when the preoperative transesophageal study has demonstrated high-grade atherosclerosis of the ascending aorta. New or worsened regional wall motion abnormalities, especially in the coronary perfusion territory supplied by the bypass graft suggest technical problems with the graft and/or coronary spasm of the graft or in the native vessel. Reports have also suggested that repairing or replacing the graft has led to resolution of the myocardial ischemia and salvaged left ventricular function.[39,59–61]

Non-cardiac surgery

During non-cardiac surgery the role of transesophageal echocardiography for monitoring myocardial function and ischemia is not as well defined.[62–70] Transesophageal echocardiography is extremely sensitive for detecting myocardial ischemia as new or worsening regional wall motion abnormalities which occur before ST segment changes on the standard two-lead EKG. Transesophageal echocardiography also provides estimates of pulmonary artery pressure, pulmonary capillary wedge pressure, cardiac output and left ventricular dysfunction.[71–83] Transesophageal monitoring of these parameters allows the initiation of timely and appropriate therapy to prevent postoperative myocardial ischemia and dysfunction.

Eisenberg and colleagues demonstrated new or worsening regional wall motion abnormalities in 20% of cases monitored with transesophageal echocardiography.[70] In 40%, transesophageal echocardiography demonstrated ischemic events before any changes in systolic blood pressure and heart rate and determined the incremental value of transesophageal echocardiography over 12-lead EKG for detecting myocardial ischemia. Although 39% of cases suggested intraoperative myocardial ischemia, the incremental value of transesophageal echocardiography monitoring over routine two-lead EKG monitoring was small. Although myocardial ischemia occurs frequently during non-cardiac surgery, ischemic events do not predict the occurrence of postoperative myocardial infarction.

However, intraoperative transesophageal echocardiography is used in selected high-risk cases to monitor for ischemia, as an adjunct to monitoring hemodynamics, and for detecting air or atheromatous debris associated with cerebrovascular or pulmonary complications during neurological and orthopedic procedures.[83–85]

Intra aortic balloon pump

Intra aortic balloon pumps traditionally have been inserted and positioned with fluoroscopic guidance. In emergent cases or in the operating room, when fluoroscopy is not available, intra aortic balloon pump positioning during insertion can be guided with transesophageal echocardiography.

During cannulation of the femoral artery, the transesophageal probe is advanced into the stomach to visualize the aorta in cross-section at 0°. Once the aorta is visualized, the transducer array is rotated to 90° producing a longitudinal view of the aorta, and the probe is advanced as far as possible to visualize as much of the distal aorta in the abdomen as possible. In many patients the aorta may be visualized to the depth of the right kidney or just below the celiac plexus. Confirmation of proper placement of the guidewire within the aorta is made by observing a bright echo artifact within the aortic lumen. If the guidewire is not readily visualized, the probe should be rotated in a counter-clockwise direction to visualize the inferior vena cava to look for the presence of the guidewire. Agitated saline can be injected through the femoral sheath to visualize echocardiographic contrast in the aortic lumen to confirm cannulation of the appropriate vessel. A forceful injection of contrast will be visualized in the aorta to the mid-abdominal level with low blood flow states. Advancement of the guidewire may be followed up to the aortic arch with slow withdrawal and rotation of the transesophageal probe within the esophagus. The guidewire should be freely moving within the aortic lumen. The transesophageal probe is withdrawn to the level of the left subclavian artery, at which level the guidewire is easily demonstrated and oscillates as the balloon catheter is advanced over it. The balloon catheter is demonstrated as an increase in the size of the artifact as it reaches the aortic arch. After removal of the guidewire, the balloon tip is less well-visualized, but can be positioned 1–2 cm distal to the origin of the left subclavian artery. If the balloon tip is not well seen after removal of the guidewire, agitated saline may be infused through the balloon to document its position. During pulsation the balloon should appear freely expanding and contracting in its entire length. The development of aortic regurgitation should be excluded during balloon pumping.

Port-access and minimally invasive cardiac surgery

The development of endovascular cannulas and catheters for performing cardiopulmonary bypass has permitted smaller surgical incisions and in some patients has eliminated the need for sternotomy. During port-access (Heart-Port) surgery, venous return from the patient is directed to the cardiopulmonary console through the placement of a venous cannula in the femoral vein, which is passed through the inferior vena cava to reach and drain the right atrium. Oxygenated blood from the cardiopulmonary console is returned to the circulation via a triple lumen endoaortic cannula, which is inserted through the femoral artery and passed into the ascending aorta. At the distal portion, near the tip of the endoaortic cannula, is a large balloon which when inflated serves as an internal cross-clamp by occluding the ascending aorta. When the balloon is inflated, an infusion port distal to the balloon of the endoaortic cannula delivers cardioplegia in an antegrade manner to the coronary arteries. The remaining port serves as an aortic vent and provides a means to measure aortic pressure. A further catheter is inserted via the internal jugular vein and provides access for a coronary sinus catheter for retrograde cardioplegia and a port for venting the pulmonary artery. During port-access surgery transesophageal echocardiography has been utilized alone or as an adjunct to fluoroscopy for the placement of endovascular catheters.[86–97]

The coronary sinus catheter is usually the first catheter to be placed, because it is usually the most difficult catheter to position.[93–97] The catheter is inserted in the right internal jugular vein. The coronary sinus is visualized with transesophageal echocardiography from the distal esophagus in the four-chamber view. The probe is laterally flexed to the right, with mild clockwise rotation to visualize the coronary sinus in the near vertical orientation. In this view the distal portion of the vessel is closest to the apex in the image sector. The catheter may be seen entering the right atrium from where it is advanced towards the ostia of the coronary sinus and upon engaging the coronary sinus the catheter is advanced about 3 cm into the vessel. If the position of the catheter is in question, fluoroscopy may be required and radiographic contrast utilized to visualize the radiographic outline of the coronary sinus. In addition, cardioplegia solution can be visualized in the coronary sinus as a mosaic flow pattern upon initiation of retrograde cardioplegia, once cardiopulmonary bypass is initiated. The position of the coronary sinus catheter may also be confirmed by visualization of a ventricularized waveform recording obtained from the catheter when appropriately positioned in the coronary sinus.

The ostia of the coronary sinus can be visualized in a modified bicaval view, with rightward rotation and flexion of the probe. The coronary sinus may also be visualized from the deep transgastric view at 100°–125°, with the right ventricular apex towards the apex of the image sector and the right atrium in the far field towards the right of the image. In this plane the coronary sinus is visualized in the center of the image in an almost horizontal orientation and is the optimal view for advancing the coronary sinus catheter from jugular access.

For placement of the venous cannula, the inferior vena cava is visualized in long axis from the distal gastric probe position. The probe is rotated directly posterior to visualize the descending aorta in cross-section at 0° at the level of the diaphragm, with the depth of the image sector set to 16 cm. The transducer is rotated to 90° in order to visualize the aorta in long axis and the probe is slowly advanced with mild retroflexion to visualize the maximum extent of the aorta obtainable from within the abdomen. The transesophageal probe is then rotated counterclockwise until the inferior vena cava is demonstrated lying inferior within the image sector and parallel to the aorta at the level of the superior pole of the right kidney. Color flow Doppler demonstrates low velocity flow in the inferior vena cava in the opposite direction to aortic flow, with numerous branches at the level of the liver. The guide wire is visualized as it traverses the inferior vena cava and followed while the probe is slowly withdrawn with minor manipulation of the probe to keep the inferior vena cava central in the image sector until it enters the right atrium. The guide wire is then passed into the right atrium to the origin of the superior vena cava. The venous cannula is then passed over the wire, which is well-visualized echocardiographically and the tip of the cannula is placed near the origin of the superior vena cava. After positioning the venous cannula, the position of the coronary sinus catheter is re-confirmed as it may be displaced with insertion of the venous cannula.

Cannulation of the femoral artery and advancement of the guidewire follows the same principles as insertion of an intra aortic balloon pump. Fluoroscopy is not required as long as there is no significant peripheral vascular disease. The aorta is visualized from the distal stomach as described for the inferior vena cava. The guide wire is easily seen in the aortic lumen and should pass freely through the aorta. The guide wire is followed with withdrawal of the probe to the level of the aortic arch. The endoaortic clamp catheter is passed over the wire to the level of the aortic arch and the position of the transesophageal probe is changed to the mid-esophageal window visualizing the ascending aorta at 90°–110°. The tip of the endoaortic clamp should be at the level of the sinuses of Valsalva and not pass through the aortic valve plane to avoid trauma to the valve leaflets. When the endoaortic clamp balloon is inflated, the balloon should lie above the sinotubular junction and below the origin of the innominate artery. When the balloon is fully inflated it should not move during the cardiac cycle. When cardioplegia is infused through the catheter, it is visualized echocardiographically as contrast fills the sinuses of Valsalva. During the procedure the endoaortic clamp is monitored since it tends to migrate either forward toward the aortic valve or retrograde towards the take off of the great vessels. Migration of the aortic clamp catheter requires readjusting its position intra-operatively.

The postoperative transesophageal echocardiographic examination after port access should include assessment of ventricular function, evaluation for the presence of air, and assessment of the presence of trauma to the aorta and aortic valve that may have occurred with the endoaortic clamp.

Mechanical support devices

Despite improvements in the medical therapy of heart failure, a proportion of patients with congestive heart failure may benefit from mechanical support.[98–100] Ventricular assist devices are beneficial as a bridge to heart transplantation or as short-term therapy to rest the heart and recover a degree of contractile function. Ventricular assist devices are also used when weaning from cardiopulmonary bypass is not possible following cardiac surgery due to advanced heart failure. Ventricular assist devices restore normal hemodynamics and improve end-organ blood flow by unloading the diseased ventricle and reducing myocardial work. Transesophageal echocardiography has had an increasingly important role during implantation and follow-up of patients with ventricular assist devices.

Transesophageal echocardiography may be utilized to determine the need for implantation of a ventricular assist device in cases of heart failure following cardiac surgery.[103–105] Initially, echocardiography provides an overall assessment of the failing heart, and eliminates the presence of correctible causes of heart failure such as critical valvular disease, ischemia, undiagnosed congenital heart disease (cardiac shunts) and tachyarrhythmias. Intracardiac shunts must be repaired at the time of implantation to avoid right-to-left shunting during unloading of the left ventricle by the ventricular assist device which would cause further oxygen desaturation and worsening heart failure. The best clinical outcome after cardiac surgery following placement of ventricular assist devices have been reported when the use of the device is instituted early in the management of heart failure.

During implantation of the ventricular assist device, the placement of the atrial cannula and arterial graft sites are assessed echocardiographically. Blood flow lines are positioned in the left atrium or left atrial appendage and the aorta for left ventricular assist device placement. Lines are also positioned in the right atrium and the main pulmonary artery for right ventricular assist placement. Cannulas utilized for both atria are directly inserted into the atrial cavities, and may be visualized echocardiographically, normally extending approximately 2 cm into the atrial cavity. The left atrium is typically cannulated from behind the heart near the inter-atrial groove, through the left atrial appendage or in the roof of the left atrium between the aorta and the superior vena cava. The right atrium is cannulated in the mid-free wall or through the right atrial appendage. Cannulas are attached to the great vessels either directly or via a graft. If a graft is utilized it is sewn directly to the aorta or the pulmonary artery in an end to side anastomosis. The aortic graft is typically sewn to the anterolateral surface of the ascending aorta above the aortic valve and sinus of Valsalva. The pulmonary artery graft is sewn to the upper portion of the main pulmonary artery lateral to the aortic graft.

During implantation of the blood flow lines, prior to initiating the ventricular assist device, transesophageal echocardiography may be used to identify the site of anastomosis and detect air in the cardiac chambers. After initiation of flow with the ventricular assist device, the presence of air in the lines should be excluded with color flow Doppler. Flow through the cannula is observed with color flow Doppler as a high velocity jet entering the respective cardiac structure. When flow is not detected with color Doppler, obstruction of the lines by kinking or thrombus should be excluded.

Kinking of the lines is a frequent problem with ventricular assist devices, especially when four lines are present for biventricular support which frequently occurs after closure of the chest wall. When the left atrial cannula is inserted in the atrial groove it may compromise vena cava flow by external compression of the vena cava or by displacement of the atrial septum when the cannula is inserted too deep within the atrial cavity, causing the atrial septum to bow towards the right atrium and obstruct flow. The atrial cannula should extend approximately 2 cm into the atrial cavity, and should be assessed immediately before and after initiating support because the cannula may creep further into the cavity under the influence of blood flowing through it. The right atrial cannula should be positioned in the right atrium so as not to interfere with the orifice of the vena cava, coronary sinus or tricuspid valve. Flow through pulmonary artery cannula should be directed towards both the right and left pulmonary artery equally.

After initiation of flow through the ventricular assist device, the heart should be unloaded with a reduction in ventricular and atrial cavity dimension. Ventricular assist devices are exquisitely preload sensitive, which may be easily assessed echocardiographically by determining the volumes or the dimensions of the cardiac chambers. The ventricular assist device should be adjusted to provide maximum performance which can be achieved by optimizing the volume status assessed echocardiographically by cardiac chamber dimensions.

Transesophageal echocardiography may be utilized to follow-up patients on a daily or every other day basis until criteria are met for weaning from the assist device. When low flow is indicated on the device console alarm, obstruction of the bloodlines, decreased volume status due to bleeding and cardiac tamponade should be excluded.

When cardiac output and hemodynamics are maintained by flows less than 2 liters/minute with the assist device, weaning is attempted and guided by transesophageal echocardiography.[102] The flow of the ventricular assist device is reduced by 0.5 liter/minute intervals every 5 minutes as tolerated, and cardiac function is continuously monitored by transesophageal echocardiography. In patients with biventricular support, the right ventricular assist device is weaned first. Weaning failure is demonstrated by ventricular dilatation, the development of regional wall motion abnormalities, deterioration in function or the detection of significant atrioventricular regurgitation. In the setting of hypotension, with small ventricular chamber dimensions, transesophageal echocardiography may be used to guide the administration of fluids.

Pericardiocentesis

Echocardiographic imaging has been used for diagnosis and management of pericardial effusions.[106–110] Transthoracic echocardiography or transesophageal echocardiography when imaging is not diagnostic from the transthoracic approach, are extremely reliable for diagnosing pericardial effusion, estimating the quantity of effusion, determining the location of the effusion. In cases of hemodynamic instability suggesting pericardial tamponade, echocardiographic and Doppler findings are helpful for determining the need for pericardial drainage.[111–113] Echocardiographic-guided pericardiocentesis as described by the Mayo Clinic, is a safer technique than blind-needle pericardiocentesis from the subxyphoid approach.[114–129] Echocardiographic guidance during pericardiocentesis is associated with less injury of the vital organs such as liver, lung and cardiac laceration that is associated with the blind-subxyphoid needle approach.

Transthoracic two-dimensional echocardiography is the procedure of choice for directing pericardiocentesis in patients diagnosed with pericardial effusion. Pericardiocentesis may be indicated for diagnostic purposes to evaluate the etiology of the effusion as well as to relieve pericardial tamponade. In patients with pericardial effusion, transthoracic echocardiography determines the entry site for needle puncture including defining the direction of the needle insertion necessary to reach the effusion avoiding damage to other vital structures. In essence, the needle insertion site is determined by the transducer position and angulation, which demonstrates the largest area of the pericardial effusion closest to the chest wall. Continuous echocardiographic monitoring demonstrates the reduction of the pericardial fluid during drainage.

Transesophageal echocardiography has a more limited role during pericardiocentesis, and is usually reserved for cases when transthoracic echocardiographic imaging is technically inadequate. Transesophageal echocardiography cannot determine the site for needle insertion in the same manner as can be performed with the transthoracic technique. Despite this shortcoming, transesophageal echocardiography is frequently used in emergent or critically ill patient situations to demonstrate the presence of pericardial effusion and/or pericardial tamponade as a result of accident/trauma, postbypass surgery, after suspected cardiac perforation during cardiac interventional procedures.[130–135] Transesophageal echocardiography may be useful during attempted pericardiocentesis when, pericardial fluid is not obtained with transthoracic imaging, so called 'dry tap'. During pericardiocentesis, the needle position may be demonstrated by transesophageal echocardiography, as a typical metallic artifact in the vicinity of the pericardium near the right cardiac border when the needle is inserted from the traditional approach from the subxyphoid or parasternal area. When the needle position is questionable, saline contrast or echocardiographic contrast injected through the needle may help identify its position respective to the pericardial space or the cardiac chamber.[136–140] Transesophageal echocardiography in addition to identifying an effusion may also be helpful in determining the approximate site of suspected cardiac perforation during intervention, especially when the catheter or perforating device is left in place and visualized emanating from the cardiac chamber.

Biopsy

Percutaneous myocardial biopsy and intracardiac biopsy of cardiac masses have been performed with increasing frequency over the past 10 years.[141,142] The technique of myocardial biopsy as directed by transthoracic two-dimensional echocardiography is well-described.[143–147] Recently transesophageal echocardiography has been utilized in conjunction with fluoroscopy during the intracardiac biopsy for cardiac masses or tumors.[148–157]

Although intracardiac tumors occur rarely, improvements in cardiac imaging techniques have permitted their diagnosis with increased frequency premortem. Because of increased life expectancy, increased survival from cancer therapies, and rise of certain tumors such as cardiac lymphoma associated with cardiac transplantation and HIV infection, the frequency in diagnosis of cardiac tumors has increased. Cardiac tumors are classified as primary, emanating from the myocardium or pericardium or secondary tumors metastasizing to the heart from other organs in the body. Transesophageal echocardiography has greatly improved the detection and characterization of cardiac masses and tumors. Although most cardiac tumors are benign, both benign and malignant cardiac tumors are typically found in the right heart chambers. The standard methods for diagnosing cardiac neoplasm has been open thoracotomy and/or cardiopulmonary bypass utilized for attempted resection or open biopsy. A substantial number of patients may not be candidates for this aggressive approach or may not require this especially if tissue biopsy suggests that only chemotherapy or radiotherapy is required. The percutaneous approach performing an intracardiac biopsy with bioptome provides an ideal method for securing tissue for diagnosis.

Transesophageal echocardiography and fluoroscopy guided biopsy provides a much less aggressive approach for obtaining tissue diagnosis. Many reports describe the successful biopsy of cardiac tumors utilizing the transesophageal method, including biopsy of left-sided tumors with a low risk of complication, and good yield of diagnostic tissue in adults and children.[148–157]

During the intracardiac biopsy the transesophageal probe is inserted following the placement of lines. In our experience, the procedure is well tolerated and does not require general anesthesia as long as the duration of the procedure is limited to approximately 30 minutes. The cardiac chamber containing tumor or mass is visualized, and the safest site for biopsy is determined. For left-sided biopsy, a transseptal puncture is required which may be guided with transesophageal imaging. The cardiac tumor or mass is assessed for mobility or friability. As the bioptome is passed into the appropriate chamber its direction toward the mass is guided by transesophageal visualization. Since the bioptome is stiff it may be necessary to modify the shape of the bioptome so that the catheter can be directed toward the mass without damaging the surrounding cardiac structures. Usually the bioptome artifact is visualized in direct continuity with the cardiac mass and frequently the mass will be seen moving with the biopsy forceps after it is engaged and retracted with the bioptome. With a reasonable degree of certainty the cardiac mass may be biopsied from multiple sites. Although perforation of the cardiac chamber or embolization of the mass have not been reported if complications occur such as the development of pericardial effusion they should be readily detected during the biopsy procedure.

Electrophysiological procedures

The identification of certain cardiac anatomical landmarks has become vital to the accurate placement of electrode catheters during electrophysiological procedures. Echocardiography has greatly enhanced the ability to visualize cardiac structures in conjunction with fluoroscopy during electrophysiologic studies.[158–168] The major advantage of the addition of echocardiography to fluoroscopy is in limiting the radiation exposure to both the patient and operator during generally long electrophysiologic procedures. Echocardiography allows the precise localization of cardiac anatomy that correlates with the site of origin of a variety of cardiac arrhythmias. In addition to the anatomical site, echocardiography demonstrates adequate contact between cardiac tissue and the electrode catheter and also monitors movement of the catheter during the cardiac cycle.

Echocardiography may permit rapid recognition of electrophysiological complications such as cardiac perforation with pericardial effusion with or without cardiac tamponade. Tissue swelling or edema produced in the surrounding tissue following ablation may produce deformity of the cardiac structures, intracardiac thrombus and evolving obstruction of the great vessel orifices may also be demonstrated. Initially transesophageal echocardiography was utilized during electrophysiological procedures, however, recently intracardiac echocardiographic catheters have been developed with catheter tipped transducers in the range of 5–15 MHz that provide the penetration necessary to provide intracardiac imaging during the electrophysiological procedure.[168–171] Until these systems are widely available, transesophageal echocardiography may continue to be utilized in some laboratories to direct electrophysiological procedures, as both techniques demonstrate similar information. Intracardiac echocardiography has the advantage however of being better tolerated by the patient specifically requiring less sedation then transesophageal especially during long electrophysiology procedures.

The trans-septal puncture is frequently utilized to map the left atrium and ablate the focal of left-sided arrhythmia.[158,159] During the procedure, the region of the fossa ovalis of the atrial septum is visualized in the four-chamber view obtained from either the lower esophagus or in the bicaval view from the upper esophagus. During imaging the angle and or the direction of the needle may be viewed in multiple planes to confirm the catheter tip position. The catheter position is to be monitored during insertion to avoid the ostium of the coronary sinus, inferior vena cava, tricuspid apparatus and the aorta to avoid perforation of the cardiac structures and visualize possible left atrial appendage thrombus. The trans-septal catheter tip is advanced until contact with the atrial septum is demonstrated by indenting the atrial septal wall toward the left atrium, until perforation is detected with the catheter appearing in the left atrium.

The most frequent cardiac anatomical sites that may be utilized for electrophysiological mapping or ablation include the crista terminalis, the isthmus of the muscular atrioventricular septum, the coronary sinus, the ostia of the pulmonary veins and the mitral and tricuspid annulus. The origin of the crista terminalis is best visualized in the bicaval view and is represented as a prominent fold near the junction of the ostia of the superior vena cava and the right atrial appendage. The extent of the crista prominence may be followed along the wall of the atrium in a direction towards the inferior vena cava. In sinus node and atrial tachycardia ablation procedures, the catheter is placed in sites along the crista terminalis, which are difficult to appreciate, by fluoroscopy alone. With direct visualization provided with echocardiography the catheters may be directed to avoid both vena cavae orifices.

Other sites of mapping and ablation include the isthmus or the posterior portion of the muscular atrioventricular septum which includes the area between the inferior vena cava and the tricuspid annulus or the angle between the coronary sinus and the mitral annulus, which are visualized in two- and four-chamber views obtained by the lower esophageal or deep transgastric windows. The ostia of all four pulmonary veins may be visualized as discussed in Chapter 6, which is frequently necessary for mapping and ablation of atrial fibrillation.

Reports have also described echocardiographic visualization of lesions during radiofrequency ablation.[172–177] During ablation, echocardiography detects micro-bubble formation at the ablation site in approximately 30% of cases. Bubble formation indicates boiling at the site with increased temperature produced at the lesion site and is associated with larger lesions following ablation. The appearance of bubbles may also be associated with coagulation at the catheter tip and thrombus formation.[173] In addition to ablation, thrombus formation may occur due to the prolonged placement of the catheters during the procedure. Swelling of the tissues and obstruction of blood flow may occur either due to narrowing of the orifice or venous thrombosis. Ablation near the pulmonary vein orifice may be associated with pulmonary vein stenosis and may produce pulmonary venous hypertension following the procedure and has been demonstrated by transesophageal echocardiography.[172]

Closure devices

Since 1989 there has been increased interest in closure of septal defects with umbrella-type devices deployed through catheters in the cardiac catheterization laboratory.[178–184] In the United States, the Food and Drug Administration has begun the approval of several occluder type devices for the closure of atrial septal defects and patent foramen ovale. Although initially utilized for closure of ventricular septal defects as well, this procedure has largely been abandoned at the present time due to the unacceptable results for congenital lesions at the time of this writing.[185–187] At present, several manufacturers have developed occluder devices that are currently undergoing clinical trials in the United States and elsewhere.

The Amplatzer septal occluder device has obtained FDA approval for atrial septal defect and patent foramen ovale

and the CardioSEAL device has limited approval at the present time. Each device is available in a variety of sizes. The Amplatzer device is self-expanding and consists of a double disc made of nitinol wire, woven into two discs connected with a small connecting waist. The CardioSEAL device is the descendent of the Bard Clamshell device, which was successful as an occluder but developed metal fatigue. The CardioSEAL/ StarFlex device consists of two umbrellas with four radial support arms. The devices have both been successfully deployed for atrial septal defect closure in clinical trials, and more recently for patent foramen ovale closure in patients with associated neurological events. The efficacy for patent foramen ovale closure with these devices is still under investigation.

Transesophageal echocardiography has been utilized in most patients for deployment of septal occluder devices. Numerous reports in the literature have described the utility of transesophageal echocardiography during septal device closure irrespective of the type of occluder device utilized.[188–202] To limit the length of the transesophageal examination and discomfort to the patient, the probe is generally placed following venous access, insertion of the lines and after conscious sedation. In rare cases general anesthesia is required. The presence and precise location of the atrial septal defect has been established prior to the procedure and thus a full examination is not required which serves to limit the duration of the procedure. After placement of the probe the atrial septum is visualized from the mid-to-upper esophagus window allowing visualization of the defect in the perpendicular plane. An appreciation of the geometrical shape of the defect is made from viewing the defect from 0° to 180°. The diameter is measured in the view that demonstrates the largest dimension. Color flow Doppler with imaging from 0° to 180°, eliminates the presence of multiple defects, which were not initially demonstrated. Saline echocardiographic contrast may be utilized in conjunction with color flow Doppler for determining shunt flow sites, but is usually not necessary. The diameter of the shunt jet with color flow Doppler at the level of the atrial septum should correlate with the diameter measured with two-dimensional imaging. Echocardiography may underestimate the diameter of the defect due to the 'T artifact' of the defect, which may be present at the margin of the defect by two-dimensional imaging. The geometric shape of the septal defect may cause difficulties in determining the diameter of the defect especially if it is elliptical in shape when the largest diameter may not be detected. In addition, the circumference of the septal defect may vary during periods of maximum shunting during different phases of the cardiac cycle.

At present secundum atrial septal defects with a maximum diameter of 30 mm and patent foramen ovale are considered for device closure. After assessing the diameter of the defect, the location of the septal defect is determined in relationship to the other cardiac structures such as the atrioventricular valves, superior and inferior vena cava, coronary sinus, prominent eustachian valve and Thebesian valve and the right upper and lower pulmonary veins.[203–208] Ideally a 4–5 mm rim of atrial septal tissue is required surrounding at least 75% of the defect, free from the surrounding cardiac structures, to allow adequate seating of the occluder device.

During the procedure the guide wire is placed across the defect and is visualized near the orifice of the left upper pulmonary vein. A balloon filled with contrast and saline is advanced over the wire and inflated within the left atrial cavity. The balloon is pulled back to the atrial septum occluding the defect with the balloon. Color Doppler is then utilized to confirm that the defect is occluded and there are no other sites of shunt denoting multiple defects that need to be addressed.

In addition to color flow Doppler, saline contrast may be utilized. If multiple defects are present the distance from the primary defect must be determined so that the appropriate size occluder device may be chosen that covers all the defects. Occasionally multiple occluder devices have been utilized for multiple defects. The balloon is then pulled through the defect and the deformity of the balloon is noted and measured providing the stretched diameter of the septal defect. This measurement may be made with fluoroscopy or transesophageal echocardiography. The total diameter of the entire atrial septum is measured and is compared to the size of the occluder device that is chosen so as not to deploy an occluder device that would be too big for the atria.

The occluder device is passed into the left atrium over the guidewire and the cardiac chambers are visualized for the presence of air that could be introduced by the catheter system. The device is opened in the left atrium as it is passed out of the sheath. The left atrial appendage, the pulmonary vein orifice and mitral valve are observed to prevent the occluder device from interfering with these structures when it expands. The occluder device is then withdrawn to the atrial septum with an orientation for the device that is approximately parallel to the atrial septal plane. The occluder device is pulled back to the defect and fully deployed. In devices that possess metal supporting struts or arms, it is important that they are positioned on the appropriate side of the defect. Struts that pass through the defect should be noted and the device repositioned. Protrusion of the supporting arm through the defect frequently occurs with defects that exhibit a small antero-superior rim. The occluder device should be repositioned so that it covers the entire septal defect when possible, which becomes easier to appreciate as experience is gained with the technique. Many reports have addressed complications of malposition during deployment of the occluder device all of which are easily recognized with transesophageal imaging.[209–213] Once the occluder device is

deployed color flow Doppler and saline echocardiographic contrast may be utilized to determine that the shunt has been eliminated.

Small shunts may be detected following full deployment of the occluder device especially with larger defects that may disappear over time during the endothelialization process of healing. In the reports available there are no individual factors that predict residual defects and subsequent shunting.[214–219] Shunts greater than 14 mm have been observed to be frequently associated with residual shunting. A small residual shunt, usually less then 2 mm is observed in almost half of the cases reported, as demonstrated by small bubbles crossing the occluder device area with intravenous injection of saline contrast. Despite these small residual shunts, the echocardiographic signs of right ventricular volume overload usually resolve within 6–12 months along with decreases in right ventricular end-diastolic dimension that frequently normalizes with the resolution of septal wall motion abnormalities in most cases. In cases of patent foramen ovale with good position of the occluding device, total resolution of the shunt should be expected.

Transesophageal echocardiography and cardiac trauma

Transesophageal echocardiography is frequently requested for the initial evaluation of the patient who has sustained thoracic trauma and multiple injuries. Echocardiography is indicated when there is a high index of suspicion for cardiac injury in the setting of hemodynamic compromise demonstrated by diminished peripheral perfusion or hypotension. The use of transesophageal echocardiography in adult and pediatric patients has been well-described in the literature and is well-tolerated during the evaluation of severely injured patients.[220–224] The major indication for transesophageal echocardiography is the evaluation of the aorta for transection, which is described in Chapter 5. The indication for aortic evaluation coupled with the fact that transthoracic echocardiographic examination is difficult to perform with thoracic injury and thus is responsible for poor quality images leaves transesophageal echocardiography as the imaging technique of first choice. In addition to aortic transection, transesophageal echocardiography may detect myocardial contusion, injury to the great vessels or coronary arteries, rupture of the myocardium or valves, hemorrhagic pericardial effusions and/or tamponade, pleural effusions, and pulmonary vein rupture.[225–232]

Cardiac injury may be produced as a result of blunt trauma, rapid deceleration and penetrating injuries to the chest wall.[233–244] With deceleration trauma, the heart may be compressed between the sternum and the vertebral column. In addition, chest trauma may generate high intracardiac or intraventricular pressure, which may precipitate rupture of the myocardium including the ventricular or atrial septum or free wall and cardiac valves.

Echocardiographically, cardiac injury substantiated with elevated CPK-MB fractions may be defined as concussion if the two-dimensional echocardiogram is normal or as contusion if the two-dimensional echocardiogram is abnormal.[242–244] Echocardiographically cardiac injury of the myocardium presents as a new regional wall motion abnormality frequently demonstrated as akinesis or dyskinesis with or without cardiac dilatation. Most studies have suggested that the right ventricle is the most vulnerable to injury, probably due to its anterior anatomical position. Although injuries are frequently suggested by the elevation of specific cardiac enzymes most studies have shown that CPK-MB is an insensitive and nonspecific indicator of cardiac injury. Early studies of troponin have been encouraging for the identification of cardiac injury, however further studies need to be performed.

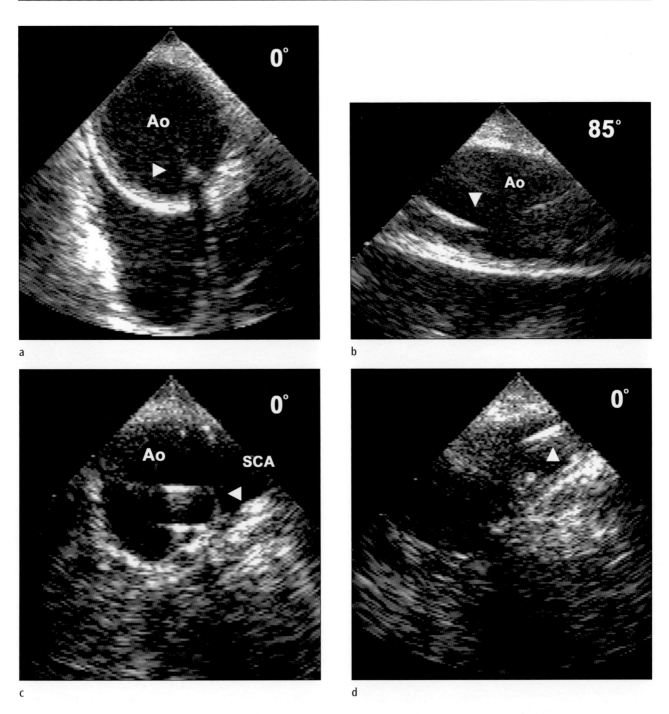

Case 10.1

Intra aortic balloon pump. During cannulation of the femoral artery, the transesophageal probe is advanced into the stomach to visualize the aorta in cross-section at 0°. Once the aorta is visualized, the transducer array is rotated to 90° producing a longitudinal view of the aorta, and the probe is advanced as far as possible to visualize as much of the distal aorta in the abdomen as possible. (a) Confirmation of proper placement of the guidewire within the aorta is made by observing a bright echo artifact within the aortic lumen (arrow). (b) If the guidewire is not readily visualized, the probe should be rotated in a counter-clockwise direction to visualize the inferior vena cava to look for the presence of the guidewire (arrow). Advancement of the guidewire may be followed up to the area of the aortic arch with slow withdrawal of the transesophageal probe within the esophagus, and the guidewire should appear to be moving freely within the aortic lumen. (c) The transesophageal probe is withdrawn to the level of the subclavian artery. The guidewire will be easily demonstrated at this level, which oscillates as the balloon catheter is advanced over the guidewire. (d) The end of the guidewire should be approximated and if the wire enters one of the great vessels (arrow), it can be withdrawn appropriately.

continued

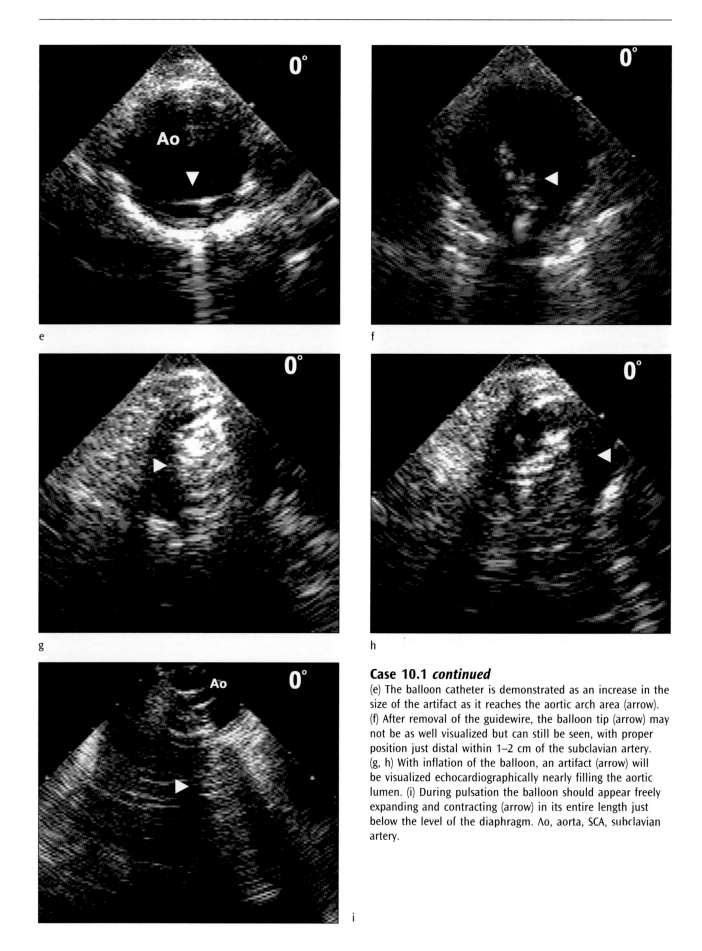

Case 10.1 *continued*

(e) The balloon catheter is demonstrated as an increase in the size of the artifact as it reaches the aortic arch area (arrow). (f) After removal of the guidewire, the balloon tip (arrow) may not be as well visualized but can still be seen, with proper position just distal within 1–2 cm of the subclavian artery. (g, h) With inflation of the balloon, an artifact (arrow) will be visualized echocardiographically nearly filling the aortic lumen. (i) During pulsation the balloon should appear freely expanding and contracting (arrow) in its entire length just below the level of the diaphragm. Ao, aorta, SCA, subclavian artery.

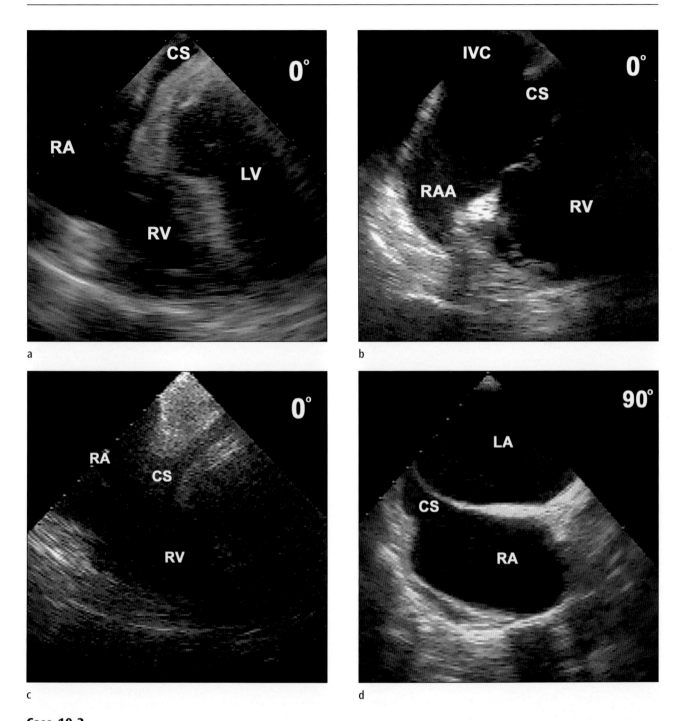

Case 10.2

Coronary sinus cannulation during minimally invasive surgery. (a) The coronary sinus is visualized with transesophageal echocardiography (TEE) from the distal esophageal probe position visualizing the four-chamber view. The probe is laterally flexed to the right, with mild rightward rotation of the probe to visualize the coronary sinus in a near vertical orientation (b, c). In this view the distal portion of the vessel is closest to the apex in the image sector. (d) The coronary sinus may also be visualized in a modified bicaval view with rightward rotation and flexion of the probe. In this view a smaller segment of the coronary sinus is visualized compared to the four-chamber view.

continued

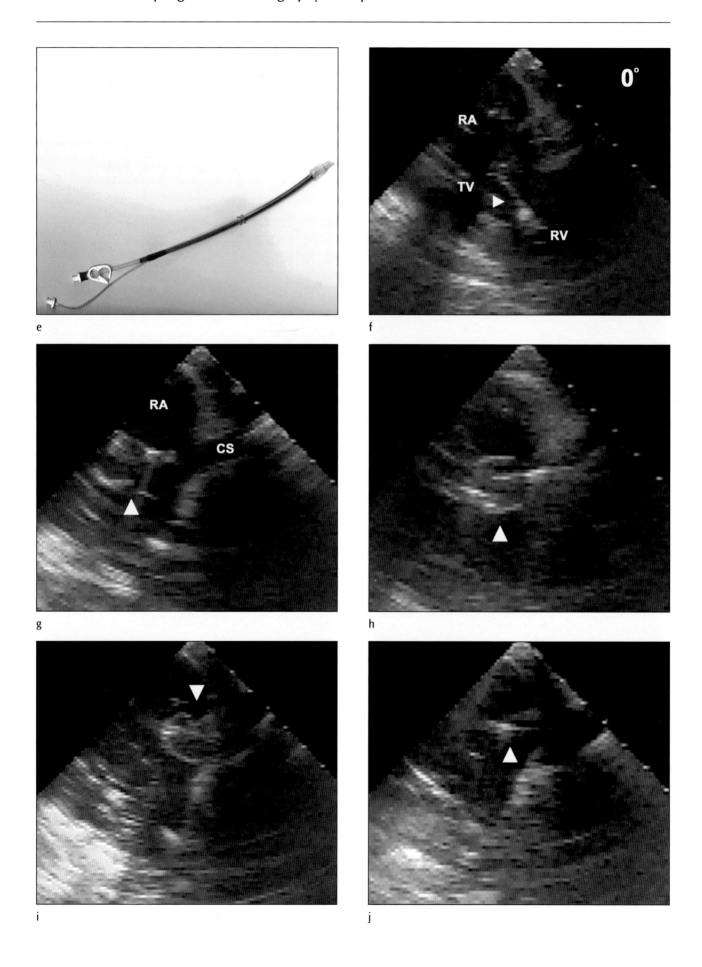

e

f

g

h

i

j

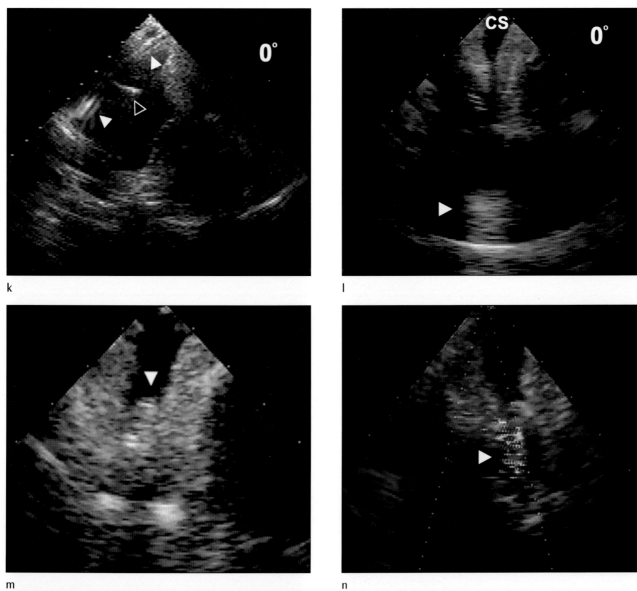

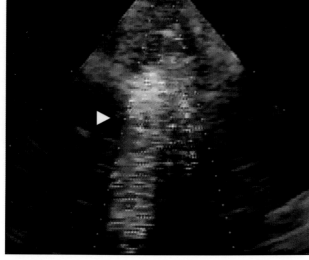

Case 10.2 *continued*

(e) Photograph of a coronary sinus cannula. There are two infusion ports on the proximal end with a self-inflating balloon and monitoring port on the distal end. The catheter may be seen entering the right atrium and is advanced towards the ostia of the coronary sinus in a direction opposite the right atrial appendage. The cannula frequently finds the tricuspid valve orifice, which is readily identified during echocardiographic visualization (f, g), and requires manipulation of the cannula towards the coronary sinus. As the balloon inflates it is easily recognized (arrow) during insertion (h–j), upon engaging the coronary sinus the catheter is advanced approximately 3 cm into the vessel (k–m). Cardioplegia solution should be visualized in the coronary sinus as a mosaic flow pattern (arrow) within the coronary sinus upon initiation of retrograde cardioplegia, once cardiopulmonary bypass is initiated (n, o). RA, right atrium; CS, coronary sinus; RV, right ventricle; IVC, inferior vena cava; RAA, right atrial appendage; LA, left atrium; TV, tricuspid valve; LV, left ventricle.

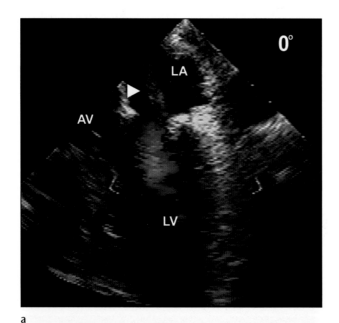

a

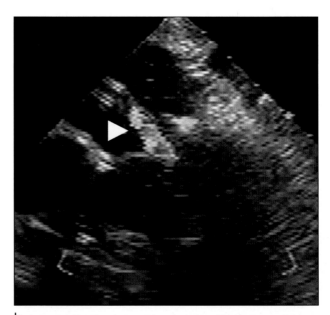

b

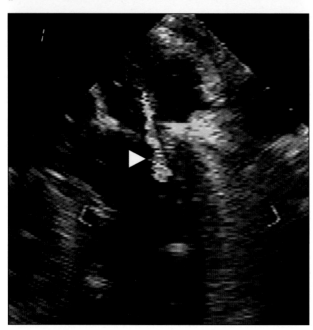

c

Case 10.3

Left ventricular venting catheter. Catheters are frequently utilized during various types of cardiac surgery, to vent the left ventricle and should be recognized echocardiographically. (a–c) Left ventricular vent lying across the mitral valve following a reparative procedure. The catheter is initially visualized in the left atrium and when it is actively attached to suction, flow is demonstrated within the vent catheter as a mosaic flow pattern (arrow). LA, left atrium; LV, left ventricle; AV, aortic valve.

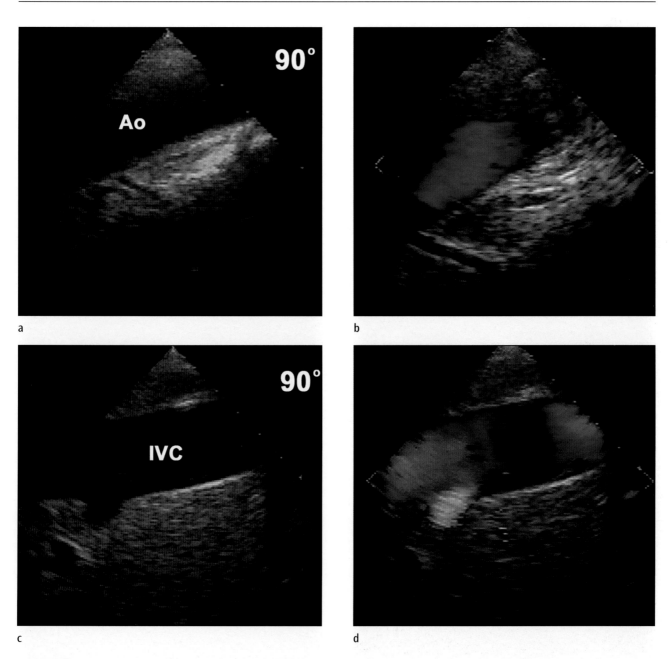

Case 10.4

Port access surgery. For placement of the venous cannula the inferior vena cava is visualized in long-axis from the distal gastric probe position. The transesophageal probe is rotated directly posterior to visualize the descending aorta in cross-section at 0° at a level that approximates the level of the diaphragm with the depth of the image sector set to approximately 16 cm. (a) The transducer is rotated to 90° in order to visualize the aorta in long-axis and the probe is slowly advanced with mild retroflexion to visualize the maximum extent of the aorta obtainable within the abdomen. (b) The transesophageal probe is then rotated in a counterclockwise manner until the inferior vena cava is demonstrated lying inferior within the image sector and in the same direction parallel to the aorta at an approximate level of the superior pole of the right kidney. (c, d) Color flow Doppler demonstrates low velocity flow in the inferior vena cava in the opposite direction of the aortic flow, with numerous branches at the level of the liver.

continued

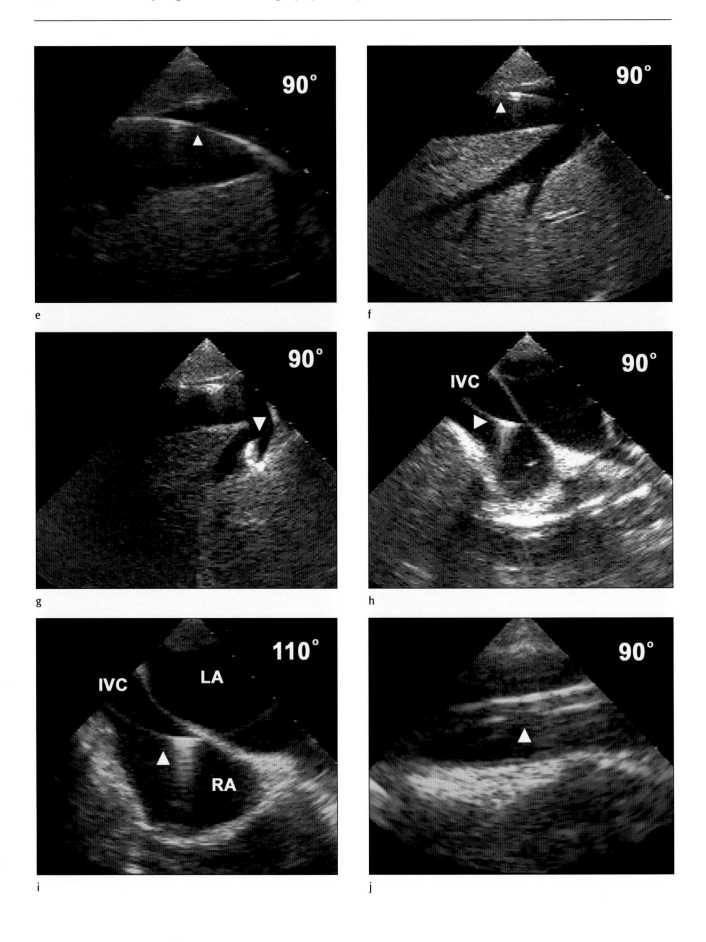

k

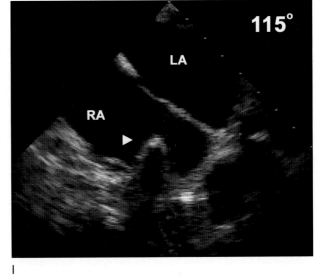

l

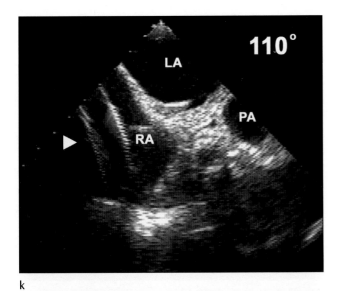

m

Case 10.4 *continued*

(e–g) The guide wire (arrow) is visualized as it traverses the inferior vena cava and followed while the probe is slowly withdrawn with minor manipulation of the probe to keep the inferior vena cava central in the image sector and until it is seen entering the right atrium. If the guidewire enters a branch of the hepatic veins it may be withdrawn under echocardiographic guidance. (h, i) The guidewire is passed into and through the right atrium to the ostium of the superior vena cava. (j–m) The endovascular venous cannula (arrow) is then passed over the wire, which is well-visualized echocardiographically and the tip of the cannula is placed near the origin of the superior vena cava. The surgeon may try to detect the cannula as it enters the right atrium with palpation (arrow, surgeon's finger) to assist in cannula positioning, and the surgeon's palpating finger (arrow) is seen indenting the atrial wall (l, m). Ao, aorta; IVC, inferior vena cava; LA, left atrium; RA, right atrium; PA, pulmonary artery.

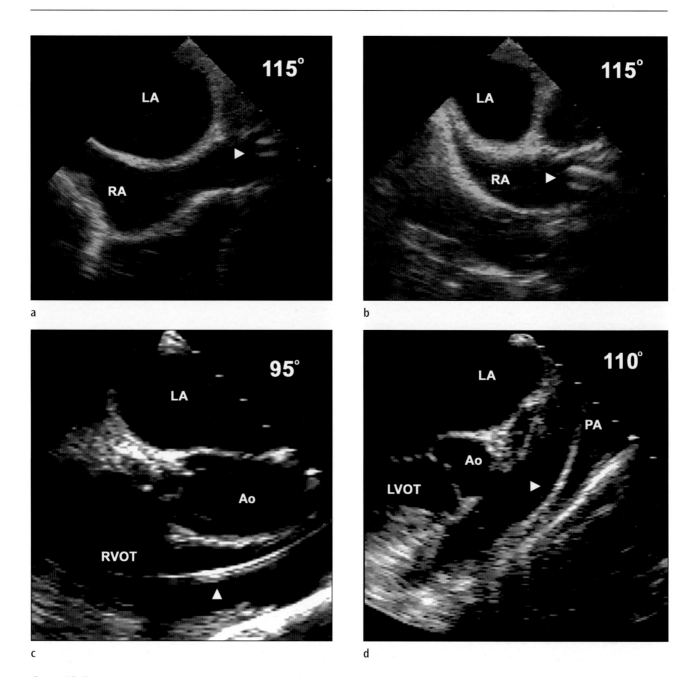

Case 10.5

Port access surgery. A pulmonary artery vent cannula may be utilized and is placed in the right atrium from the internal jugular approach and appears similar to a Swan Ganz catheter. Introducing cannula (arrow) visualized in the superior vena cava (a, b). The pulmonary artery vent cannula is positioned in the main pulmonary artery, so that the tip of the cannula is visualized in the main pulmonary artery (c, d). LA, left atrium; RA, right atrium; RVOT, right ventricular outflow tract; Ao, aorta; LVOT, left ventricular outflow tract; PA, pulmonary artery.

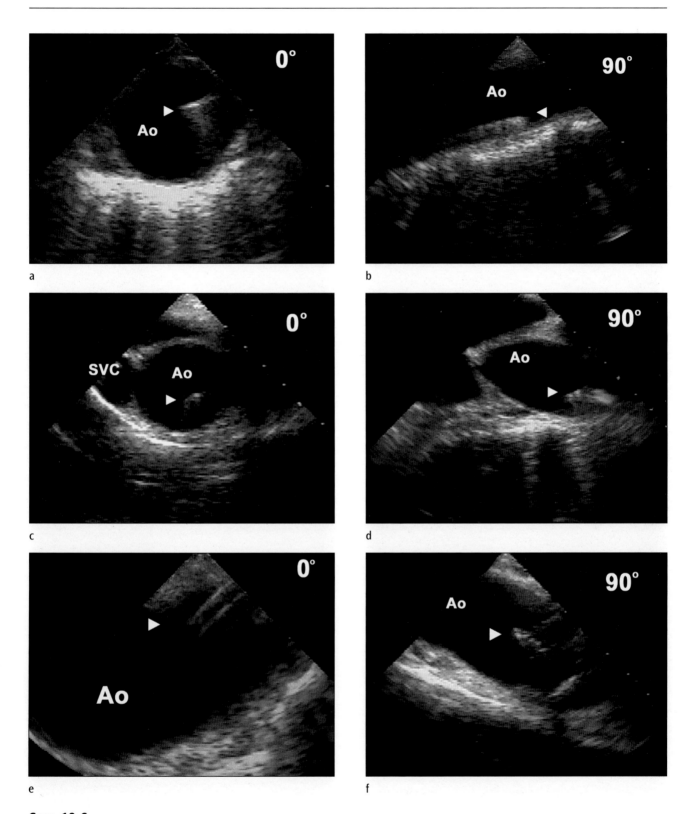

Case 10.6

Port access surgery. Cannulation of the femoral artery and the aorta is visualized from the distal stomach as described for the inferior vena cava. (a–c) The guidewire is well-visualized in the aortic lumen and should appear to be freely passing through the aorta. The guidewire (arrow) is followed with withdrawal of the probe to the level of the aortic arch. (d) The endoaortic clamp catheter is passed over the wire to the level of the aortic arch and the position of the transesophageal probe is changed to the mid-esophageal window visualizing the ascending aorta at 90°–110°. (e, f) Echocardiographic demonstration of the tip of the endoaortic clamp (arrow). Ao, aorta; SVC, superior vena cava.

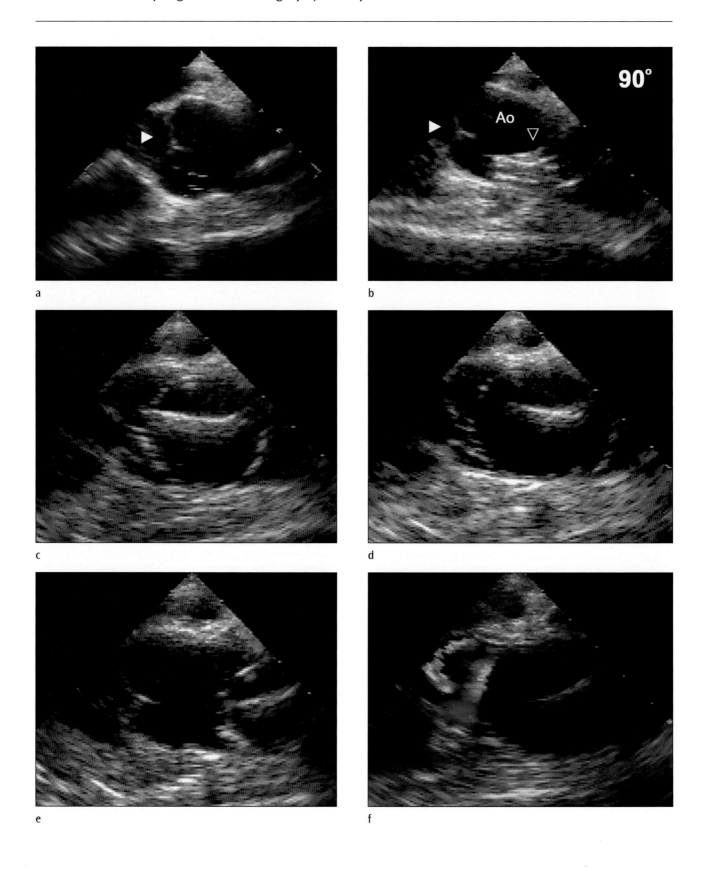

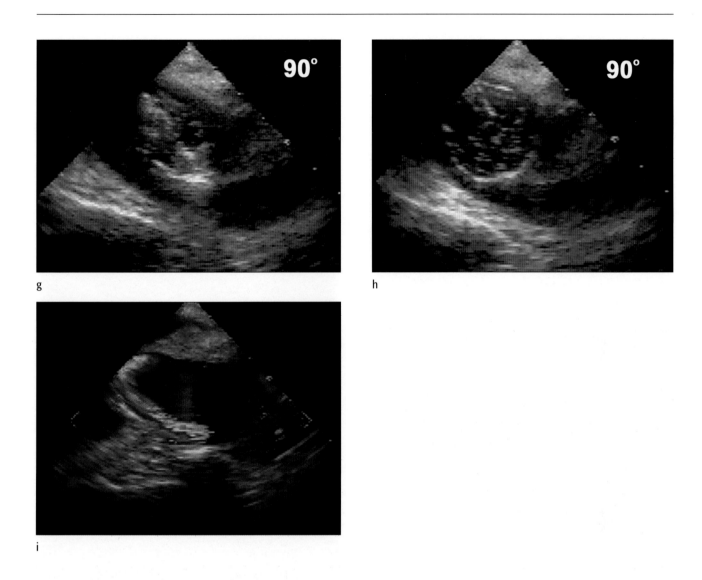

g

h

i

Case 10.7

Port access surgery. The tip of the endoaortic clamp should approximate the level of the sinus of Valsalva and not pass through the aortic valve plane as to eliminate the possibility of producing trauma to the valvular cusps. When the endoaortic clamp balloon is inflated (arrow), the balloon should lie above the sinotubular junction and below the origin of the innominate artery (a–e). When the balloon is fully inflated it should not exhibit motion during the cardiac cycle. When cardioplegia is infused through the catheter, it is visualized echocardiographically as contrast filling the sinus of Valsalva, and with full cardiac arrest the closed aortic valve constrains the extent of the echocardiographic contrast (c). During the procedure the endoaortic clamp is monitored since it tends to migrate either forward toward the aortic valve (f, g) or in a retrograde fashion towards the take off of the great vessels (h). Frequent re-positioning of the endoaortic cannula may be necessary under echocardiographic guidance during the procedure to place the cannula in the proper position (i) to allow the proper occlusion of the aorta and adequate infusion of cardioplegia. Ao, aorta.

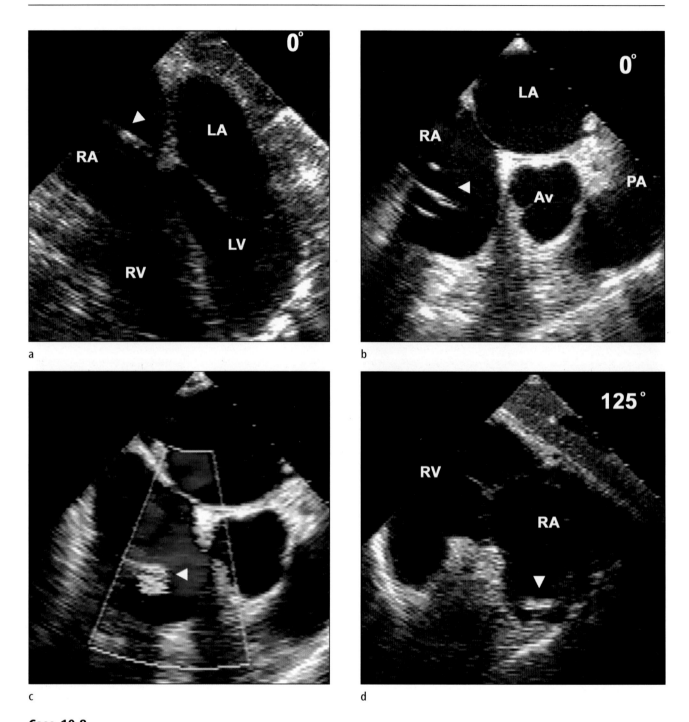

Case 10.8

During implantation of the ventricular assist device, the placement of the atrial cannula and arterial graft sites are assessed echocardiographically. (a–f) Demonstration of the right heart cannulation sites. (a–f) Right atrial cannula visualized from multiple windows demonstrating anatomy, position and normal color flow Doppler. The right atrium is cannulated in the mid free wall or through the right atrial appendage.

continued

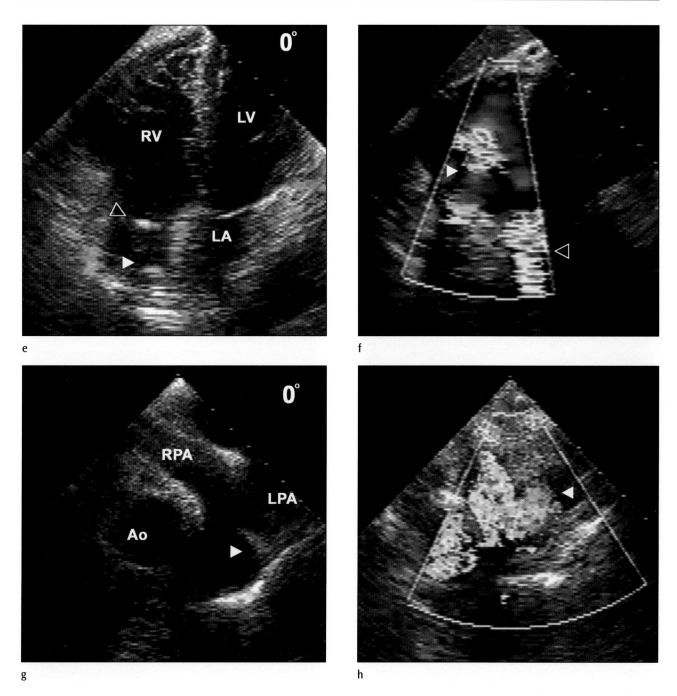

e

f

g

h

Case 10.8 *continued*

(g, h) The pulmonary artery is visualized from the upper esophageal window with the cannula (arrow) sewn to the main pulmonary artery and with the addition of color flow normal flow is demonstrated from both cannulas. (h) Color flow Doppler demonstrates flow from the pulmonary artery cannula emptying into both pulmonary artery branches equally.

continued

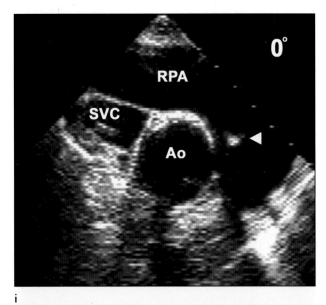

i

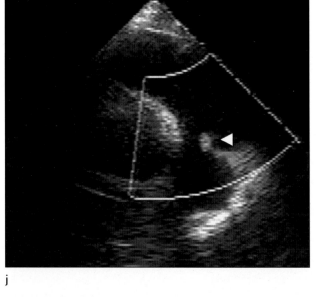

j

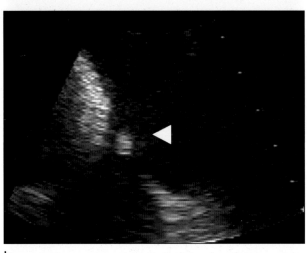

k

Case 10.8 *continued*

(i–k) A small clot is seen emanating from the anastomosis of the pulmonary artery cannula (arrow), zoom mode, (k).
RA, right atrium; RV, right ventricle; LA, left atrium; LV, left ventricle; PA, pulmonary artery.

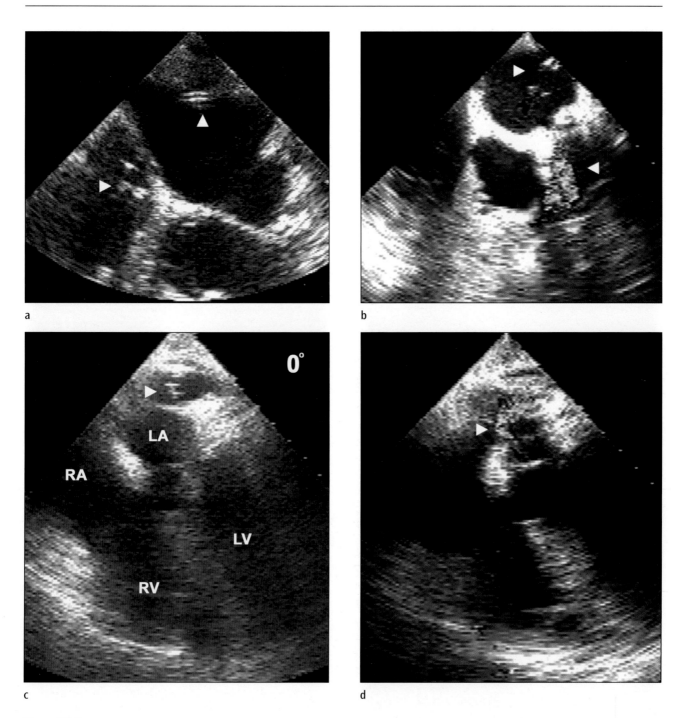

Case 10.9

Biventricular assist device demonstrating left heart cannulation sites. The left atrium is typically cannulated from behind the heart near the interatrial groove, through the left atrial appendage or in the dome of the left atrium (the area between the aorta and the superior vena cava). (a–d) The aortic graft is typically sewn to the anterolateral surface of the ascending aorta above the aortic valve and sinus of Valsalva.

continued

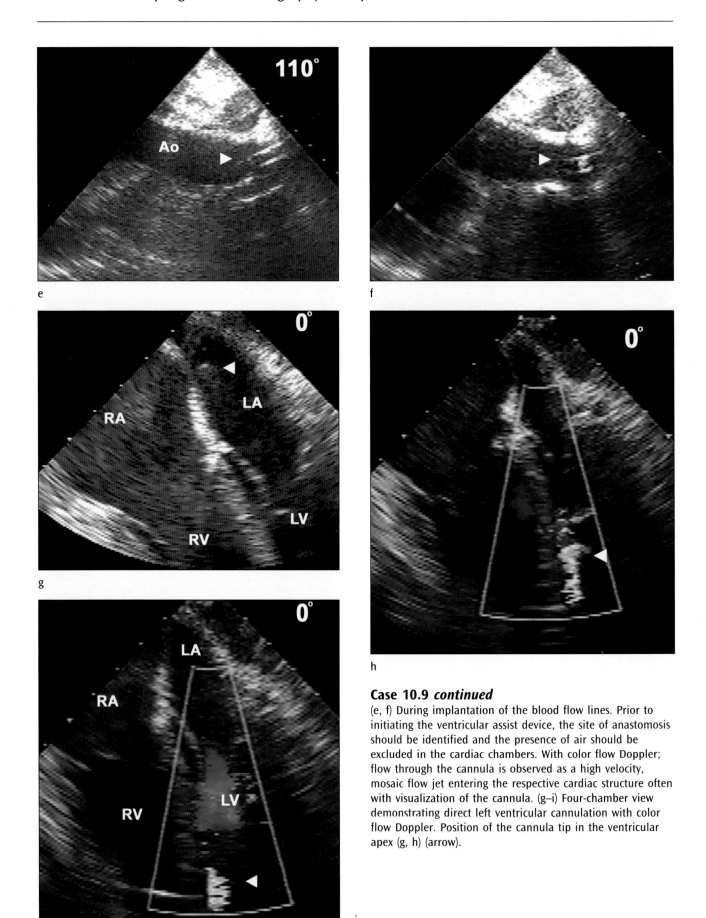

Case 10.9 *continued*

(e, f) During implantation of the blood flow lines. Prior to initiating the ventricular assist device, the site of anastomosis should be identified and the presence of air should be excluded in the cardiac chambers. With color flow Doppler; flow through the cannula is observed as a high velocity, mosaic flow jet entering the respective cardiac structure often with visualization of the cannula. (g–i) Four-chamber view demonstrating direct left ventricular cannulation with color flow Doppler. Position of the cannula tip in the ventricular apex (g, h) (arrow).

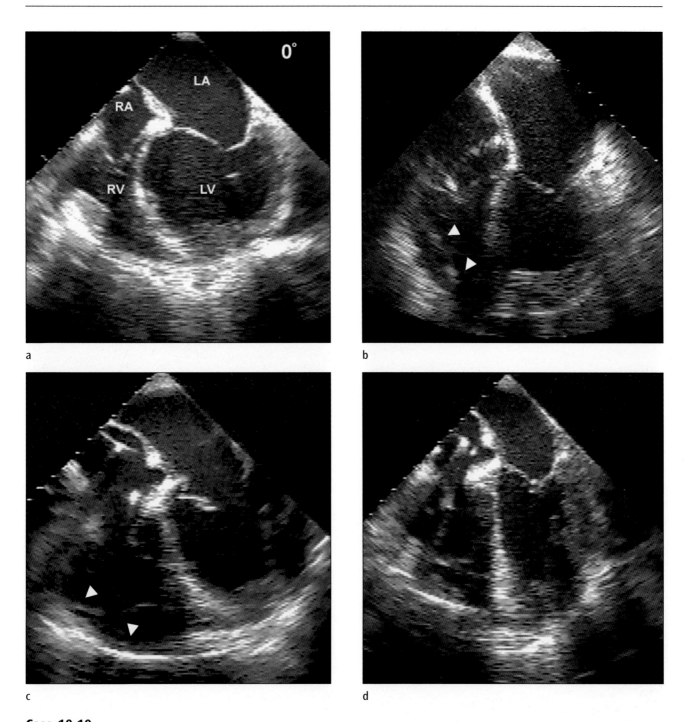

Case 10.10

Right ventricular failure post CABG. Echocardiographic monitoring following placement of a left ventricular assist device demonstrates progressive dilatation and worsening of right ventricular wall motion secondary to ensuing right ventricular failure with left heart assist only. Note the full unloading affect of the left ventricular assist device to the left ventricle denoted by small left atrial and especially left ventricular dimensions. The right heart failure produced decreased cardiac output, which necessitated placement of a right-sided assist device and biventricular support. (a–d) Four-chamber views over time demonstrating progressive right ventricular enlargement and dysfunction (arrows) with decreasing left ventricle size with maximum unloading of the left heart with insertion of left ventricular assist device only. RA, right atrium; RV; right ventricle; LA, left ventricle; LV, left ventricle.

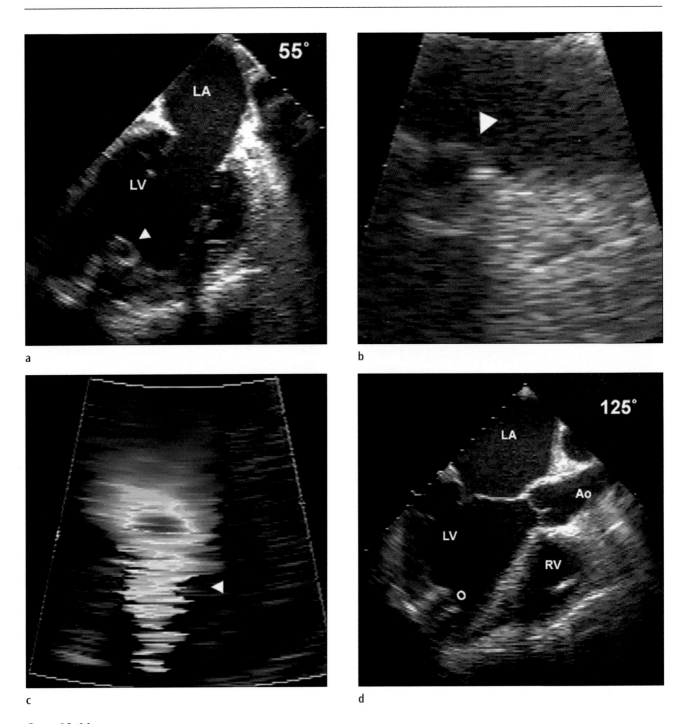

Case 10.11

Thoratec® ventricular assist device. In situations that may result in prolonged ventricular assistance or as a bridge to transplant, a Thoratec® ventricular assist device may be utilized. A cannula with a tip shaped like a top hat is sewn directly to the left ventricular apex to unload the left ventricle instead of placing a left atrial cannula. A separate cannula is sewn in an end-to-side anastomosis to the aorta in a similar fashion to other ventricular assist devices. Echocardiographic visualization demonstrates the left ventricular and aortic cannulas and flow at the ventricular apex and the aorta. With continuous wave Doppler the flows should be identical in both areas, and left ventricular dimensions should decrease with institution of ventricular assistance. To ensure maximum support the cannulas and associated flow may be visualized in multiple planes in order to detect dysfunction or interference with surrounding cardiac anatomy. (a–c) Two-dimensional image of the left ventricle at 55° illustrating the apical cannula, (b) magnified view of the cannula, (c) color Doppler of flow through the cannula. (d, e) Two-dimensional image of the left ventricle at 125° with associated color flow Doppler image of flow through the apical cannula.

continued

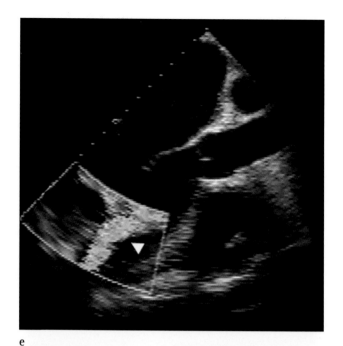

e

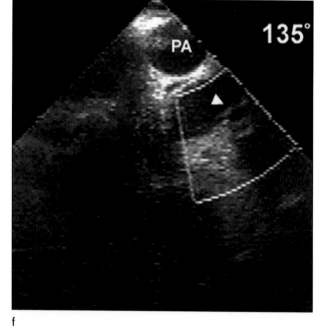

f

Case 10.11 *continued*

(f, g) Two-dimensional image of the ascending aorta obtained from the mid-esophageal window at 135°. The probe is slightly withdrawn after visualizing the proximal aortic root to visualize the most distal portion of the ascending aorta, (g) color flow Doppler demonstrating flow through the aortic cannula.

continued

g

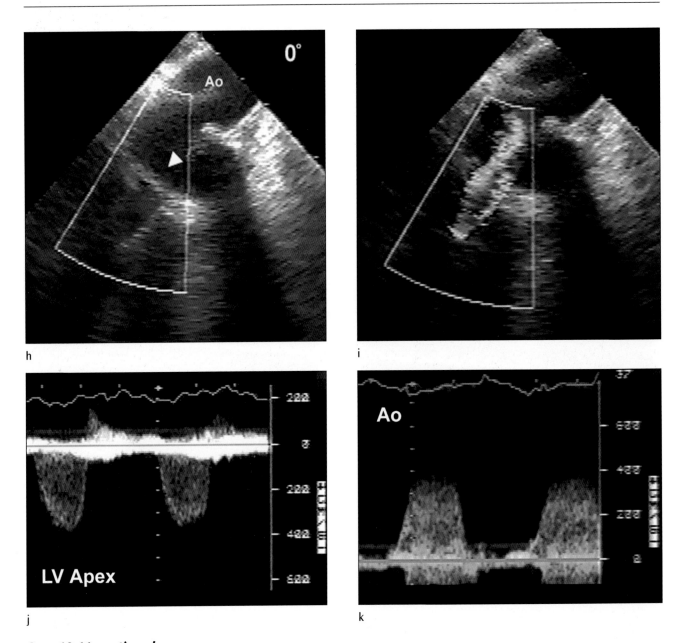

Case 10.11 *continued*

(h, i) Views of the ascending aorta from the upper esophageal window viewing the area of the proximal aortic arch. The aortic cannula is visualized in the ascending aorta and flow is visualized in the cannula filling the aorta. These views allow continuous wave Doppler interrogation of the apical cannula flow (j) and ascending aortic cannula flow (k) with the flows being nearly equal. LA, left atrium; LV, left ventricle; RV, right ventricle; PA, pulmonary artery; Ao, aorta.

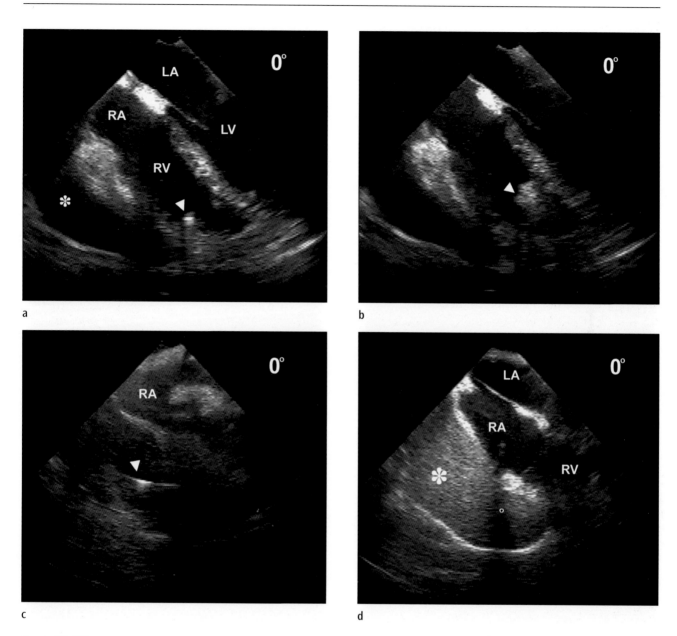

Case 10.12

Pericardiocentesis. Transesophageal echocardiography (TEE) may be beneficial during pericardiocentesis especially in difficult cases. (a) Pericardiocentesis attempted with needle insertion from the subxyphoid approach. Four-chamber view from the lower esophageal window, demonstrates the tip of the needle (arrow) in the right ventricle. (b) Injection of contrast demonstrating abnormal needle position within the right ventricular cavity. (c) Reinsertion of the position of the pericardiocentesis needle (arrow) to the area of the roof of the right atrium with echocardiographic guidance. (d) Injection of contrast demonstrates proper needle position within the pericardial sac as contrast (star) highlights the pericardial effusion.

continued

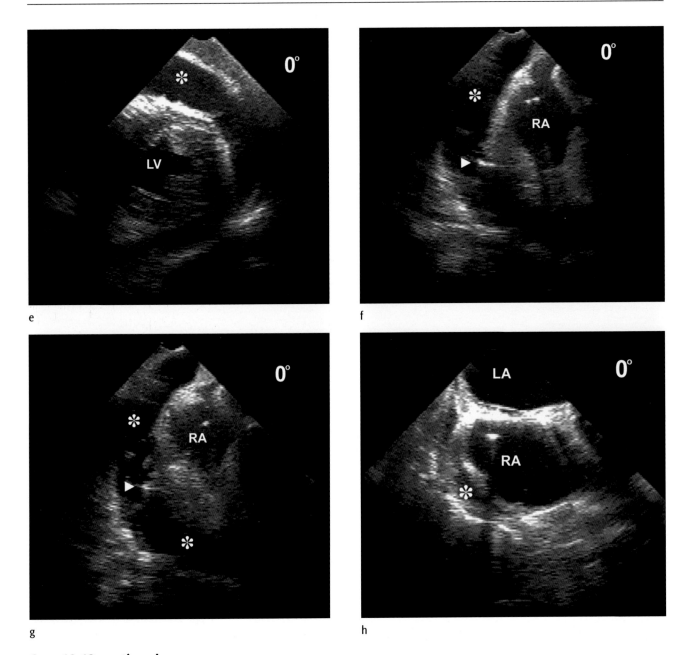

Case 10.12 *continued*

(e–h) Echocardiographic monitoring of the removal of pericardial effusion (star). The pericardiocentesis catheter is denoted as an echocardiographic artifact (arrow) in multiple views. RA, right atrium; LA, left atrium; RV, right ventricle; LV, left ventricle.

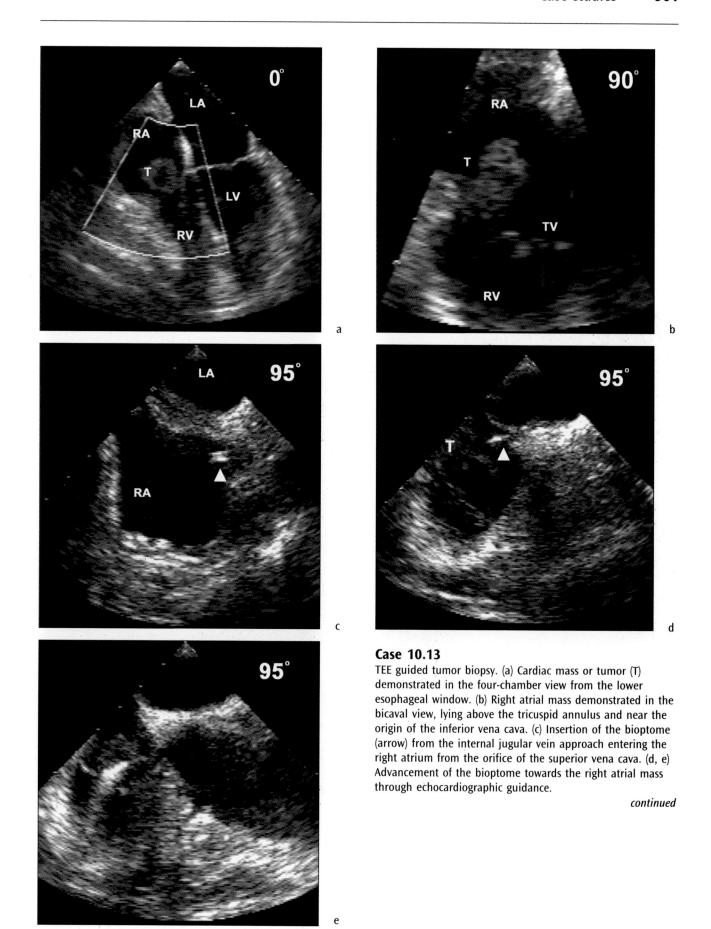

Case 10.13

TEE guided tumor biopsy. (a) Cardiac mass or tumor (T) demonstrated in the four-chamber view from the lower esophageal window. (b) Right atrial mass demonstrated in the bicaval view, lying above the tricuspid annulus and near the origin of the inferior vena cava. (c) Insertion of the bioptome (arrow) from the internal jugular vein approach entering the right atrium from the orifice of the superior vena cava. (d, e) Advancement of the bioptome towards the right atrial mass through echocardiographic guidance.

continued

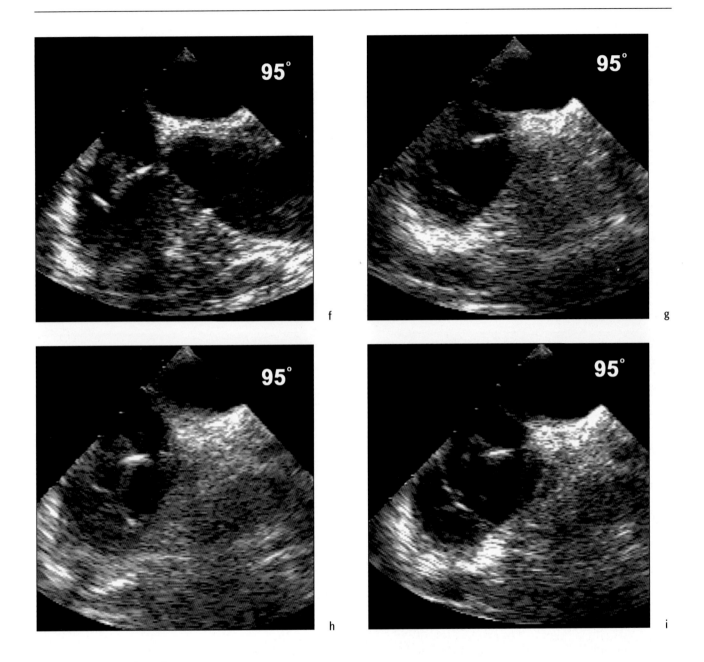

Case 10.13 *continued*

(h, i) Tumor fragment in the jaws of the bioptome (arrow) upon withdrawal of the catheter. RA, right atrium; LA, left atrium; RV, right ventricle; LV, left ventricle; T, tumor; TV, tricuspid valve.

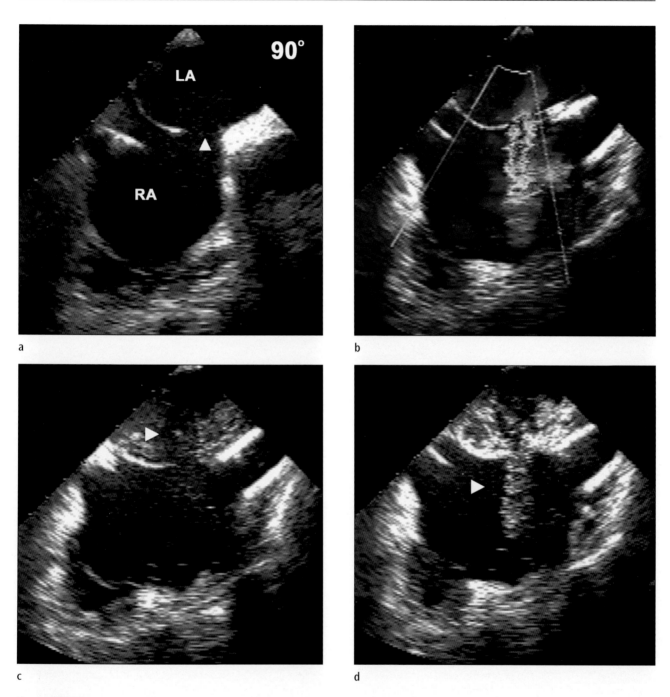

a   b

c   d

Case 10.14

Atrial septal defect device closure. (a) Secundum atrial septal defect as demonstrated in the bicaval view at 90° from the upper esophageal window. The geometrical shape of the defect may be appreciated by viewing the defect from 0° to 180°. The diameter is measured in the view that demonstrates the largest dimension and reported. (b) Color Doppler of the atrial septal defect depicting significant shunt flow through the defect. (c–i) Deployment of the closure device in an atrial septal defect. During the procedure the guide wire is placed across the defect and is visualized ending near the orifice of the left upper pulmonary vein. A balloon filled with contrast and saline is advanced over the wire and inflated within the left atrial cavity. (c) The balloon is pulled back to the atrial septum occluding the defect with the balloon. Saline contrast (arrow) is injected into the left atrium to help determine proper balloon occlusion of the defect. The balloon is then pulled through the defect and the deformity of the balloon is noted and measured providing the stretch diameter of the septal defect. The occluder device is then passed into the left atrium over the guidewire. The device is opened in the left atrium as it is passed out of the sheath. The left atrial appendage, the pulmonary vein orifice and mitral valve are observed to prevent the occluder device from entangling or interfering with these structures when it expands. The occluder device is then withdrawn to the atrial septum with an orientation for the device that is roughly parallel to the atrial septal plane.

continued

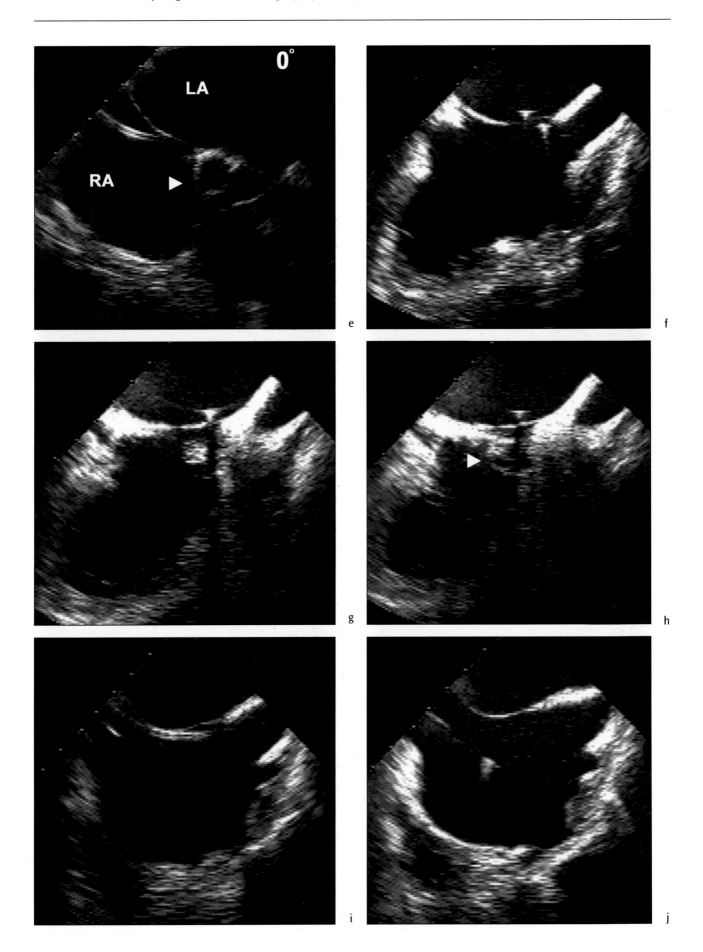

Case 10.14 *continued*

(f–i) The occluder device is pulled back to the defect and fully deployed. J. Following deployment of the device the results are assessed with interrogation of the atrial septum with two-dimensional imaging and color flow Doppler. LA, left atrium; RA, right atrium.

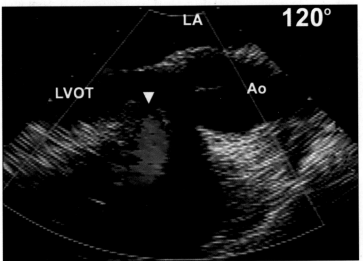

a

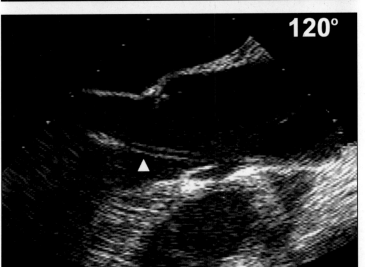

b

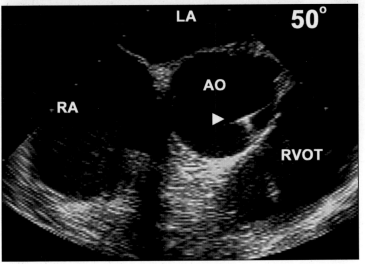

c

Case 10.15

Ventricular septal defect device closure.
(a) Color flow Doppler demonstration of a membranous ventricular septal defect in the longitudinal view of the left ventricular outflow tract at 120° from the mid-esophageal window. The diameter of the defect is estimated by observing the largest diameter of the color flow shunt jet. (b, c) The closure device deployment catheter (arrow) is passed through the aorta and guided into the left ventricle with transesophageal echocardiography and fluoroscopy.

continued

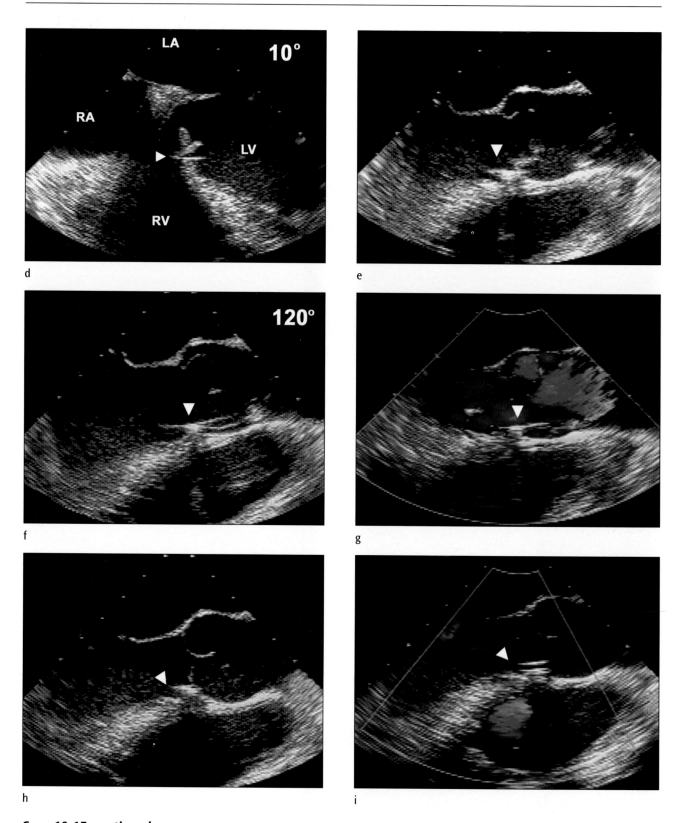

Case 10.15 *continued*

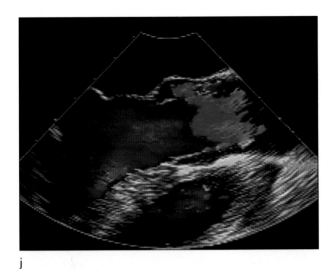

Case 10.15 continued

(d–f) The closure device is deployed in the ventricular septal defect. D. The supporting arms are demonstrated in the defect in the four-chamber view emanating within the septal defect. (g–j) Following deployment of the closure device the defect is interrogated with two-dimensional imaging and color flow Doppler to determine proper positioning of the device free from interfering with surrounding cardiac structures and obliteration of the shunt. LA, left atrium; LVOT, left ventricular outflow tract; Ao, aorta; RVOT, right ventricular outflow tract; RA, right atrium; RV, right ventricle; LV, left ventricle.

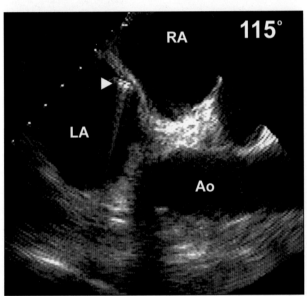

a

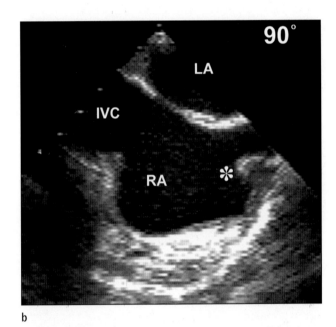

b

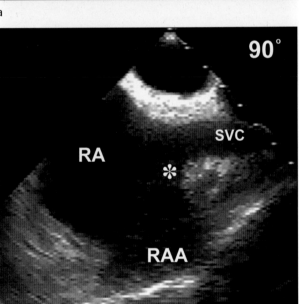

c

Case 10.16

Echocardiographic guidance of electrophysiology procedures. TEE may be utilized for guidance of catheter placement during electrophysiology procedures. Echocardiographic guidance is frequently utilized to guide atrial transseptal puncture to allow access for left atrial mapping or ablation. (a) Two-dimensional image from the left atrium demonstrating the transseptal catheter after penetrating the atrial septum in the ideal position. (b–e) TEE views for frequent ablation and mapping sites (stars) include the crista terminalis, near the origin of the (b, c) superior vena cava or (d, e) inferior vena cava.

continued

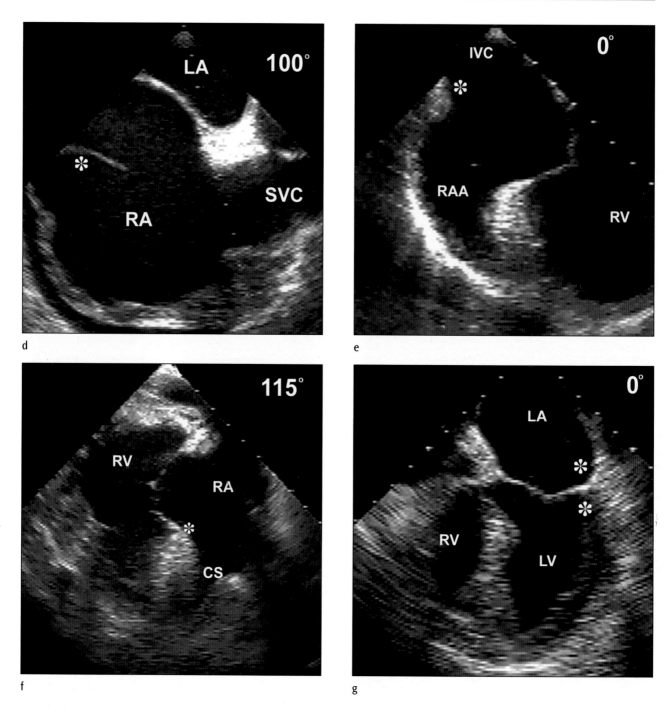

Case 10.16 *continued*

(f) Mapping may involve cannulation of the coronary sinus. (f) Deep transgastric view of the isthmus area located between the tricuspid annulus and the ostium of the coronary sinus. (g) Sites of lateral bypass tracts.

continued

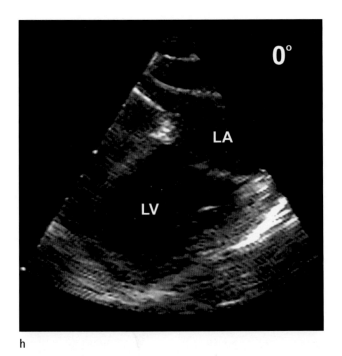

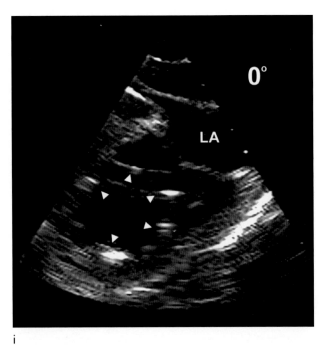

h

i

Case 10.16 *continued*

(h, i) Newer electrode catheters include 64-electrode basket demonstrated in the left ventricle of a pig. Normal pig two-chamber view (h). The electrode basket (arrow) is monitored for position as well as confirming avoidance of cardiac structures that would interfere with hemodynamics. LA, left atrium; RA, right atrium; LV, left ventricle; RV, right ventricle; CS, coronary sinus; IVC, inferior vena cava; SVC, superior vena cava; CT, crista terminalis; PMV, posterior mitral leaflet; Ao, aorta; RAA, right atrial appendage.

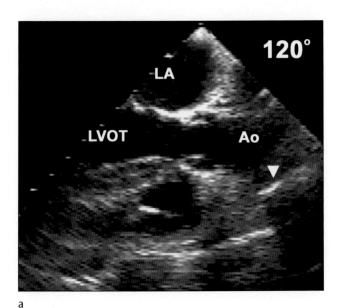

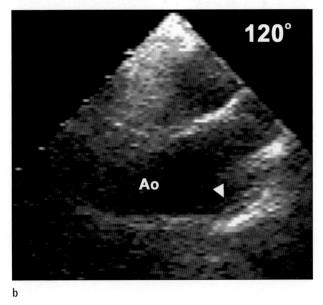

a

b

Case 10.17

Aorta evaluation pre-CABG. Inspection of the aorta is beneficial before cardiac surgery to evaluate the presence of arteriosclerotic plaque and debris that may be a source of embolus or stroke during the surgical procedure. The site of aortic cross clamping is usually above the sinotubular junction and below the innominate artery. (a–c) Aortic plaque demonstrated in the ascending aorta (arrow) obtained from the mid-esophageal window in a longitudinal projection (a), mild withdrawal of the probe with image magnification to visualize the distal ascending aorta (b).

continued

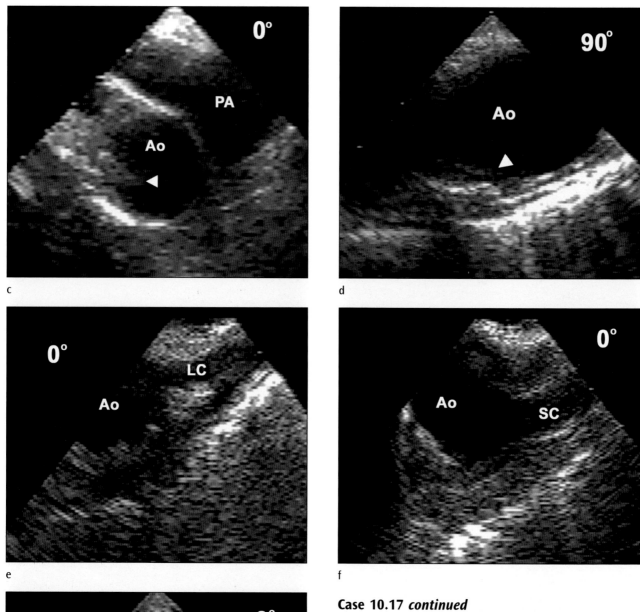

c

d

e

f

g

Case 10.17 *continued*

Short-axis view of the ascending aorta from the upper esophageal window (c) and distal ascending aorta from the upper esophageal window following visualization of the aortic arch (d). Plaque is identified as a bright echogenic region associated with shadowing behind the plaque. Frequently after demonstrating the presence of atherosclerotic plaque in this area of the aorta, the surgeon may request epicardial imaging to evaluate the precise placement of the cross clamp site. The presence of atherosclerotic plaque in severe atherosclerotic disease often involves the take-off of the great vessels which may also be flow limiting during cardiopulmonary bypass. Visualization of the left carotid orifice demonstrating plaque with narrowing at the ostia (e) with thickening of the ostia noted of the left subclavian artery (f), and mild thickening of the intima (arrow) noted in the proximal descending thoracic aorta (g). LVOT, left ventricular outflow tract; LA, left atrium; Ao, aorta; PA, pulmonary artery; LC, left carotid; SC, left subclavian artery.

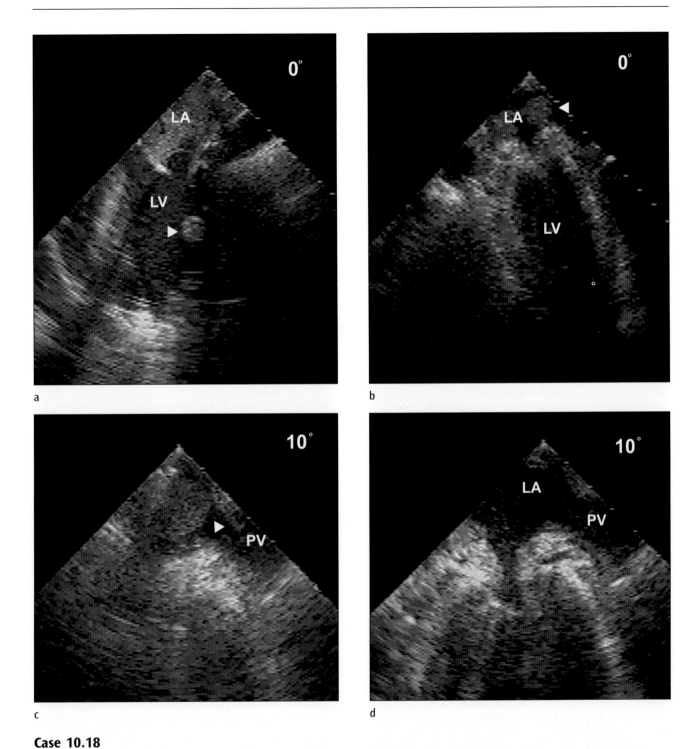

Case 10.18

Displaced left ventricular thrombus pre-CABG. (a) In a patient who presented with a mobile left ventricular thrombus prior to coronary artery bypass surgery the thrombus (arrow) became dislodged during arresting of the heart before the institution of cardiopulmonary bypass and traveled through the left atrium (b) and became lodged in a pulmonary vein orifice (c) during echocardiographic surveillance. The clot was successfully discovered and removed surgically (d) limiting the potential of a postoperative complication that could have been unrecognized. LV, left ventricle; LUPV, left upper pulmonary vein; LA, left atrium; PV, pulmonary vein.

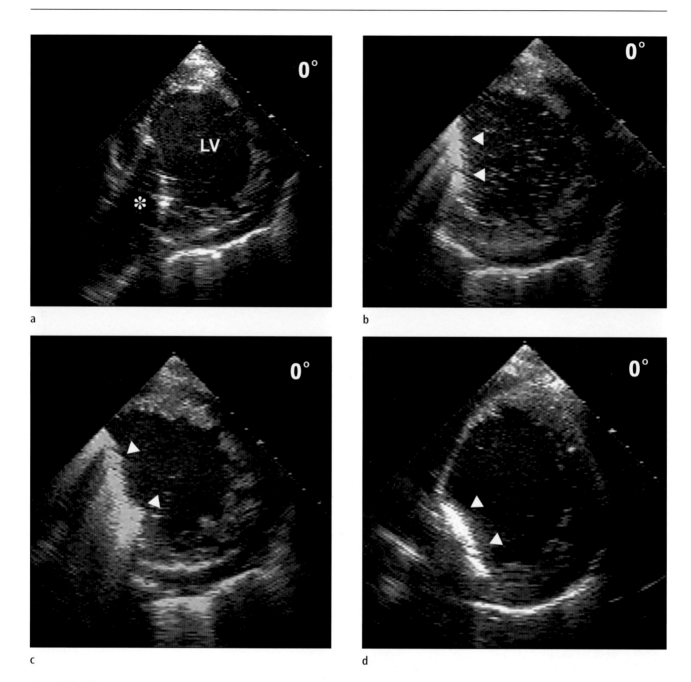

Case 10.19

Postoperative air. Air is frequently detected in the heart following open-heart surgical procedures including coronary artery bypass surgery even when the cardiac chambers are not opened. Transesophageal echocardiographic visualization of the heart is helpful in detecting the presence of air in the cardiac chambers before and shortly after cardiopulmonary bypass is terminated. Typical echocardiographic artifact demonstrating air in the apex of the left ventricle which is the highest point of the heart with the patient supine lying on the operative table, transgastric short-axis view of the left ventricle (a–e) and four-chamber lower esophageal view of the left ventricle (f). Note the small air bubbles that are demonstrated moving with the cardiac cycle. (g) Air embolism to the right coronary artery frequently may occur during a surgical procedure since the ostia of the right coronary artery (arrow) also is a high point with the patient in the supine position and the chest open. Arrows point to microbubbles in the myocardium. RV, right ventricle; LV, left ventricle; LA, left atrium; Ao, aorta.

continued

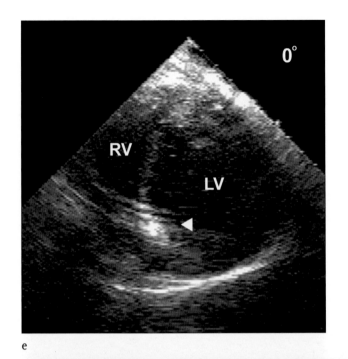

e

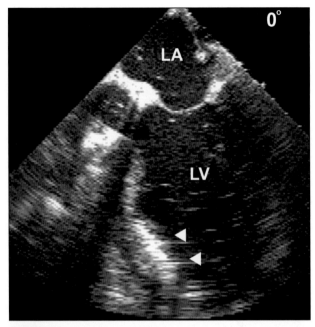

f

Case 10.19 *continued*

g

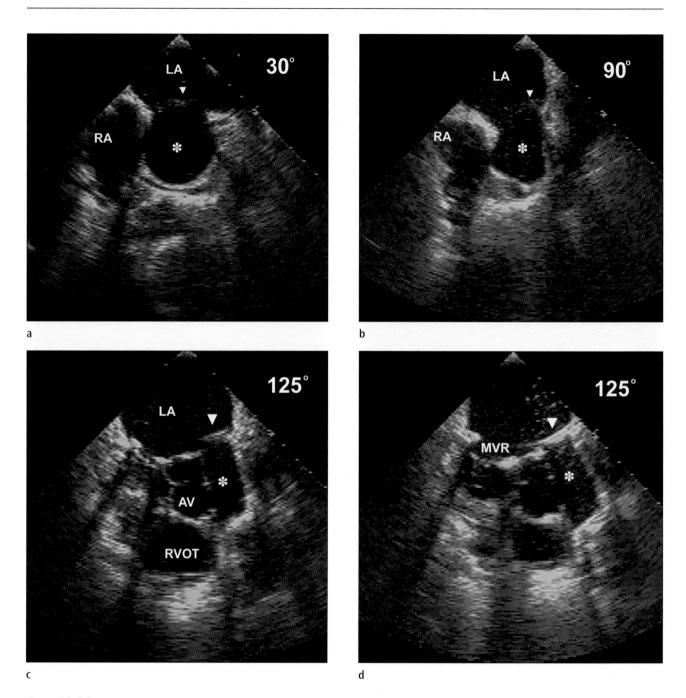

Case 10.20

Postoperative air. Although air usually rises to the highest point within the cardiac chambers, surface tension may allow large air pockets to form in the atria especially when they have been opened for valvular cases. (a–d) Transgastric short-axis views of the left ventricle demonstrating a large air bubble (star) in the left ventricle with numerous small bubbles (arrow) filling the left ventricular cavity. Note the large area of ghosting that actually shimmers echocardiographically with cardiac motion (a). Large air pocket (star) in the left atrium demonstrated in multiple standard views immediately following mitral valvular surgery. LV, left ventricle; RA, right atrium; LA, left atrium; MVR, mitral valve prosthesis; AV, aortic valve; RVOT, right ventricular outflow tract.

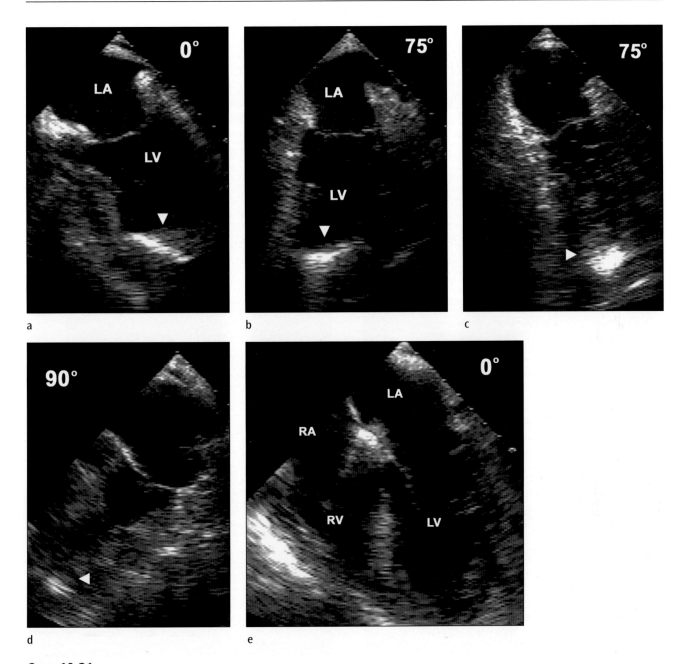

Case 10.21

Postoperative air with needle removal. Air is removed from the left ventricle either through a venting catheter or by insertion of a large bore needle into the left ventricular apex. (a, b) Air pocket (arrow) in the apex of the left ventricle demonstrated in multiple standard views. (c, d) Needle artifact noted at the apex of the left ventricle with disruption of the air pocket by the needle producing multiple small bubbles (arrow). (e) Final result following removal of air in the left ventricular apex. LA, left atrium; LV, left ventricle; RA, right atrium; RV, right ventricle.

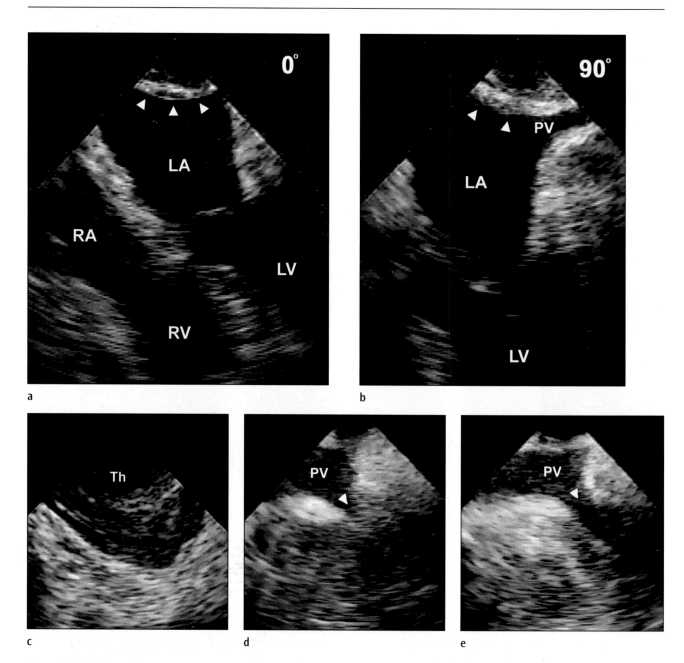

Case 10.22

Postoperative oblique sinus hematoma. Hematoma formation within the pericardial cavity is a rare complication that may occur following open-heart surgeries. Hematoma formation may be large and frequently occur or settle in the most dependent portions of the pericardial cavity. Numerous reports have described hemodynamic compromise similar to cardiac tamponade as a result of the hematoma producing external compression of the cardiac structures, which may interfere with hemodynamics. (a–f) A large hematoma collection in a patient following routine coronary artery bypass surgery that formed in the oblique sinus and compressed the pulmonary veins. (a, b) Echocardiographic visualization of indentation (arrows) of the left atrium and pulmonary vein in a patient exhibiting sign of pericardial tamponade in the first postoperative day. Note the lack of pericardial effusion, which was the indication for the transesophageal examination. (c–e) Magnification of the thrombus in the oblique sinus, which appears to be collapsing the pulmonary vein (arrow) during the respiratory cycle.

continued

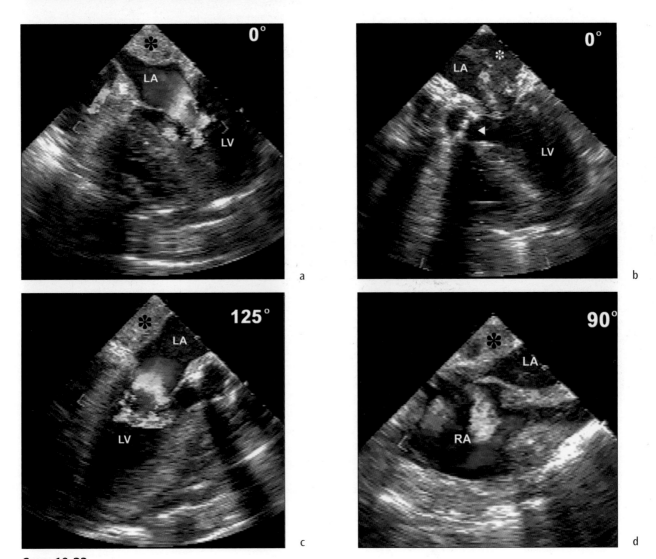

Case 10.22 *continued*

(f) Pulsed-wave Doppler flow demonstrating the obliteration of pulmonary venous flow emptying into the left atrium correlating with the visual demonstration of the collapsing pulmonary vein. The patient was taken back to surgery and the hematoma was successfully evacuated. RA, right atrium; LA, left atrium; RV, right ventricle; LV, left ventricle; PV, pulmonary vein; Th, hematoma.

Case 10.23

Postoperative hematoma. Postoperative hematoma severely compressing both the left and right atrium 2 days following an aortic valve replacement secondary to persistent bleeding from the aortic aortotomy site. (a–d) Large echogenic masses representing hematoma (star) producing indentation of both the left and right atrium obtained from multiple views in a patient with low cardiac output. LA, left atrium; LV, left ventricle; RA, right atrium.

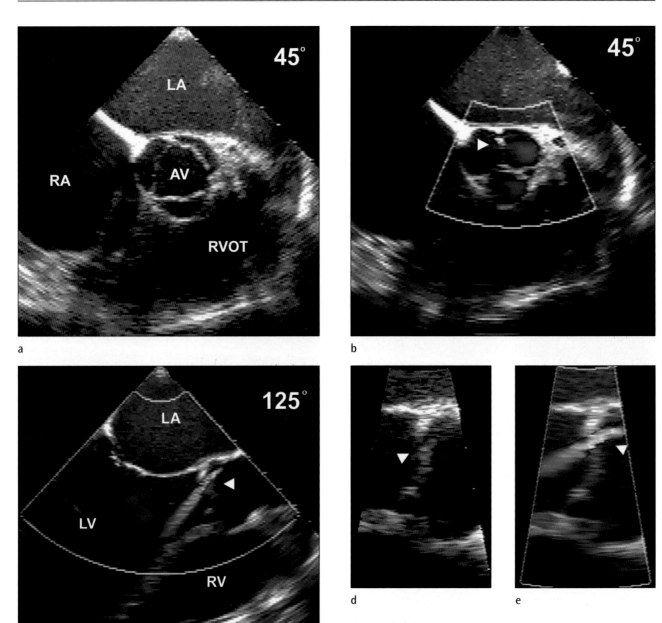

a

b

c

d   e

Case 10.24

Postoperative aortic valve perforation. Immediately during the postoperative echocardiographic evaluation a perforation was detected in the non-coronary sinus of the aortic valve. (a–e) Two-dimensional and color Doppler echocardiographic demonstration of new aortic valve insufficiency following routine coronary bypass surgery. Magnified views demonstrating the aortic cusp perforation (arrow) and the associated small aortic insufficiency jet (arrow). LA, left atrium; LV, left ventricle; Ao, aorta; RV, right ventricle; RA, right atrium; AV, aortic valve; RVOT, right ventricular outflow tract.

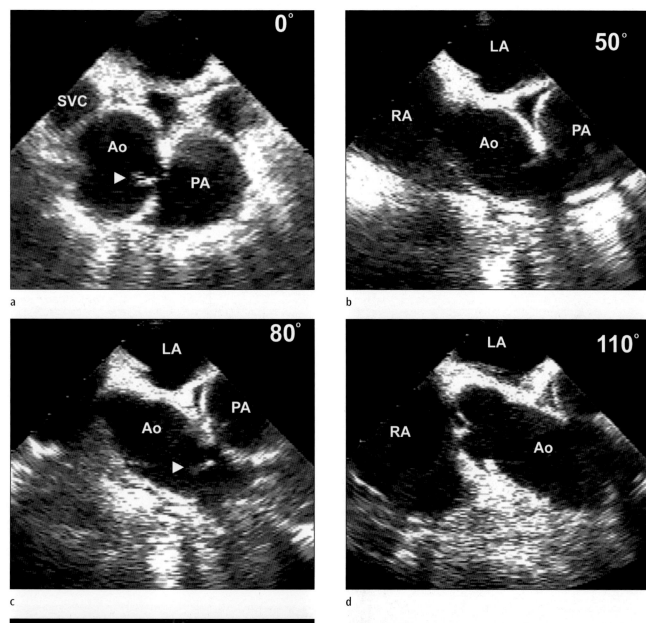

Case 10.25

Aortic transection ascending aorta (grade 1). Aortic intimal disruption is frequently demonstrated in trauma cases. The most frequent site of aortic transection is the aortic isthmus but may occur in other areas of the thoracic aorta necessitating a detailed echocardiographic evaluation of the entire aorta. (a–d) Multiple views of the ascending aorta demonstrating a grade 1 aortic intimal disruption (arrow) in the lumen of the distal ascending aorta adjacent to the main pulmonary artery. (e) View of the distal ascending aorta and the proximal aortic arch obtained from the upper esophageal window demonstrating atherosclerotic plaque without signs of distal extension. LA, left atrium; LV, left ventricle; Ao, aorta; PA, pulmonary artery; RA, right atrium; SVC, superior vena cava; Asc Ao, ascending aorta.

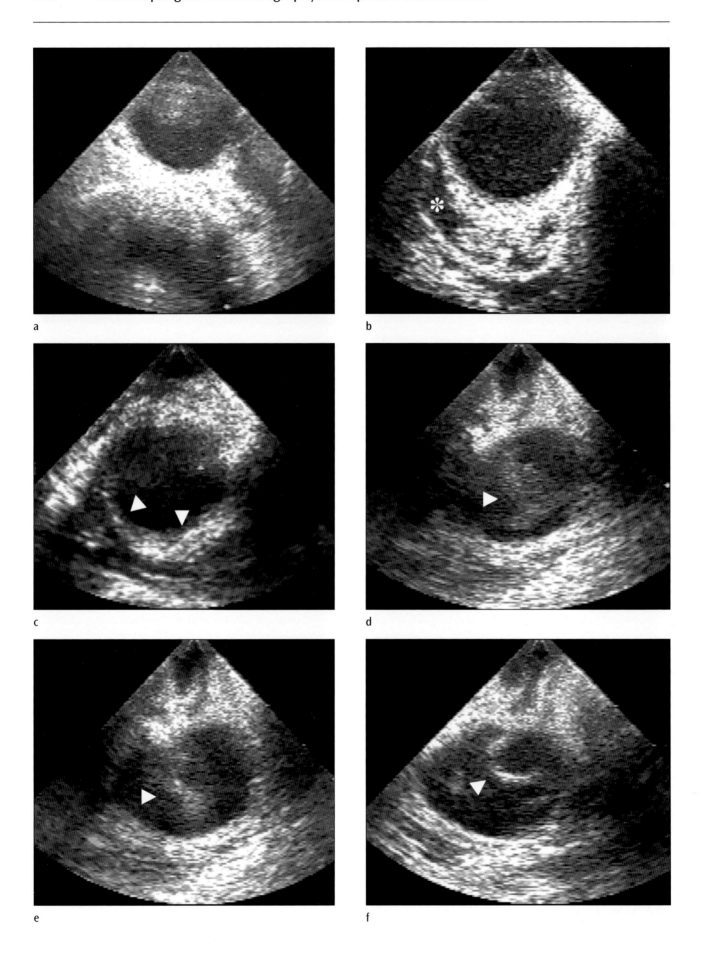

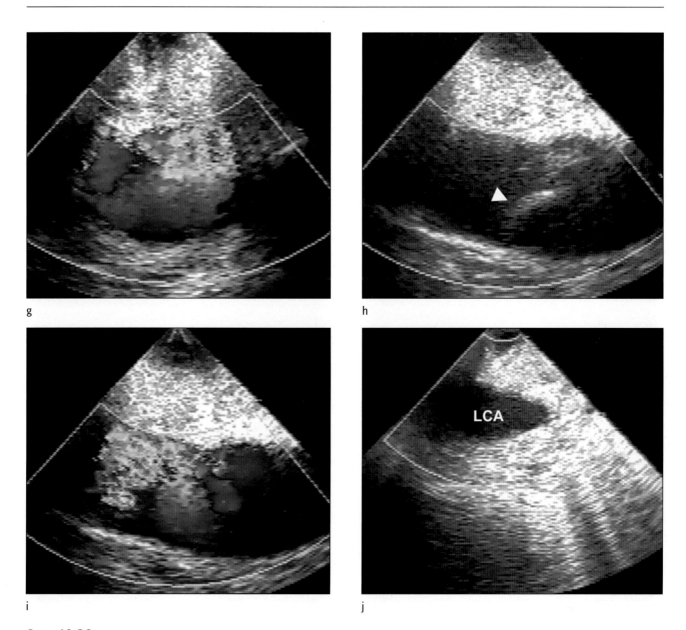

g

h

i

j

Case 10.26

Aortic transection (grade III). Transesophageal demonstration of a partial aortic transection with advential hematoma following a motor vehicle accident. (a–f) Multiple serial short-axis slices of the descending aorta obtained with withdrawal of the probe from the level of the diaphragm to the proximal descending aorta just distal to the aortic arch. (g–i) Longitudinal images of the proximal descending aorta distal to the great vessels highlighting the typical flow disturbance produced by the transection. Transesophageal echocardiography is useful for demonstrating transection and its complications that may occur with the great vessels. Complicating the transection of the aorta, a hematoma produced external compression of the subclavian artery and complete occlusion of the left carotid artery at its take off from the aortic arch (j). In addition a complete transection (arrow) occurred within the left subclavian artery near the origin from the aorta, which produced a pulseless left arm (k–n). Post-op the patient exhibited a CVA despite surgical repair of the great vessels. LCA, left carotid artery; LSA, left subclavian artery.

continued

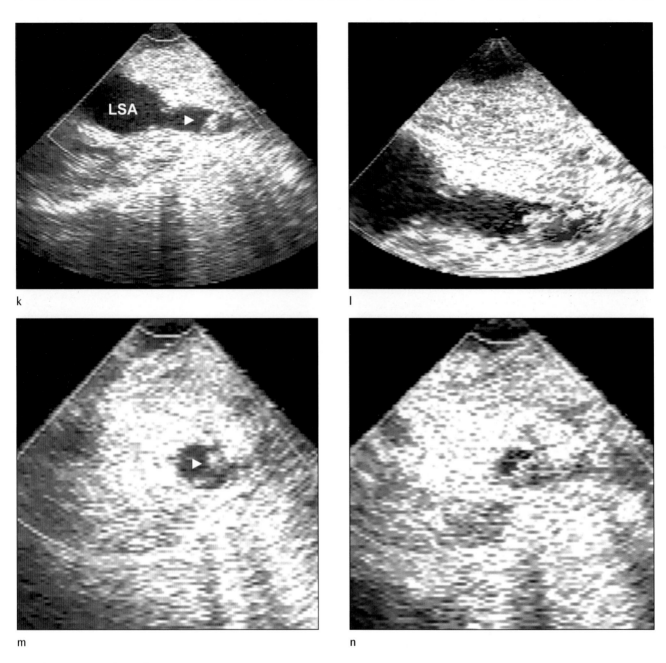

Case 10.26 *continued*

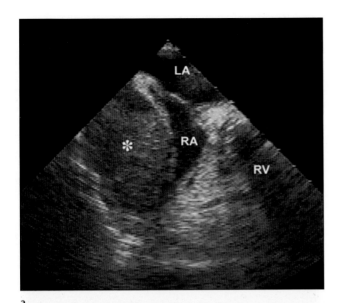

a

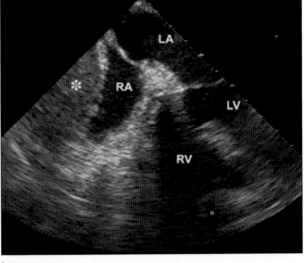

b

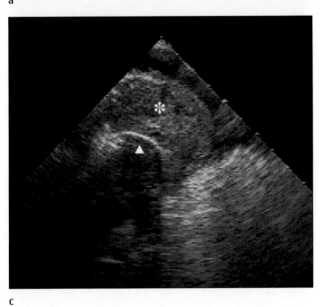

c

Case 10.27

Mediastinal hematoma associated with aortic transection. Large hematomas are demonstrated in multiple views with transesophageal echocardiography. (a, b) Right atrial compression in produced by a large hematoma (star) collecting near the roof and lateral border of the right atrium. (c) In addition a hematoma (star) formed in the transverse sinus surrounding the proximal ascending aorta (arrow). RA, right atrium; LA, left atrium; RV, right ventricle; LV, left ventricle.

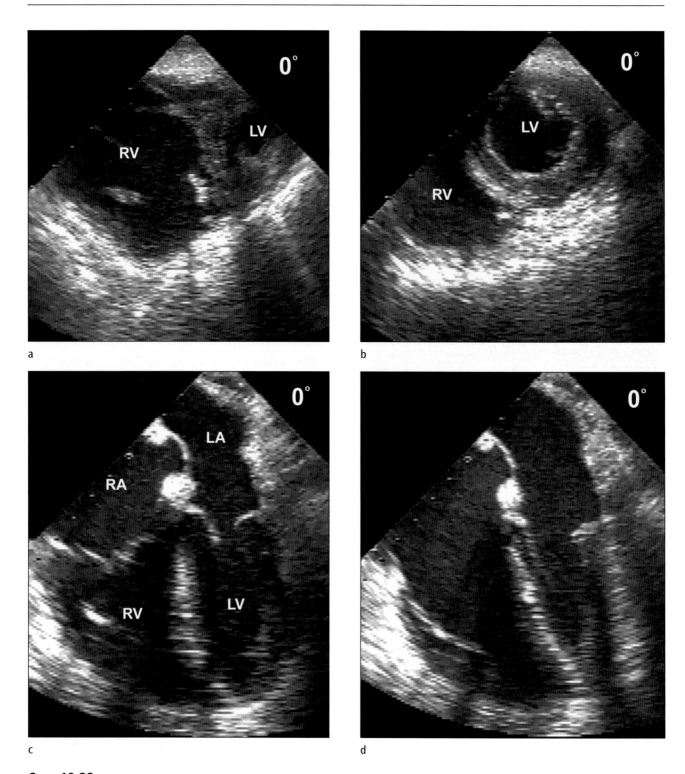

Case 10.28

Right ventricular contusion. Myocardial concussion or contusion is frequently associated with trauma produced to the thorax. Myocardial injury occurs with rise in cardiac enzyme, which is associated with the development of new regional wall motion abnormalities. Due to its anterior orientation in the chest the right ventricle is most vulnerable to myocardial injury. (a–d) Right ventricular contusion demonstrated in transgastric and lower esophageal views illustrating extreme right ventricular dilatation with akinesis. Diastolic four-chamber frame and systolic frame demonstrating akinetic right ventricular wall motion (arrows). RV, right ventricle; LV, left ventricle; RA, right atrium; LA, left atrium.

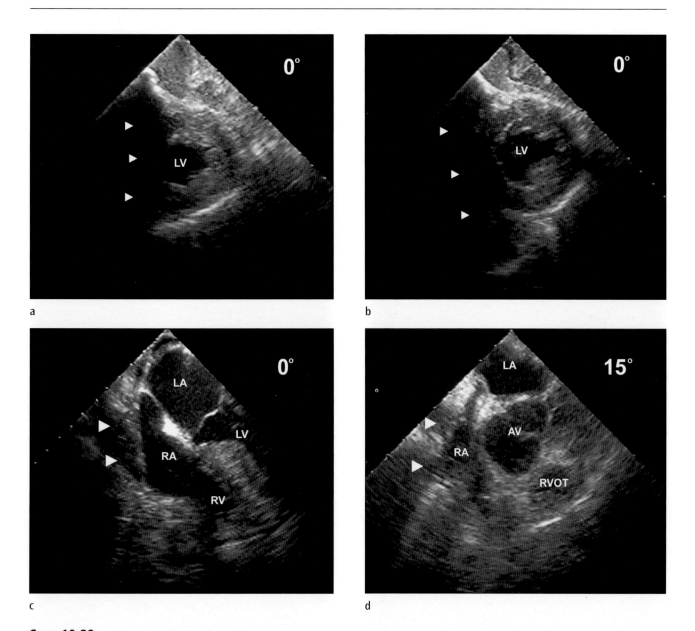

a   b

c   d

Case 10.29

Pneumothorax. Transesophageal evaluation of a thoracic trauma patient with widened mediastinum on chest X-ray. TEE was performed in routine manner, however, visualization of the heart was poor from the standard transgastric window. Air artifact obscured the right heart and portions of the ventricular septum suggesting a left pneumothorax that occurred following the initial chest X-ray (a, b). Collapse (arrow) of the right atrium and right ventricle suggesting tension produced by the pneumothorax (c, d). All findings disappeared following resolution of the pneumothorax permitting a detailed examination of the cardiac structures. LV, left ventricle; RA, right atrium; LA, left atrium; RV, right ventricle; LV, left ventricle; AV, aortic valve; RVOT, right ventricular outflow tract.

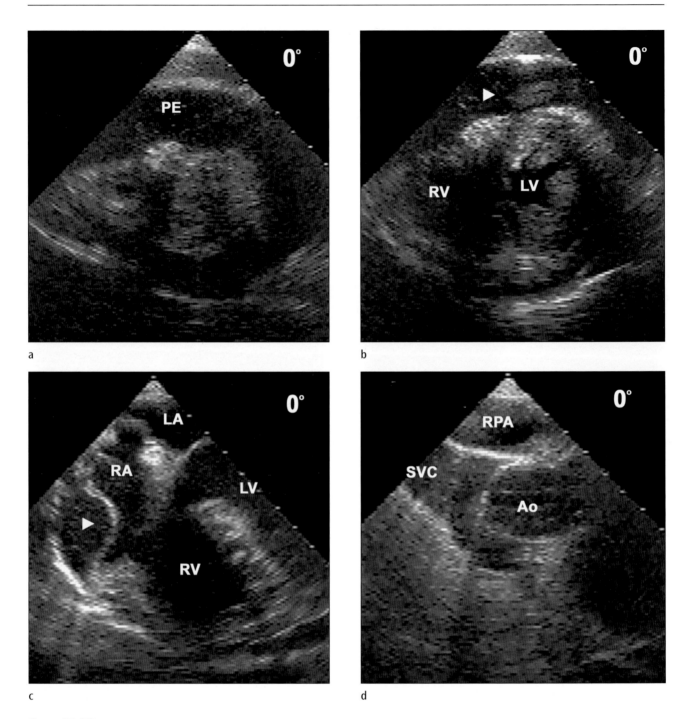

Case 10.30

Traumatic pulmonary vein rupture. A rare complication of cardiac thoracic injury is rupture of the pulmonary vein. Pulmonary artery rupture is a devastating consequence of thoracic injury and requires a rapid diagnosis. It appears that any of the pulmonary veins may rupture and produce echocardiographic findings of a large hemorrhagic pericardial effusion with pericardial tamponade. (a–f) Multiple standard transesophageal views demonstrating a large pericardial effusion, with non-specific tissue debris (arrow) at the origin of the pulmonary vein on the surface of the heart and within the left atrium near the ostia, which were demonstrated as pulmonary vein, rupture at the time of surgical repair. RA, right atrium; Ao, ascending aorta; RVOT, right ventricular outflow tract; LV, left ventricle; LA, left atrium; AV, aortic valve; RV, right ventricle.

continued

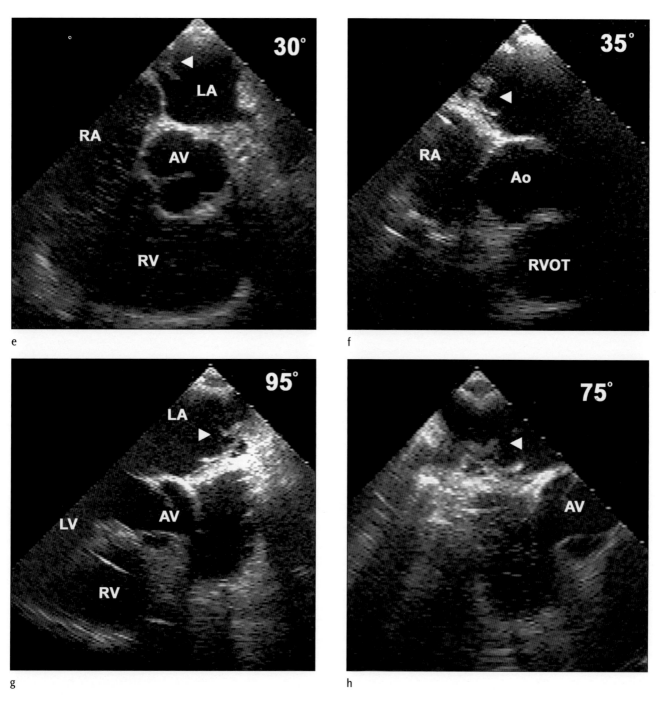

e

f

g

h

Case 10.30 *continued*

continued

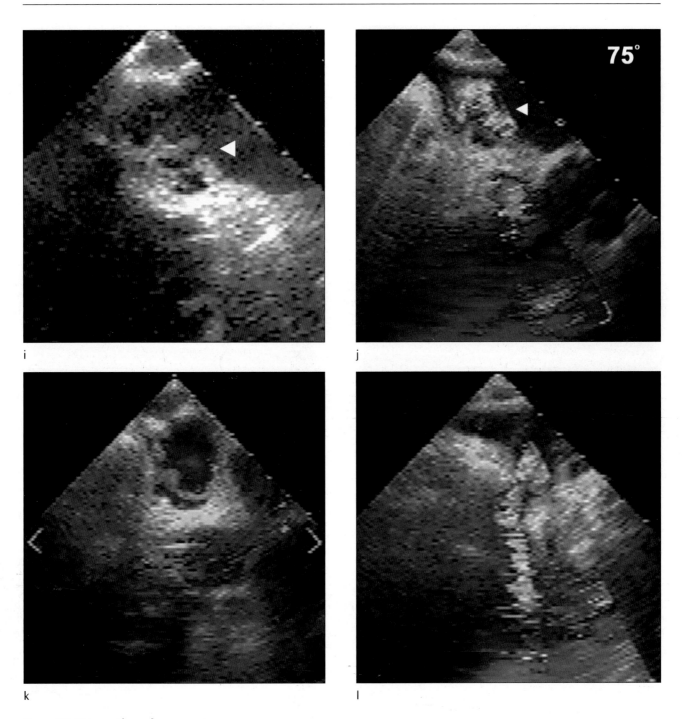

Case 10.30 *continued*

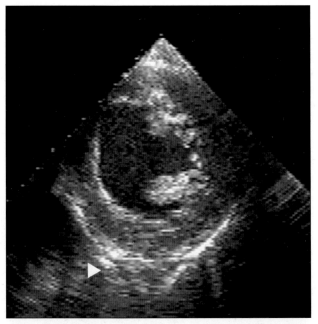

a

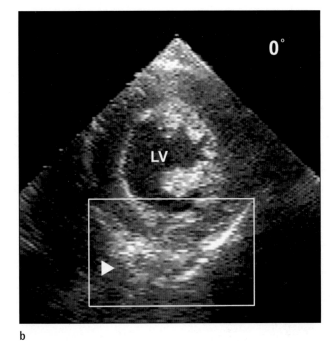

b

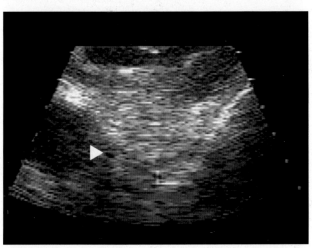

c

Case 10.31

Traumatic left anterior descending rupture. Rupture of the coronary arteries has also been described in the traumatic literature usually from post mortem examination. (a–c) TEE demonstration of a hematoma on the surface of the anterior wall of the left ventricle following blunt chest trauma sustained during a fall. Non-specific mass-producing a distortion to the surface of the anterior wall near the ventricular septum without a significant pericardial effusion. (c) Magnification of the hematoma demonstrating a confluent echogenicity to the mass which is different that the surrounding myocardium. In addition to the lack of a significant pericardial effusion, there was only a mild area of hypokinesis noted in the ventricular septum and anterior walls. LV, left ventricle.

References

1. Practice guidelines for perioperative transesophageal echocardiography: a report by the American Society of Anesthesiologists and Society of Cardiovascular Anesthesiologists Task Force on Transesophageal Echocardiography. *Anesthesiology* 1996;84:986–1006.

2. Sheikh KH, de Bruijn NP, Rankin JS, et al. The utility of transesophageal echocardiography and Doppler color flow imaging in patients undergoing cardiac valve surgery. *J Am Coll Cardiol* 1990;15:363–72.

3. Stewart WJ, Currie PJ, Salcedo EE, et al. Intraoperative Doppler color flow mapping for decision-making in valve repair for mitral regurgitation: technique and results in 100 patients. *Circulation* 1990;81:556–66.

4. Stewart WJ, Thomas JD, Klein AL, et al. Ten-year trend in utilization of 6430 intraoperative echos. *Circulation* 1995;92(suppl 1):I–514.

5. Grimm RA, Stewart WJ. The role of intraoperative echocardiography in valve surgery. *Cardiol Clin* 1998;16:477–89.

6. Oh CC, Click RL, Orszulak TA, et al. Role of intraoperative transesophageal echocardiography in determining aortic annulus diameter in homograft insertion. *J Am Soc Echocardiogr* 1998;11:638–42.

7. Kraker PK, Davis E, Barash PG. Transesophageal echocardiography and the perioperative management of valvular heart disease. *Curr Opin Cardiol* 1997;12:108–13.

8. Ramamoorthy C, Lynn AM, Stevenson JG. Pro: transesophageal echocardiography should be routinely used during pediatric open cardiac surgery. *J Cardiothorac Vasc Anesth* 1999;13:629–31.

9. McGowan FX Jr, Laussen PC. Con: transesophageal echocardiography should not be used routinely for pediatric open cardiac surgery. *J Cardiothorac Vasc Anesth* 1999;13:632–4.

10. Hickey PR. Transesophageal echocardiography in pediatric cardiac surgery. *Anesthesiology* 1992;77:610–11.

11. Kallmeyer IJ, Collard CD, Fox JA, et al. The safety of intraoperative transesophageal echocardiography: a case series of 7200 cardiac surgical patients. *Anesth Analg* 2001;92:1126–30.

12. Stoddard MF, Longaker RA. The safety of transesophageal echocardiography in the elderly. *Am Heart J* 1993;125:1358–62.

13. Daniel WG, Erbel R, Kasper W, et al. Safety of transesophageal echocardiography. A multicenter survey of 10,419 examinations. *Circulation* 1991;83:817–21.

14. Ofili EO, Rich MW. Safety and usefulness of transesophageal echocardiography in persons aged greater than or equal to 70 years. *Am J Cardiol* 1990; 66:1279–80.

15. Pearson AC, Castello R, Labovitz AJ. Safety and utility of transesophageal echocardiography in the critically ill patient. *Am Heart J* 1990;119:1083–9.

16. Hulyalkar AR, Ayd JD. Low risk of gastroesophageal injury associated with transesophageal echocardiography during cardiac surgery. *J Cardiothorac Vasc Anesth* 1993;7:175–7.

17. Greene MA, Alexander JA, Knauf DG, et al. Endoscopic evaluation of the esophagus in infants and children immediately following intraoperative use of transesophageal echocardiography. *Chest* 1999;116:1247–50.

18. Owall A, Stahl L, Settergren G. Incidence of sore throat and patient complaints after intraoperative transesophageal echocardiography during cardiac surgery. *J Cardiothorac Vasc Anesth* 1992;6:15–16.

19. Andropoulos DB, Stayer SA, Bent ST, et al. The effects of transesophageal echocardiography on hemodynamic variables in small infants undergoing cardiac surgery. *J Cardiothorac Vasc Anesth* 2000;14:133–5.

20. Deutsch HJ, Curtius JM, Leischik R, et al. Diagnostic value of transesophageal echocardiography in cardiac surgery. *Thorac Cardiovasc Surg* 1991;39:199–204.

21. Pepi M, Barbier P, Doria E, et al. Multiplane transesophageal echocardiography for the monitoring of cardiac surgery. *Cardiologia* 1994;39:557–63.

22. Pepi M, Barbier P, Doria E, et al. Intraoperative multiplane vs. biplane transesophageal echocardiography for the assessment of cardiac surgery. *Chest* 1996;109:305–11.

23. Murphy PM. Pro: intraoperative transesophageal echocardiography is a cost-effective strategy for cardiac surgical procedures. *J Cardiothorac Vasc Anesth* 1997;11:246–9.

24. Bryden KE, Hall RI. Con: transesophageal echocardiography is not a cost-effective monitor during cardiac surgery. *J Cardiothorac Vasc Anesth* 1997;11:250–2.

25. Loick HM, Scheld HH, Van Aken H. Impact of perioperative transesophageal echocardiography on cardiac surgery. *Thorac Cardiovasc Surg* 1997; 45:321–5.

26. Couture P, Denault AY, McKenty S, et al. Impact of routine use of intraoperative transesophageal echocardiography during cardiac surgery. *Can J Anaesth* 2000;47:20–5.

27. Michel-Cherqui M, Ceddaha A, Liu N, et al. Assessment of systematic use of intraoperative transesophageal echocardiography during cardiac surgery in adults: a prospective study of 203 patients. *J Cardiothorac Vasc Anesth* 2000;14:45–50.

28. Schmidlin D, Schuepbach R, Bernard E, et al. Indications and impact of postoperative transesophageal echocardiography in cardiac surgical patients. *Crit Care Med* 2001;29:2143–8.

29. Kato M, Nakashima Y, Levine J, et al. Does transesophageal echocardiography improve postoperative outcome in patients undergoing coronary artery bypass surgery?. *J Cardiothorac Vasc Anesth* 1993;7:285–9.

30. Shintani H, Nakano S, Matsuda H, et al. Efficacy of transesophageal echocardiography as a perioperative monitor in patients undergoing cardiovascular surgery. Analysis of 149 consecutive studies. *J Cardiovasc Surg* 1990;31:564–70.

31. Bryan AJ, Barzilai B, Kouchoukos NT. Transesophageal echocardiography and adult cardiac operations. *Ann Thorac Surg* 1995;59:773–9.

32. Cicek S, Demirkilic U, Tatar H. Intraoperative echocardiography: techniques and current applications. *J Card Surg* 1993;8:678–92.

33. Deutsch HJ, Curtius JM, Leischik R, et al. Diagnostic value of transesophageal echocardiography in cardiac surgery. *Thorac Cardiovasc Surg* 1991;39:199–204.

34. Currie PJ. Transesophageal echocardiography: intraoperative applications. *Echocardiography* 1989;6:403.

35. Benson MJ, Cahalan MK. Cost–benefit analysis of transesophageal echocardiography in cardiac surgery. *Echocardiography* 1995;12:171–83.

36. Davila-Roman VG, Barzilai B. Perioperative ultrasonic imaging in cardiac surgery. *Curr Opin Cardiol* 1992;7:300–5.

37. Marschall K, Kanchuger M, Kessler K, et al. Superiority of transesophageal echocardiography in detecting aortic arch atheromatous disease: identification of patients at increased risk of stroke during cardiac surgery. *J Cardiothorac Vasc Anesth* 1994; 8:5–13.

38. Katz ES, Tunick PA, Rusinek H, et al. Protruding aortic atheromas predict stroke in elderly patients undergoing cardiopulmonary bypass: experience with intraoperative transesophageal echocardiography. *J Am Coll Cardiol* 1992;20:70–7.

39. Mendelson LS, Maniet AR, Steers JC et al. Is there utility for transesophageal echocardiography during routine coronary artery surgery? *Circulation* 1996;94:I–455.

40. Sousa RC, Garcia-Fernandez MA, Moreno M, et al. The contribution and usefulness of routine intraoperative transesophageal echocardiography in cardiac surgery. An analysis of 130 consecutive cases. *Rev Port Cardiol* 1995;14:15–27.

41. Asakura T, Aoki K, Tadokoro M, et al. Transesophageal echocardiography as an early postoperative monitoring patients after cardiovascular surgery: analysis of 500 consecutive studies. *Kyobu Geka* 1996; 49:261–6.

42. Sheikh KH, Bengtson JR, Rankin JS, et al. Intraoperative transesophageal Doppler color flow imaging used to guide patient selection and operative treatment of ischemic mitral regurgitation. *Circulation* 1991;84:594–604.

43. Click RL, Abel MD, Schaff HV. Intraoperative transesophageal echocardiography: 5-year prospective review of impact on surgical management. *Mayo Clin Proc* 2000;75:241–7.

44. Mizuno T, Toyama M, Tabuchi N, et al. Thickened intima of the aortic arch is a risk factor for stroke with coronary artery bypass grafting. *Ann Thorac Surg* 2000;70:1565–70.

45. Davila-Roman VG, Phillips KJ, Daily BB, et al. Intraoperative transesophageal echocardiography and epiaortic ultrasound for assessment of atherosclerosis of the thoracic aorta. *J Am Coll Cardiol* 1996;28:942–7.

46. Trehan N, Mishra M, Dhole S, et al. Significantly reduced incidence of stroke during coronary artery bypass grafting using transesophageal echocardiography. *Eur J Cardio-Thorac Surg* 1997;11:234–42.

47. Andropoulos DB, Stayer SA, Bent ST, et al. A controlled study of transesophageal echocardiography to guide central venous catheter placement in congenital heart surgery patients. *Anesth Analg* 1999;89:65–70.

48. Diehl JT, Ramos D, Dougherty F, et al. Intraoperative, two-dimensional echocardiography-guided removal of retained air. *Ann Thorac Surg* 1987;43:674–5.

49. Wake PJ, Ali M, Carroll J, et al. Clinical and echocardiographic diagnoses disagree in patients with unexplained hemodynamic instability after cardiac surgery. *Can J Anaesth* 2001;48:778–83.

50. Adsumelli RS, Shapiro JR, Shah PM, et al. Hemodynamic effects of chest closure in adult patients undergoing cardiac surgery. *J Cardiothorac Vasc Anesth* 2001;15:589–92.

51. Leslie D, Hall TS, Goldstein S, Shindler D. Mural left atrial thrombus: a hidden danger accompanying cardiac surgery. *J Cardiovasc Surg* 1998;39:649–50.

52. Leung JM, O'Kelly BF, Mangano DT. Relationship of regional wall-motion abnormalities to hemodynamic indices of myocardial oxygen supply and demand in patients undergoing CABG surgery. *Anesthesiology* 1990;73:802–14.

53. Leung JM, Levine EH. Left ventricular end-systolic cavity obliteration as an estimate of intraoperative hypovolemia. *Anesthesiology* 1994;81:1102–9.

54. Buffington CW, Coyle RJ. Altered load dependence of postischemic myocardium. *Anesthesiology* 1991;75:464–74.

55. Aoyagi S, Tayama E, Nishimi M, et al. Aortic dissections complicating open cardiac surgery: report of three cases. *Surg Today* 2000;30:1022–5.

56. Katz ES, Tunick PA, Colvin SB, et al. Aortic dissection complicating cardiac surgery: diagnosis by intraoperative biplane transesophageal echocardiography. *J Am Soc Echocardiogr* 1993;6:217–22.

57. Sakakibara Y, Matsuda K, Sato F, et al. Aortic dissection complicating cardiac surgery in a patient with calcified ascending aorta. *Jpn J Thorac Cardiovasc Surg* 1999;47:625–8.

58. Varghese D, Riedel BJ, Fletcher SN, et al. Successful repair of intraoperative aortic dissection detected by transesophageal echocardiography. *Ann Thorac Surg* 2002;73:953–5.

59. Leung JM, O'Kelly B, Browner WS, et al. Prognostic importance of postbypass regional wall-motion abnormalities in patients undergoing coronary artery bypass graft surgery. SPI Research Group. *Anesthesiology* 1989;71:16–25.

60. Comunale ME, Body SC, Ley C, et al. The concordance of intraoperative left ventricular wall-motion abnormalities and electrocardiographic S–T segment changes: association with outcome after coronary revascularization. Multicenter Study of Perioperative Ischemia (McSPI) Research Group. *Anesthesiology* 1998;88:945–54.

61. Al-Tabbaa A, Gonzalez RM, Lee D. The role of state-of-the-art echocardiography in the assessment of myocardial injury during and following cardiac surgery. *Ann Thorac Surg* 2001;72:S2214–18.

62. Gewertz BL, Kremser PC, Zarins CK, et al. Transesophageal echocardiographic monitoring of myocardial ischemia during vascular surgery. *J Vasc Surg* 1987;5:607–13.

63. Hong Y, Orihashi K, Oka Y. Intraoperative monitoring of regional wall motion abnormalities for detecting myocardial ischemia by transesophageal echocardiography. *Echocardiography* 1990;7:323–32.

64. Corda DM, Caruso LJ, Mangano D. Myocardial ischemia detected by transesophageal echocardiography in a patient undergoing peripheral vascular surgery. *J Clin Anesth* 2000;12:491–7.

65. Smith JS, Cahalan MK, Benefiel DJ, et al. Intraoperative detection of myocardial ischemia in high-risk patients: electrocardiography versus two-dimensional transesophageal echocardiography. *Circulation* 1985;72:1015–21.

66. Shively B, Watters T, Benefiel D, et al. The intraoperative detection of myocardial infarction by transesophageal echocardiography. *J Am Coll Cardiol* 1986;7(suppl A):2A.

67. Ellis JE, Shah MN, Briller JE, et al. A comparison of methods for the detection of myocardial ischemia during noncardiac surgery: automated ST-segment analysis systems, electrocardiography, and transesophageal echocardiography. *Anesth Analg* 1992;75:764–72.

68. Kozmary SV, Lampe GH, Benefiel D, et al. No finding of increased myocardial ischemia during or after carotid endarterectomy under anesthesia with nitrous oxide. *Anesth Analg* 1990;71:591–6.

69. London MJ, Tubau JF, Wong MG, et al. The 'natural history' of segmental wall motion abnormalities in patients undergoing noncardiac surgery. S.P.I. Research Group. *Anesthesiology* 1990;73:644–55.

70. Eisenberg MJ, London MJ, Leung JM, et al. Monitoring for myocardial ischemia during noncardiac surgery. A technology assessment of transesophageal echocardiography and 12-lead electrocardiography. The Study of Perioperative Ischemia Research Group. *JAMA* 1992;268:210–16.

71. Deutsch HJ, Curtius JM, Leischik R, et al. Reproducibility of assessment of left-ventricular function using intraoperative transesophageal echocardiography. *Thorac Cardiovasc Surg* 1993;41:54–8.

72. Feinberg MS, Hopkins WE, Davila-Roman VG, Barzilai B. Multiplane transesophageal echocardiographic Doppler imaging accurately determines cardiac output measurements in critically ill patients. *Chest* 1995;107:769–73.

73. Royse CF, Barrington MJ, Royse AG. Transesophageal echocardiography values for left ventricular end-diastolic area and pulmonary vein and mitral inflow Doppler velocities in patients undergoing coronary artery bypass graft surgery. *J Cardiothorac Vasc Anesth* 2000;14:130–2.

74. Royse CF, Royse AG, Soeding PF, Blake DW. Shape and movement of the interatrial septum predicts change in pulmonary capillary wedge pressure. *Ann Thorac Cardiovasc Surg* 2001;7:79–83.

75. Kawahito S, Kitahata H, Tanaka K, et al. Pulmonary arterial pressure can be estimated by transesophageal pulsed Doppler echocardiography. *Anesth Analg* 2001;92:1364–9.

76. Nomura T, Lebowitz L, Koide Y, et al. Evaluation of hepatic venous flow using transesophageal echocardiography in coronary artery bypass surgery: an index of right ventricular function. *J Cardiothorac Vasc Anesth* 1995;9:9–17.

77. Troianos CA, Porembka DT. Assessment of left ventricular function and hemodynamics with transesophageal echocardiography. *Crit Care Clin* 1996;12:253–72.

78. Hogue CW Jr, Platin M, Barzilai B, Kaiser LR. Intraoperative use of transesophageal echocardiography with pulsed-wave Doppler evaluation of ventricular filling dynamics during pericardiotomy. *Anesthesiology* 1991;75:701–4.

79. Mishra M, Chauhan R, Sharma KK, et al. Real-time intraoperative transesophageal echocardiography—how useful? Experience of 5,016 cases. *J Cardiothorac Vasc Anesth* 1998;12:625–32.

80. Connor BG. Transesophageal echocardiography and monitoring applications. *J Clin Monitor* 1995;11:396–405.

81. Matsumoto M, Oka Y, Strom J, et al. Application of transesophageal echocardiography to continuous intraoperative monitoring of left ventricular performance. *Am J Cardiol* 1980;46:95–105.

82. Muhiudeen IA, Kuecherer HF, Lee E, et al. Intraoperative estimation of cardiac output by transesophageal pulsed Doppler echocardiography. *Anesthesiology* 1991;74:9–14.

83. Suriani RJ, Cutrone A, Feierman D, Konstadt S. Intraoperative transesophageal echocardiography during liver transplantation. *J Cardiothorac Vasc Anesth* 1996;10:699–707.

84. Black S, Muzzi DA, Nishimura RA, Cucchiara RF. Preoperative and intraoperative echocardiography to detect right-to-left shunt in patients undergoing neurosurgical procedures in the sitting position. *Anesthesiology* 1990;72:436–8.

85. Topol EJ, Humphrey LS, Borkon AM, et al. Value of intraoperative left ventricular microbubbles detected by transesophageal two-dimensional echocardiography in predicting neurologic outcome after cardiac operations. *Am J Cardiol* 1985;56:773–5.

86. Moises VA, Mesquita CB, Campos O, et al. Importance of intraoperative echocardiography during coronary artery surgery without cardiopulmonary bypass. *J Am Soc Echocardiogr* 1998;11:1139–44.

87. Applebaum RM, Cutler WM, Bhardwaj N, et al. Utility of transesophageal echocardiography during PortAccess minimally invasive cardiac surgery. *Am J Cardiol* 1998;82:183–8.

88. Siegel LC, St Goar FG, Stevens JH, et al. Monitoring considerations for port-access cardiac surgery. *Circulation* 1997;96:562–8.

89. Secknus MA, Asher CR, Scalia GM, et al. Intraoperative transesophageal echocardiography in minimally invasive cardiac valve surgery. *Am Soc Echocardiogr* 1999;12:231–6.

90. Coddens J, Callebaut F, Hendrickx J, et al. Case 5—2001. Port-access cardiac surgery and aortic dissection: the role of transesophageal echocardiography. *J Cardiothorac Vasc Anesth* 2001;15:251–8.

91. Ceriana P, Pagnin A, Locatelli A, et al. Monitoring aspects during port-access cardiac surgery. *J Cardiovasc Surg* 2000;41:579–83.

92. Schulze CJ, Wildhirt SM, Boehm DH, et al. Continuous transesophageal echocardiographic (TEE) monitoring during port-access cardiac surgery. *Heart Surg Forum* 1999;2:54–9.

93. Kronzon I, Tunick PA, Jortner R, et al. Echocardiographic evaluation of the coronary sinus. *J Am Soc Echocardiogr* 1995;8:518–26.

94. Clements MD, Wright SJ, deBruijin N. Coronary sinus catheterization made easy for PortAccess minimally invasive cardiac surgery. *J Cardiothorac Vasc Anesth* 1998;12:96–101.

95. Hasel R, Barash PG. Dilated coronary sinus on prebypass transesophageal echocardiography. *J Cardiothorac Vasc Anesth* 1996;10:432–5.

96. Plotkin IM, Collard CD, Aranki SF, et al. Percutaneous coronary sinus cannulation guided by transesophageal echocardiography. *Ann Thorac Surg* 1998;66:2085–7.

97. Menasche P, Kural S, Fauchet M, et al. Retrograde coronary sinus perfusion: a safe alternative for ensuring cardioplegic delivery in aortic valve surgery. *Ann Thorac Surg* 1982;34:647–58.

98. Goldstein DJ, Oz MC, Rose EA. Implantable left ventricular assist devices. *New Engl J Med* 1998;339:1522–33.

99. Nakatani S, McCarthy PM, Kottke-Marchant K, et al. Left ventricular echocardiographic and histologic changes: impact of chronic unloading by an implantable ventricular assist device. *J Am Coll Cardiol* 1996;27:894–901.

100. Levin HR, Oz MC, Catanese KA, et al. Transient normalization of systolic and diastolic function after support with a left ventricular assist device in a patient with dilated cardiomyopathy. *J Heart Lung Transplant* 1996;15:840–2.

101. Mandarino WA, Gorcsan J III, Gasior TA, et al. Estimation of left ventricular function in patients with a left ventricular assist device. *ASAIO* 1995;41:M544–7.

102. Muller J, Wallukat G, Weng Y-G, et al. Weaning from mechanical cardiac support in patients with idiopathic dilated cardiomyopathy. *Circulation* 1997;96:542–9.

103. Simon P, Owen AN, Moritz A, et al. Transesophageal echocardiographic evaluation in mechanically assisted circulation. *Eur J Cardiothorac Surg* 1001;5:492–7.

104. Brack M, Olson JD, Pedersen WR, et al. Transesophageal echocardiography in patients with mechanical circulatory assistance. *Ann Thorac Surg* 1991;52:1306–9.

105. Shapiro GC, Leibowitz DW, Oz MC, et al. Diagnosis of patent foramen ovale with transesophageal echocardiography in a patient supported with a left ventricular assist device. *J Heart Lung Transplant* 1995;14:594–7.

106. Feigenbaum H, Zaky A, Grabhorn L. Cardiac motion in patients with pericardial effusion: a study using ultrasound cardiography. *Circulation* 1966;34:611–19.

107. Kronzon I, Cohen ML, Winer HE. Diastolic atrial compression: a sensitive echocardiographic sign of cardiac tamponade. *J Am Coll Cardiol* 1983;2:770–5.

108. Armstrong WF, Schilt BF, Helper DJ, et al. Diastolic collapse of the right ventricle with cardiac tamponade: an echocardiographic study. *Circulation* 1982;65:1491–6.

109. Martin RP, Rakowski H, French J, Popp RL. Localization of pericardial effusion with wide angle phases array echocardiography. *Am J Cardiol* 1978;42:904–12.

110. Himelman RB, Kircher B, Rockey DC, et al. Inferior vena cava plethora with blunted respiratory response: a sensitive echocardiographic sign of cardiac tamponade. *J Am Coll Cardiol* 1988;12:1470–7.

111. Krikorian JG, Hancock EW. Pericardiocentesis. *Am J Med* 1978;65:808–14.

112. Spodick DH. The technique of pericardiocentesis. When to perform it and how to minimize complications. *J Crit Illn* 1995;10:807–12.

113. Wong B, Murphy J, Change CJ, et al. The risk of pericardiocentesis. *Am J Cardiol* 1979;44:1110–14.

114. Goldberg BB, Pollack HM. Ultrasonically guided pericardiocentesis. *Am J Cardiol* 1973;31:490–3.

115. Callahan JA, Seward JB, Tajik AJ, et al. Pericardiocentesis assisted by two-dimensional echocardiography. *J Thorac Cardiovasc Surg* 1983;85:877–9.

116. Callahan JA, Seward JB, Nishimura RA, et al. Two-dimensional echocardiographic-guided pericardiocentesis: experience in 117 consecutive patients. *Am J Cardiol* 1985;55:476–9.

117. Callahan JA, Seward JB, Tajik AJ. Cardiac tamponade: pericardiocentesis directed by two-dimensional echocardiography. *Mayo Clin Proc* 1985;60:344–7.

118. Berger BC. Pericardiocentesis using echocardiography. *Cardiovasc Clin* 1985;15:269–79.

119. Pandian NG, Brockway B, Simonetti J, et al. Pericardiocentesis under two-dimensional echocardiographic guidance in loculated pericardial effusion. *Ann Thorac Surg* 1988;45:99–100.

120. Tsang TS, Freeman WK, Sinak LJ, Seward JB. Echocardiographically guided pericardiocentesis: evolution and state-of-the-art technique. *Mayo Clin Proc* 1998;73:647–52.

121. Tsang TSM, Freeman WK, Barnes ME, et al. Rescue echocardiographically guided pericardiocentesis for cardiac perforation

complicating catheter-bases procedures: the Mayo Clinic experience. *J Am Coll Cardiol* 1998;32:1345–50.

122. Tsang TS, Barnes ME, Hayes SN, et al. Clinical and echocardiographic characteristics of significant pericardial effusions following cardiothoracic surgery and outcomes of echo-guided pericardiocentesis for management: Mayo Clinic experience, 1979–1998. *Chest* 1999;116:322–31.

123. Drummond JB, Seward JB, Tsang TS, et al. Outpatient two-dimensional echocardiography-guided pericardiocentesis. *J Am Soc Echocardiogr* 1998;11:433–5.

124. Salem K, Mulji A, Lonn E. Echocardiographically guided pericardiocentesis – the gold standard for the management of pericardial effusion and cardiac tamponade. *Can J Cardiol* 1999;15:1251–5.

125. Maggiolini S, Bozzano A, Russo P, et al. Echocardiography-guided pericardiocentesis with probe-mounted needle: report of 53 cases. *J Am Soc Echocardiogr* 2001;14:821–4.

126. Armstrong G, Cardon L, Vilkomerson D, et al. Localization of needle tip with color Doppler during pericardiocentesis: in vitro validation and initial clinical application. *J Am Soc Echocardiogr* 2001;14:29–37.

127. Meliones JN, Snider AR, Beekman RH, et al. Echocardiographic detection of pericardiocentesis-induced subepicardial and intramyocardial hematoma. *Am J Cardiol* 1989;64:820–1.

128. Tsang TS, El-Najdawi EK, Seward JB, et al. Percutaneous echocardiographically guided pericardiocentesis in pediatric patients: evaluation of safety and efficacy. *J Am Soc Echocardiogr* 1998;11:1072–7.

129. Suehiro S, Hattori K, Shibata T, et al. Echocardiography-guided pericardiocentesis with a needle attached to a probe. *Ann Thorac Surg* 1996;61:741–2.

130. Wang JY, Lin YF. Usefulness of pericardiostomy with guidance of transesophageal echocardiography in a CAPD patient with pericardial tamponade. *Perit Dial Int* 1999;19:594.

131. Sohn DW, Shin GJ, Oh JK, et al. Role of transesophageal echocardiography in hemodynamically unstable patients. *Mayo Clin Proc* 1995;70:925–31.

132. Chen TH, Chan KC, Cheng YJ, et al. Bedside pericardiocentesis under the guidance of transesophageal echocardiography in a 13-month-old boy. *J Formosan Med Assoc* 2001;100:620–2.

133. Friedrich SP, Berman AD, Baim DS, Diver DJ. Myocardial perforation in the cardiac catheterization laboratory: incidence, presentation, diagnosis, and management. *Cathet Cardiovasc Diagn* 1994;32:99–107.

134. Seggewis H, Schmidt HK, Mellwig KP, et al. Acute pericardial tamponade after percutaneous transluminal coronary angioplasty (PTCA). A rare life threatening complication. *Z Kardiol* 1993;82:721–6.

135. Hsin ST, Luk HN, Lin SM, et al. Detection of iatrogenic cardiac tamponade by transesophageal echocardiography during vena cava filter procedure. *Can J Anaesth* 2001;47:638–41.

136. O'Sullivan J, Heads A, Hunter S. Microbubble image enhancement and pericardiocentesis. *Int J Cardiol* 1993;42:95–6.

137. Betts TR, Radvan JR. Contrast echocardiography during pericardiocentesis. *Heart* 1999;81:329.

138. Chandraratna PAN, Reid CL, Nimalasuriya A, et al. Application of 2-dimensional contrast studies during pericardiocentesis. *Am J Cardiol* 1983;52:1120–2.

139. Weisse AB, Desai RR, Rajihah G, et al. Contrast echocardiography as an adjunct in haemorrhagic or complicated pericardiocentesis. *Am Heart J* 1996;131:822–5.

140. Chiang HT, Lin M. Pericardiocentesis guided by two-dimensional contrast echocardiography. *Echocardiography* 1993;10:465–9.

141. Gosalakkal JA, Sugrue DD. Malignant melanoma of the right atrium: antemortem diagnosis by transvenous biopsy. *Br Heart J* 1989; 62:159–60.

142. Flipse TR, Tazelaar HD, Holmes DR Jr. Diagnosis of malignant cardiac disease by endomyocardial biopsy. *Mayo Clin Proc* 1990; 65:1415–22.

143. Pierard L, El Allaf D, D'Orio V, et al. Two-dimensional echocardiographic guiding of endomyocardial biopsy. *Chest* 1984;85:759–62.

144. Pennestri F, Loperfido F, Salvatori MP, et al. 2-dimensional echocardiography in performing myocardial biopsy. *Cardiologia* 1982;27:1141–5.

145. Grande AM, De Pieri G, Pederzolli C, et al. Echo-guided endomyocardial biopsy in heterotopic heart transplantation. *J Cardiovasc Surg* 1998;39:223–5.

146. Grande AM, Minzioni G, Martinelli L, et al. Echo-controlled endomyocardial biopsy in orthotopic heart transplantation with bicaval anastomosis. *G Ital Cardiol* 1997;27:877–80.

147. Deckers JW, Hare JM, Baughman KL. Complications of transvenous right ventricular endomyocardial biopsy in adult patients with cardiomyopathy: a seven-year survey of 645 consecutive diagnostic procedures in a tertiary referral center. *J Am Coll Cardiol* 1992;19:43–7.

148. Seward JB, Khandheria BK, Oh JK, et al. Transesophageal echocardiography: technique, anatomic correlations, implementation, and clinical applications. *Mayo Clin Proc* 1988;63:649–80.

149. Scott PJ, Ettles DF, Rees MR, Williams GJ. The use of combined transoesophageal echocardiography and fluoroscopy in the biopsy of a right atrial mass. *Br J Radiol* 1990;63:222–4.

150. Starr SK, Pugh DM, O'Brien-Ladner A, Stites S, Wilson DB. Right atrial mass biopsy guided by transesophageal echocardiography. *Chest* 1993;104:969–70.

151. Van Camp G, Abdulsater J, Cosyns B, Liebens I, Vandenbossche JL. Transesophageal echocardiography of right atrial metastasis of a hepatocellular carcinoma. *Chest* 1994;105:945–7.

152. Weston MW. Comparison of costs and charges for fluoroscopic- and echocardiographic-guided endomyocardial biopsy. *Am J Cardiol* 1994;74:839–40.

153. Hammoudeh AJ, Chaaban F, Watson RM, Millman A. Transesophageal echocardiography-guided transvenous endomyocardial biopsy used to diagnose primary cardiac angiosarcoma. *Cathet Cardiovasc Diagn* 1996;37:347–9.

154. Malouf JF, Thompson RC, Maples WJ, Wolfe JT. Diagnosis of right atrial metastatic melanoma by transesophageal echocardiographic-guided transvenous biopsy. *Mayo Clin Proc* 1996;71:1167–70.

155. Savoia MT, Liguori C, Nahar T, et al. Transesophageal echocardiography-guided transvenous biopsy of a cardiac sarcoma. *J Am Soc Echocardiogr* 1997;10:752–5.

156. Burling F, Devlin G, Heald S. Primary cardiac lymphoma diagnosed with transesophageal echocardiography-guided endomyocardial biopsy. *Circulation* 2000;101:E179–81.

157. McCreery CJ, McCulloch M, Ahmad M, deFilippi CR. Real-time 3-dimensional echocardiography imaging for right ventricular endomyocardial biopsy: a comparison with fluoroscopy. *J Am Soc Echocardiogr* 2001;14:927–33.

158. Tucker KJ, Curtis AB, Murphy J, et al. Transesophageal echocardiographic guidance of transseptal left heart catheterization during radiofrequency ablation of left-sided accessory pathways in humans. *Pacing Clin Electrophysiol* 1996;19:272–81.

159. Hahn K, Gal R, Sarnoski J, et al. Transesophageal echocardiographically guided atrial transseptal catheterization in patients with normal-sized atria: incidence of complications. *Clin Cardiol* 1995;18:217–20.

160. Lee MS, Evans SJ, Blumberg S, et al. Echocardiographically guided electrophysiologic testing in pregnancy. *J Am Soc Echocardiogr* 1994;7:182–6.

161. Kantoch MJ, Frost GF, Robertson MA. Use of transesophageal echocardiography in radiofrequency catheter ablation in children and adolescents. *Can J Cardiol* 1998;14:519–23.

162. Hamilton K, Castillo M, Arruda M, Jackman W. Echocardiographic demonstration of coronary sinus diverticula in patients with Wolff–Parkinson–White syndrome. *J Am Soc Echocardiogr* 1996;9:337–43.

163. Gill JS, de Belder M, Ward DE. Right ventricular outflow tract ventricular tachycardia associated with an aneurysmal malformation: use of transesophageal echocardiography during low-energy, direct-current ablation. *Am Heart J* 1994;128:620–3.

164. Saxon LA, Stevenson WG, Fonarow GC, et al. Transesophageal echocardiography during radiofrequency catheter ablation of ventricular tachycardia. *Am J Cardiol* 1993;72:658–61.

165. Goldman AP, Irwin JM, Glover MU, et al. Use of transesophageal echocardiography (TEE) aided radiofrequency ablation of Wolff–Parkinson–White accessory pathways. *Pacing Clin Electrophysiol* 1992;15:244.

166. Goli VD, Prasad R, Hamilton K, et al. Transesophageal echocardiographic evaluation for mural thrombus following radiofrequency catheter ablation of accessory pathways. *Pacing Clin Electrophysiol* 1991;14:1992–7.

167. Goldman AP, Irwin JM, Glover MU, Mick W. Transesophageal echocardiography to improve positioning of radiofrequency ablation catheters in left-sided Wolff–Parkinson–White syndrome. *Pacing Clin Electrophysiol* 1991;14:1245–50.

168. Epstein LM. The utility of intracardiac echocardiography in interventional electrophysiology. *Curr Cardiol Rep* 2000;2:329–34.

169. Marchlinski FE, Ren JF, Schwartzman D, et al. Accuracy of fluoroscopic localization of the Crista terminalis documented by intracardiac echocardiography. *J Interven Card Electrophysiol* 2000;4:415–21.

170. Lesh MD, Kalman JM, Karch MR. Use of intracardiac echocardiography during electrophysiologic evaluation and therapy of atrial arrhythmias. *J Cardiovasc Electrophysiol* 1998;9(8 suppl):S40–7.

171. Kalman JM, Olgin JE, Karch MR. Lesh MD. Use of intracardiac echocardiography in interventional electrophysiology. *Pacing Clin Electrophysiol* 1997;20(9 pt 1):2248–62.

172. Yu WC, Hsu TL, Tai CT, et al. Acquired pulmonary vein stenosis after radiofrequency catheter ablation of paroxysmal atrial fibrillation. *J Cardiovasc Electrophysiol* 2001;12:887–92.

173. Farah A, Khan F, Machado C. Thrombus formation at the site of radiofrequency catheter ablation. *Pacing Clin Electrophysiol* 2000;23(4 Pt 1):538–40.

174. Sparks PB, Jayaprakash S, Vohra JK, et al. Left atrial 'stunning' following radiofrequency catheter ablation of chronic atrial flutter. *J Am Coll Cardiol* 1998;32:468–75.

175. Voci P, Tritapepe L, Critelli G. Iatrogenic pneumohemomediastinum mimicking cardiac tamponade: a complication of catheter ablation procedure. *Pacing Clin Electrophysiol* 1997;20:138–9.

176. Le Groupe de Rythmologie de la Societe Francaise de Cardiologie. Complications of radiofreqency ablation: a French experience. *Arch Mal Coeur Vaiss* 1996;89:1599–605.

177. Horowitz LN. Safety of electrophysiologic studies. *Circulation* 1986;73:II28–31.

178. Formigari R, Santoro Giuseppe Rossetti L, et al. Comparison of three different atrial septal defect occlusion devices. *Am J Cardiol* 1998;28:690–2, A9.

179. Pedra CAC, Pihkala J, Lee KJ, et al. Transcatheter closure of atrial septal defects using the Cardio-Seal implant. *Heart* 2000;84:320–6.

180. Lee CH, Kwok OH, Fan K, et al. Transcatheter closure of atrial septal defect using Amplatzer septal occluder in Chinese adults. *Catheter Cardiovasc Interv* 2001;53:373–7.

181. Onorato E, Pera I, Lanzone A, et al. Transcatheter treatment of coronary artery disease and atrial septal defect with sequential implantation of coronary stent and Amplatzer septal occluder: preliminary results. *Catheter Cardiovasc Interv* 2001;54:454–8.

182. Acar P, Saliba Z, Bonhoeffer P, et al. Influence of atrial septal defect anatomy in patient selection and assessment of closure with the CardioSEAL device; a three-dimensional transoesophageal echocardiographic reconstruction. *Eur Heart J* 2000;21:573–81.

183. Zahn EM, Wilson N, Cutright W, Latson LA. Development and testing of the Helex septal occluder, a new expanded polytetrafluoroethylene atrial septal defect occlusion system. *Circulation* 2001;104:711–16.

184. Sievert H, Babic UU, Hausdorf G, et al. Transcatheter closure of atrial septal defect and patent foramen ovale with ASDOS device (a multi-institutional European trial). *Am J Cardiol* 1998;82:1405–13.

185. Thanopoulos BD, Tsaousis GS, Konstadopoulou GN, Zarayelyan AG. Transcatheter closure of muscular ventricular septal defects with the Amplatzer ventricular septal defect occluder: initial clinical applications in children. *J Am Coll Cardiol* 1999;33:1395–9.

186. Amin Z, Gu X, Berry JM, et al. New device for closure of muscular ventricular septal defects in a canine model. *Circulation* 1999;100:320–8.

187. Bilgic A, Celiker A, Ozkutlu S, et al. Transcatheter closure of secundum atrial septal defects, a ventricular septal defect, and a patent arterial duct. *Turk J Pediatr* 2001;43:12–18.

188. Latiff HA, Samion H, Kandhavel G, et al. The value of transesophageal echocardiography in transcatheter closure of atrial septal defects in the oval fossa using the Amplatzer septal occluder. *Cardiol Young* 2001;11:201–4.

189. Hijazi Z, Wang Z, Cao Q, et al. Transcatheter closure of atrial septal defects and patent foramen ovale under intracardiac echocardiographic guidance: feasibility and comparison with transesophageal echocardiography. *Catheter Cardiovasc Interv* 2001;52:194–9.

190. Salaymeh KJ, Taeed R, Michelfelder EC, et al. Unique echocardiographic features associated with deployment of the Amplatzer atrial septal defect device. *J Am Soc Echocardiogr* 2001;14:128–37.

191. Cheung YF, Leung MP, Lee J, Yung TC. An evolving role of transesophageal echocardiography for the monitoring of interventional catheterization in children. *Clin Cardiol* 1999;22:804–10.

192. Zhu W, Cao QL, Rhodes J, Hijazi ZM. Measurement of atrial septal defect size: a comparative study between three-dimensional transesophageal echocardiography and the standard balloon sizing methods. *Pediatr Cardiol* 2000;21:465–9.

193. Ussia GP, Momenah TS, Ursell P, et al. Evaluation of the morphology of the oval fossa for placement of devices. *Cardiol Young* 2000;10:502–9.

194. Ewert P, Daehnert I, Berger F, et al. Transcatheter closure of atrial septal defects under echocardiographic guidance without X-ray: initial experiences. *Cardiol Young* 1999;9:136–40.

195. Banerjee A, Bengur AR, Li JS, et al. Echocardiographic characteristics of successful deployment of the Das AngelWings atrial septal defect closure device: initial multicenter experience in the United States. *Am J Cardiol* 1999;83:1236–41.

196. Minich LL, Snider AR. Echocardiographic guidance during placement of the buttoned double-disk device for atrial septal defect closure. *Echocardiography* 1993;10:567–72.

197. Mazic U, Gavora P, Masura J. The role of transesophageal echocardiography in transcatheter closure of secundum atrial septal defects by the Amplatzer septal occluder. *Am Heart J* 2001;142:482–8.

198. Tseng HC, Hsiao PN, Lin YH, et al. Transesophageal echocardiographic monitoring for transcatheter closure of atrial septal defect. *J Formos Med Assoc* 2000;99:684–8.

199. Masura J, Gavora P, Formanek A, Hijazi ZM. Transcatheter closure of secundum atrial septal defects using the new self-centering Amplatzer septal occluder: initial human experience. *Cathet Cardiovasc Diagn* 1997;42:388–93.

200. Hellenbrand WE, Fahey JT, McGowan FX, et al. Transesophageal echocardiographic guidance of transcatheter closure of atrial septal defect. *Am J Cardiol* 1990;66:207–13.

201. Cooke JC, Gelman JS, Harper RW. Echocardiologists' role in the deployment of the Amplatzer atrial septal occluder device in adults. *J Am Soc Echocardiogr* 2001;14:588–94.

202. Pedra CA, Pihkala J, Lee KJ, et al. Transcatheter closure of atrial septal defects using the CardioSEAL implant. *Heart* 2000;84:320–6.

203. Demkow M, Ruzyllo W, Konka M, et al. Transvenous closure of moderate and large secundum atrial septal defects in adults using the Amplatzer septal occluder. *Catheter Cardiovasc Interv* 2001;52:188–93.

204. Aeschbacher BC, Chatterjee T, Meier B. Transesophageal echocardiography to evaluate success of transcatheter closure of large secundum atrial septal defects in adults using the buttoned device. *Mayo Clin Proc* 2000;75:913–20.

205. Podnar T, Martanovic P, Gavora P, Masura J. Morphologic variations of secundum-type atrial septal defects: feasibility for percutaneous closure using Amplatzer septal occluders. *Catheter Cardiovasc Interv* 2001;53:386–91.

206. McMahon CJ, Pignatelli RH, Rutledge JM, et al. Steerable control of the eustachian valve during transcatheter closure of secundum atrial septal defects. *Catheter Cardiovasc Interv* 2000;51:455–9.

207. Kaulitz R, Peuster M, Jux C, et al. Transcatheter closure of various types of defects within the oval fossa using the double umbrella device (CardioSEAL)-feasibility and echocardiographic follow-up. *Cardiol Young* 2001;11:214–22.

208. Carano N, Hagler DJ, Agnetti A, Squarcia U. Device closure of fenestrated atrial septal defects: use of a single Amplatzer atrial septal occluder after balloon atrial septostomy to create a single defect. *Catheter Cardiovasc Interv* 2001;52:203–7.

209. Celiker A, Bilgic A, Ozkutlu S, et al. A late complication with the CardioSEAL ASD occluder device and need for surgical revision. *Catheter Cardiovasc Interv* 2001;54:335–8.

210. Cooke JC, Gelman JS, Harper RW. Cobrahead malformation of the Amplatzer septal occluder device: an avoidable compilation of percutaneous ASD closure. *Catheter Cardiovasc Interv* 2001;52:83–5.

211. Mazic U, Gavora P, Masura J. 'Cobra-like' deformation of an Amplatzer septal occluder. *Pediatr Cardiol* 2001;22:253–4.

212. La Rosee K, Deutsch HJ, Schnabel P, et al. Thrombus formation after transcatheter closure of atrial septal defect. *Am J Cardiol* 1999;84:356–9.

213. Fabricius AM, Krueger M, Falk V, et al. Floating thrombus on an ASD occluder device in a patient with hemophilia A. *Thorac Cardiovasc Surg* 2001;49:312–13.

214. Rosenfeld HM, van der Velde ME, Sanders SP, et al. Echocardiographic predictors of candidacy for successful transcatheter atrial septal defect closure. *Catheter Cardiovasc Diagn* 1995;34:29–34.

215. Momenah TS, McElhinney DB, Brook MM, et al. Transesophageal echocardiographic predictors for successful transcatheter closure of defects within the oval fossa using the CardioSEAL septal occlusion device. *Cardiol Young* 2000;10:510–18.

216. Cowley CG, Lloyd TR, Bove EL, et al. Comparison of results of closure of secundum atrial septal defect by surgery versus Amplatzer septal occluder. *Am J Cardiol* 2001;88:589–91.

217. Boutin C, Musewe NN, Smallhorn JF, et al. Echocardiographic follow-up of atrial septal defect after catheter closure by double-umbrella device. *Circulation* 1993;88:621–7.

218. Cao QL, Du ZD, Joseph A, et al. Immediate and six-month results of the profile of the Amplatzer septal occluder as assessed by transesophageal echocardiography. *Am J Cardiol* 2001;88:754–9.

219. Acar P, Bonhoeffer P, Saliba Z, et al. Three-dimensional reconstruction by transesophageal echocardiography of Amplatzer and CardioSEAL prosthetic devices after percutaneous closure and atrial septal defects. *Arch Mal Coeur Vaiss* 2000;93:539–45.

220. Weiss RL, Brier JA, O'Connor W, et al. The usefulness of transesophageal echocardiography in diagnosing cardiac contusions. *Chest* 1996;109:73–7.

221. Sousa RC, Garcia-Fernandez MA, Moreno M, et al. Value of transesophageal echocardiography in the assessment of blunt chest trauma: correlation with electrocardiogram, heart enzymes, and transthoracic echocardiogram. *Rev Port Cardiol* 1994;13:833–43.

222. Brooks SW, Young JC, Cmolik B, et al. The use of transesophageal echocardiography in the evaluation of chest trauma. *J Trauma* 1992;32:761–5.

223. Shapiro MJ, Yanofsky SD, Trapp J, et al. Cardiovascular evaluation in blunt thoracic trauma using transesophageal echocardiography (TEE). *J Trauma* 1991;31:835–9.

224. Potkin RT, Werner JA, Trobaugh GB, et al. Evaluation of noninvasive tests of cardiac damage in suspected cardiac contusion. *Circulation* 1982;66:627–31.

225. Dodd DA, Johns JA, Graham TP Jr. Transient severe mitral and tricuspid regurgitation following blunt chest trauma. *Am Heart J* 1987;114:652–4.

226. Rosenthal A, Parisi LF, Nadas AS. Isolated interventricular septal defect due to nonpenetrating trauma. *N Engl J Med* 1970;283:338–41.

227. Pickard LR, Mattox KL, Beall AC Jr. Ventricular septal defect from blunt chest injury. *J Trauma* 1980;20:329–31.

228. Pretre R, Faidutti B. Surgical management of aortic valve injury after nonpenetrating trauma. *Ann Thorac Surg* 1993; 56:1426–31.

229. Cherng WJ, Bullard MJ, Chang HJ, Lin FC. Diagnosis of coronary artery dissection following blunt chest trauma by transesophageal echocardiography. *J Trauma* 1995;39:772–4.

230. Allen RP, Liedtke AJ. The role of coronary artery injury and perfusion in the development of cardiac contusion secondary to nonpenetrating chest trauma. *J Trauma* 1979;19:153–6.

231. Kumpuris AG, Casale TB, Mokotoff DM, et al. Right bundle-branch block. Occurrence following nonpenetrating chest trauma without evidence of cardiac contusion. *JAMA* 1979;242:172–3.

232. Berman RW, Rook GD, Bronsther B, Abrams MW. Traumatic nonpenetrating ventricular septal defect: recovery under conservative management. *J Pediatr Surg* 1966;1:275–83.

233. Kaye P, O'Sullivan I. Myocardial contusion: emergency investigation and diagnosis. *Emerg Med J* 2002;19:8–10.

234. Kram HB, Appel PL, Shoemaker WC. Increased incidence of cardiac contusion in patients with traumatic thoracic aortic rupture. *Ann Surg* 1988;208:615–18.

235. Olsovsky MR, Wechsler AS, Topaz O. Cardiac trauma. Diagnosis, management and current therapy. *Angiology* 1997;48:423–32.

236. Miura H, Taira O, Hiraguri S, et al. Blunt thoracic injury. *Jpn J Thorac Cardiovasc Surg* 1998;46:556–60.

237. Mohl W, Simon P, Neumann F. Intraoperative echocardiography in cardiac emergencies. *Echocardiography* 1990;7:193–200.

238. Kettunen P, Nieminen M. Creatine kinase MB and M-mode echocardiographic changes in cardiac contusion. *Ann Clin Res* 1985;17:292–8.

239. Mori F, Zuppiroli A, Ognibene A et al. Cardiac contusion in blunt chest trauma: a combined study of transesophageal echocardiography and cardiac troponin I determination. *Ital Heart J* 2001;2:222–7.

240. Tiao GM, Griffith PM, Szmuszkovicz JR, Mahour GH. Cardiac and great vessel injuries in children after blunt trauma: an institutional review. *J Pediatr Surg* 2000;35:1656–60.

241. Bromberg BI, Mazziotti MV, Canter CE, et al. Recognition and management of nonpenetrating cardiac trauma in children. *J Pediatr* 1996;128:536–41.

242. King RM, Mucha P Jr, Seward JB, et al. Cardiac contusion: a new diagnostic approach utilizing two-dimensional echocardiography. *J Trauma* 1983;23:610–14.

243. Miller FA Jr, Seward JB, Gersh BJ, et al. Two-dimensional echocardiographic findings in cardiac trauma. *Am J Cardiol* 1982;50:1022–7.

244. Beggs CW, Helling TS, Evans LL, et al. Early evaluation of cardiac injury by two-dimensional echocardiography in patients suffering blunt chest trauma. *Ann Emerg Med* 1987;16:542–5.

Index

Page numbers in italics refer to illustrations; numbers followed by 't' indicate tables